# New Horizons in Predictive Toxicology
## Current Status and Application

**RSC Drug Discovery Series**



*Titles in the Series:*

1: Metabolism, Pharmacokinetics and Toxicity of Functional Groups: Impact of Chemical Building Blocks on ADMET
2: Emerging Drugs and Targets for Alzheimer's Disease; Volume 1: Beta-Amyloid, Tau Protein and Glucose Metabolism
3: Emerging Drugs and Targets for Alzheimer's Disease; Volume 2: Neuronal Plasticity, Neuronal Protection and Other Miscellaneous Strategies
4: Accounts in Drug Discovery: Case Studies in Medicinal Chemistry
5: New Frontiers in Chemical Biology: Enabling Drug Discovery
6: Animal Models for Neurodegenerative Disease
7: Neurodegeneration: Metallostasis and Proteostasis
8: G Protein-Coupled Receptors: From Structure to Function
9: Pharmaceutical Process Development: Current Chemical and Engineering Challenges
10: Extracellular and Intracellular Signaling
11: New Synthetic Technologies in Medicinal Chemistry
12: New Horizons in Predictive Toxicology: Current Status and Application

*How to obtain future titles on publication:*
A standing order plan is available for this series. A standing order will bring delivery of each new volume immediately on publication.

*For further information please contact:*
Book Sales Department, Royal Society of Chemistry, Thomas Graham House, Science Park, Milton Road, Cambridge, CB4 0WF, UK
Telephone: +44 (0)1223 420066, Fax: +44 (0)1223 420247, Email: books@rsc.org
Visit our website at http://www.rsc.org/Shop/Books/

# *New Horizons in Predictive Toxicology*
## *Current Status and Application*

Edited by

**Alan G. E. Wilson**
*Lexicon Pharmaceuticals Inc., The Woodlands, Texas, USA*

RSC Publishing

RSC Drug Discovery Series No. 12

ISBN: 978-1-84973-051-8
ISSN: 2041-3203

A catalogue record for this book is available from the British Library



Published by The Royal Society of Chemistry,
Thomas Graham House, Science Park, Milton Road,
Cambridge CB4 0WF, UK

Registered Charity Number 207890

For further information see our web site at www.rsc.org

# Foreword

Developments in toxicology over the past 50 years have been driven primarily by burgeoning regulatory requirements to demonstrate the safety of drugs, pesticides and other chemicals. The approach used throughout this period has relied primarily on the application of standardised *in vivo* tests in laboratory rodents although the number of tests required to be performed has increased considerably.

This methodology has served to protect consumer and public health. However, it is probably not sustainable in its present form for the following reasons:

1) The number of chemicals requiring testing under recently introduced legislation has increased substantially (for example, the REACH regulations in the EU). Therefore, more cost effective methods are needed;
2) Public and political pressures are leading to restrictions on the use of experimental animals for testing purposes;
3) A number of challenges, for example, prediction of vulnerable members of the population and the impact of co-exposure to several/many chemicals are not adequately addressed by the current methods.

There have been major advances in scientific understanding of the traditional pathways leading to human diseases and the initiation of the toxic effects of chemicals. These innovations enable a more predictive, less prescriptive approach to the characterisation of the risk from individual chemicals and combinations of chemicals. Toxicologists should also draw on high-throughput methods developed for other purposes, such as genomics informatics. These methods enable multiple endpoints to be determined and the data generated to be processed efficiently.

RSC Drug Discovery Series No. 12
New Horizons in Predictive Toxicology: Current Status and Application
Edited by Alan G. E. Wilson

Published by the Royal Society of Chemistry, www.rsc.org

There is an urgent need for a thorough debate on what could be achieved through these exciting recent developments and on the necessary steps required to facilitate their adoption in toxicology. This book will inform the debate. It focuses on a very important issue: how current understanding of mechanisms/modes of action in the more common target organs can enhance the prediction of toxic effects without necessary recourse to a standard raft of toxicity tests. It also reviews the utility of various model systems for this purpose.

The comprehensive nature of the chapters and the fact that they follow a largely common format allows an extremely useful overview of the current status of predictive toxicology and its potential developments. It should be regarded as essential reading for anyone interested in the future of toxicological risk assessment.

Prof. Jim Bridges
Emeritus Professor of Toxicology and Environmental Health,
The University of Surrey, Guildford, Surrey, GU2 7XH, UK
Chair of the EU Scientific Committee on Emerging and
Newly Identified Health Risks

# *Preface*

When first approached by the Royal Society of Chemistry in regard to editing this book, my immediate response was: what could such a book add to the literature that would make a difference, and shift the current paradigm on the role of predictive approaches in the identification of chemical toxicities to ensure human safety? The outcome ended up being very satisfying and I greatly appreciate the contribution of the authors to this book. The hope is that this book may play a part in the on-going process of transforming the current way toxicity is assessed. In this book the reader will see expert discussion of the variety of approaches for toxicity prediction including *in silico*, *in vitro* and *in vivo*. A number of key toxicities, target organs and mechanisms are highlighted. Our current approaches have limitations and the utility of animal data does not always ensure the safety of a chemical or pharmaceutical in humans. Our quest is not an easy one, but is a critical one, and one that recalls the often used quote: "Prediction is very difficult, especially about the future", (Neils Bohr and later to Yogi Berra).

Predictive toxicology is often thought of in terms of *in silico* computational approaches. However, the concept of predictive toxicology has broader implications and in this context the chapters in this book discuss *in silico*, *in vitro*, and *in vivo* approaches that are being developed and applied in regard to toxicity prediction; and how these approaches may be integrated into modeling and simulation approaches for human hazard and risk assessment. *Ultimately, it will be how we use and evaluate all of the data and approaches* that will assist in making the breakthrough that is needed in assessing risks and improving human safety of chemicals, and thereby reducing the attrition of drug candidates due to safety issues, and the potential human health hazards associated with chemical exposures.

The hope is that the reader will find that this book provides an expert and comprehensive discussion on the current status and future directions of

RSC Drug Discovery Series No. 12
New Horizons in Predictive Toxicology: Current Status and Application
Edited by Alan G. E. Wilson

Published by the Royal Society of Chemistry, www.rsc.org

predictive toxicology and its application. It covers areas of *in silico*, *in vitro* and *in vivo* approaches, and how they are being used and integrated to improve toxicity prediction and risk assessment of chemicals. The various chapters in this book also reflect the growing need for improvements in our technologies and abilities to predict toxicities of pharmaceutical and industrial chemicals to ensure product safety and the protection of public health. It brings together leading experts in the fields of toxicology and risk assessment to discuss their views on the current status of toxicity prediction as well as their visions of the future needs and challenges.

Alan G. E. Wilson, Editor
Lexicon Pharmaceuticals Inc.
The Woodlands, Texas, USA

# *Contents*




RSC Drug Discovery Series No. 12
New Horizons in Predictive Toxicology: Current Status and Application
Edited by Alan G. E. Wilson



Published by the Royal Society of Chemistry, www.rsc.org

# Acknowledgements

I would like to personally thank all of the authors for taking the time to contribute to this book, the Royal Society of Chemistry for their patience, and a special thanks goes to Ayako Takei, President of ICaRuS Japan for her expert and diligent review and editing of the chapters. And finally, to the reader, I hope you will find this book of value to you in pursuing safer chemicals and as much fun to read as it was to compile.

This book is dedicated to Julia, and the memory of Mary.

RSC Drug Discovery Series No. 12
New Horizons in Predictive Toxicology: Current Status and Application
Edited by Alan G. E. Wilson

Published by the Royal Society of Chemistry, www.rsc.org

CHAPTER 1

# *Introduction and Overview*

ALAN G. E. WILSON

Lexicon Pharmaceuticals Inc., Drug Metabolism, Pharmacokinetics, Toxicology and Pathology, 8800 Technology Forest Place, The Woodlands, Texas 77381-1160, USA

## 1.1 Introduction

This book provides an expert and comprehensive discussion on the current status and future directions of predictive toxicology and its applications. It covers areas of *in silico*, *in vitro* and *in vivo* approaches, and how they are being used and integrated to improve toxicity prediction and risk assessment of chemicals. The various chapters in this book also reflect the growing need for improvements in our technologies and ability to predict the toxicities of pharmaceutical and industrial chemicals to ensure product safety and the protection of public health. It brings together leading experts in the fields of toxicology and risk assessment to discuss their views on the current status of toxicity prediction as well as their visions of the future needs and challenges.

It is becoming increasingly critical to identify potential toxicities early in the development of new chemical entities, be they for the pharmaceutical or chemical industries. It is quite apparent, however, that our current approaches have limitations and the utility of animal data may not always ensure the safety of a chemical or pharmaceutical in humans. Ultimately, it will be how we use and evaluate all of the data and approaches that will assist in making the breakthroughs that are needed in assessing risks and improving human safety of chemicals, and thereby reducing attrition of drug candidates due to safety issues and potential human health hazards associated with chemical exposures.

RSC Drug Discovery Series No. 12
New Horizons in Predictive Toxicology: Current Status and Application
Edited by Alan G. E. Wilson

Published by the Royal Society of Chemistry, www.rsc.org

## 1.2 The Growing Need for Improvement in Toxicity Prediction

### 1.2.1 Global Regulatory Initiatives

In recent years we have seen the introduction of several initiatives by regulatory agencies to improve the safety assessment of pharmaceutical and industrial chemicals. For example, the European Commission (EC) introduced legislation in 2003 for a new chemical management system, REACH (Registration, Evaluation, Authorisation and Restriction of Chemicals).[1] In 2004, the US Food and Drug Administration (FDA) launched the Critical Path Initiative, which is focused on improving drug and medical device development, the quality of data generated during development, and the outcomes of clinical use. The major focus of these initiatives is to ensure reasonable product safety, while also facilitating the translation into commercial products.[2] Thus, these separate regulatory initiatives highlight a common theme of ensuring that we are maximizing our ability to predict the safety of pharmaceutical and industrial chemicals in humans.

There have also been a number of initiatives by regulatory agencies to improve our abilities in toxicity prediction, and to facilitate the development and validation of computational *in silico* approaches. In the European Union (EU), efforts have been ongoing for a number of years to develop quantitative structure–activity relationships (QSARs) and other models to aid in toxicity prediction, and the implementation of REACH is expected to accelerate the process to develop important data sources to further improve these models.[3] Similarly, the US FDA has been engaged in a number of programs focused on developing *in silico* models for various toxicities, and has a long-standing interest in, and much experience of, working with industry on the evaluation of *in silico* approaches of toxicity prediction. In addition, in 2007 the US Environmental Protection Agency (EPA) initiated ToxCast™, a project in computational toxicology.[4] ToxCast™ is designed to apply high-throughput screening (HTS) data to building computational models to forecast the potential human toxicity of environmental chemicals.[4] The hazard predictions obtained with ToxCast™ are expected to provide the US EPA regulatory programs with science-based information helpful in prioritizing chemicals for higher tier toxicological evaluations, leading to a more efficient use of resources, and expediting the process to evaluate existing environmental chemicals.

### 1.2.2 Industrial Initiatives

For the pharmaceutical industry, safety issues remain a major concern and a cause of late-stage attrition, low success rate and withdrawal of products from the market.[5,6] Only about 30% of possible drugs that have acceptable animal testing make it into Phase III of clinical testing, with approximately 30% of those failing in Phase III.[7] Discovering safety issues late in development is potentially devastating financially for a company. It is therefore imperative that potential safety issues are identified early. Thus, the current focus and urgency in the pharmaceutical industry is to shorten the timelines for all aspects of drug discovery and to improve the ability to filter out potential safety issues earlier. We are therefore seeing an increasing interest and focus on predictive approaches. These predictive approaches are generally employed early in drug discovery often before efficacy screening. It is expected that these approaches will gain increasing importance in the coming years in allowing early identification of potential toxicity issues. In addition, the continuing understanding and advancement of, "*-omics*" (*i.e.*, genomics, transcriptomics, proteomics, metab(ol)onomics) technologies are expected to identify biomarkers that will assist in the prediction of different toxicities.

In the case of industrial chemicals, the extent of environmental exposure and potential safety issues of many chemicals to which humans might be exposed, has not been well studied. Thus, in recent years we have seen an increasing focus on the need to improve our ability to more accurately screen for potential safety issues and improve the translation of safety data to humans. In order to expedite the process for assessing risks and ensuring the human safety of the chemicals already in market, it is imperative to improve our technologies and ability to predict their toxicities. The pressure to reduce the use of experimental animals further enhances the needs to innovate our strategies for predicting toxicity of chemicals in humans.[8]

### 1.2.3 Paradigm Shift in Toxicity Testing

Current toxicity testing relies primarily on determining the potential for adverse responses in animals (typically rodents, dogs and/or non-human primates) exposed to high doses of a test agent. *In vivo* animal toxicity testing has been considered the benchmark to identify potential adverse effects of chemicals. However, the standard *in vivo* approach typically provides little information on the mode and mechanism of toxicity. Such information is frequently critical for understanding interspecies differences in toxicological responses, and in the translation of animal data to humans. *In vivo* studies are also expensive, time-consuming and require large numbers of animals. Hence, for a number of years we have seen global interest and initiatives to reduce, replace and refine animal testing (the three Rs) from both the standpoint of animal welfare and out of economical necessity.[8]

The National Research Council (NRC) of the National Academy of Sciences (NAS) issued its landmark report *Toxicity Testing in the 21st Century: a Vision and a Strategy*[9] in 2007. The report's vision for assessing the potential adverse effects of chemicals on human health shifts the focus from overt effects such as pathological changes in animals, to upstream effects on biological pathways. The new framework is centered on human biology and a computational systems approach, and proposes a shift from *in vivo* animal testing to human-cell based *in vitro* testing. This new paradigm suggests the possibility of accelerating the human hazard assessment of environmental chemicals by replacing the current framework based on extrapolating experimental animal data to humans, with the evaluation of the *in vitro* effects in human cellular systems on the toxicity pathways leading to the human diseases. The NRC report presented an ambitious vision for the future of toxicity testing with the hope that advances in new technologies would make toxicity testing quicker, less expensive, and more directly relevant to human exposure.

The excitement over the NRC vision has led to a general emphasis on "21$^{st}$ Century Toxicology"—a phrase drawn from the report's title and intended to encompass multiple approaches to toxicity testing that harness modern advances in biology and technology. In order to realize the new vision and strategy of toxicity testing proposed by the NRC, the regulatory agencies in the US are providing leadership on the improvement of our toxicity prediction approaches. In 2007, the National Institute of Health (NIH) Chemical Genomics Center (NCGC) of the National Human Genome Research Institute (NHGRI), the National Institute of Environmental Health Sciences (NIEHS) National Toxicology Program (NTP), and the US EPA, collaborated on a new high-throughput toxicity screening initiative entitled Tox21.[10]

Tox21 is a collaborative effort between federal agency partners striving to develop a new paradigm of predictive toxicology by pursuing seven enabling objectives:

1) Research, develop, validate, and translate innovative chemical testing methods that characterize toxicity pathways;
2) Investigate ways to use new tools to identify chemically induced biological activity mechanisms;
3) Prioritize which chemicals need more extensive toxicological evaluation;
4) Develop models that can be used to more effectively predict how chemicals will affect biological responses;
5) Identify chemicals, assays, computational platforms, and targeted testing needed for the innovative testing methods;
6) Complete acquisition in 2010 for a library of more than 10 000 chemicals for quantitative high-throughput screening (qHTS) at the NCGC; and
7) Implement Phase II of EPA's ToxCast™ program, which will include the screening of a 700-compound subset of the 10 000-compound library in various mid- and high-throughput assays.

The goal of Tox21 is to develop automated, high-throughput molecular and cell-based approaches for determining the potential human toxicity of the thousands of chemicals currently in use in the US. These early high-throughput screening approaches can also be used in the early phases of drug discovery, and are expected to gain increasing importance in the coming years by facilitating earlier prediction and identification and prediction of toxicity issues. In 2010, the FDA also joined the Tox21 collaboration and is expected to provide additional expertise and chemical information including human clinical data to improve our ability in toxicity prediction. The data generated from the innovative chemical testing methods used by the Tox21 partnership will be publicly available for making decisions about protecting human health and the environment.

## 1.3 Technologies for Toxicity Prediction

The goal of toxicity testing is to develop data that can provide adequate protection of public health from the potential adverse effects of exposure to chemicals, drugs, biologics, *etc*. This goal provides a clear standard for judging the performance of prospective screening assays. An obvious approach for the initial screening of toxicity amongst a large number of environmental chemicals or drug candidates is to combine predictions from different high-throughput assays, and the integration of bioassay results with *in silico* models such that more accurate weight-of-evidence assessment can be generated. However, for any predictive technology to add value it will be critical that the relevance to humans is fully understood. Whilst no preclinical approach is expected to be totally predictive of potential human health hazards, the strategic application of *in silico* in conjunction with *in vitro*, and *in vivo* animal studies heralds the possibility and opportunity for improving toxicity prediction and human safety assessment.

### 1.3.1 Computational Modeling Approaches

We have seen over the past decade a continuing interest and focus on the development and application of *in silico* approaches for the prediction of toxicity. For even with the application of high-throughput screening for *in vitro* toxicity testing, such testing may still be precluded by cost, timing or other practical considerations. Consequently, the results from *in vitro* assays are increasingly being integrated with computer modeling to predict compound toxicity for untested or poorly studied chemicals.[11,12]

Despite their initial promise over the past decade or so, the application of *in silico* technology for toxicity prediction has now settled down to a more reasonable and rational strategy for developing and applying *in silico* approaches.[11,13] Encouragingly, in recent years we have seen increasing focus and improvement in the utility of *in silico* and computational modeling and simulation approaches.[11,12] These range from QSAR approaches to the increasing focus on more integrated and more sophisticated systems biology approaches.

Publicly and commercially available toxicity databases represent invaluable sources of toxicology information and cover a diverse array of chemicals of widely differing chemical structures and properties, and toxicity endpoints. Such information is an important resource for the development and validation of computational toxicity modeling.

The sophistication of our modeling and simulation technologies has improved dramatically over the past decade. The utility of Pharmacokinetic/Pharmacodynamic (PK/PD), Toxicokinetic/Toxicodynamic (TK/TD), Physiologically-Based Pharmacokinetic (PBPK) models is well documented and, as mentioned earlier, we are seeing increasing focus on integrative systems biology approaches. The continued advancement of modeling and simulation approaches is critical for both the integration of data generated in the assessment of a chemical's toxicity, and also to the critical issue of improving the risk assessment process. This integration of predictive toxicology approaches will become increasingly critical as industrial chemicals advance and change (*e.g.*, nanoparticles) and as new pharmaceutical entities are discovered and developed.

### 1.3.2 *In Vitro* Approaches

Traditionally, *in vitro* testing has been positioned as a screening and triaging approach for *in vivo* higher tier testing or for mechanistic investigations. With the new vision presented by NRC's *Toxicity Testing in the 21st Century*,[9] the role of *in vitro* assays in toxicity prediction may change dramatically in the future.

*In vitro* toxicity assays are conducted primarily with cells or cell lines, ideally from humans or transfected prokaryotic cells.[10]

### 1.3.3 "-omics" Technologies

We are seeing an increasing focus on the application of "omics" technologies (proteomics, genomics, metabon(l)omics) in the generation of predictive biomarkers of potential adverse events. To date, this work has been largely focused on a retrospective analysis of the correlation between biomarkers and toxicity. However, increasingly, we are seeing the utility of biomarkers for a particular toxicity emerging and it is reasonable to assume that the rate of the identification of robust and reliable safety biomarkers will accelerate in coming years.

### 1.3.4 *In Vivo* Animal Models

The reliability of animal models for toxicity prediction is also an area for continued focus and much needed improvement. The reliability of the typical rodent and canine models for assessment of toxicity and establishment of safe exposure levels or dosing is far from foolproof. In this book you will find an extensive discussion of the utility of the current animal models for various toxicities and target mediated toxicities. The future increase in genetically modified models (*i.e.*, animal knockouts, transgenics, humanized) will further add to the critical need to improve our armamentarium and the robustness of the animal models we use for the extrapolation to, and assessment of, human safety and risk.

### 1.3.5 Integrative Approaches

As previously discussed, there is now increasing focus on integrating *in silico*, *in vitro* and *in vivo* animal data into a more holistic assessment of human safety and risk. As discussed in several chapters, various approaches are being utilized to better assess toxicity issues earlier and integrate these with modeling approaches. In recent years we have seen increasing focus on the use of biologically based modeling approaches and this is being further extended as data on toxicity biomarkers becomes more widely available. In this book there is discussion of how such data is being generated, and integrated into biologically based modeling approaches.

## 1.4 Future Perspective

It is well established that the prediction of human safety and risk issues from *in silico*, *in vitro* and animal *in vivo* data is fraught with high uncertainty and significant challenges. Safety issues remain a major cause of attrition in drug failure[5] and the prediction of safety from exposure to environmental and industrial chemicals is no less challenging. In time, we will gain a much clearer insight into the key regulatory pathways and processes and the consequences of perturbation of these for human safety. This book provides a discussion of the current assessment of the state-of-the-art-and-science in the prediction of toxicity and outlines the many challenges that lie ahead. The chapters discuss the various technologies currently available to predict toxicities of chemicals by leading experts in the fields of computational modeling, *in vitro* testing, "-omics" technologies, *in vivo* animal models, and integrative approaches.

Clearly the challenge is daunting, however, as mentioned, the integration of data from a variety of sources heralds the possibility of improving our ability to predict toxicity and significantly improve our ability to identify human safety and risk issues, and reduce the risk to humans from exposure to industrial, occupational and pharmaceutical chemicals.

## References

1. European Commission, Corrigendum to Regulation (EC) No. 1907/2006 of the European Parliament and of the Council of 18 December 2006 concerning the Registration, Evaluation, Authorisation and Restriction of Chemicals (REACH), establishing a European Chemicals Agency, amending Directive 1999/45/EC and repealing Council Regulation (EEC) No 793/93 and Commission Regulation (EC) No 1488/94 as well as Council Directive 76/769/EEC and Commission Directives 91/155/EEC, 93/67/EEC, 93/105/EC and 2000/21/EC, Official Journal of the European Union, 2007, L136, 3–282.
2. J. Woodcock and R. Woosley, *Annu. Rev. Med.*, 2008, **59**, 1–12.
3. A. P. Worth, A. Bassan, J. de Brujin, A. Gallegos Saliner, T. Netzeva, G. Patlewicz, M. Pavan, I. Tsakovska and S. Eisenreich, *SAR QSAR Environ. Res.*, 2007, **18**, 111–125.
4. R. S. Judson, K. A. Houch, R. J. Kavlock, T. B. Knudsen, M. T. Martin, H. M. Mortensen, D. M. Reif, D. M. Rotroff, I. Shah, A. M. Richard and D. J. Dix, *Environ. Health Perspect.*, 2009, **118**, 485–492.
5. I. Kola and J. Landis, *Nat. Rev. Drug Discovery*, 2004, **3**, 711–715.
6. D. Schuster, C. Laggner and T. Langer, *Curr. Pharm. Des.*, 2005, **11**, 3545–3559.

7. J. A. DiMasi and H. G. Grabowski, *J. Clin. Oncol.*, 2007, **25**, 209–216.
8. J. Zurlo, D. Rudacille and A. M. Goldberg, *Environ. Health Perspect.*, 1996, **104**, 878–880.
9. Committee on Toxicity Testing and Assessment of Environmental Agents, National Research Council, *Toxicity Testing in the 21st Century: a Vision and a Strategy,* The National Academies Press, Washington, DC, 2007.
10. Memorandum of Understanding on High Throughput Screening, Toxicity Pathway Profiling and Biological Interpretation of Findings, http://www.epa.gov/ncct/Tox21/.
11. C. Helma, in *Predictive Toxicology*, ed. C. Helma, Taylor & Francis, Boca Raton, FL, 2005, pp. 1–9.
12. J. C. Dearden, *J. Comput.-Aided Mol. Des.*, 2003, **17**, 119–127.
13. A. G. E. Wilson, X. Liu and J. A. Kramer, *Future Med. Chem.*, 2009, **1**, 1201–1205.

CHAPTER 2

# In Silico *Tools for Toxicity Prediction*

MARK T. D. CRONIN

School of Pharmacy and Chemistry, Liverpool John Moores University, Byrom Street, Liverpool, L3 3AF, UK

## 2.1 Introduction

*In silico* techniques for toxicity prediction encompass a wide variety of approaches.[1] The approaches vary from forming a simple relationship between a structural fragment and a toxicological event through to complex multivariate relationships between descriptors and toxicity values. The conceptual basis for this variety of approaches is described by Worth and Mostrag-Szlichtyng (see Chapter 4) and elsewhere (*e.g.*, Madden[2]). In addition to regulatory use (as described by Worth[3]), there is great interest in the use of these techniques to predict the toxicity of products such as pharmaceuticals.[4–6]

To make *in silico* approaches usable for the practical purpose of toxicity prediction, it is helpful to have them formalised into tools. Such tools are usually software algorithms that, generally speaking, lead the user through an input of the chemical structure to various process(es) (automated or manual) to make a prediction of toxicity. Some software is freely available or on a not-for-profit basis; other programs are developed on a commercial basis. Whilst there may be a natural bias towards freely available tools, it must be remembered that nothing is free and that the development of such a tool will require funding at some point—this is often through governmental agencies or *via* public grants (*e.g.*, European Union Framework Programmes). The advantages of commercial software, however, are that they are often better developed, more user-friendly and better supported in terms of help and technical

RSC Drug Discovery Series No. 12
New Horizons in Predictive Toxicology: Current Status and Application
Edited by Alan G. E. Wilson

Published by the Royal Society of Chemistry, www.rsc.org

assistance. The purpose of this chapter is to provide an overview of the tools available for toxicity prediction, with a particular emphasis (although not exclusively) on freely available tools. Due to the nature of this expanding field, this chapter cannot provide an exhaustive overview of every technique, and therefore the reader should pay special attention to the techniques described in Worth and Mostrag-Szlichtyng (see Chapter 4) as well as elsewhere.[1,4–6]

## 2.2 Structure–Activity Relationships (SARs) and Structural Alerts

Structure–activity relationships are qualitative in nature. They relate a fragment of a molecule to a particular activity or functionality. This, therefore, makes them amenable to the prediction of categoric (yes/no) toxicity endpoints. To achieve this, fragments within a molecule that are associated with a toxicity endpoint must be identified. This is normally assumed to be from human expert judgement, thus a toxicologist may be have the knowledge that a certain fragment is associated with a toxic effect. For instance, aromatic amines are known to (often) be mutagenic. Thus, if such a fragment is observed in a further molecule it may be assumed to also be mutagenic. This collation, or harvesting, of the knowledge of experts into a computational approach has been termed an "expert system". It should be noted, however, that somewhat confusingly, many predictive systems in toxicology and QSAR in general are termed "expert system"; of these a large proportion go beyond the collation of experts' knowledge.

### 2.2.1 *In Silico* Tools for SARs and Structural Alerts to Predict Toxicity

Whilst being the simplest approach to modelling toxicity, the development of expert systems for toxicological endpoints is possibly the most time-consuming to achieve. This is because it requires the extraction of knowledge of expert toxicologists and translation of that knowledge into usable and succinct chemistry-based computer code, ideally supported by evidence from study reports or the peer-reviewed literature. This "manual" collation of data is in contrast to the relatively more rapid statistical methods to develop models. The software below describes some of the approaches that have been taken to derive and present SARs.

#### *2.2.1.1 DEREK Nexus*

One of the better developed knowledge-based expert systems is DEREK Nexus from Lhasa Ltd, Leeds, England (more information is available from https://www.lhasalimited.org/derek_nexus/). DEREK Nexus follows on from the DEREK for Windows software—incorporating a number of strategic updates and improvements. DEREK Nexus applies the knowledge of toxicological experts to identify substructures or fragments of a molecule that may cause toxicity in humans, other mammals and bacteria. This can be used to identify the potential hazard associated with a compound.

The DEREK Nexus software contains "rules" for a number of toxicity endpoints, the best developed knowledge bases are those for mutagenicity/carcinogenicity and skin sensitisation. There are a multitude of other endpoints covered by DEREK Nexus.[7] It is of interest that the creation of the DEREK Nexus rulebase has largely been a collaborative effort, with membership of Lhasa Ltd allowing for development of the rulebase. This has enabled Lhasa Ltd to draw upon a unique collection of toxicologists and experts to assemble the knowledge in the rulebase.

As a qualitative system to identify toxic hazard, it is difficult, or even misleading, to consider performance statistics for the predictive capability of DEREK Nexus. Some of these are reviewed by Dearden,[7] but must be treated with caution. There is also an on-going debate as to whether the absence of an alert from a molecule is an indication that the molecule is non-toxic.[8] In the author's opinion, the absence of an alert gives an indication that toxicity may be less likely, but unless an endpoint is very well characterised in DEREK Nexus—note that some endpoints such as skin sensitisation are well characterised—it is only an indication rather than a prediction. To increase confidence, the use of multiple or consensus modelling may be advantageous.[8]

#### *2.2.1.2 Other Knowledge-Based Expert Systems*

There are a small number of additional knowledge-based expert systems for toxicity prediction. These include:

1) The Oncologic™ expert system from the US Environmental Protection Agency (US EPA). Oncologic™ predicts cancer-causing potential by applying the rules of SAR analysis, mimicking the decision logic of human experts, and incorporating knowledge of how chemicals cause cancer in animals and humans. This software is freely downloadable from http://www.epa.gov/oppt/sf/pubs/oncologic.htm.
2) ToxAlert/HazardExpert Pro from Compudrug Inc. These programs include knowledge-based rules covering toxicity endpoints such as oncogenicity, mutagenicity, teratogenicity, neurotoxicity and cell toxicity. More information is available from: www.compudrug.com.

### 2.2.2 SARs and Knowledge-Based Expert Systems—Conclusions

SARs, structural fragments and structural alerts are powerful methods to identify the hazard associated with a chemical. They are particularly powerful when they capture the knowledge of expert toxicologists and can apply this easily. They are, however, time-consuming and labour intensive to create due to the manual nature of the definition of the structural alert. The following recommendations regarding the use of SARs and knowledge-based expert systems can be made:

1) Knowledge-based expert systems are transparent methods with which to identify the hazard associated with a chemical. They are excellent tools to garner the expertise of toxicologists.
2) The limitations of expert systems must be understood. Association with an alert does not necessarily mean any recognisable risk, this can only be established with a knowledge of the exposure, endpoint and associated information. As such, structural alerts can be used to screen out potentially hazardous compounds, or prioritise compounds for further testing or investigation.
3) Structural alerts and SARs must be well defined in terms of chemistry. Thus any mitigating fragments that may increase or decrease toxicity must be defined. However, too fine a definition means that the alert will be relevant to only a very small number of compounds; too broad a definition means that too many compounds may be identified. An appropriate balance is required.
4) Structural alerts and SARs must be supported by strong evidence. This could be from sources such as study results or peer-reviewed publications.
5) Structural alerts and SARs are highly amenable to computerisation, the expert systems described in this section (DEREK Nexus, Oncologic™, HazardExpert as well as others) are excellent examples of what may be achieved.
6) Structural alerts and SARs are relatively mature for certain endpoints *e.g.*, skin sensitisation and mutagenicity. They require further development for other human health endpoints, especially chronic and organ specific toxicities.

## 2.3 Category Formation and Read-Across

The basis of category formation is described in Chapter 4. This is a general process of identifying a suitable means forming a group of compounds related in some, significant manner to the target compound. There are a variety of possible approaches to achieve this, however, the best method to form robust categories is on a mechanistic basis. Following grouping of compounds, the category can be populated with toxicological data and information and read-across attempted.[9]

### 2.3.1 *In Silico* Tools for Category Formation and Read-Across

At its simplest level, the general process of category formation and read-across can be performed manually. For instance, it was possible to form a simple category based on structural analogues for long-chain alcohols.[10,11] However, there is a need for computerisation for a number of reasons including:

1) the anticipated greater throughput to cope with *e.g.*, REACH;
2) the greater variety of chemical structures leading to increased difficulty to obtain analogues through structural similarity;
3) the need for more advanced methods to group compounds (the profilers) that go beyond structural similarity and incorporate a greater mechanistic emphasis;
4) the need to seamlessly search for toxicological data and information;
5) the requirement for reporting formats suitable for regulatory use;
6) and numerous other reasons.

With these, and many other criteria in mind, the Organisation for Economic Cooperation and Development (OECD) has been co-ordinating the development of the OECD QSAR Toolbox.

#### *2.3.1.1 OECD QSAR Toolbox*

The OECD QSAR Toolbox incorporates information and tools from various sources into a logical workflow. Crucial to this workflow is grouping chemicals into chemical categories. The OECD QSAR Toolbox allows for the input of a chemical structure and then progression through the workflow by identifying relevant structural characteristics and/or potential mechanisms or modes of toxic action of the target chemical. This is achieved by the application of what are termed "profilers". It should be noted that some profilers are based around chemistry and therefore could be considered to span across endpoints (*e.g.*, protein reactivity as described Enoch *et al.*[12]) whilst others more closely related to a particular endpoint (*e.g.*, DNA reactivity summarised by Enoch and Cronin[13]). When the relevant structural characteristics have been identified, other chemicals that (potentially) share the same structural characteristics and/or mechanism or mode of action are identified. These compounds (target and structural/mechanistic analogues) form a group or category. Experimental data from the databases within the Toolbox, or the user's own databases, can then be used to populate the category. Read-across, trend analysis or even simple QSAR can be performed within the category to make an assessment of toxicity. Predictions can be captured through appropriate reporting formats.

The Toolbox is freely downloadable from www.qsartoolbox.org. It is gaining acceptance for regulatory use due to its transparency and mechanistic basis, not to mention its low cost. The formation of categories and use of software such as the OECD QSAR Toolbox will come to the fore as we tackle more complex human health and environmental endpoints such as chronic toxicity.

#### 2.3.1.2 *Other* In Silico *Tools for Category Formation and Read-Across*

There are a number of other methods that may be employed to form chemical categories, including the following:

1) The Analog Identification Methodology (AIM) from the US EPA is available on-line at: http://www.epa.gov/oppt/sf/tools/aim.htm. AIM is free to use and identifies closely related chemical structures for which experimental data may be available in the public domain to help users in their efforts to determine the potential hazard(s) of the untested material. As such, AIM allows for the entry of a compound structure *via* the internet interface. Following entry of a structure, AIM gives a list of analogues that share structural features with the target compound and also obtains experimental data in publicly available, readily accessible data sources.
2) Toxtree is an open-source application provided free of charge from the European Commission's Computational Toxicology Group in the Institute for Health and Consumer Protection at the Joint Research Centre (JRC) in Ispra, Italy. It is available for download from: http://ecb.jrc.ec.europa.eu/qsar/qsar-tools/index.php?c=TOXTREE. Part, or all, of the software has been implemented into the OECD QSAR Toolbox. Toxtree assigns the target chemical into categories and predicts various kinds of toxic effect by applying decision-tree approaches. The current decision trees have implemented the original and extended Cramer classification schemes; the Verhaar scheme to assign a compound to aquatic mechanisms and modes of action; rulebases to determine skin and eye irritation and corrosion; the Benigni–Bossa rulebase for mutagenicity and carcinogenicity; the ToxMic rulebase for the *in vivo* micronucleus assay; structural alerts for identification of Michael Acceptors; the START rulebase for persistence/biodegradation potential.[14,15]
3) ToxMatch is also provided free of charge from the EC's JRC.[15,16] It is available for download from: http://ecb.jrc.ec.europa.eu/qsar/qsar-tools/index.php?c=TOXMATCH. Toxmatch allows the user to apply several chemical similarity indices to facilitate the grouping of chemicals into categories and read-across. This includes the ability to compare datasets based on various structural and descriptor-based similarity indices as well as the means to calculate pairwise similarity between compounds or aggregated similarity of a compound to a set. Thus ToxMatch assists the user to identify structurally similar compounds.
4) There are numerous other methods to create categories and perform read-across. It can, of course, be performed manually. In addition, in theory any structure-searchable toxicity database could also be used to create categories and read-across.

### 2.3.2 *In Silico* Tools for Category Formation and Read-Across—Conclusions

The grouping of chemicals together and "reading across" of activity is one of the simplest methods to predict toxicity. It has been used in a regulatory setting for a number of years, however interest in this technique has grown rapidly in the past five years due to the reality of supplying data to meet regulations such as REACH; its transparency allowing for ease of use and regulatory acceptance; the development of the freely available and highly successful OECD QSAR Toolbox; and the realisation that predicting chronic human effects is unlikely to be achieved by QSAR statistical methods. The following recommendations for chemical grouping methods to allow for read-across can be made:

1) The use of category formation should not lose sight of the need for a rational and, preferably, mechanistic basis for forming a group of compounds.
2) Read-across should consider likely physico-chemical and structural factors that modulate activity such as absorption, reactivity and enzyme binding.
3) Without doubt, currently the best computational tool for category formation and read-across is the OECD QSAR Toolbox. This freely available tool is remarkably well developed and provides an excellent platform for these activities. It is supported by comprehensive training material.
4) There are two challenges for the further development of category formation and read-across for the prediction of chronic toxicity:
   i) The development of better profilers for chronic toxicity.
   ii) The inclusion of more toxicological data into the publicly available databases.

## 2.4 Quantitative Structure–Activity Relationships (QSARs)

A quantitative structure–activity relationship (QSAR) attempts to relate the biological activity (in this case toxicity) of a series of compounds to their structural physico-chemical properties (see Chapter 4; Cronin and Madden;[1]Madden[2]). QSARs take many forms, from relatively simple linear regression analyses based on a single descriptor, through to highly multivariate and non-linear approaches such as support vector machines and self-organising maps. A description of what constitutes a QSAR is provided in Chapter 4. In terms of toxicity prediction, ideally a QSAR should be based around a single recognisable mechanism of action and descriptor(s) that can be related directly to the effect and mechanism. Such a scenario gives the user confidence in the application of such a model. It is, however, often difficult to obtain especially for chronic toxicities with varied and even unknown mechanisms of action.

### 2.4.1 Tools for Compiling QSARs

There are thousands of published QSARs in the literature. Ideally, an interested user does not want to have to search the literature for the QSAR, calculate the descriptors and reformulate the QSAR. In addition to the practicalities of use, there has been a desire to use reporting formats (see Chapter 4; Cronin[17]) for regulatory use of QSARs. Clearly it is wasteful to reformulate the reporting format every time a QSAR is used. Because of these, and many other good reasons, there has been an increasing emphasis on developing databases of QSAR models. A small number of examples of such databases are given below.

#### *2.4.1.1 JRC QSAR Model Database*

The EC JRC are developing a database of (Q)SAR models (*i.e.*, an inventory of information on the models);[14,15] the JRC QSAR Model Database is freely accessible from the website: http://ecb.jrc.ec.europa.eu/qsar/qsar-tools/index.php?c=QRF. The JRC QSAR database is based around the QSAR Model Reporting Format (QMRF). The QMRF is a harmonised template for summarising and reporting key information on (Q)SAR models, including the results of any validation studies. The information is structured according to the OECD (Q)SAR validation principles. Developers and users of (Q)SAR models can submit JRC information on (Q)SARs using a QMRF template. The JRC performs a quality control (*i.e.*, adequacy and completeness of the documentation) of the QMRFs submitted. It should be noted that this is not a validation process or assessment of the quality of the QSAR itself, merely an assessment of the description of the model and its level of documentation. At first sight, this may seem self-defeating—why compile models and then not be critical of them? However the purpose here is to build an inventory with documentation suitable for regulatory use (especially for REACH) and then allow the user to assess the validity of any prediction they make using the model. Thus, properly documented summaries of (Q)SARs (*i.e.*, robust summaries) are included in the JRC QSAR Model Database, but not recommendations as to the "best QSARs". Inclusion of a model in the QSAR Model Database does not imply acceptance or endorsement by the JRC or the European Commission. More information on the nature of QMRFs is provided in Worth and Mostrag-Szlichtyng (see Chapter 4) and by Cronin.[17]

#### *2.4.1.2 Bio-Loom*

A more comprehensive compilation of historical QSAR models is the Bio-Loom database from BioByte (http://www.biobyte.com/bb/prod/bioloom.html). This QSAR database is derived around searches for biological activities. There are hundreds of searchable biological activity types, both targets (*e.g.*, enzyme inhibition) and results (*e.g.*, effects). These searches lead to thousands of active structures, many of which have been carefully studied *via* QSAR. It should be noted that the majority of targets and effects are related to pharmacological activity, rather than directly to toxicity. In order to create the QSARs, Bio-Loom calculates hydrophobic and molecular refractivity parameters *via* their software programmes CLOGP and CMR. It also has BioByte's entire access to the Thor Masterfile database, which includes over 60 000 measured log *P* and log *D* values (in many solvent systems), as well as 14 000 p$K_a$s, including associated references. An interesting example of this approach is reported by Juranić *et al.*[18] for rat acute toxicity. In terms of regulatory use, whilst this is a useful resource, the models are not available with "ready-made" QMRFs. These would have to be written by the user.

### *2.4.1.3 The QSAR DataBank (QDB)*

There are a number of other approaches to creating databases of QSARs. An interesting example is given by the University of Tartu in Estonia. Their QSAR DataBank (QDB) gives a strategy and platform for recording QSARs and is available from http://qsardb.org/StartingPage. Importantly the QDB sets out the type of information that is essential to record and describe each QSAR. QDB defines six types of domain objects which have attributes that define their identity and interrelations with other domain objects. Different types of domain objects have different attributes. Some attributes are common to all types, some of them are not. The domain objects are given additional description by attaching documents to them. QDB defines a limited set of system document attachments. Applications are free to define and use any number of extension document attachments. The domain objects with document attachments include the:

1) Compound: chemical substance with a known structure utilising structure files.
2) Property: experimentally measured or perceived characteristics of compounds. This includes the units of biological activity and reference.
3) Descriptor: theoretically derived characteristics of compounds.
4) Model: the mathematical relationship between one or more descriptors and a property. This may be a statistical or data mining model in Predictive Model Markup Language (PMML).
5) Prediction: execution of a model on a set of compounds.
6) Workflow: step-by-step instructions for (re)producing predictions.

The QDB is in its infancy and needs to be populated with a broader selection of QSARs. However, it provides a framework within which we can develop a searchable database populated with structures, data and models. The use of largely open-source software also makes it attractive.

### *2.4.1.4 Other Databases of QSAR Models*

The databasing field and its interaction with chemoinformatics is fast moving, and there are likely to be other sources of databasing opportunities arising in the future.

### 2.4.2 Tools for Compiling QSARs—Conclusions

For a variety of reasons, attempts have been made to create databases of QSAR models. On the surface this may seem a relatively straightforward process, particularly for regression-based models. However, it is clear that thought must be given to what is required and how the database will be used. In terms of a usable product, the Bio-Loom database sets that standard, however it is a commercial product and little biased towards toxicological endpoints. The JRC QSAR Model Database and QDB approach the problem with different philosophies; the former with regulatory use in mind, the latter to create an open-access database. The user must decide what their priorities are in order to obtain the greatest utility from whatever product they choose. In summary, the following conclusions can be made:

1) The development of databases of QSAR models for toxicity is to be encouraged.
2) The current databases of QSAR models for toxicity are currently in their infancy.
3) A database for QSAR models for toxicity requires the correct database structure to capture the relevant information (as QDB), a suitable searchable graphical interface (as Bio-Loom) and regulatory significance (as the JRC QSAR Model Database). The user will have to define which is their priority.
4) For regulatory use of a QSAR model for toxicity, the ability to create suitable documentation (*e.g.*, the QMRF) to ensure the validity of the prediction, is extremely valuable.
5) The next generation of databases should allow for seamless integration with software for descriptor calculation and model deployment—see Section 2.6 on *in silico* workflows.

## 2.5 QSAR-Derived and Related Expert Systems for Toxicity Prediction

The increase in availability of toxicity datasets from various sources, as well as better data manipulation and handling capabilities, has allowed for, and stimulated growth in the development of expert systems for toxicity prediction based on QSAR-type modelling approaches. This a fast-moving field, with rapid development of models and techniques. The philosophy of most expert systems is to develop quantitative models for toxicity, allowing the user to enter a chemical structure and obtain a result. The expert system usually "takes care" of the practicalities of running a QSAR, *i.e.*, descriptor calculation and running of the statistical model. This certainly makes life easier for the user who therefore requires less expertise to use individual models. A downside of this automation, and also necessary commercial sensitivity, is that the models and datasets may be hidden, reducing transparency of how the prediction is made.

### 2.5.1 QSAR-Derived and Related Expert Systems for Toxicity Prediction—*In Silico* Tools

There is a great variety of expert systems for toxicity prediction. These allow the user to input a structure and be led directly to a prediction of toxicity, often with some indication regarding issues such as whether the target molecular is within the chemical space, or applicability domain, of the model. A comprehensive review of expert systems is given by Dearden,[7] the current chapter can only serve to provide a relatively limited overview. The following is a non-comprehensive selection of expert systems available.

#### *2.5.1.1 Caesar*

The Caesar models for toxicity prediction arose from a European Union project.[19] The models are freely available from: www.caesar-project.eu. The Caesar project developed new QSAR models specifically for REACH to address the following endpoints (the citations give details of the models): bioconcentration in fish;[20] skin sensitisation;[21] mutagenicity;[22] carcinogenicity;[23] developmental toxicity.[24] These endpoints were chosen not only due to their relevance to REACH, but also as a result of their anticipated high animal use.

The models are developed from a number of multivariate approaches. These describe the molecules in terms of 2D descriptors and then use statistical analysis to predict toxicity, or identify the most similar compounds to the target. The software allows for molecules to be entered singly or in batch by a variety of processes. Caesar assesses the reliability of the results and whether the compound is within the applicability domain of the model (in Caesar version 2.0). The latter is a useful check, and applicability domain is assessed using a further free tool based on: a chemometric check; searching fragments for outliers; use of a similarity index; concordance of the prediction with experimental values; and the uncertainty of the prediction.

#### *2.5.1.2 ADMET Predictor™*

ADMET Predictor™ is marketed by Simulations Plus, more information is available from http://www.simulations-plus.com/Default.aspx. The program contains a number of predictive models for the following endpoints, amongst others: œstrogen and androgen receptor binding; maximum recommended therapeutic dose (MRTD); skin and respiratory sensitisation; chromosomal aberration; phospholipidosis; reproductive/developmental toxicity; rat acute toxicity; carcinogenicity in rats and mice; hERG-encoded $K^+$ channel affinity; human liver adverse effects. Models are created in ADMET Predictor™ by calculation of descriptors for physico-chemical properties and structure. Descriptors are selected to best represent the endpoint. The models are then created using a variety of machine-learning methods including Kohonen Self-Organising Maps, artificial neural network ensembles, support vector machines, Kernel Partial Least Squares (PLS) and Ordinary PLS, as well as multiple linear regression. Excellent performance statistics are reported by the developers. An issue with this approach will be the lack of QMRFs for these models, as well as understanding the models and their transparency for regulatory use.

#### 2.5.1.3 ACD/ToxSuite

ACD/ToxSuite is a collection of software modules that predict probabilities for basic toxicity endpoints.[25–27] The endpoints predicted include hERG inhibition, genotoxicity, acute toxicity, eye and skin irritation, endocrine disruption. More information is available from http://www.acdlabs.com/products/pc_admet/tox/tox/. The software allows for structure input and the prediction of toxicity with a reliability index. Up to five similar compounds from within the training set with literature data and references are displayed to assist with comprehension of the prediction.[28] The ACD/ToxSuite modules use a number of approaches to produce the models including fragmental Partial Least Squares (PLS) with 100 bootstraps to yield baseline predictions that are automatically corrected for non-linear effects in local chemical spaces—a combination called Global, Adjusted Locally According to Similarity (GALAS) modelling methodology.

#### 2.5.1.4 Other QSAR-Derived and Related Expert Systems for Toxicity Prediction

There are an increasing number of other systems for toxicity prediction, a non-exhaustive list is provided below:

1) A number of programs, and an even wider selection of endpoints modelled, are available from MultiCASE Inc. More than 180 modules covering various areas of toxicology and pharmacology are supplied. These are modelled by the well established Computer Automated Structure Evaluation (CASE) technology.[29] The software is widely used and it is stated to be applicable for regulatory use.[30]
2) LAZAR (LAZy structure–Activity Relationships) has been developed by Prof. Christoph Helma of the University of Freiburg, Germany. Models for a number of endpoints including those relating to liver toxicity, mutagenicity, carcinogenicity and maximum recommended daily dose are freely available from: http://lazar.in-silico.de/. The endpoint is predicted from a similarity searching methodology based on molecular fragments.[31]
3) TerraBase Inc. market a number of QSAR prediction modules relating to health-related toxicity. They are models of mouse and rat oral and intravenous acute toxicity, œstrogen receptor binding and skin irritation. The computation of each toxicity endpoint uses molecular fragments in a neural network type of approach.[32]

4) TOPKAT (TOxicity Prediction by Komputer Assisted Technology) is a QSAR-based system for the prediction of toxicity, marketed commercially by Accelrys Inc.; it is incorporated into their Discovery Studio suite as DS-TOPKAT and more information is available from http://accelrys.com/solutions/scientific-need/predictive-toxicology.html. TOPKAT has a long history as a successfully developed predictive toxicology approach, current endpoints predicted include: carcinogenicity, mutagenicity, acute and chronic toxicity as well as skin sensitisation and skin and eye irritation.

### 2.5.2 QSAR-Derived and Related Expert Systems for Toxicity Prediction—Conclusions

There is a wide variety of QSAR-derived expert systems to predict toxicity—this is now a mature field which allows for the rapid development of new models. These should be seen as complementary to the other approaches to predict toxicity *i.e.*, SARs and read-across. The following recommendations can be made:

1) QSAR-Derived and related expert systems provide rapid and user-friendly platforms to predict toxicity. They are usually professionally developed and well supported in terms of support and guidance.
2) The user of a QSAR-derived expert system must have some knowledge and expertise in the science behind the modelling approach.
3) The available expert systems are seldom designed for regulatory use—they provide little automation of reporting formats and may be considered as non-transparent by some regulatory agencies.
4) There is no one "best" expert system that can be recommended. The user must weigh up their individual merits and benefits.
5) A criticism of the highly automated approaches to predict toxicity can be that they lose sight of the mechanistic basis and of toxicity prediction.

## 2.6 Workflows to Develop and Use QSARs

There are likely to be many instances when a QSAR developer will want to save their model and use it (and allow others to use it) at a later date. Whilst we have databases of QSARs (see Section 2.4) these do not form usable models *i.e.*, they are not incorporated with the appropriate software to calculate descriptors. Similarly, bespoke (or commercially sensitive) models will not usually be available through the expert systems described in Section 2.5. Therefore, there has been interest in using further software to link together the different elements of toxicity prediction *i.e.*, entry of chemical structure, calculation of descriptors, searching of databases, modelling, storage of models *etc.* A useful overview of chemoinformatic tools is provided by Muchmore *et al.*[33] Their use and the generic process of developing a QSAR and modelling approach is termed a 'workflow', and is described in more detail by Bassan and Worth.[34]

### 2.6.1 Workflow Tools to Develop and Use QSARs

Recently software is becoming available that can manage computational workflows. Whilst workflows include a number of chemistry applications, the applications available for use in the workflows go far beyond chemistry and toxicology into other areas such as business operations and banking. The following describe two of the more commonly applied software platforms for developing computational workflows that are amenable to toxicity prediction.

#### *2.6.1.1 KNIME*

KNIME, the Konstanz Information Miner, is a user-friendly, open-source data analytics, reporting and integration platform. KNIME integrates various components for machine learning and data mining through its modular data pipelining concept. The graphical user interface allows for the assembly of nodes for data pre-processing, modelling and data analysis and visualisation. The workflow software is freely available from http://www.knime.org/. The philosophy of KNIME is described by Berthold *et al.*[35] and various applications of it in pharmaceutical drug development are detailed by Patel *et al.*[36] and Geldenhuys *et al.*[37]

On the technical side, KNIME integrates various other open-source projects, *e.g.*, machine-learning algorithms from Weka, the statistics package R, as well as LibSVM, JFreeChart, ImageJ, and the Chemistry Development Kit. KNIME is implemented in Java but also allows for wrappers calling other code in addition to providing nodes that allow the developer to run Java, Python, Perl and other code fragments. This means that computational workflows can be developed for toxicity prediction and shared openly between interested parties.

#### *2.6.1.2 Pipeline Pilot*

Pipeline Pilot is developed and marketed by Accelrys Inc. (http://accelrys.com/products/pipeline-pilot/). It is an informatics platform that allows access to data stored in databases, automates the scientific analysis of those data, and enables researchers to explore, visualise and report research results rapidly. Pipeline Pilot has an integrated set of applications for modelling and simulation, formed into a number of "component collections". The use of Pipeline Pilot is gaining popularity with pharmaceutical companies and the use of workflows to predict toxicity (in this case Ames mutagenicity) is described by Hansen *et al.*[38]

The "component collections" in Pipeline Pilot are wide ranging. Within the chemistry collection, there are a number of modules *e.g.*, the Chemistry Component Collection is able to analyse, profile, and manage the compounds in databases with chemically intelligent filters and learning. The ADMET Component Collection calculates predicted absorption, distribution, metabolism, excretion and toxicity (ADMET) properties for collections of molecules. The collection includes models for human intestinal absorption, aqueous solubility, blood–brain barrier penetration, plasma protein binding, cytochrome P450 2D6 inhibition, and hepatotoxicity. The Cheminformatics Component

Collection allows the user to build database-focused search and browse applications using Pipeline Pilot. The collection is comprised of two sub-systems: List Management and Query Services—a database search and hit list management system, and Pipeline Pilot Chemistry Cartridge—enabling the storage and searching of chemical structures and reactions.

### 2.6.2 Workflows to Develop and Use QSARs—Conclusions

There is an increase in all areas of research and development in the use of computational workflows. The area of toxicity prediction can utilise this technology to its advantage to store and disseminate models. The following recommendations can be drawn:

1) Workflows should be considered for developing, storing and distributing toxicity models. They should simplify the process of modelling and allow for the use of models.
2) Use of workflows does require some training, which is recommended for any user.
3) KNIME is a free-to-use open-source workflow technology, however it was not developed specifically for chemistry applications (although does integrate them). Pipeline Pilot may require some payment to obtain full applications, but is developed with chemistry applications in mind.
4) All workflows require good components to work successfully *e.g.*, descriptor calculators and modelling software. Care must be taken to obtain high-quality components.
5) As workflows are developed for toxicity prediction, there should be an effort to distribute them in a co-ordinated manner.

## 2.7 Conclusions

There are a large number of *in silico* tools to predict toxicity. An increasing number are freely available, although there are some distributed on a commercial basis. The freely available tools have, generally, been developed with public money to help with regulatory use of predictive toxicology—a particular driver in the past decade has been the European Union's REACH regulation; the next decade will require solutions to the new generation of chemicals legislation in the US and Japan, in addition to the challenge of the European Union's Cosmetic Regulation, amongst many other pieces of global legislation. Commercial tools have traditionally been focussed towards product (especially drug) development. However, as use of these *in silico* tools becomes more widespread, these distinctions are being lost.

Some *in silico* tools for toxicity prediction are very simplistic, often based around little more than the presence of a particular molecular fragment to identify hazard or group chemicals together. Other *in silico* tools are more complex, involving multivariate modelling of large toxicological databases. There is no "ideal" or "best" *in silico* tool for toxicity prediction. It is true to say that the simpler the model the better, but the user of any approach should make a pragmatic decision with regard to the models they may have available, the endpoint, the chemical and the need and use of the prediction *i.e.*, the use of the model and application is performed in a context-dependent manner. It is the user's responsibility to ensure the validity of any prediction of toxicity, the process to achieving this is well described by Cronin[17] and Worth and Mostrag-Szlichtyng (see Chapter 4).

## Acknowledgements

This project was sponsored by Defra through the Sustainable Arable Link Programme. This work also was supported by the EU 6[th] Framework Integrated Project OSIRIS (http://www.osiris-reach.eu; Contract No. GOCE-ET-2007-037017).

## References

1. *In Silico Toxicology: Principles and Applications*, ed. M. T. D. Cronin and J. C. Madden, Royal Society of Chemistry, Cambridge, 2010.
2. J. C. Madden, in *In Silico Toxicology: Principles and Applications*, ed. M. T. D. Cronin and J. C. Madden, Royal Society of Chemistry, Cambridge, 2010, p. 11.
3. A. P. Worth, in *Recent Advances in QSAR Studies. Methods and Applications*, ed. T. Puzyn, J. Leszczynski and M. T. D. Cronin, Springer, Dordrecht, 2010, p. 367.
4. L. G. Valerio Jr, *Toxicol. Appl. Pharmacol.*, 2009, **241**, 356.
5. S. Boyer, *Altern. Lab. Anim.*, 2009, **37**, 467.
6. C. Yang, L. G. Valerio and K. B. Arvidon, *Altern. Lab. Anim.*, 2009, **37**, 523.
7. J. C. Dearden, in *In Silico Toxicology: Principles and Applications*, ed. M. T. D. Cronin and J. C. Madden, Royal Society of Chemistry, Cambridge, 2010, p. 478.
8. C. M. Ellison, J. C. Madden, P. Judson and M. T. D. Cronin, *Mol. Informat.*, 2010, **29**, 97.
9. S. J. Enoch, in *Recent Advances in QSAR Studies. Methods and Applications*, ed. T. Puzyn, J. Leszczynski and M. T. D. Cronin, Springer, Dordrecht, 2010, p. 209.
10. C. Schäfers, U. Boshof, H. Juerling, S. E. Belanger, H. Sanderson, S. D. Dyer, A. M. Nielsen, A. Willing, K. Gamon, Y. Kasai, C. V. Eadsforth, P. R. Fisk and A. E. Girling, *Ecotox. Environ. Saf.*, 2009, **72**, 996.
11. S. E. Belanger, H. Sanderson, P. R. Fisk, C. Schäfers, S. M. Mudge, A. Willing, Y. Kasai, A. M. Nielsen, S. D. Dyer and R. Toy, *Ecotox. Environ. Saf.*, 2009, **72**, 1006.
12. S. J. Enoch, T. W. Schultz and M. T. D. Cronin, *Crit. Rev. Toxicol.*, 2011, **41**, in press.

13. S. J. Enoch and M. T. D. Cronin, *Crit. Rev. Toxicol.*, 2011, **40**, 728.
14. M. Pavan and A. P. Worth, *SAR QSAR Environ. Res.*, 2007, **18**, 515.
15. A. Mostrag-Szlichtyng, J. M. Z. Comenges and A. P. Worth. *Exp. Opin. Drug Metab. Toxicol.*, 2010, **6**, 785.
16. G. Patlewicz, *SAR QSAR Environ. Res.*, 2008, **19**, 785.
17. M. T. D. Cronin, in *In Silico Toxicology: Principles and Applications*, ed. M. T. D. Cronin and J. C. Madden, Royal Society of Chemistry, Cambridge, 2010, p. 275.
18. I. O. Juranić, B. J. Drakulić, S. D. Petrović, D. Ž. Mijin and M. V. Stanković, *Chemosphere*, 2006, **62**, 641.
19. E. Benfenati, *Chem. Cent. J.*, 2010, **4**, I1.
20. A. Lombardo, A. Roncaglioni, E. Boriani, C. Milan and E. Benfenati, *Chem. Cent. J.*, 2010, **4**, S1.
21. Q. Chaudhry, N. Piclin, J. Cotterill, M. Pintore, N. R. Price, J. R. Chrétien and A. Roncaglioni, *Chem. Cent. J.*, 2010, **4**, S5.
22. T. Ferrari and G. Gini, *Chem. Cent. J.*, 2010, **4**, S2.
23. N. Fjodorova, M. Vračko, M. Novič, A. Roncaglioni and E. Benfenati, *Chem. Cent. J.*, 2010, **4**, S3.
24. A. Cassano, A. Manganaro, T. Martin, D. Young, N. Piclin, M. Pintore, D. Bigoni and E. Benfenati, *Chem. Cent. J.*, 2010, **4**, S4.
25. D. Zmuidinavicius, P. Japertas, A. Petrauskas and R. Didziapetris, *Curr. Top. Med. Chem.*, 2003, **3**, 1301.
26. R. Didziapetris, K. Lanevskij and P. Japertas, *Chem. Res. Toxicol.*, 2008, **21**, 2450.
27. J. Dapkunas, A. Sazonovas and P. Japertas, *Chem. Biodivers.*, 2009, **6**, 2101.
28. A. Sazonovas, P. Japertas and R. Didziapetris, *SAR QSAR Environ. Res.*, 2010, **21**, 127.
29. G. Klopman, *J. Am. Chem. Soc.*, 1984, **106**, 7315.
30. R. D. Saiakhov and G. Klopman, *Toxicol. Mech. Meth.*, 2008, **18**, 159.
31. C. Helma, *Mol. Diversity*, 2006, **10**, 147.
32. K. L. E. Kaiser, S. P. Niculescu and T. W. Schultz, *SAR QSAR Environ. Res.*, 2002, **13**, 57.
33. S. W. Muchmore, J. J. Edmunds, K. D. Stewart and P. J. Hajduk, *J. Med. Chem.*, 2010, **53**, 4830.
34. A. Bassan and A. P. Worth, *QSAR Comb. Sci.*, 2008, **27**, 6.
35. M. R. Berthold, N. Cebron, F. Dill, T. R. Gabriel, T. Kotter, T. Meinl, P. Ohl, C. Sieb, K. Thiel and B. Wiswedel, *Data Anal. Mach. Learning Applic.*, 2008, **319**, 326.
36. H. Patel, M. J. Bodkin, B. N. Chen and V. J. Gillet, *J. Chem. Inf. Model.*, 2009, **49**, 1163.
37. W. J. Geldenhuys, A. S. Darvesh, M. O. Funk, C. J. Van der Schyf and R. T. Carroll, *Bioorg. Med. Chem. Lett.*, 2010, **20**, 5295.
38. K. Hansen, S. Mika, T. Schroeter, A. Sutter, A. ter Laak, T. Steger-Hartmann, N. Heinrich and K. R. Müller, *J. Chem. Inf. Model.*, 2009, **49**, 2077.

CHAPTER 3

# *Development of an Evaluation Support System for Estimating Repeated-Dose Toxicity of Chemicals Based on Chemical Structure*

MAKOTO HAYASHI*[a,b] AND YUKI SAKURATANI[b]

[a] Biosafety Research Center, Foods, Drugs and Pesticides, 582-2, Shioshinden, Iwata, Shizuoka 437-1213, Japan; [b] National Institute of Technology and Evaluation, Chemical Management Center, 2-49-10, Nishihara, Shibuya-ku, Tokyo 151-0066, Japan

## 3.1 Introduction

In Japan, industrial chemicals are regulated by the Chemical Substances Control Law (CSCL) for the prevention of environmental pollution caused by chemical substances that exhibit a risk of impairing human health or interfering with the inhabitation and/or growth of flora and fauna. This law mandates prior examination of the hazardous properties of new chemical substances which are intended to be manufactured in or imported into Japan.

The safety evaluations of chemicals designated as "existing chemicals" under CSCL have been continuously conducted by the government since implementation of CSCL. As a result, various test data for existing chemicals were

RSC Drug Discovery Series No. 12
New Horizons in Predictive Toxicology: Current Status and Application
Edited by Alan G. E. Wilson

Published by the Royal Society of Chemistry, www.rsc.org

accumulated for certain endpoints such as biodegradation, bioconcentration, genotoxicity, repeated (mainly 28 days) dose toxicity and ecotoxicity. The test data for the existing chemicals under CSCL are disclosed on the websites of public institutions:[1,2]

Based on the test data for new and existing chemicals, the activities for developing evaluation methods by (quantitative) structure–activity relationship [(Q)SAR] and the category approach[3] have been conducted under governmental initiatives.[4–8] These methods are utilized in the prioritization of untested existing chemicals or the preparation of the reference information in the examination of new chemicals.

Repeated dose toxicity (RDT) testing is one of the important endpoints of CSCL. However, a reliable and satisfactory (Q)SAR or category approach method for evaluating the RDT of chemicals still remains undeveloped. Generally, the purpose of RDT is to determine values such as the no-observed-effect level (NOEL), no-observed-adverse-effect level (NOAEL), lowest observed effect level (LOEL), and lowest observed adverse effect level (LOAEL). These values are determined by experts in the field based on test data of various endpoints related to hematology, blood biochemistry, and histopathology. Therefore, it is difficult to directly correlate the NOEL and other parameters with chemical structure since all these parameters are influenced by many toxicological events. In order to make an *in silico* evaluation of RDT for target chemicals from their chemical structure, a comprehensive collaboration of experts possessing a variety of knowledge on the analogue chemicals is necessary.

The project, "Development of hazard assessment techniques using structure–activity relationship methods",[9] sponsored by New Energy and Industrial Technology Development Organization (NEDO) in Japan, aims to develop the "Hazard Evaluation Support System Integrated Platform (HESS)"[10] for providing decision support information to experts to evaluate the RDT of chemicals by the category approach (project period: 2007–2011). This chapter contains an overview of HESS and describes the methodology for evaluating RDT by the category approach developed in this project. The trial version of the system has been developed and will be available in 2012.

## 3.2 Overview of the Hazard Evaluation Support System Integrated Platform (HESS)

As shown in Figure 3.1, HESS has two main databases. One is the Toxicity Knowledge Information Database containing RDT test reports and toxicity mechanism information. The other is the Metabolism Knowledge Information Database containing metabolic maps and Adsorption, Distribution, Metabolism, and Excretion (ADME) information. HESS has two support tools for estimating the RDT of chemicals by using information from these databases—the Bayesian Net RDT Prediction Model and the Category Approach Support Function. HESS is designed to be compatible with the Organisation for

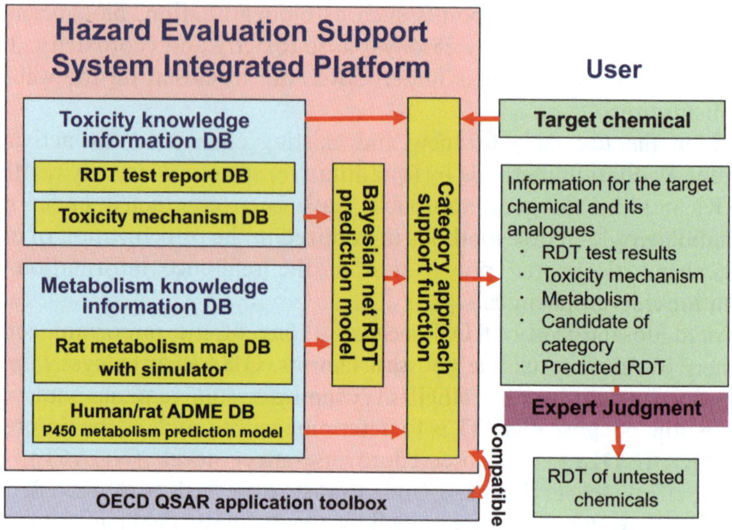


**Figure 3.1** Structure of the Hazard Evaluation Support System Integrated Platform (HESS).

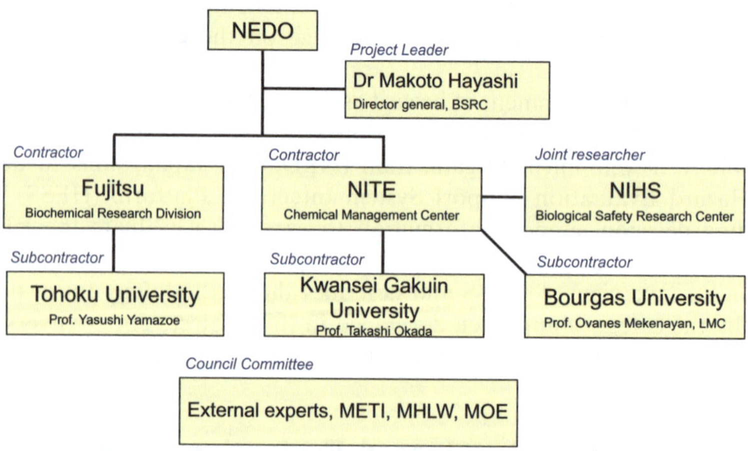


**Figure 3.2** Organization of the "Development of hazard assessment techniques using structure–activity relationship methods" project.

Economic Co-operation and Development (OECD) (Q)SAR Application Toolbox.[11]

Figure 3.2 shows the organizational structure of the project. The project leader is Dr Makoto Hayashi who is the Director General of Biosafety Research Center, Foods, Drugs and Pesticides (BSRC) and former Head of the Division of Genetics and Mutagenesis, National Institute of Health Sciences (NIHS). The main contractors of the project are National Institute of

Technology and Evaluation (NITE) and Fujitsu Limited. NITE, in a joint research effort with NIHS, is primarily responsible for the collection and systemization of toxicity and metabolism information. Fujitsu Limited is primarily responsible for building the database systems. A group of experts led by Prof. Takashi Okada of Kwansei Gakuin University and a group of experts led by Prof. Yasushi Yamazoe of Tohoku University are responsible for development of the Bayesian Net RDT Prediction system and development of the metabolism prediction method, respectively.

HESS is not designed to be an "automatic prediction system". Rather, the aim is to provide support for experts such as toxicologists, pathologists and risk assessors in making toxicological decisions. Therefore, it is very important for the system to be easy to use by such experts. As such, the system is being developed primarily by toxicologists, pathologists and risk assessors. This is the most important feature of our project and is largely different from other projects in which systems are developed primarily by IT experts.

The other important feature of this project is its international focus. Since this system is designed to be compatible with the OECD (Q)SAR Application Toolbox and is intended to be used internationally, Professor Menkenyan's team from the Laboratory of Mathematical Chemistry (LMC) of Bourgas Prof. Assen Zlatarov University, responsible for building the OECD (Q)SAR Application Toolbox system, was invited to join the project. Accordingly, the project is coordinating closely with OECD activities.

In addition, recommendations from regulatory authorities are also being taken into consideration in the development of HESS. External experts in relevant fields and members of three ministries [The Ministry of Economy, Trade and Industry (METI); The Ministry of Health, Labour and Welfare (MHLW); and The Ministry of Environment (MOE)] are participating in the supporting committee of the project.

The following is an overview of each part of HESS:

### 3.2.1 Repeated-Dose Toxicity Test Report Database

This database contains RDT test reports (mainly 28-day RDT using rats with oral administration) for about 500 chemicals. The test data for the existing chemicals under CSCL comprise the main part of the database (about 300 chemicals). All these tests were conducted in compliance with GLP principles under the auspices of the Japanese government (MHLW, METI and NITE). In addition, other RTD test reports with detailed data and high reliability are included in the system (*e.g.*, US National Toxicology Program (NTP) data,[12] data from journal papers, *etc.*).

In this database, test report information is organized and stored in a uniform format in order to facilitate comparison of test data between chemicals. The data for hematological examinations, blood chemical examinations and histopathological examinations are grouped into individual data tables and incorporated into the RDT Test Report Database. In these group tables, the data showing statistically significant differences from the control group are noted with a mark. However, it is difficult to compare the data among test reports using different statistical analyses methods because the statistically significant differences depend on the analysis method used.[13] Therefore, in this database, data determined to be a toxicological effect by experts are marked differently.

Histopathological terms used in the test reports generally differed between the various laboratories. In order to make searches of histopathological findings more complete and effective, we developed a thesaurus as part of the database search engine.[14]

### 3.2.2 Toxicity Mechanism Database

The purpose of the database is to provide the rationale for the categorization of toxicity at repeated dose levels. This database contains information from about 220 original papers that suggests the mechanism of the toxicological effects observed in the collected RDT test reports of about 70 chemicals. The toxicity mechanism information covers molecular level mechanisms, cellular level mechanisms and biological level mechanisms and contains *in vitro, in vivo* and *ex vivo* test results, signal transfer pathways, *etc.* We expect the database to provide appropriate information for use with the adverse outcome pathways (AOP).

### 3.2.3 Rat Metabolism Map Database with Metabolic Simulator

This database contains metabolic maps for about 680 chemicals with repeated dose toxicity test reports. All parental chemicals and metabolites in the database can be searched by chemical structure, and the database can be used for investigating metabolites that cause toxicological effects. In addition, a simulator for estimating metabolites in rat liver has been built based on the metabolic maps.

### 3.2.4 Human/Rat ADME Database (P450 Metabolism Prediction Model)

This database contains information from about 280 original papers related to ADME information on humans and rats for about 80 chemicals with RDT test reports. A model for predicting metabolites of human P450 (CYP2E1, *etc.*) based on the substrate structure was developed. The prediction results for about 100 chemicals with repeated dose toxicity tests are also included in the database. This database can be used for comparing species differences in toxicity between humans and rats based on their different metabolisms.

### 3.2.5 Bayesian Net RDT Prediction Model

In this model, causality of toxicity is expressed as a network of conditional probabilities (Bayesian network) to predict the probability for a chemical to induce a specified toxicity.[15] Detailed repeated dose toxicity test data (hematological examinations, blood chemical examinations and histopathological examinations) were analyzed by the cascade model,[16] a data mining method to extract structure alerts used in the Bayesian Net RDT Prediction Model.[17] The model was built using the expertise of toxicologists and pathologists.

### 3.2.6 Category Approach Support Function

Chemicals considered to have the same AOP in RDT tests were categorized based on information in the Toxicity Knowledge Information Database and the Metabolism Knowledge Information Database. The definitions of the categories (structure, parameter, mechanism of action and metabolism boundaries) were entered in the system as a category library of 36 categories.

The system operates in the following way: When a user inputs a target chemical for evaluation, the system searches the category library for possible categories to which the target chemical belongs. Information about the target chemical and its analogues, extracted from the Toxicity Knowledge Information Database and the Metabolism Knowledge Information Database, are displayed in a format that can be easily analyzed by the system user. The user can also investigate the category to which the target chemical belongs and fill in data gaps using data from the analogue chemicals.

## 3.3 Example of the Category Approach for Evaluating Repeated-Dose Toxicity Tests

It is important to establish a methodology for applying the category approach to complex endpoints in the field of chemical management. OECD is proposing using AOP principles in applying the category approach to complex endpoints.[18] The AOP indicates the mechanistic pathway to the outcome in the test from the molecular initiating event. We also included AOP principles in applying the category approach to repeated dose toxicity tests based on the OECD proposal.[19]

The outcomes observed in repeated dose toxicity tests largely depend on the dose levels tested. They are a complex combination of the findings recognized as the effects of the test chemical. Accordingly, we described an adverse effect as a combination of findings. We also described the mechanism by which these adverse effects are induced from molecular level to *in vivo* level as the AOP for repeated dose toxicity.

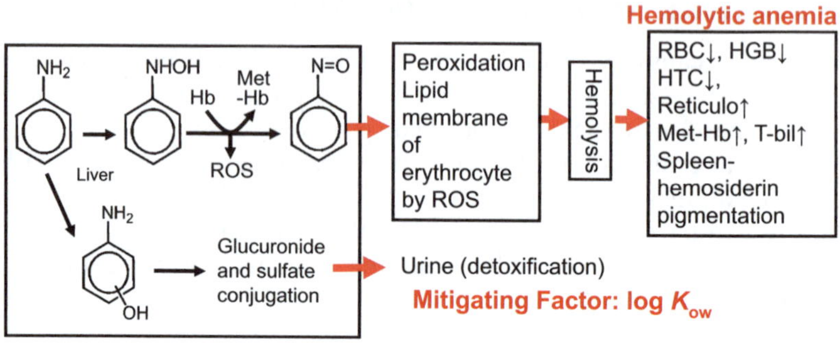


**Figure 3.3** AOP for describing the hemolytic anemia induced by anilines.

Figure 3.3 shows the AOP for describing the hemolytic anemia induced by anilines in repeated dose toxicity tests in rats. *N*-hydroxyanilines, metabolites of anilines in the liver, react with hemoglobin to produce methemoglobin (Met-Hb) and reactive oxygen species (ROS). ROS then causes peroxidation of lipids in the membranes of erythrocytes, resulting in hemolytic anemia. When hemolytic anemia is induced, hematological examinations yield the following observations: a decrease in the number of erythrocytes (RBC↓), a decrease in hemoglobin (HGB↓), a decrease in hematocrit (HTC↓) and an increase in reticulocytes (Reticulo↑). In addition, an increase in total bilirubin (T-bil↑) can be observed in blood biochemical examinations, and pigmentation of hemosiderin in the spleen is typically observed in histopathological examinations.

In order to create a category of anilines that induce hemolytic anemia, it is necessary to specify anilines that induce hemolytic anemia by the same pathway as shown in Figure 3.3. Table 3.1 shows some anilines with information related to hemolytic anemia. This information is contained in the Toxicity Knowledge Information Database and the Metabolism Knowledge Information Database. The findings related to hemolytic anemia shown in the table is obtained from RDT tests in male rats. The test for chemicals No. 4 and No. 8 is the Combined Repeat-Dose and Reproductive/Developmental Toxicity Screening test. The tests for the other chemicals are 28-day repeated dose toxicity tests.

This table shows that, as a rule, anilines with the potential to induce hemolytic anemia have a log $K_{ow} > 1$ (Nos. 1–8). On the other hand, two chemicals (amino phenols Nos. 9 and 10) with low log $K_{ow}$ values of 0.24 showed only a weak potential to induce hemolytic anemia at high-dose levels. Three chemicals, amino benzene sulfonic acids (Nos. 11–13) that had even lower log $K_{ow}$ values (negative values) lack the potential to induce hemolytic anemia even at high-dose levels. The reason aminophenols and amino benzene sulfonic acids exhibit weak or no potential to induce hemolytic anemia can be explained by their high excretion rate in urine due to their high water solubility.[20] These results indicate that a low log $K_{ow}$ value could be used as a mitigating factor in the formation of category boundaries.

**Table 3.1** Evidence related to the adverse outcome pathway in Figure 3.3 for anilines.

| No. | Structure | *Observed findings related to hemolytic anemia in the repeated dose toxicity tests for male rats (dose* $mg^{-1}\ kg^{-1}\ day^{-1}$*)* | *log* $K_{ow}$* | *Mechanism information* | | *Metabolism information* |
|---|---|---|---|---|---|---|
| | | | | *Met-Hb* | *HBI*[23–24] | |
| 1 | 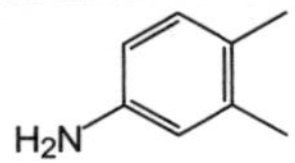 | RBC ↓ • Hgb ↓ · Hct ↓ · Ret ↑<br>Spleen pigmentation (250) | 2.17 | *in vitro*[21]<br>*in vivo*[21] | 0.7 | — |
| 2 | 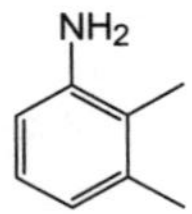 | Hgb ↓ (60)<br>RBC ↓ · Hct ↓ · Ret ↑ · MetHb ↑<br>T-Bil ↑ (300) | 2.17 | *in vitro*[21]<br>*in vivo*[21] | — | — |
| 3 | 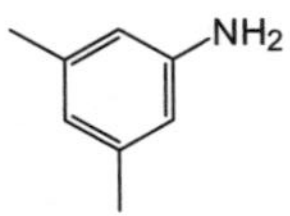 | Hgb ↓ · Hct ↓ · Ret ↑<br>Spleen pigmentation (60)<br>RBC ↓ (360) | 2.17 | *in vitro*[21]<br>*in vivo*[21] | 14 | — |
| 4 | 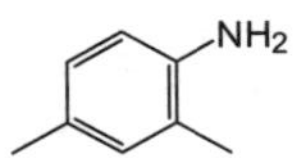 | Bil ↑ (2) Hgb ↓ (10) | 2.17 | *in vitro*[21]<br>*in vivo*[21] | 2.3 | 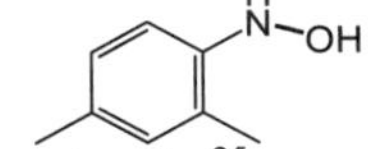<br>*in vitro*[25] |
| 5 | 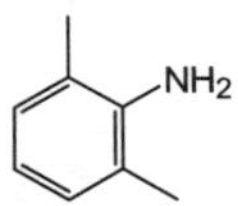 | RBC ↓ · Hgb ↓ · Ret ↑ · Met-Hb ↑<br>Spleen pigmentation (250) | 2.17 | *in vitro*[21]<br>*in vivo*[21] | 1.1 | — |
| 6 | 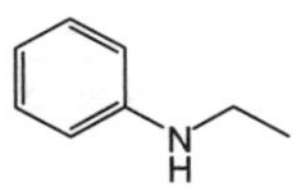 | RBC ↓ (5)<br>Hgb ↓ · Hct ↓ · Ret ↑ · Met-Hgb ↑<br>Spleen pigmentation (25) | 2.11 | — | — | — |

**Table 3.1** (*Continued*)

| *No.* | *Structure* | *Observed findings related to hemolytic anemia in the repeated dose toxicity tests for male rats (dose $mg^{-1}$ $kg^{-1}$ $day^{-1}$)* | *log $K_{ow}$** | *Mechanism information* | | *Metabolism information* |
|---|---|---|---|---|---|---|
| | | | | *Met-Hb* | *$HBI^{23–24}$* | |
| 7 | 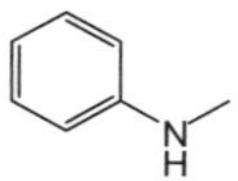 | RBC ↓ · Hgb ↓ · Hct ↓ · Ret ↑<br>Spleen pigmentation (25)<br>Bil ↑ (125) | 1.62 | — | — | 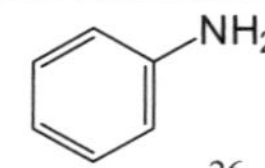<br>*in vitro*[26] |
| 8 | 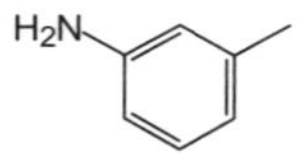 | Spleen pigmentation (30)<br>RBC ↓ · Hgb ↓ · Hct ↓ · Bil ↑ (100) | 1.62 | *in vitro*[22]<br>*in vivo*[22] | 4.9 | — |
| 9 | 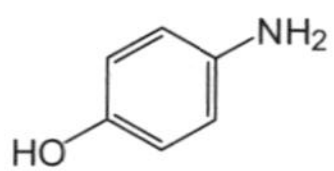 | RBC ↓ (500) | 0.24 | — | — | — |
| 10 | 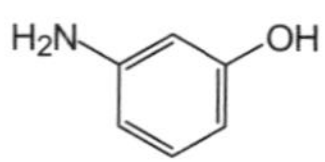 | Bil ↑ · Spleen pigmentation (720) | 0.24 | — | — | — |
| 11 | 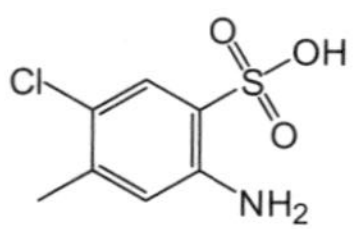 | — | –0.89 | — | — | — |
| 12 | 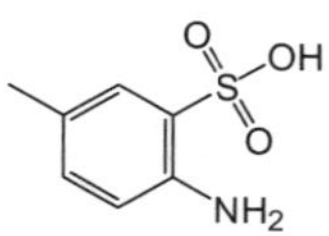 | — | –1.53 | — | — | — |
| 13 | 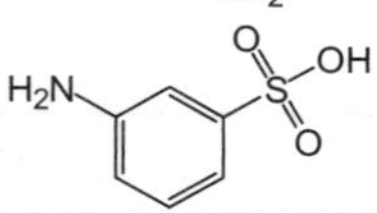 | — | –2.08 | — | — | — |

*Calculated by KOWWIN 1.67 (US EPA).

Mechanism and metabolism information can be used as supporting evidence for the pathway shown in Figure 3.3. For example, Met-Hb is not measured in many repeated dose toxicity tests, but the production of Met-Hb can be strong evidence for the pathway shown in Figure 3.3. However, such an information gap can be complemented by other studies.[21,22] For example, hemoglobin binding index (HBI)[23,24] values measured in other studies and the presence of metabolites such as *N*-hydroxy-, or nitroso-amines observed in other studies can be evidence for the pathway.

In comparison to the other anilines in the Table 3.1, 2,4-dimethylaniline (No. 4 in Table 3.1) did not show the same apparent potential to induce hemolytic anemia. This can be explained by the fact that the chemical was tested at rather low dose levels. However, the possible potential for this chemical to induce hemolytic anemia can be predicted by the pathway shown in Figure 3.3 by the supporting evidence that the production of Met-Hb was observed[21] as a result of the production of *N*-hydroxy-2,4-dimethylaniline as a metabolite[25] of the target chemical.

In the case of *N*-methylaniline (No. 7), the existence of aniline as a metabolite[26] in the *in vitro* test supported the fact that *N*-methylaniline induces hemolytic anemia. Therefore, it is suggested that the boundary of the category can be extended from primary aniline to *N*-alkyl aniline.

Based on the above discussions, chemical Nos. 1–8 in Table 3.1 can be specified as the category members inducing hemolytic anemia by the pathway shown in Figure 3.3. The boundary of the category can be defined not only by

**Table 3.2** Evidence related to the adverse outcome pathway in Figure 3.3 for untested anilines.

| *No.* | *Structure* | *Observed findings related to hemolytic anemia in the repeated dose toxicity tests for male rats (dose mg$^{-1}$ kg$^{-1}$ day$^{-1}$)* | *log* $K_{ow}$* | *Mechanism information* | | *Metabolism information* |
|---|---|---|---|---|---|---|
| | | | | *Met-Hb* | *HBI*[23,24] | |
| 14 | 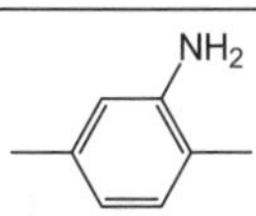 | Untested | 2.17 | *in vitro*[21]<br>*in vivo*[21] | 7.3 | — |
| 15 | 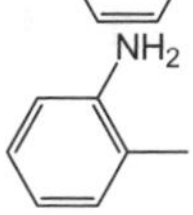 | Untested | 1.62 | — | 4.0 | 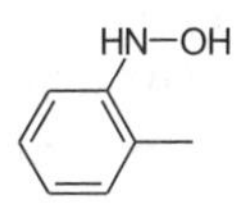<br>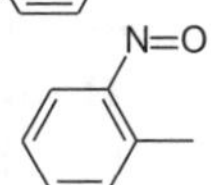<br>*in vivo*[27] |
| 16 | 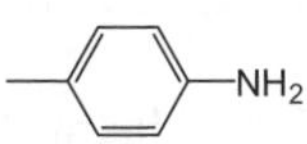 | Untested | 1.62 | — | 4.3 | 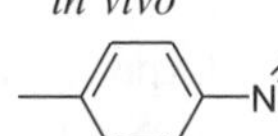<br>*in vitro*[28] |

*Calculated by KOWWIN 1.67 (US EPA).

the chemical structure but also by the activity of the chemicals. In the case of the members mentioned above, the boundary of the category can be defined as monocyclic anilines and alkylated anilines with log $K_{ow} > 1$. In HESS, the boundaries of RDT categories defined by such an approach are registered in the category library.

It is also necessary to consider AOPs using evidence other than actual RDT data in order to find an appropriate category for chemicals lacking experimental data. For example, from the structure of an untested chemical, we can predict the reactivity in the molecular initiating event in an AOP based on, for example, the nature and position of a substitution group. Table 3.2 shows examples of chemicals in a category defined by the method described above and the supporting evidence. Based on the RDT test data of the category members (Nos. 1–8 in Table 3.1), these chemicals (Nos. 14–16 in Table 3.2) can be estimated to induce hemolytic anemia at dose levels less than 250 mg $kg^{-1}$ $day^{-1}$.

## 3.4 Conclusions

In this chapter, we have given an overview of HESS and the category approach for evaluating RDT tests, as well as an example of categorization by this system. Because this system is designed to provide detailed RDT test data in conjunction with mechanism and metabolism information, the system can provide reliable information based on scientific evidence to the experts who evaluate the safety of chemicals. Completion of the final version of the system is planned for 2012.

## Acknowledgements

This work was supported by a NEDO grant for the "Development of hazard assessment techniques using structure–activity relationship methods" project.

## References

1. http://dra4.nihs.go.jp/mhlw_data/jsp/SearchPageENG.jsp.
2. http://www.safe.nite.go.jp/jcheck/Top.do.
3. OECD, Manuals for Investigation of HPV Chemicals, OECD, Paris, 2007, Ch 3.2.
4. http://kate.nies.go.jp/.
5. http://qsar.cerij.or.jp/cgi-bin/QSAR/index.cgi?e.
6. A. Hirose, E. Kamata, H. Akiyama, M. Takahashi, T. Morita, M. Ema and M. Hayasi, 6th World Congress on Alternatives & Animal Use in the Life Sciences Abstracts, Japanese Society of Alternatives to Animal Experiments, Tokyo, 2007, p. 80.
7. Y. Sakuratani, J. Yamada, K. Kasai, Y. Noguchi and T. Nishihara, *SAR QSAR Environ. Res.*, 2005, **16**, 403.
8. http://www.safe.nite.go.jp/english/kasin.html.

9. http://www.nedo.go.jp/activities/portal/p07033.html.
10. M. Hayashi, *ALTEX*, 2009, **26**, 85.
11. Guidance Document for Using the OECD (Q)SAR Application Toolbox to Develop Chemical Categories According to the OECD Guidance on Grouping of Chemicals, Organisation for Economic Cooperation and Development, Paris, 2009.
12. http://ntp.niehs.nih.gov/.
13. K. Kobayashi, Y. Sakuratani, T. Abe, S. Nishikawa, J. Yamada, A. Hirose, E. Kamata and M. Hayashi, *J. Toxicol. Sci.*, 2010, **35**, 79.
14. S. Nishikawa, T. Yamashita, T. Imai, M. Yoshida, Y. Sakuratanil, J. Yamada, A. Maekawa and M. Hayashi, *J. Toxicol. Sci.*, 2010, **35**, 295.
15. T. Okada, N. Ohmori, S. Mori, H. Horikawa, M. Yamakawa, Y. Sakuratani, T. Yamada and M. Hayashi, *ALTEX*, 2009, **26**, 86.
16. T. Okada, *J. Comput.-Aided Chem.*, 2002, **2**, 79.
17. T. Okada, M. Yamakawa, N. Ohmori, S. Mori, H. Horikawa, T. Hayashi and S. Fujishima, *Chem. Cent. J.*, 2010, **4**, 1.
18. http://www.oecd.org/document/23/0,3343,en_2649_34365_33957015_1_1_1_1,00.html.
19. Y. Sakuratani, S. Sato, S Nishikawa, J. Yamada, A. Maekawa and M. Hayashi, *ALTEX*, 2009, **26**, 80.
20. Y. Sakuratani, S. Sato, S. Nishikawa, J. Yamada, A. Maekawa and M. Hayashi, *SAR QSAR Environ. Res.*, 2008, **19**, 681.
21. D. Cauchon and K. Krishnan, *J. Appl. Toxicol.*, 1997, **17**, 397.
22. M. Kiese, *Pharmacol. Rev.*, 1966, **18**, 1091.
23. G. Sabbioni, *Environ. Health Perspect.*, 1993, **99**, 213.
24. G. Sabbioni, *Environ. Health Perspect.*, 1994, **102**, S6.
25. T. Nohmi, R. Miyata, K. Yoshikawa, M. Nakadate and M. Ishidate, *Biochem. Pharmacol.*, 1983, **32**, 735.
26. R. Kato, M. Takayanagi and T. Ohshima, *Jpn. J. Phamcol.*, 1969, **19**, 53.
27. O. S. Son, D. W. Everetf and E. S. Fiala, *Xenobiotica*, 1980, **10**, 457.
28. B. Tyrakowska, S. Boeren, B. Geurtsen and I. M. C. M. Rietjens, *Drug Metabol. Disposition*, 1993, **21**, 508.

CHAPTER 4

# Towards a Common Regulatory Framework for Computational Toxicology: Current Status and Future Perspectives

ANDREW P. WORTH* AND ALEKSANDRA MOSTRAG-SZLICHTYNG

European Commission, Joint Research Centre, Institute for Health and Consumer Protection, Via E. Fermi, 21027 Ispra, VA, Italy

## 4.1 Introduction

In order to efficiently and effectively assess the risks of large numbers of existing chemicals and new chemical entities, there is an increasing emphasis in the regulatory setting on the use of so-called "non-testing" methods, either as a supplement to, or as a substitute for, traditional testing methods. In particular, alternatives to animal methods are being developed to reduce the need for animal testing in pharmacology and toxicology. Non-testing methods are based on the premise that the properties (including physicochemical properties and biological activities) of a chemical depend on its intrinsic nature and can be directly predicted from its molecular structure or inferred from the properties of similar compounds whose activities are known.

Non-testing methods include a range of predictive approaches, including Structure–Activity Relationships (SARs), Quantitative Structure–Activity Relationships (QSARs), chemical grouping and read-across, and computer-based tools based on the use of one or more of these approaches. Non-testing

RSC Drug Discovery Series No. 12
New Horizons in Predictive Toxicology: Current Status and Application
Edited by Alan G. E. Wilson

Published by the Royal Society of Chemistry, www.rsc.org

methods also include models for predicting the absorption, distribution, metabolism and elimination (ADME) characteristics of chemicals in biological organisms,[1] even though these models are not based entirely on the intrinsic properties of chemicals.

The main question for the assessor when applying non-testing methods for regulatory purposes concerns the usefulness of the approach, which can be broken down into the practical applicability of the method and the adequacy of the predictions. Considerable progress has been made at the EU and international levels to develop a harmonised framework for assessing and documenting non-testing methods and their predictions. Exactly how this framework is applied in practice will depend on the provisions of the specific legislation (*e.g.*, chemicals, pesticides, biocides, cosmetics) and the context in which the non-testing data are being used (including, for example, whether a traditional testing method is being replaced, whether additional, supporting data are available, and the consequences of making an inaccurate prediction). The general framework leaves largely open the difficult question of how to determine the adequacy of predicted data, and there is a considerable need to develop detailed guidance on how the predictions generated by non-testing methods can be translated into regulatory decisions.

This chapter introduces the conceptual basis of SARs and QSARs, collectively referred to as (Q)SARs, as well as the related approach of chemical grouping (category formation) and read-across within chemical groups (categories). The current international framework for (Q)SAR models and predictions is then described (a similar framework has been developed for category and read-across approaches). The practical applicability of this framework is illustrated by focussing on a checklist of 10 key questions, with respect to some well known software tools and their predictions of genotoxicity of two case study compounds. The purpose of these case studies is to highlight some of the scientific issues that need to be considered, as well the difficulties encountered. This leads into a discussion of what is needed to provide further guidance on the assessment of prediction adequacy.

## 4.2 Conceptual Basis of (Q)SAR Models

(Q)SARs are theoretical models that are designed to predict the physicochemical, biological (*e.g.*, toxicological) and fate properties of molecules from knowledge of chemical structure.

More specifically, a SAR is a qualitative relationship between a molecular (sub)structure and the presence or absence of a given biological activity, or the capacity to modulate a biological activity imparted by another substructure. The term substructure refers to an atom, or group of adjacently connected atoms, in a molecule. A substructure associated with the presence of a biological activity is also called a structural alert. A SAR can also be based on the ensemble of steric and electronic features considered necessary to ensure the intermolecular interaction with a specific biological target molecule, which results in the manifestation of a specific biological effect. In this case, the SAR is sometimes called a 3D SAR or pharmacophore.

A QSAR is a quantitative relationship (often a regression model) between a biological activity (which may be categorical or quantitative) and one or more molecular descriptors that describe chemical structure in numerical terms and which are used as predictors of the biological activity. A molecular descriptor is a structural or physicochemical property of a molecule, or part of a molecule. A comprehensive review of molecular descriptors has been published by Todeschini and Consonni.[2]

Guidance on the regulatory application of (Q)SARs was developed to support the implementation of the REACH legislation in Europe, and has been published by the European Chemicals Agency (ECHA).[3]

## 4.3 Chemical Grouping and Read-Across

In addition to the formalised approach of QSAR analysis, it is possible to estimate chemical properties and endpoints by using a less formalised approach based on the grouping and comparison of chemicals. The grouping approach can be used, for example, to support the results of QSAR analysis or to generate estimated data (and fill data gaps) in the absence of suitable QSARs. Guidance on the application of the grouping approach has been published by the OECD[4] and by ECHA.[3] The ECHA and OECD guidance documents are scientifically equivalent, except that the ECHA guidance makes additional references to REACH criteria and procedures. To accompany the more detailed guidance, ECHA has published a summary guide on how to report categories and read-across.[5]

The use of endpoint information for one chemical, called a "source chemical", to make a prediction of the same endpoint for another chemical, called a "target chemical", is termed "read-across". The source and target chemicals are considered to be similar in some way, usually on the basis of structural similarity. Similar compounds (analogues) are assumed to exhibit similar biological activity. In principle, read-across can be applied to predict physicochemical properties, fate, human health effects and ecotoxicity, and it can be performed in a qualitative or quantitative manner, depending on the whether the analogue data being used is categorical or numerical in nature.

The reliability of read-across depends on the selection of appropriate analogues associated with the availability of reliable experimental data. In some cases, it is only possible to identify a limited number of suitable analogues, whereas in other cases, it is possible to build up a larger and more robust chemical group, called a chemical category. A chemical category is a group of chemicals whose physicochemical and human health and/or environmental toxicological and/or environmental fate properties are likely to be similar or follow a regular pattern as a result of structural similarity (or other similarity characteristic). The presence of common behaviour or coherent trends in the chemical category is generally associated with a common underlying mechanism of action. In general, the application of read-across between analogues in a chemical category is considered to be more reliable than the application of read-across in a smaller group of analogues (in which trends are not apparent).

## 4.4 The Adequacy of (Q)SARs

The REACH guidance for applying (Q)SARs provides a flexible framework according to which it is possible to use data from (Q)SAR models instead of experimental data if each of four main conditions is fulfilled:[3]

1) the model used is shown to be scientifically valid;
2) the model used is applicable to the chemical of interest;
3) the prediction (result) is relevant for the regulatory purpose; and
4) appropriate documentation on the method and result is given.

Thus, multiple, overlapping conditions must be fulfilled to use a (Q)SAR prediction instead of data generated by a standard experimental test, as illustrated in Figure 4.1. The extent to which these conditions can be relaxed for the indirect and supporting use of (Q)SAR data, remains to be established on the basis of experience.

The following sections will explain the considerations necessary for demonstrating model validity, applicability and adequacy. The need to provide "appropriate documentation" is fulfilled by the provision of QSAR reporting formats for models and their predictions. The former type of documentation is the QSAR Model Reporting Format (QMRF) and the latter is the QSAR Prediction Reporting Format (QPRF). To accompany the more detailed guidance, ECHA has published a summary guide on how to report QSAR models.[6]

### 4.4.1 Demonstrating Validity

The first condition for using (Q)SARs is the demonstration of model validity. There is widespread agreement that models should be scientifically valid or validated if they are to be used in the regulatory assessment of chemicals.

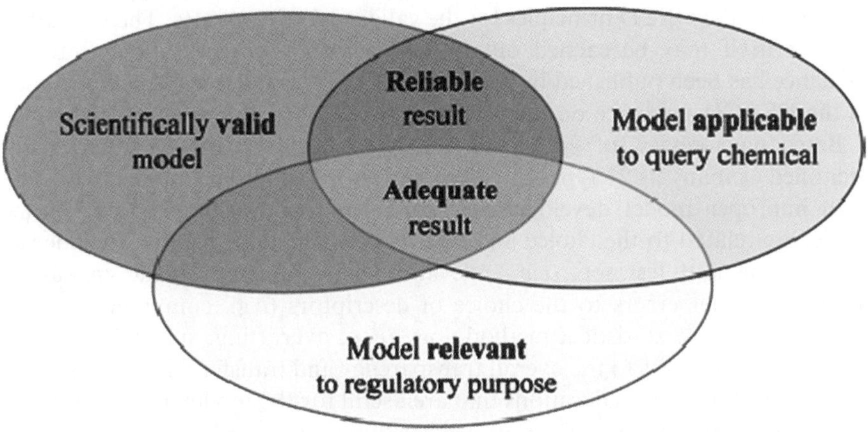


**Figure 4.1** The overlapping considerations of validity, applicability and relevance needed to demonstrate (Q)SAR adequacy.

According to the OECD Guidance Document on the Validation and International Acceptance of New or Updated Test Methods for Hazard Assessment, the term validation is defined as follows:[7]

*"... the process by which the reliability and relevance of a particular approach, method, process or assessment is established for a defined purpose."*

This wide-ranging definition is intended to cover all kinds of traditional and alternative testing methods. In the context of (Q)SARs, this definition is rather abstract and difficult to apply. A more operational definition is based on a set of five validation principles established by the OECD.[8] These principles state that in order:

*"to facilitate the consideration of a (Q)SAR model for regulatory purposes, it should be associated with the following information:*

1. *a defined endpoint;*
2. *an unambiguous algorithm;*
3. *a defined domain of applicability;*
4. *appropriate measures of goodness-of-fit, robustness and predictivity;*
5. *a mechanistic interpretation, if possible."*

The OECD validation principles identify the types of information that are considered useful for the assessment of (Q)SARs for regulatory purposes. They constitute the basis of a conceptual framework, but they do not in themselves provide criteria for the regulatory acceptance of (Q)SARs. Fixed criteria are difficult, if not impossible, to define, given the highly context-dependent and variable ways in which non-testing data may be used. The intent of each principle is explained in Table 4.1.

The assessment of (Q)SAR model validity should therefore be performed by reference to the OECD principles for the validation of (Q)SARs. The validation exercise itself may be carried out by any person or organisation. Practical guidance has been published by the OECD.[8] This guidance is also summarised in the REACH guidance on the use of (Q)SARs.[3]

Based on a review of QSARs in the scientific literature, Dearden *et al.*[9] identified as many as 21 types of common "error" which the authors associate with improper model development, assessment and documentation.[9] Some errors are related to the choice and treatment of the data that are included in the training and test sets (*e.g.*, relevance, heterogeneity, spread in values, accuracy); other errors to the choice of descriptors (*e.g.*, comprehensibility), and others to the statistical methodology (*e.g.*, overfitting, suitable choice of statistics); and others to the overall transparency and transferability. This paper provides technical considerations that are useful for the model developer, some of which are also suitable for routine checking by the model end-user.

As an example, a common technical error in the modelling of toxicological endpoints is that QSAR models should be based on molar units, rather than on

**Table 4.1** Explanation of the OECD (Q)SAR validation principles.

| *A (Q)SAR model should be ...* | *Explanation* |
|---|---|
| 1) associated with a defined endpoint. | Aims to ensure transparency in the endpoint being predicted by a given model, since a given endpoint could be determined by different experimental protocols and under different experimental conditions. The endpoint refers to any physicochemical property, biological effect (human health or ecological) environmental fate parameter that can be measured and therefore modelled. |
| 2) expressed in the form of an unambiguous algorithm. | Aims to ensure transparency in the description of the model algorithm. |
| 3) associated with a defined domain of applicability. | Recognises that (Q)SARs are reductionist models which are inevitably associated with limitations in terms of the types of chemical structures, physicochemical properties and mechanisms of action for which the models can generate reliable predictions. The principle expresses the need to justify that a given model is being used within the boundary of its limitations when making a given prediction. |
| 4) appropriate measures of goodness-of-fit, robustness and predictivity. | Expresses the need to provide two types of information: i) the internal performance of a model (as represented by goodness-of-fit and robustness), determined by using a training set; and ii) the predictivity of a model, determined by using an appropriate test set. |
| 5) associated with a mechanistic interpretation, wherever possible. | Aims to ensure that there is an assessment of the mechanistic associations between the descriptors used in a model and the endpoint being predicted, and that any association is documented. Where a mechanistic interpretation is possible, it can add strength to the confidence in the model already established on the basis of principles 1–4. The wording of this principle, while seemingly redundant in its use of "where possible" emphasises that is not always possible to provide a mechanistic interpretation of a given (Q)SAR. |

weight or concentration units. This is because physical and biological effects depend on the number of molecules present, and not on how much they weigh. However, this is often overlooked by the model developer because the underlying data, generated from guideline studies, are generally expressed in concentration or weight units. However, it is a simple exercise to convert values derived from dose–response curves (typically median values) from mg $kg^{-1}$ to molar units, and this often improves the models derived. If, however, the response is measured at a fixed weight dosage for all chemicals, then conversion is useless, because each chemical will have been tested at a different molar dose, making comparison impossible. This one example illustrates the detail that is ideally needed in a comprehensive assessment of QSAR models. In developing the QSAR reporting formats, the main challenge was to define a level of detail in reporting models and their predictions that represents a workable compromise between what is desirable scientifically and what is workable and sufficient to support the regulatory assessment of models.

Information on (Q)SAR model validity, including peer-reviewed documentation, is available from the JRC QSAR Model Database (http://qsardb.jrc.it). This database is intended to be a repository of potentially useful information on models, structured according to the internationally accepted format of the QMRF. It is not intended to be an inventory of officially accepted or adopted (Q)SAR models, since in the EU there is no formal process for their validation and acceptance.[10]

### 4.4.2 Model Overfitting—Causes, Consequences and Diagnostics

An important consideration when assessing the validity of statistically-based models concerns the problem of overfitting. This is covered by OECD validation principle 4. The goodness-of-fit of a QSAR model reflects: 1) the ability of the model predictors to account for the variance of the response in the training set; and 2) the statistical significance of the model. The optimal model should express a balance between the complexity and relevance of the applied predictors/methodology and the resulting benefits in terms of performance. According to the principle of parsimony (Occam's Razor), the optimal model should be based on the minimum necessary information and nothing more. Otherwise, it can result in one of two extremes: either the model is overfitted, *i.e.*, too complex and simply modelling noise, or the model is underfitted, *i.e.*, too simplistic and lacking vital information.[11,12] Moreover, if the model is not statistically significant, it should not be used for predictive purposes. These considerations do not apply to models that are entirely knowledge-based rather than statistically based.

There are two main causes of overfitting, resulting in a redundant level of model complexity, which does not improve (and may even diminish) the model performance. The first main cause is the improper selection of independent variables by: 1) including more predictors than are necessary to capture the variance of the response;[13] 2) using predictors that are inter-correlated (collinear); 3) using predictors that are irrelevant and correlated with the response "by chance", without being meaningful and predictive.[14–16] Another main cause of overfitting is related to the choice of modelling technique that is: 1) more complicated than necessary to find the relationships between the descriptors and the response; or 2) not suitable to describe particular dependencies.

Overfitting is undesirable for a variety of reasons. Using superfluous and/or irrelevant predictors can result in the loss of valuable information, adding random variation to the predictions (*i.e.*, prediction error) and incomplete or misleading interpretation of the modelled phenomenon. The use of collinear predictors means that the same information is being used more than once to fit the model and this leads to an overestimation of its importance. Overfitting usually results in unpredictable errors, which are related to the noise in the dataset (due to the selected variables and methods), rather the modelled property.[17] The problem of overfitting is more likely to occur, and harder for the non-specialist to diagnose, in the case of methods capable of handling large amounts of correlated information and noisy variables (*e.g.*, Support Vector Machines, Artificial Neural Networks).

To assess the goodness-of-fit of a model, the predictions for chemicals in the training set are used. However, models that are overfitted typically show worse predictivity for independent data than their internal validation statistics imply. Thus, internal validation should ideally be followed by external validation. The main indication of an overfitted model is its high internal "predictivity" (error of estimation much lower than the experimental error), accompanied by a lower (or lack of) external predictivity.

To avoid overfitting, it is necessary to apply certain statistical validation techniques providing fitness functions that allow verification of the appropriate form (relevance) of the model (in terms of the variables and methodology used) and which enable the optimal model complexity to be found. Clearly, statistical expertise is required to apply and interpret the results of such techniques.

The initial splitting of data into training and test sets is of vital importance, since it determines the data which will be used to fit the model. Ideally, both the training and test sets should cover the entire range of the considered chemical space, defined by the predictor values, on the one hand, and by the endpoint values, on the other.[18] The most popular algorithms used to design the optimal size and composition of training and test sets are: Kennard–Stone[19] Duplex,[20] D-optimal distance,[21] repeated test set technique[22] and self-organising map.[23] However, a practical problem is that high-quality data are not always sufficiently available to divide into independent training and test sets, which means that most if not all of the available data are used to train the model.

### *4.4.2.1 Regression Models*

In order to assess the predictive ability of a regression model in the absence of an external test set, a number of internal validation techniques can be used.[24] The most popular techniques are based on leave-one-out (LOO) and leave-many-out (LMO) cross-validation methods,[25] as well as bootstrap resampling.[26] Although the LOO cross-validation is probably the most widely used technique, it often provides an overly optimistic simulation of a model's predictive ability, especially when large datasets are used. In such cases, more realistic (lower) estimates of predictivity can be obtained by LMO cross-validation, which introduces a larger perturbation in the studied dataset. Similarly, the fitness statistics provided by the bootstrapping method are indicative of the model's predictivity. Models which are based on "chance correlation" can be identified by the response permutation test (Y-scrambling)[27] or the QUIK rule of Todeschini.[28]

The statistical significance of a model can be estimated by its *F*-values for a given number of degrees of freedom. The probability that the model equation is significant increases with the $F$-value. A statistically significant model ensures that the highest possible predictivity is obtained with the minimal number of predictors (Occam's razor) and that the predictors are orthogonal (uncorrelated). A model having low significance statistics may be underfitted, based on "chance correlations", noisy predictors or intercorrelated predictors, and will probably show discrepancies between its goodness-of-fit and its predictivity. In order to assess the statistical significance of each regression coefficient, a $t$-test (for a given number of degrees of freedom) should be performed. This allows identification of those predictors that significantly contribute to the explanation of the response variable and those that are meaningless. The main fitness functions performed for various types of models and possible ways of interpreting them are summarised in Table 4.2.

### *4.4.2.2 Classification Models*

The goodness-of-fit of a classification model can be assessed in terms of its Cooper statistics, namely: sensitivity, specificity, concordance (accuracy), positive/negative predictivity, as well as false positive/false negative rates. For individual classification models, the relevant Cooper statistics should be significantly greater than a pre-defined threshold (typically 50%, but a lower percentage may be acceptable if the emphasis is on positive/negative predictivity rather than sensitivity/specificity). In order to compare the performances of a number of classification models, the Receiver Operating Characteristic (ROC) curve, plotting the true positive rate against the false positives rate, is often used. In the ROC curve, a model in the top left-hand corner is ideal (fully predictive), whereas a model along the diagonal is producing predictions nor better than chance.

Methods for checking whether a model is overfitted can be automatically applied by available statistical software packages. Nevertheless, the user will need sufficient knowledge about the diagnostic rules and the underlying methods in order to interpret the statistical. Different statistical approaches may provide different statistics; for example, different values of the same statistics can result from varying the composition of the training and test sets. Thus, transparency is necessary to document the procedure of model development and validation process. However, exactly how much transparency is needed for regulatory purposes is still a matter of debate.

Apart from the statistical approaches to assess whether a QSAR model is overfitted or not, which require statistical expertise to apply and interpret, some more simple and straightforward "rules of thumb" approaches can be followed, based on the information available to the assessor. The following list is an indicative guide for the assessor:

1) to estimate the goodness-of-fit, internal predictivity and statistical significance of a model, the following statistics should be provided: $n$, $r^2$ ($R^2$), $q^2$ ($Q^2$), $R^2_{adj}$, $s$, $F$ statistics including $p$-values;
2) the ratio of chemicals ($n$) to predictors should be at least 5 : 1;[29]

**Table 4.2** Goodness-of-fit parameters for regression models.

| *Statistic* | *Definition* | *Interpretation* |
|---|---|---|
| $R^2$ (Multiple determination coefficient) | The variance of the response that is explained by the regression model. | * $R^2 = 0$: the lack of linear relationship between the response and predictors variables<br>* $R^2 = 1$: the perfect linear fit<br>* $R^2 > 0.5$: the variance explained by the model is higher than the unexplained variance.<br>The value of $R^2$ increases with additional predictors, even if they do not contribute to the explained variance in the response. |
| $R^2_{adj}$ (Adjusted multiple determination coefficient) | The variance of the model's response that is explained by the regression for respective degrees of freedom. | The value of $R^2_{adj}$ decreases if a predictor is added to the equation but does not contribute to the explanation of the variance. |
| $s$ (Standard error of estimate) | The dispersion of the observed values about the regression line. | The smaller the value of $s$, the higher the reliability of prediction. Standard error of estimate smaller than the experimental error of the biological data is indicative of an overfitted model. |
| $Q^2(Y)$ (Cross-validation coefficient) | Explained variance in prediction. | Indicates the model with the highest predictive ability. $Q^2(Y)$ does not increase after a certain degree of model complexity and indicates the zone with a balance between predictive power and reasonable fit.<br>The difference between $R^2(Y)$ and $Q^2(Y)$ should not exceed 0.3. A larger difference indicates an overfitted model, the presence of irrelevant predictors or outliers in the data. |
| $F$-value | The ratio between explained and unexplained model variance for a given number of degrees of freedom. | The regression equation/coefficients are statistically significant if the calculated $F$-value/$t$-value is greater than a tabulated value for the chosen level of significance (typically 95%) and the corresponding degrees of freedom of $F/t$ ($p$). |
| $t$-test | The ratio between estimated regression coefficient and its standard deviation for a given number of degrees of freedom. | Higher $F$-/$t$-values of a regression equation/coefficient correspond to greater statistical significance. Significance of the equation at the 95% level means that there is 5% probability that the dependence found is obtained due to chance correlations between the variables. Significance of a coefficient at the 95% level means that there is a 5% probability that the coefficient of a given variable is not significantly different from zero. |

3) for transparent mechanistic interpretation of the model, the maximal number of predictors (except group contributions and electropological state indices) should not exceed 5–6;[9]
4) the standard error of the estimate ($s$) should not be significantly less than the known experimental error for the predicted endpoint;
5) the difference between the $R^2(Y)$ and $Q^2(Y)$ values should not exceed 0.3.

### 4.4.3 Demonstrating Applicability

Assessment of model validity is a necessary but not sufficient step in assessing the adequacy of a (Q)SAR prediction. Assuming that the model of choice is considered valid, a second essential step is to demonstrate the applicability of the model to the chemical of interest. The evaluation of model applicability is related to the evaluation of the reliability of prediction for the chemical of interest, since a valid (Q)SAR is associated with at least one defined applicability domain in which the model makes estimations with a defined level of accuracy (reliability). When applied to chemicals within its applicability domain, the model is expected to give reliable results (or results with a defined level of reliability). Conversely, if a model is applied to a chemical outside its applicability domain, it is likely that the estimated result will either be unreliable or of unknown reliability.

The applicability domain of a model is a multi-faceted concept, and can be broken down into: i) a descriptor domain; ii) a structural fragment domain; iii) a mechanistic domain; and iv) a metabolic domain. In other words, the reliability of a prediction is constrained by whether the chemical of interest has: i) descriptor values within predefined ranges; ii) structural fragments that are "known" to the model; iii) its predefined mode and/or mechanism of action; and iv) the likelihood that it may undergo transformation or metabolism, and the characteristics of any products.

There is no unique measure of model reliability, and no criteria for (Q)SAR reliability have been established in regulatory guidance. Model reliability should be regarded as a relative concept, depending on the context in which the model is applied. In other words, a greater or lesser degree of reliability may be sufficient for a given regulatory application. This implies that the applicability domain can be defined to suit the regulatory context.

The assessment of whether a given model is applicable to a given chemical can be broken down into the following specific questions:

1) is the chemical of interest within the scope of the model, according to the defined applicability domain of the model?
2) is the defined applicability domain suitable for the regulatory purpose?
3) how well does the model predict chemicals that are similar to the chemical of interest?
4) is the model estimate reasonable, taking into account other information?

The importance of having an explicit definition of the model domain becomes apparent when addressing question 1). In practice, there is often limited information concerning the descriptor, structural fragment, mechanistic, and metabolic domains.

The second question arises because most currently available models were not tailor-made for current regulatory needs and inevitably incorporate biases which may or may not be useful, depending on the context of prediction. A model can be (deliberately or inadvertently) biased toward certain classes of chemicals), or toward a certain type of prediction (*e.g.*, a model optimised to correctly identify positives at the expense of correctly identifying negatives). Such biases do not affect the validity of the model, but they do affect its applicability for specific purposes. Information on these biases can therefore help the user determine whether the model is suitable.

The third question provides a simple way of checking whether a model is appropriate by checking its predictive capability for one or more analogues that are similar to the one of interest and for which measured values exist. This is effectively using a read-across argument to support the reliability of the (Q)SAR prediction.

A more generic check, expressed by question 4), is whether the predicted value seems "reasonable", based on any other information available. This is an appeal to an expert judgement, supported with argumentation.

The judicious application of these questions to assess the applicability of a (Q)SAR model is by no means straightforward, and needs specialised expertise. Software applications that generate (Q)SAR estimates vary in the extent and manner to which they incorporate and report applicability domain considerations.

### 4.4.4 Demonstrating Adequacy

The preceding two sections explain that in order for a (Q)SAR result to be adequate for a given regulatory purpose, the estimate should be generated by a valid model, and the model should be applicable to the chemical of interest with the necessary level of reliability. Fulfilment of these two conditions is necessary but not sufficient for demonstrating adequacy. At present, there is no detailed and firm guidance on how to demonstrate adequacy, but some general considerations are offered in the REACH guidance.[4] This is partly a reflection of the fact that more experience is needed at the regulatory level to expand on existing guidance, but also that the concept of adequacy, by its very nature, means that only general considerations will be possible. In any case, to demonstrate the adequacy of a QSAR estimate generated by a valid and applicable model some additional argumentation is required.

One argument is that the model endpoint should be relevant to the regulatory purpose. For some models, in which the model predicts directly the regulatory endpoint (*e.g.*, an acute toxicity $LD_{50}$ value), the relevance is self-evident. However, in the case of many QSAR models, and especially a new generation of QSAR models that are focusing on predicting lower level mechanistic endpoints,[30] an additional extrapolation is needed to relate the modelled endpoint (*e.g.*, nucleophilic reactivity towards DNA or proteins) to the endpoint of regulatory interest (*e.g.*, mutagenicity or sensitisation).

The relevance and reliability of a given prediction need to be assessed in relation to a particular regulatory purpose, taking into account the availability of other information in the context of a weight-of-evidence assessment. In other words, the question is whether the totality of information is sufficient to reach a regulatory conclusion, and if not, what additional information (possibly including new test data) is needed to reduce the uncertainty and increase confidence in the conclusion. This should take account of the "severity" of the decision (the "principle of proportionality") as well as the possible consequences of reaching a "wrong" conclusion ("principle of caution or conservativeness"). Thus, the amount and quality of information that is required depends on the uncertainty in the data, the severity of the regulatory decision, and the consequence of being wrong. It follows that the determination of adequacy is based not only on scientific argumentation, but also on a policy decision. For this reason, it is impossible, to develop absolute criteria for assessing adequacy that are acceptable in all regulatory decision-making contexts.

## 4.5 Proposed Checklist for Assessing the Adequacy of (Q)SARs in Risk Assessment

Although absolute criteria cannot be meaningfully formulated for assessing the adequacy of (Q)SAR predictions for regulatory purposes, it is possible to highlight a minimal set of important questions that can applied in a practical manner by the risk assessor. For illustrative purposes, a checklist of 10 questions is proposed in Table 4.3. Questions 1–6 are related to the model, whereas questions 7–10 are related to the model prediction. This set of questions is not intended to be definitive—individual questions could be skipped or additional questions could be added, depending on the needs of a particular regulatory framework and the context in which the predictions are being used.

## 4.6 Application of the Checklist to Selected Software Models for Genotoxicity Prediction

To illustrate the application of the checklist, the 10 questions have been applied to the predictions of genotoxicity for two case study chemicals, methylparathion and sodium nitroguaiacolate, obtained with four popular software tools (the first two are publicly available and the second two are commercial): Caesar,[31] Toxtree,[32] ToxBoxes (now called ACD/ToxSuite),[3] and DEREK for Windows.[34] These tools were selected for illustrative purposes. Many other software tools also make predictions of genotoxicity, and there is a vast literature of published models, as reviewed elsewhere.[35,36]

**Table 4.3** Checklist of questions to help establish the adequacy of a (Q)SAR prediction.

| *No.* | *Question* | *Interpretation* |
|---|---|---|
| 1 | Is the predicted endpoint clearly defined? | If the endpoint is not clearly defined, the use of the prediction will be open to different interpretations, and thus of questionable value. |
| 2 | If the predicted endpoint is clearly defined ("yes" to Q1), does it represent a direct information requirement under the legislation of interest, or is it related to one of the information requirements? | If the predicted endpoint corresponds directly with an information requirement, it may be possible to use the prediction instead of experimental data. Alternatively, if the predicted endpoint is indirectly related to an information requirement, it may be useful as supporting information. |
| 3 | If the model is statistically based (as opposed to knowledge-based), is the model training set fully available? | If the model training set of a statistically based model is not fully available (*e.g.*, because the data are proprietary), it will be impossible for another practitioner to independently reproduce the model, which may reduce confidence in the model estimates. However, this may not be an issue if the model is coded into a software tool. This does not apply to knowledge-based models, which are based on human knowledge and do not have a clearly identified training set. |
| 4 | Is the method used to develop the model documented or referenced (*e.g.*, in a scientific paper or QMRF) | If the details of model development are not documented, it will be impossible for another practitioner to independently develop and confirm the model, which may reduce confidence in the model estimates. Even if the method is documented, it will require a QSAR specialist to determine whether the documentation is sufficiently detailed to reproduce the model. |
| 5 | Is information available (in terms of statistical properties) concerning the performance of the model, including its goodness-of-fit, predictivity, robustness and error of prediction (uncertainty)? | The statistical properties of a model can provide evidence of its usefulness in a given context (*e.g.*, the need to minimise false negatives) and can also be used to assess whether the model has been overfitted (see question 7). |
| 6 | If the model is statistically based (as opposed to knowledge-based), does examination of the available statistics indicate that the model may have been overfitted? | The overfitting of statistically based models is undesirable because it can result in unpredictable errors. This consideration does not apply to knowledge-based models.<br>Overfitted statistical models typically show worse predictivity (outside their training sets) than their internal validation statistics imply. Several simple diagnostics exist, for example:<br>i) the model estimation error (uncertainty of prediction) should not be significantly less than the known experimental error.<br>ii) the ratio of data points (chemicals) to variables (descriptors) should be at least 5 : 1. |

**Table 4.3** (*Continued*)

| *No.* | *Question* | *Interpretation* |
|---|---|---|
| 7 | Does the model training set contain the chemical of interest? | If the model training set contains the chemical of interest, then a prediction is not needed because some experimental data is available for direct use. |
| 8 | Does the model make reliable predictions for analogues of the chemical structure of interest? | The generation of reliable predictions for analogues of the chemical of interest increases confidence in the prediction. In the case of a software tool, it should be indicated whether the software automatically identifies analogues and their associated data within the model training set. In the case of a literature model, it should be considered whether suitable analogues can be identified in the training set (if available). |
| 9 | Is the model prediction substantiated with argumentation based on the applicability domain of the model? | Confidence in a prediction is increased if information is available concerning the applicability domain of the model, and thus whether the model is applicable to the chemical of interest. The applicability domain can include physicochemical and structural space, as well as mechanistic and metabolic considerations. |
| 10 | Can the model prediction be easily reproduced? | Not all model predictions can be easily reproduced, depending on the complexity and transparency of the model development process, and the availability of a user-friendly software tool implementing the model.<br>If the model is a simple SAR (structural alert) it should be possible to apply it by visual inspection. However, some differences of expert interpretation may arise.<br>If the model is a QSAR in the form of a transparent mathematical formula, it will be possible to apply it in a spreadsheet (*e.g.*, Excel).<br>If the model is implemented in the form of a freely or commercially available software tool, it is possible for different users to verify the same result (even if the model development process is not transparent), thereby increasing confidence in the prediction. |

The results are given in Tables 4.4–4.7. Many of the questions are straightforward to answer, provided that the background documentation is available (QMRF, software manual and/or research publications). However, a few noteworthy points are elaborated in the following paragraphs:

**Table 4.4** Application of the checklist of questions to Caesar (genotoxicity prediction).

| *No* | *Question (Q) and answer (A)* |
|---|---|
| Q1 | Is the predicted endpoint clearly defined? |
| A1 | Yes, the endpoint is Ames (*S. typhimurium*) mutagenicity |
| Q2 | If the predicted endpoint is clearly defined ("yes" to Q1), does it represent a direct information requirement under the legislation of interest, or is it related to one of the information requirements? |
| A2 | Yes, genotoxicity test data are required under most types of chemicals legislation (*e.g.*, industrial chemicals, pesticides, biocides) |
| Q3 | If the model is statistically based (as opposed to knowledge-based), is the model training set fully available? |
| A3 | Yes, the training and test set will be soon available from the JRC QSAR model database |
| Q4 | Is the method used to develop the model documented or referenced (*e.g.*, in a scientific paper or QMRF) |
| A4 | Yes, a QMRF is in preparation, based on the following publications:[50,51]<br>T. Ferrari, G. Gini and E. Benfenati, Support vector machines in the prediction of mutagenicity of chemical compounds, *Proc. NAFIPS'09*, Cincinnati, USA, pp. 1–6.<br>T. Ferrari and G. Gini, A new multistep model to predict mutagenicity from statistic analysis and relevant structural alerts, *Chem. Cent. J.*, **4**, S2. |
| Q5 | Is information available (in terms of statistical properties) concerning the performance of the model, including its goodness-of-fit, predictivity, robustness and error of prediction (uncertainty)? |
| A5 | Yes. Information on the accuracy (82.1%), sensitivity (90.6%) and specificity (71.4%) are provided in the QMRF. |
| Q6 | If the model is statistically based (as opposed to knowledge-based), does examination of the available statistics indicate that the model may have been overfitted? |
| A6 | The model is statistically based but should not be overfitted because the ratio of chemicals (3380) to descriptors (42) is 80.5. |
| Q7 | Does the model training set contain the chemical of interest? |
| A7 | The model training set includes some pesticides including methylparathion but not sodium nitroguaiacolate. |
| Q8 | Does the model make reliable predictions for analogues of the chemical structure of interest? |
| A8 | Yes, the Caesar software gives the chance to examine, for each compound submitted, the six most similar compounds found in the model training set. For these compounds the experimental value for the selected endpoint is shown, together with the prediction made by the model. The similarity measure employed by the Caesar software takes into account functional group similarity, constitutional similarity, ring similarity and fingerprint similarity.<br>For methylparathion (correctly predicted by the software), the similar structures obtained are: methylparathion (input structure contained in the training set), |

**Table 4.4** (*Continued*)

| No | Question (Q) and answer (A) |
|---|---|
| | aminofenitrothion, 1-ethenoxy-4-nitrobenzene, fenitrooxon, *o*-nitroanisole, *N*-hydroxy-*N*-(4-nitrophenyl)acetamide. All of them are predicted correctly by the software. For nitroguaiacolate (wrongly predicted by the software) the similar structures obtained are: *o*-nitroanisole, 1-ethoxy-3-nitrobenzene, 2,5-dinitrophenol, *p*-nitrosoanisole, 2-methoxy-1,3,5-trinitrobenzene, 1-ethenoxy-4-nitrobenzene. All of them are predicted correctly by the software. |
| Q9 | Is the model prediction substantiated with argumentation based on the applicability domain of the model? |
| A9 | Yes, Caesar addresses the applicability domain in several ways, namely by: i) checking whether the compound of interest falls in the descriptors space—if the compound is out of domain, this is noted in the output; ii) providing a similarity score (1 = identity) for the structure-based comparison with analogues; iii) visual representation of the most similar compounds; iv) by revealing the known and predicted the known and predicted toxicities for the analogues, thereby indicating the prediction error. Thus Caesar provides an assessment based on both the input (descriptor) space and the output (toxicological endpoint) space. |
| Q10 | Can the model prediction be easily reproduced? |
| A10 | Yes, the software is accessible in the form of a freely accessible web platform (http://www.caesar-project.eu) and is easy to use, even for non-specialists. |

**Table 4.5** Application of the checklist of questions to Toxtree.

| No | Question (Q) and answer (A) |
|---|---|
| Q1 | Is the predicted endpoint clearly defined? |
| A1 | No. The software makes generic predictions of genotoxicity using two rulebases: 1) the Benigni–Bossa rulebase is a decision tree for estimating both the genotoxic and non-genotoxic carcinogenicity potentials of chemicals, based on the rules published in the EC report "The Benigni–Bossa rulebase for mutagenicity and carcinogenicity – a module of Toxtree", by Benigni *et al.* (2008).[52] The present list of SAs (over 30) refers mainly to genotoxic carcinogenicity, and also includes a number of SAs for potential non-genotoxic carcinogens. In addition to the SAs, the module performs discriminant QSAR analyses for i) the mutagenic activity in the *S. typhimurium* TA100 strain (Ames test) of aromatic amines (QSAR6) and α,β-unsaturated aldehydes (QSAR13), and ii) the carcinogenicity in rodents of aromatic amines (QSAR8). The underlying mechanism(s) for the triggering of an alert for genotoxic carcinogenicity are not clearly defined, as these may include different possible mechanisms of genotoxicity (*e.g.*, Ames mutagenicity, chromosomal aberration, chromosomal instability, *etc.*) which may be linked to carcinogenicity. 2) the *in vivo* micronucleus assay plug-in, for the prediction of the outcome of this assay in rodents, is based on the SAs published in the EC report "Development of structural alerts for the *in vivo* micronucleus assay in rodents", in Benigni *et al.* (2009)[53] and Benigni *et al.* (2010).[54] |

**Table 4.5** (*Continued*)

| *No* | *Question (Q) and answer (A)* |
|---|---|
| | Thus, except for the QSAR model estimates of the Ames test and the SA-based predictions for the *in vivo* micronucleus assay, the predictions of (non)genotoxic carcinogenicity are intended in a broad sense, rather than representing specific mechanisms of genotoxic damage. |
| Q2 | If the predicted endpoint is clearly defined ("yes" to Q1), does it represent a direct information requirement under the legislation of interest, or is it related to one of the information requirements? |
| A2 | Yes, genotoxicity test data are required under most types of chemicals legislation (*e.g.*, industrial chemicals, pesticides, biocides) |
| Q3 | If the model is statistically based (as opposed to knowledge-based), is the model training set fully available? |
| A3 | Yes, in the case of the QSAR models included in the Benigni–Bossa rulebase, the training sets are described in Benigni *et al.* (2008).[52] |
| Q4 | Is the method used to develop the model documented or referenced (*e.g.*, in a scientific paper or QMRF) |
| A4 | Yes, described in Benigni *et al.* (2008, 2009).[34,52] |
| Q5 | Is information available (in terms of statistical properties) concerning the performance of the model, including its goodness-of-fit, predictivity, robustness and error of prediction (uncertainty)? |
| A5 | Yes. Measures of performance include $r^2$ values and external predictivity values (Benigni *et al.*, 2009).[53] In addition, the included SAs have been tested against the Istituto di Sanità carcinogenicity and mutagenicity database (ISSCAN), resulting in 70% and 78% accuracy, respectively. |
| Q6 | If the model is statistically based (as opposed to knowledge-based), does examination of the available statistics indicate that the model may have been overfitted? |
| A6 | There is no evidence of overfitting. The included QSAR models have been tested using external test sets, which resulted in high predictive accuracy (Benigni *et al.*, 2009).[53] |
| Q7 | Does the model training set contain the chemical of interest? |
| A7 | No, parathion-methyl (true positive mutagen) and sodium nitroguaiacolate (false positive mutagen) are not included in the QSAR training sets. |
| Q8 | Does the model make reliable predictions for analogues of the chemical structure of interest? |
| A8 | The software does not provide information on analogues. |
| Q9 | Is the model prediction substantiated with argumentation based on the applicability domain of the model? |
| A9 | Yes. The QSAR models are applicable to aromatic amines and alpha,beta-unsaturated aldehydes, with a few specified exceptions. The SAs are considered to be generally applicable. |
| Q10 | Can the model prediction be easily reproduced? |
| A10 | Yes, the software is freely available from the JRC and easy to use, even for non-specialists. Software and supporting documents are available at: http://ihcp.jrc.ec.europa.eu/our_labs/computational_toxicology<br>The software is based on qualitative SARs (structural alerts) and (in the case of the Benigni–Bossa module) QSARs in form of transparent mathematical formulas. These algorithms can therefore be reprogrammed into a different software platform. |

**Table 4.6** Application of the checklist of questions to ToxBoxes.

| *No* | *Question (Q) and answer (A)* |
|---|---|
| Q1 | Is the predicted endpoint clearly defined? |
| A1 | Two models are available: a fragment-based model predicts Ames test results, whereas the genotoxicity hazards module is a knowledge-based expert system containing 27 known "genotoxicophore" fragments collected from literature. |
| Q2 | If the predicted endpoint is clearly defined ("yes" to Q1), does it represent a direct information requirement under the legislation of interest, or is it related to one of the information requirements? |
| A2 | Yes, genotoxicity test data are required under most types of chemicals legislation (*e.g.*, industrial chemicals, pesticides, biocides) |
| Q3 | If the model is statistically based (as opposed to knowledge-based), is the model training set fully available? |
| A3 | The Ames model training set is available through the software. The data consist of Ames test results obtained with various *S. typhimurium* and *E. coli* bacteria strains. |
| Q4 | Is the method used to develop the model documented or referenced (*e.g.*, in a scientific paper or QMRF) |
| A4 | No, not adequately. The software manual gives some general information about the model, but not a detailed description of model development. No research papers are cited. |
| Q5 | Is information available (in terms of statistical properties) concerning the performance of the model, including its goodness-of-fit, predictivity, robustness and error of prediction (uncertainty)? |
| A5 | No, information not available. |
| Q6 | If the model is statistically based (as opposed to knowledge-based), does examination of the available statistics indicate that the model may have been overfitted? |
| A6 | The model is statistically based but no information relating to overfitting could be found. |
| Q7 | Does the model training set contain the chemical of interest? |
| A7 | The training set includes parathion-methyl, but not sodium nitroguaiacolate. |
| Q8 | Does the model make reliable predictions for analogues of the chemical structure of interest? |
| A8 | Yes, the ToxBoxes software provides a list of the five most similar structures from its training set. Some general information on the similarity measure is provided—it is calculated using Tanimoto and fingerprint Max2 similarity.<br>For methylparathion, the five most similar structures identified are: methylparathion (the input structure), fenitrothion, parathion, hydroxymethylfenitrothion and fenitrooxon. The second compound (a non-mutagen) and the third (with an inconclusive Ames result) are predicted as indeterminate (probability of positive Ames test between 0.3 and 0.7), whereas the fourth and fifth (the known mutagens) are predicted correctly.<br>For nitroguaiacolate five similar structures are identified, including one false positive (FP), three true positives (TP) and one true negative (TN): *m*-nitroanisole (FP), *o*-nitroanisole (TP), *p*-nitroanisole (TP), 2,5-dimethoxy-4-nitroazobenzene (TP), and 3-methyl-4-nitrophenol (TN). |
| Q9 | Is the model prediction substantiated with argumentation based on the applicability domain of the model? |
| A9 | Yes, the software calculates a Reliability Index for every prediction, which takes account of the applicability domain. |
| Q10 | Can the model prediction be easily reproduced? |
| A10 | Yes, the software is very easy to use, even for non-specialists. |

**Table 4.7** Application of the checklist of questions to DEREK for Windows.

| *No* | *Question (Q) and answer (A)* |
|---|---|
| Q1 | Is the predicted endpoint clearly defined? |
| A1 | Yes. DEREK provides predictions for mutagenicity, genotoxicity, chromosome damage and carcinogenicity (among other endpoints). The user can select the species and the endpoint of interest.<br>DEREK v.11 contains 87 alerts for mutagenicity, 4 for genotoxicity, 74 for chromosome damage and 56 for carcinogenicity. |
| Q2 | If the predicted endpoint is clearly defined ("yes" to Q1), does it represent a direct information requirement under the legislation of interest, or is it related to one of the information requirements? |
| A2 | Yes, genotoxicity test data are required under most types of chemicals legislation (*e.g.*, industrial chemicals, pesticides, biocides) |
| Q3 | If the model is statistically based (as opposed to knowledge-based), is the model training set fully available? |
| A3 | Not applicable (knowledge-based predictions). DEREK rules are not built from the automated analysis of training sets. The alerts are created by experts who compare the toxicity of compounds from various different sources (proprietary, public domain and freely available) and knowledge of the mechanism of action where known. The software gives additional information in the alert description (comments, references, examples). |
| Q4 | Is the method used to develop the model documented or referenced (*e.g.*, in a scientific paper or QMRF) |
| A4 | Yes. A QMRF for the genotoxicity module is available in the JRC QSAR model database. There are also numerous papers which describe the development and use of DEREK for different endpoints. The documentation which is supplementary to the software is very readable. Users receive support from the support centre of Lhasa Ltd. The original publication is: M. Sanderson and C. Earnshaw, *Hum. Exp. Toxicol.*, 1991, **10**, 261. |
| Q5 | Is information available (in terms of statistical properties) concerning the performance of the model, including its goodness-of-fit, predictivity, robustness and error of prediction (uncertainty)? |
| A5 | Not applicable. |
| Q6 | If the model is statistically based (as opposed to knowledge-based), does examination of the available statistics indicate that the model may have been overfitted? |
| A6 | Not applicable. |
| Q7 | Does the model training set contain the chemical of interest? |
| A7 | Not applicable. |
| Q8 | Does the model make reliable predictions for analogues of the chemical structure of interest? |
| A8 | The software does not identify a set of most similar analogues, but the case of most alerts, examples with experimental data are provided. |
| Q9 | Is the model prediction substantiated with argumentation based on the applicability domain of the model? |
| A9 | There is no defined applicability domain but all predictions are well supported with explanations, references, and examples. If boundary conditions exist for an alert, these are clearly noted. |
| Q10 | Can the model prediction be easily reproduced? |
| A10 | Yes, the software is commercially available and is easy to use. |

The predicted endpoint is not always defined in detail; for example, sometimes a generic prediction of genotoxic potential is made but the underlying mechanistic effect may not be clearly identified (*e.g.*, Ames mutagenicity, chromosome aberration). In the case of expert systems, the predictions are likely to be based on heterogeneous datasets of expert conclusions based on data from multiple test methods: the conclusions for genotoxic potential are likely to vary between assessors and over time, especially when the criteria for assessing the raw data have changed or were not clear in the first place. In the case of statistical models, this is a source of variability in the training set, which will inevitably affect the reliability of prediction.

The question of model overfitting is not applicable to all types of models, especially knowledge-based models which encode human knowledge and statistical models that employ instance-based (nearest neighbour) learning algorithms. However, in general this consideration is applicable to statistically based models.

Comparing the prediction for the chemical of interest with predictions made for similar chemicals helps to assign confidence to the prediction, even when information on the statistical characteristics or the mechanistic basis of the model are missing. Some software tools (*e.g.*, Caesar, ToxBoxes) provide information on analogues. In such cases, it is recommended to consider the analogues provided by the software since these are likely to reflect the applicability domain of the model. However, additional and/or different analogues might also be considered. Other software tools (*e.g.*, Toxtree) do not provide any information on analogues, so in these cases, the user needs to use other resources to find analogues. It is useful to know whether the selected analogues are in the training set of the model. This does not mean that they are not appropriate choices. On the contrary, if the model training set contains analogues of the chemical of interest, this increases confidence that the model is applicable since it covers the same chemical space.

At present, there is no firm guidance on how to select an appropriate set of analogues—it is left largely to expert judgement. However, a few rules-of-thumb can be proposed:

1) at least two analogues should be selected, including both known positives and negatives;
2) in general, 2–5 analogues should be sufficient for the evaluation;
3) the experimental data for the analogues selected should be reliable and appropriate (*e.g.*, same effect/endpoint) for the comparison;

Computer-based search tools can be used to find analogues. Freely available tools include PubChem,[37] ChemSpider,[38] AMBIT[39] and AIM.[40] These tools do not always provide links to relevant and reliable experimental data. Freely downloadable tools such as the OECD QSAR Toolbox[41] and Toxmatch[42] can also be used (provided that a suitable dataset is already included or imported in the software). While these tools can assist the user in finding analogues, it is still necessary to judge whether the analogues are appropriate (or which analogues are most appropriate). Worked examples on how to use AMBIT and Toxmatch are given in Jeliazkova *et al.*[43]

## 4.7 Use of Analogue Data in the Assessment of Predictions

An illustration of the use of analogue data is provided by predictions for methylparathion and sodium nitroguaiacolate. Methylparathion is a well-predicted chemical, in the sense that all software tools correctly predict it to be a mutagen (or indeterminate in the case of ToxBoxes). Conversely, sodium nitroguaiacolate is a poorly predicted chemical, in the sense that all software tools incorrectly predict it to be a mutagen (or indeterminate in the case of ToxBoxes). In other words, methylparathion is usually a true positive in mutagenicity prediction, whereas sodium nitroguaiacolate is usually a false positive.

The main question considered here is whether a judicious choice of analogues and their associated mutagenicity data would lead an assessor to trust the prediction for the true positive, but doubt the prediction for the false positive. A selection of analogues for methylparathion and sodium nitroguaiacolate is given in Tables 4.8 and 4.9, respectively. These analogues were chosen merely to illustrate the process, and are not necessarily the most appropriate analogues for the assessment of the two pesticides.

For methylparathion, four analogues were identified (Table 4.8), including a non-mutagen (fenitrothion) and three mutagens (fenitrooxon, hydroxymethylfenitrothion 4-aminofenitrothion).

For sodium nitroguaiacolate, five analogues were identified (Table 4.9), including two mutagens (*o*-nitroanisole, *p*-nitroanisole) and three non-mutagens (*m*-nitroanisole, 3-methyl-4-nitrophenol, *m*-nitrophenetole).

### 4.7.1 Caesar Predictions

In the case of methyl parathion, Caesar generates correct predictions for the three mutagens, and also correctly identifies the non-mutagen (Table 4.4). Thus, the predicted mutagenicity of methylparathion would probably be considered reliable (all four predictions correct). In the case of sodium nitroguaiacolate, the predictions the two mutagens were correct but the predictions for the three non-mutagens were incorrect (including 1-ethoxy-3-nitrobenzene which is in the training set). Thus the prediction for sodiumm nitroguaiacolate would probably be considered unreliable on the basis of weight-of-evidence (three out of five incorrect) and the fact the model does not correctly predict a known non-mutagen in its training set. In other words, this interpretation of Caesar predictions would lead to the right conclusions for both chemicals.

**Table 4.8** Methylparathion and some of its analogues.

| *Chemical and experimental mutagenicity* | *Structure* | *Toxtree* | *ToxBoxes* | *DEREK* | *Caesar* |
|---|---|---|---|---|---|
| Methylparathion<br>Dimethoxy-(4-nitrophenoxy)-thioxophosphorane<br>CAS 298-00-0<br>S=P(Oc1ccc(cc1)[N+]([O-])=O)(OC)OC<br>Mutagen | 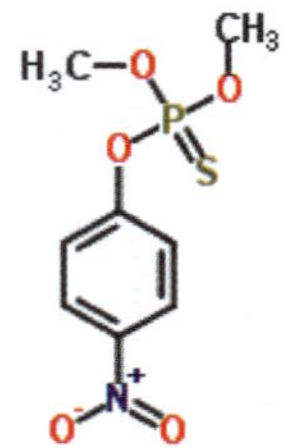 | Mutagen (TP) | IND<br>($p=0.631$)<br>In TS | Mutagen (TP) | Mutagen (TP)<br>In TS |
| Fenitrothion<br>Dimethoxy-(3-methyl-4-nitrophenoxy)-thioxophosphorane<br>CAS 128-14-5<br>S=P(Oc1cc(c(cc1)[N+]([O-])=O)C)(OC)OC<br>Non-Mutagen | 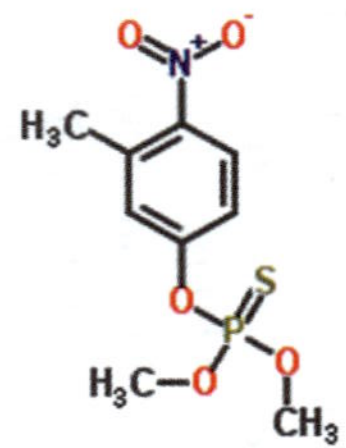 | Mutagen (FP) | IND<br>($p=0.668$)<br>In TS | Mutagen (FP) | Non-Mutagen<br>(TN) |
| Fenitrooxon<br>Dimethyl (3-methyl-4-nitrophenyl)phosphate<br>CAS 2255-17-6<br>[O-][N+](=O)c1c(cc(OP(=O)(OC)OC)cc1)C<br>Mutagen | 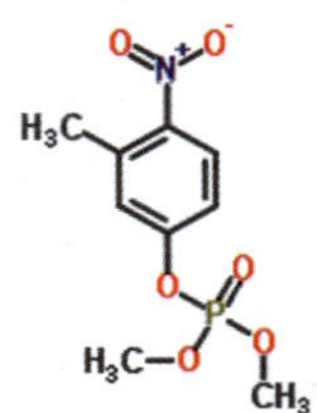 | Mutagen (TP) | Mutagen (TP)<br>($p=0.889$)<br>In TS | Mutagen (TP) | Mutagen (TP)<br>In TS |

| | | | | | |
|---|---|---|---|---|---|
| Hydroxymethylfenitrothion<br>Phosphorothioic acid<br>(5-Dimethoxyphosphinothioyloxy-2-nitrophenyl)methanol<br>CAS 59417-73-1<br>S=P(Oc1cc(c(cc1)[N+]([O-])=O)CO)(OC)OC<br>Mutagen | 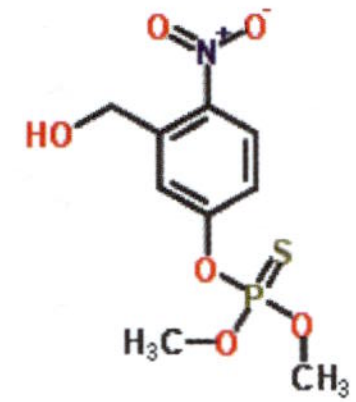 | Mutagen (TP) | Mutagen (TP)<br>($p = 0.796$)<br>In TS | Mutagen (TP) | Mutagen (TP) |
| 4-Aminofenitrothion<br>4-Dimethoxyphosphinothioyloxy-2-methylaniline<br>CAS 13306-69-9<br>S=P(Oc1ccc(c(c1)C)N)(OC)OC<br>Mutagen | 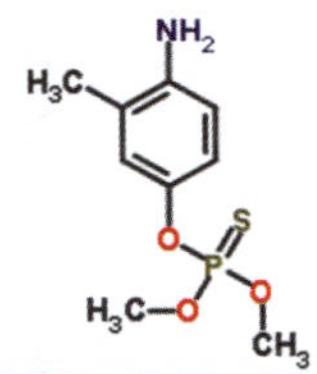 | Mutagen (TP) | Mutagen (TP)<br>($p = 0.762$) | Mutagen (TP) | Mutagen (TP)<br>In TS |

$p$ = probability of positive Ames test result; IND = indeterminate; FN = false negative; TN = true negative; TP = true positive; FP = false positive; In TS = compound in model training set

**Table 4.9** Sodium nitroguaiacolate and some of its analogues.

| *Chemical and experimental mutagenicity* | *Structure* | *Toxtree* | *ToxBoxes* | *DEREK* | *Caesar* |
|---|---|---|---|---|---|
| Nitroguaiacolate<br>2-Methoxy-5-nitrophenolate<br>CAS 67233-85-6<br>[Na + ].[O-]c1cc(ccc1OC)[N + ]([O-])=O<br>Non mutagen | 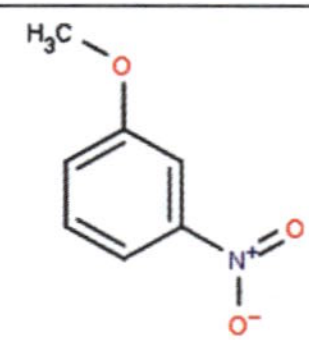 | Mutagen (FP) | IND<br>($p = 0.643$) | Mutagen<br>(FP) | Mutagen (FP) |
| *m*-Nitroanisole<br>1-Methoxy-3-nitrobenzene<br>CAS 555-03-3<br>COc1cccc(c1)[N + ]([O-])=O<br>Non Mutagen | 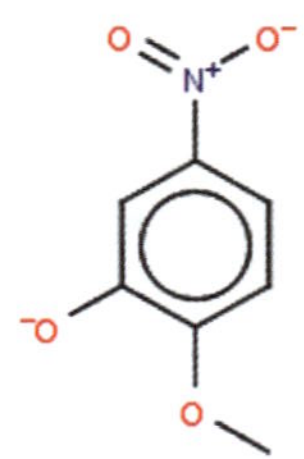 | Mutagen (FP) | Mutagen (FP)<br>($p = 0.738$)<br>In TS | Mutagen (FP) | Mutagen (FP)<br>In TS |
| *o*-Nitroanisole<br>1-Methoxy-2-nitrobenzene<br>CAS 91-23-6<br>COc1c(cccc1)[N + ](=O)[O-]<br>Mutagen | 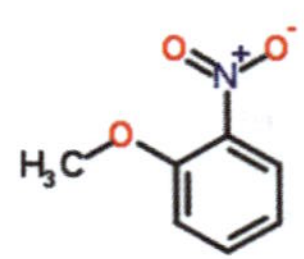 | Mutagen (TP) | Mutagen (TP)<br>($p = 0.738$)<br>In TS | Mutagen (TP) | Mutagen (TP)<br>In TS |

| | | | | | |
|---|---|---|---|---|---|
| *p*-Nitroanisole<br>1-Methoxy-4-nitrobenzene<br>CAS 100-17-4<br>COc1ccc(cc1)[N + ]([O-])=O<br>Mutagen | 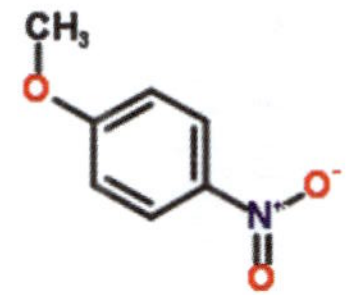 | Mutagen (TP) | Mutagen (TP)<br>($p=0.955$)<br>In TS | Mutagen (TP) | Mutagen (TP)<br>In TS |
| 3-Methyl-4-nitrophenol<br>CAS 2581-34-2<br>O=[N + ]([O-])c1c(cc(O)cc1)C<br>Non-Mutagen | 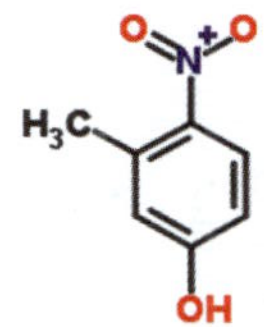 | Mutagen (FP) | Non-Mutagen (TN)<br>($p=0.193$) | Non-Mutagen (TN) | Mutagen (FP)<br>In TS |
| 1-Ethoxy-3-nitrobenzene<br>*m*-Nitrophenetole<br>CAS 621-52-3<br>CCOc1cc(ccc1)[N + ](=O)[O-]<br>Non-Mutagen | 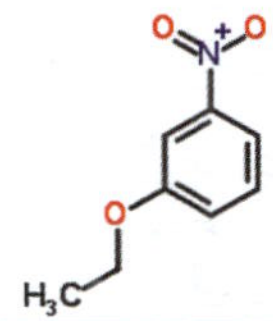 | Mutagen (FP) | Mutagen (TP)<br>($p=0.717$) | Mutagen (FP) | Mutagen (FP)<br>In TS |

$p$ = probability of positive Ames test result; IND = indeterminate; FN = false negative; TN = true negative; TP = true positive; FP = false positive; In TS = compound in model training set.

### 4.7.2 Toxtree Predictions

In the case of methylparathion, comparison of the known and predicted mutagenicities reveals that Toxtree makes the correct predictions for the three mutagens, but incorrectly predicts the non-mutagen to be a mutagen (Table 4.5). On the basis of a weight-of-evidence (three out of four predictions correct), this might be considered sufficient supporting evidence to rely on the mutagenicity prediction for methylparathion. The false positive prediction for fenitrothion, as opposed to fenitrooxon for example, might be related to the fact that the latter is the phosphoryl derivative (bearing the P=O functionality) of the former (bearing the P=S functionality). It is known that phosphoryl derivatives are more toxic than the corresponding thiophosphoryl compounds because they bind more strongly to (and act as more potent inhibitors of) certain enzymes, such as acetyl cholinesterase. However, the Toxtree rulebase does not capture the difference between the phosphoryl and thiophosphoryl groups.

In the case of sodium nitroguaiacolate, the Toxtree predictions for the three non-mutagens were incorrect, whereas the predictions of the two mutagens were correct (Table 4.5). Thus, in this case, the prediction for sodium nitroguaiacolate might be doubted purely on the basis of weight-of-evidence (three out of five predictions incorrect), and this would be the right conclusion.

Overall, comparison of the Toxtree predictions with the data for the above-mentioned analogues indicates that Toxtree tends to overpredict mutagenicity, which is consistent with the global statistics—a positive predictivity of 73% and a negative predictivity of 82%.[44] This means that in general greater confidence should be assigned to a negative prediction than a positive prediction. In terms of the underlying (Benigni–Bossa) rulebase, this indicates that the structural alerts act as a coarse-grain filter that tend to overpredict because they are unable to capture subtle differences in molecular substructures and/or properties.

### 4.7.3 ToxBoxes Predictions

The application of ToxBoxes (Table 4.6) is interesting since it appears to perform very well on the basis of a global statistical analysis—positive and negative predictivities of 93%.[44] However, the apparent high predictivity of the model could be due to its large training set, which contains an unknown overlap with any test set. When ToxBoxes is applied to methylparathion and sodium nitroguaiacolate, it gives indeterminate predictions, which means that further information would be sought. The generation of indeterminate predictions is not necessarily a weakness in a model. On the contrary, it could be seen as a strong point, since it would avoid reliance on an incorrect prediction.

### 4.7.4 DEREK Predictions

In the case of methylparathion, DEREK generates correct predictions for the three mutagenic analogues, but incorrectly predicts the non-mutagenic analogue to be a mutagen (Table 4.7). Thus, the predicted mutagenicity of methylparathion might be considered reliable on the basis of weight-of-evidence (three out of four correct), and this would lead to the right conclusion. In the case of sodium nitroguaiacolate, the predictions for the two mutagenic analogues were correct whereas the predictions for two of the three non-mutagens were incorrect (unlike Toxtree, DEREK correctly predicts the non-mutagenicity of 3-methyl-4-nitrophenol). On the basis of marginal weight-of-evidence (three out of five correct), the predicted mutagenicity of sodium nitroguaiacolate might be considered reliable, but this would lead to the wrong conclusion.

### 4.7.5 Comments on the Assessment of (Q)SAR Predictions

In practice, the argumentation would be supplemented with additional information. Available information on the underlying toxicological mechanisms of action could also be considered in the assessment. For example, chemicals that are structural analogues but are known to act by a different mechanism of action would not be suitable choices. Unfortunately, such detailed information is rarely available. Furthermore, if the raw experimental data are available, these could be analysed in more depth. In this example, the conclusions of the assessor (mutagenic or non-mutagenic) are adopted without question, but it is possible that a more in-depth analysis might result in differences of opinion based on the raw data. Clearly, this level of analysis requires toxicological expertise and is more time-consuming.

## 4.8 Conclusions

In this chapter, the conceptual basis of (Q)SAR analysis and related non-testing methods has been explained. The current regulatory framework for documenting and assessing the validity of (Q)SAR models, and the adequacy of (Q)SAR predictions, has been described, and some of the scientific issues encountered when applying the framework illustrated *via* case studies on the genotoxicity prediction. Two examples were given that illustrate that these issues are not trivial: i) the interpretation of different diagnostics of model fit and predictivity, which requires a reasonable level of statistical expertise; and ii) the selection of suitable analogues to fill a data gap by read-across or to substantiate a QSAR prediction, which requires expertise in chemistry and biology (toxicology) and access to a range of computational tools and databases.

It is argued that the framework developed for REACH is sufficiently flexible to be applied in the risk assessment of all types of chemicals and products, irrespective of the legislation under which they are regulated (industrial chemicals, biocides, pesticides *etc.*). However, there is a need to develop and share experience within industry and the regulatory authorities on the use of computational models predictions for regulatory purposes. In addition, more detailed guidance is needed on how to evaluate models and interpret their predictions. The best way of achieving this is probably through the development of detailed case studies that illustrate the amount and type of information needed.

The QSAR model reporting formats (QMRF and QPRF) were developed on the basis of consensus with the main stakeholders (industry and authorities). They capture a level of resolution that is a compromise between scientific rigour and practicality. However, it is not always clear how much detail should be included under the different headings, and what kind of information is pertinent for models developed by different methodological approaches—in addition to traditional QSAR modelling based on (multiple) linear regression, there is an increasing use of "novel" model-building methods such as Support Vector Machines,[45] artificial neural networks, instance-based learning[46] and consensus modelling.[47] If models based on such methods are to gain acceptance, they need to be understandable to the assessor, and described with a sufficient level of transparency to form the basis for regulatory decision making. Furthermore, and more generally, in the regulatory assessment of chemicals, there should be greater emphasis on the development of models that are suitable for specific regulatory purposes, rather than trying to understand whether existing models (developed for other reasons) might be useful.

It is noteworthy that the current reporting formats focus on the result of the modelling process in the case of the QMRF (*i.e.*, the model validation characteristics) and its application to a chemical of interest in the case of the QPRF (*i.e.*, the characteristics of the prediction), rather than on the modelling and prediction process itself. It has been argued that the acceptability of (Q)SAR predictions could be improved through the development of principles and standards for Good Computer Modelling Practice (GCMP), analogous to the principles of Good Laboratory Practice (GLP).[48]

At present, there is also little guidance on how to supplement (Q)SAR and read-across predictions with information on biokinetics and mechanisms of action, in order to develop weight-of-evidence-based arguments for the replacement of (animal) testing. Therefore, further efforts are needed to develop strategies for integrating different kinds of experimental and non-testing information and guidance is needed on how to report this in a transparent and consistent manner.[49]

In conclusion, despite the tremendous amount of progress made in the development of chemoinformatic and (Q)SAR methodologies, there is still a considerable need to gain and share experience in the practical application of these tools, with a view to improving the scientific robustness, transparency and consistency of chemical risk assessments in which data gaps are filled by computational modelling.

## Acknowledgements

Some of this work was carried out under the terms of a contract awarded by the European Food Safety Authority (EFSA) to the European Commission's Joint Research Centre (JRC). EFSA contract number: SLA/EFSA-JRC/2009-01.

# References

1. A. Mostrag-Szlichtyng and A. P. Worth, *Review of QSAR Models and Software Tools for predicting Biokinetic Properties,* JRC Technical Report EUR 24377 EN, Publications Office of the European Union, Luxembourg, 2010.
2. R. Todeschini and V. Consonni, *Handbook of Molecular Descriptors*, Wiley-VCH, Weinheim, Germany, 2009.
3. ECHA, *Guidance on Information Requirements and Chemical Safety Assessment,* European Chemicals Agency, Helsinki, 2008, ch. R6.
4. *Guidance on Grouping of Chemicals.* ENV/JM/MONO(2007)28, Organisation for Economic Cooperation and Development, Paris, 2007.
5. ECHA, *Practical guide 6: How to report categories and read-across*, European Chemicals Agency, Helsinki, 2010.
6. ECHA, *Practical guide 5: How to report (Q)SARs*, European Chemicals Agency, Helsinki, 2010.
7. *Guidance Document on the Validation and International Acceptance of New or Updated Test Methods for Hazard Assessment.* ENV/JM/MONO(2005)14, Organisation for Economic Cooperation and Development, Paris, 2005.
8. *Guidance Document on the Validation of (Quantitative) Structure Activity Relationship [(Q)SAR] Models.* ENV/JM/MONO(2007)2, Organisation for Economic Cooperation and Development, Paris, 2007.
9. J. C. Dearden, M. T. D. Cronin and K. L. E. Kaiser, *SAR QSAR Environ. Res.*, 2009, **20**, 241.
10. A. P. Worth, in *Recent Advances in QSAR Studies: Methods and Applications*, ed. T. Puzyn, J. Leszczynski and M. Cronin, Springer, Heidelberg, Germany, 2010, p. 367.
11. D. M. Hawkins, *J. Chem. Inform. Comput. Sci.*, 2003, **44**, 1.
12. P. Gramatica, *QSAR Comb. Sci.*, 2007, **26**, 694.
13. O. Aptula, N. Jeliazkova, T. W. Schultz and M. T. D. Cronin, *QSAR Comb. Sci.*, 2005, **24**, 385.
14. J. G. Topliss and R. P. Edwards, *J. Med. Chem.*, 1979, **22**, 1238.
15. S. Wold and W. J. Dunn, *J. Chem. Inform. Comput. Sci.*, 1983, **23**, 6.
16. M. Clark and R. D. Cramer III, *Quant. Struct.–Act. Relat.*, 1993, **12**, 137.
17. V. Tetko, I. Sushko, A. K. Pandey, H. Zhu, A. Tropsha, E. Papa, T. Öberg, R. Todeschini, D. Fourches and A. Varnek, *J. Chem. Inf. Model.*, 2008, **48**, 1733.
18. M. Daszykowski, B. Walczak and D. L. Massart, *Anal. Chim. Acta*, 2002, **468**, 91.
19. R. Kennard and L. Stone, *Technometrics*, 1969, **11**, 137.
20. R. Snee, *Technometrics*, 1977, **19**, 415.
21. R. Cook and C. Nachtsheim, *Technometrics*, 1980, **22**, 315.
22. R. Boggia, M. Forina, P. Fossa and L. Mosti, *Quant. Struct.–Act. Relat.*, 1997, **16**, 201.
23. T. Kohonen, *Neurocomputing*, 1998, **21**, 1.
24. R. Cramer, J. Bunce, D. Patterson and I. Frank, *Quant. Struct.–Act. Relat.*, 1988, **7**, 18.

25. D. W. Osten, *J. Chemom.*, 1988, **2**, 39.
26. R. Wehrens, H. Putter and L. Buydens, *Chemom. Intell. Lab. Syst.,* 2000, **54**, 35.
27. F. Lindgren, B. Hansen, W. Karcher, M. Sjöström and L. Eriksson, *J. Chemom.*, 1996, **10**, 521.
28. R. Todeschini, V. Consonni and A. Maiocchi, *Chemom. Intell. Lab. Syst.*, 1999, **46**, 13.
29. G. Topliss and R. J. Costello, *J. Med. Chem.*, 1972, **15**, 1066.
30. M. T. D. Cronin, F. Bigot, S. J. Enoch, J. C. Madden, D. W. Roberts and J. Schwöbel, *Altern. Lab. Anim.*, 2009, **37**, 513.
31. http://www.caesar-project.eu.
32. http://ihcp.jrc.ec.europa.eu/our_labs/computational_toxicology.
33. http://www.acdlabs.com/products/admet/tox/.
34. http://www.lhasalimited.org.
35. R. Benigni, T. Netzeva, E. Benfenati, C. Bossa, R. Franke, C. Helma, E. Hulzebos, C. Marchant, A. Richard, Y. Woo and C. Yang, *J. Environ. Sci. Health C*, 2007, **25**, 53.
36. R. Serafimova, M. Fuart Gatnik and A. Worth, *Review of QSAR Models and Software Tools for predicting Genotoxicity and Carcinogenicity,* JRC Technical Report EUR 24427 EN, Publications Office of the European Union, Luxembourg, 2010.
37. http://pubchem.ncbi.nlm.nih.gov/.
38. http://www.chemspider.com.
39. http://ambit.sourceforge.net/intro.html.
40. http://www.epa.gov/oppt/sf/tools/aim.htm.
41. http://www.oecd.org.
42. http://ihcp.jrc.ec.europa.eu/our_labs/computational_toxicology.
43. N. Jeliazkova, J. Jaworska and A. Worth, in *In Silico Toxicology: Principles and Applications*, ed. M. T. D. Cronin and J. C. Madden, The Royal Society of Chemistry, Cambridge, 2010, p. 408.
44. JRC, *Applicability of QSAR analysis to the evaluation of the toxicological relevance of metabolites and degradates of pesticide active substances for dietary risk assessment*, a report prepared by the European Commission's Joint Research Centre for the European Food Safety Authority, Parma, Italy, 2010.
45. R. Burbidge, M. Trotter, B. Buxton and S. Holden, *Comput. Chem.*, 2001, **26**, 5.
46. Helma, *Mol. Diversity*, 2006, **10**, 147.
47. M. Hewitt, M. T. D. Cronin, J. C. Madden, P. H. Rowe, C. Johnson, A. Obi and S. J. Enoch, *J. Chem. Inf. Model.*, 2007, **47**, 1460.
48. P. N. Judson, *Qual. Assur. J.*, 2009, **12**, 120.
49. Bassan and A. P. Worth, in *Computational Toxicology: Risk Assessment for Pharmaceutical and Environmental Chemicals*, ed. S. Ekins, John Wiley & Sons, New York, 2007, vol. 1, p. 751.
50. T. Ferrari and G. Gini, *Chem. Cent. J.*, 2010, **4**, S2.
51. T. Ferrari, G. Gini and E. Benfenati, *Proc. NAFIPS'09*, Cincinnati, USA, 2009, pp. 1–6.

52. R. Benigni, C. Bossa, N. Jeliazkova, T. Netzeva and A. Worth, *The Benigni/Bossa rulebase for mutagenicity and carcinogenicity – a module of Toxtree*, JRC Technical Report EUR 23241 EN, Publications Office of the European Union, Luxembourg, 2008.
53. R. Benigni, C. Bossa, O. Tcheremenskaia and A. Worth, *Development of structural alerts for the* in vivo *micronucleus assay in rodents*, JRC Technical Report EUR 23844 EN, Publications Office of the European Union, Luxembourg, 2009.
54. R. Benigni, C. Bossa and A. Worth, *Mutagenesis*, 2010, **25**, 335.

CHAPTER 5

# Information, Informatics and Modeling in Predictive Toxicology

SCOTT BOYER,[*,a] DANIEL MUTHAS[a] AND NIGEL GREENE[b]

[a] AstraZeneca R&D, Computational Toxicology, Global Safety Assessment, Mölndal, Sweden; [b] Pfizer Global Research and Development, Groton, CT 06340, USA

## 5.1 Introduction

The practice of modern toxicology has and continues to generate enormous amounts of data. Since much of the toxicology information that has been generated in the past 70 years has been to evaluate the safety of commercial products such as pesticides, industrial chemicals, cosmetics and pharmaceuticals, a great deal of the data are still unavailable to the public. This situation is improving however mostly due to improving informatics infrastructure, better mechanisms for data sharing and above all, more standard ways of expressing the basic foundations of toxicology—dose, species, exposure, relevant toxicological endpoints and chemical composition of the compound(s) of interest.

In this chapter we will review the various data sources ranging from public to commercial, including the tools that are available to analyze and interrogate these data. As expected, the data are spread out among literally hundreds of

RSC Drug Discovery Series No. 12
New Horizons in Predictive Toxicology: Current Status and Application
Edited by Alan G. E. Wilson

Published by the Royal Society of Chemistry, www.rsc.org

sources. The challenge of the past two decades, and indeed the foreseeable future, is not only the synthesis of toxicology information into meaningful data structures that can be more easily accessed and exploited, but also the linking of that information out to chemical and biological information available in other sources. All scientific disciplines face this challenge and thus many of the solutions discussed in this chapter are indeed borrowed from other areas.

We will first discuss the various public data sources in an attempt to give a current view of the breadth of safety-related information from both public sources and commercial suppliers. We then go on to discuss the current state-of-the-art in analysis and data mining to make the most of these data, including some of the issues around data quality. Finally we will review the actual use of these data and tools to make decisions in industrial and regulatory settings.

## 5.2 Sources of Toxicology Data

### 5.2.1 Public Sources of Toxicology Data

Ideally, there would be a single source of toxicology data that is accumulated and standardized, with an interface that allows searching by effect, species and chemical structure.

Such a source does not exist yet but here we present a representative group of the data sources from which much of the publically available data of toxicological relevance can be retrieved. Table 5.1 gives a list of public data sources that can be of use in the evaluation of the safety of drug candidates. The table

**Table 5.1** Public toxicologically relevant data sources.

| | | *Searchable by...* | | |
|---|---|---|---|---|
| *Name* | *Source* | *Endpoint* | *Chemical structure* | *Species* |
| ToxNet | http://toxnet.nlm.nih.gov/index.html | Y | Y | Y |
| DSSTox | http://www.epa.gov/ncct/dsstox/ | Y | Y | Y |
| ACToR | http://actor.epa.gov/actor/faces/Download.jsp | Y | Y | Y |
| RTECS | http://www.cdc.gov/niosh/rtecs/default.html | Y | Y | Y |
| CTD | http://ctd.mdibl.org | N | N | Y |
| GENETOX | http://www.nlm.nih.gov/pubs/factsheets/genetxfs.html | Y | Y | Y |
| DART | http://www.nlm.nih.gov/pubs/factsheets/dartfs.html | Y | Y | Y |
| KEGG | http://www.kegg.jp/kegg/drug/ | N | N | Y |
| DITOP | http://bioinf.xmu.edu.cn/databases/ADR/search.php | Y | N | Y |
| T3DB | http://www.t3db.org | N | N | Y |
| CTD | http://ctd.mdibl.org/ | Y/N | N | Y |
| ToxCast | http://www.epa.gov/ncct/toxcast/ | N | Y | Y |
| Tox21 | http://www.epa.gov/ncct/Tox21/ | N/A | N/A | N/A |

gives an indication of whether species, specific endpoint and chemical structure information is included.

First on the list is TOXNET,[1–3] maintained by the US National Library of Medicine. As the name implies, TOXNET is a network of scores of data sources assembled under a single user interface. TOXNET is searchable by chemical structure via the ChemIDPlus[4] function and within ChemIDPlus one can search for either structural similarity or substructure and the interface covers essentially all of the data sources in TOXNET. An additional, very useful, source of structured data is the DSSTox initiative[5] which does not formally offer a search interface but rather offers a number of structured data sources that are endpoint-specific and downloadable in a standard format. DSSTox is maintained by the United States Environmental Protection Agency (USEPA) and is one of the data sources included in the ACToR compilation.[6] ACToR includes a very large number of databases, primarily focused on environmental endpoints befitting the mission of the EPA. One quite useful data source worth noting is the Registry of Toxic Effects of Chemical Substances (RTECS),[7] maintained by the US Centers for Disease Control and National Institute for Occupational Safety and Health (NIOSH) that is available for searching via TOXNET/ChemIDPlus. RTECS results cannot be accessed *via* TOXNET directly however and the user will need to obtain a license, but TOXNET will alert the user to the fact that results do exist in RTECS.

There are a few endpoints that are of particular interest and worth mentioning specifically here. The first is GENE-TOX,[8,9] which as the name implies, contains endpoints and chemical structure data relevant to genetic toxicology endpoints. Another endpoint-specific data source is the DART database[10] which contains developmental toxicity data that could be of high value for drug discovery organizations. These two endpoints are mentioned specifically as they represent two of the endpoints in preclinical drug safety evaluation which will almost invariably end project progression if they are observed and thus worth special attention.

With regard to biological aspects of public data of toxicological relevance there are several sources that are available. For general biological pathways the KEGG database[11] is widely regarded as the standard and represents a good starting point from which new custom pathways can be annotated or broad searches for gene function can begin. A relative newcomer in the area of tying biological, toxicological and drug data together is the Drug-Induced Toxicity of Proteins (DITOP) database.[12] One can search DITOP by protein, drug or toxicity. DITOP does not allow for searching by chemical structure, and a name must be used. A rather unique resource is the toxin and toxin-targets database (T3DB)[13] which lists known toxin–target interactions and, like DITOP, is searchable by protein or chemical name only. With regard to toxicogenomics, one of the primary public sources is the Comparitive Toxicogenomics Database (CTD).[14–16] Finally, it is worth mentioning ToxCast,[17] the initial evaluation of chemical libraries and toxicologically relevant endpoints that is the basis for further, more drug-related, compound evaluations in the project named Tox21.[18] Both ToxCast and Tox21 have the potential to significantly enhance our understanding of patterns of biological changes in a variety of systems induced by well-characterized *in vivo* toxicants.

There are, of course, a great number of public data sources for toxicological data and the list in Table 5.1 is a sample of the major sources and tools. As one searches in these sources, other, related data sources are almost always uncovered. No matter what the public source used, one must be aware that searching by chemical structure in any of these sources in their public interfaces implies that the chemical structure is not only exposed to the public domain, but also presumably stored on the servers of the host institution and may represent a public disclosure of a potentially proprietary chemical structure. Caution should be exercised and if a data source is found to be particularly useful, it may be worthwhile bringing it inside the company firewall to search on it without risk of disclosure.

### 5.2.2 Proprietary Sources of Toxicology Data

The potential of organizing toxicology data for commercial resale has not been lost on several organizations. There are now several sources of toxicological data offered for sale. The data can take the shape of chemical structure–activity fields in which the only information given is chemical structure and a Positive or Negative activity. More common are compilations of chemical structures with literature or 'public' data that have varying degrees of toxicological relevance. We will review a list of these tools and attempt to give a general overview of the data types that can be expected from these sources. The data types will, of course, dictate the types of queries that can be made against them and thus will determine which one the user will find useful in a given situation. The types of commercial data sources can be categorized in five distinct groups: 1) Those that give chemical structure–toxicity data lists intended for building structure–activity relationships, 2) those that list general toxicity findings in multiple species in which one can search for either effect or chemical structure, 3) data sources that list chemical structure–pharmacology relationships, some of which could be highly relevant for assessing toxicological/safety risk, 4) bioinformatics tools that include data of toxicological/ safety relevance and finally, 5) data sources that contain toxicology data that may not be available in any of the other sources. The sources that we have chosen to review here can be found in Table 5.2 and their features are reviewed below. The following five sections will briefly review commercial data sources from the perspective of the types of data they offer, the various sources of the data and any particular features of each source, such as the types of analysis one can do, or that are features of the package. One core feature of all commercial data sources that differentiate them from the open public data sources listed above is the act of annotation of the data. Annotation in this context can take many forms, but the various sources below have added value to the datasets *via* varying degrees of annotation and quality control. This may take the form of selecting only datasets of a minimum quality standard or by putting effort into understanding, categorizing and selecting data that are of a certain minimum quality.

**Table 5.2** Commercial toxicologically relevant data sources.

| *Name* | *Source* | *Endpoints* | *Source of information* |
|---|---|---|---|
| | *Chemical structure–activity data* | | |
| MCASE | http://www.multicase.com/ | Toxicity | Public and FDA |
| LeadScope | http://www.leadscope.com/toxicity_databases/ | Toxicity | Public and FDA |
| VITIC | https://www.lhasalimited.org/vitic/ | Toxicity | Public and internal industrial data |
| | *Toxicology data searchable by chemical structure* | | |
| RTECS | http://www.cdc.gov/niosh/rtecs/default.html | Toxicity | Public and National Toxicology Program |
| GVKBio MBT | www.gvkbio.com/database_pdf/Mechanism_Based_Toxicity.pdf | Toxicity | Public |
| | *Structure–pharmacological activity data sources* | | |
| BioPrint | http://www.cerep.fr/Cerep/Users/pages/ProductsServices/bioprintservices.asp | Pharmacology, drug side-effects | Public and proprietary |
| GVKBio | http://www.gvkbio.com/ | Pharmacology | Public and patents |
| Aureus Pharma | http://www.aureus-sciences.com/aureus/web/guest/databases | Pharmacology, pharmacokinetics | Public |
| WOMBAT | http://www.sunsetmolecular.com/index.php?option=com_content&view=article&id=15&Itemid=10 | Pharmacology, pharmacokinetics | Public |

| | | | |
|---|---|---|---|
| | *Toxicologically relevant 'systems biology' sources* | | |
| Ingenuity Pathway Analysis | http://www.ingenuity.com/products/pathways_analysis.html | General biology pharmacology toxicology | Public |
| GeneGo MetaCore | http://www.genego.com/metacore.php | General biology pharmacology toxicology | Public |
| ToxWiz | http://www.camcellnet.com/products.php?id=14&smenu=sub1 | General biology pharmacology toxicology | Public |
| Pathway Studio | http://www.ariadnegenomics.com/pathwaystudio | General biology pharmacology | Public |
| | *General data sources* | | |
| Pharmapendium | http://www.info.pharmapendium.com/ | General biology pharmacology toxicology | Public and regulatory documents |
| BioWisdom SIP | http://www.biowisdom.com/tag/sip/ | General biology pharmacology toxicology | Public |
| SciFinder | http://www.cas.org/products/scifindr/index.html | Pharmacology chemical properties | Public |
| AERS | http://www.fda.gov/Drugs/GuidanceComplianceRegulatoryInformation/surveillance/AdverseDrugEffects/ucm082193.htm | Drug side-effects | Public |

#### 5.2.2.1 Chemical Structure–Activity Data

The basis for effective SAR and QSAR analyses is that the chemical database containing chemical structures linked to activity data is considered to be obtained in a standard (enough) way, so that the user can consider the results to be comparable. This is not a simple task with all of the experimental systems that have been used to assess the various aspects of safety. In most cases, the endpoints, even relatively well-defined measurements such as Ames assays, represent toxicological mechanisms that are diverse. This must be kept in mind when attempting to model these data and even more importantly in attempting to interpret results of predictions such model can give.

Since the level of data analysis and quality control is very high for datasets intended for modeling, the sources of these data are few. Groups like MultiCase[19] offer a large number of data sets that cover a variety of toxicological endpoints. The data offered by MultiCase are predominantly public data that have been rather carefully quality controlled. In addition, models built on these data are available in the software package. These models are trained on additional data obtained from the FDA thereby giving a measure of access to otherwise invisible data. A systematic study on whether the addition of these extra data from the FDA actually helps the predictive models has yet to be published, however. Like MultiCase the software package offered by Leadscope[20] offers databases that have been annotated from a variety of sources, including FDA-curated data. Both MultiCase and Leadscope offer each of the datasets as an individual item without obligation to license the entire collection. The licensing conditions are different so it is best to check with these vendors regarding what limitations exist. Finally, another source of highly curated structure–toxicity data is the Vitic project, sponsored by Lhasa, Ltd.[21] Vitic is a very different model from Leadscope or MultiCase in that they offer the possibility of sharing data. Submission of a certain amount of data to the intermediates and excipients data sharing groups then enables a participating organization to have access to all or parts of the larger, community-derived data set. There is also a possibility of buying the regular database without sharing, but then you cannot access the shared data.

#### 5.2.2.2 General Toxicology Findings Searchable by Chemical Structure

Toxicology is a very complicated science with a concomitantly complex data history. Very few agreed terms exist for toxicological endpoints and thus study outcomes, whether *in vivo* or *in vitro* are sometimes very difficult to compare. This limitation notwithstanding, one must be aware as best one can of the existing data that relates a chemical structure to any possible toxicology. With this in mind, two data sources are of possible utility in making general searches of annotated toxicology data that are linked to chemical structure. The first is the RTECS[7,22] database. A short review of RTECS was presented above and for the purposes of this section it is worth adding that RTECS can be obtained as a simple database file against which one can make chemical structure-based searches. The greatest value of RTECS may be in the ability to run substructure searches to explore the underlying toxicology of various functional groups or ring systems. The data in RTECS is a mixture of annotated literature data and data taken directly from studies performed at the National Center for Toxicological Research (NCTR). Another data source that is organized in a similar fashion to RTECS is the Mechanism-Based Toxicity (MBT)[23] database offered by GVKBio.[24] The data are annotated from the literature and sensibly organized to allow searching by chemical structure or substructure. As stated above, both RTECS and MBT suffer from the variety of terms used for what may be the same toxicological finding but in both sources the chemical structure-based search capacity makes them worth the effort if one is to perform a proper due diligence on a particular chemical feature.

### *5.2.2.3 Chemical Structure–Pharmacological Data*

The data sources listed above have been collected with the express purpose of annotating toxicological outcomes to chemical structure. Since some safety issues are a result of the action of a chemical structure on a protein that results in a pathophysiologial effect, the assessment of the safety of a given chemical structure should include a search of the known pharmacological activity of similar structures or substructures. Several public initiatives to annotate pharmacological data to chemical structure exist, the most prominent among those being perhaps PUBCHEM[25,26] and ChemSpider.[27] Several commercial data collections also exist which offer some level of either analysis functionality, a greater level of confidence in the annotated data or unique data collections not available in the public data sources.

One unique source of pharmacology data is the BioPrint database[28,29] which offers a defined set of substances (mostly drugs) measured against a defined set of assays. BioPrint, and its use in assessing unintended pharmacology and its consequences will be discussed in a later section as its unique 'full matrix' of pharmacological activity offers unique opportunities for investigating pharmacology-toxicology relationships. The next three data sources contain data annotated from the open literature and/or drug or chemical registration documents (regulatory submission or patents). They are GVKBio,[24] Aureus Pharma Pharmacology database[30] and WOMBAT.[31,32] All three of these sources appear to be well annotated with unique value added to each in different areas. One feature of these kinds of datasets is that although they are annotated from roughly the same sources, they do not necessarily contain the same data.[33,34] All three data sources offer not only pharmacological data coupled to structure but also pharmacokinetic data, when it is available.

### *5.2.2.4 Toxicologically Relevant 'Systems Biology' Sources*

While the above-named sources can give quite comprehensive information on the possible pharmacological activity of a given compound very little information is available in these sources linking pharmacological target to possible physiological functions that could manifest themselves as an adverse effect. This coupling is naturally an absolute requirement when attempting to interpret the toxicological consequences of a predicted or measured pharmacological effect. There are a few tools in this area that have made attempts at annotating these associations from the literature and then, to varying degrees, building some toxicological knowledge into the mix. The tools of particular note are Ingenuity Pathway Analysis from Ingenuity (IPA),[35] GeneGos suite of MetaCore, MetaDrug and ToxHunter,[36] ToxWiz from Cambridge Cell Networks,[37] the Safety Information Programme (SIP) from BioWisdom[38] and Pathway studio from Ariadne Genomics.[39] As with the pharmacology data sources, each of these tools has advantages and disadvantages. Analysis of toxicogenomic data along with pharmacology data is reasonably easy in IPA and MetaCore/ToxHunter for instance, while Toxwiz is interesting due to its almost exclusive focus on toxicology/adverse effects and SIP gives the user the possibility of incorporating additional data from in house studies, for example. A comprehensive comparison is not possible here, but one aspect that is quite critical is that all of the above-named sources do offer reasonably generous pilot test periods and also well-organized training and user support programmes so those wishing to test them for their particular circumstances can easily do so.

#### *5.2.2.5 General Data Sources*

Some additional data sources are worth mentioning here even though they do not fit into any of the above categories. The first is the commonly used chemistry literature search tool SciFinder.[40] SciFinder contains a few special search functions that do narrow searches to those which have been identified (by their annotation process) to contain toxicologically relevant information. Our experience has been that most users are not aware that this kind of specific search is possible. The second source is Pharmapendium.[41] Pharmapendium contains well-organized data predominantly (as the name implies) focused on drugs and their preclinical and clinical data, including links to some regulatory submissions, such as the Summary Basis of Approval, which gives a summary of the preclinical and clinical safety findings for drugs. Thirdly is the adverse event reporting system (AERS)[42] from FDA. AERS is a database used to monitor post-marketing safety, to which healthcare professionals, patients and manufactures report any found adverse event. All AERS terms are standardized according to Medical Dictionary for Regulatory Activities terminology (MedDRA).

### 5.2.3 Data from the Pharmaceutical Industry

Thus far we have reviewed and compared data sources from either public or commercial organizations. However, the single richest source of relevant and high-quality data is without question the pharmaceutical industry itself. It is not surprising, however, that nearly all of these data are kept within the companies themselves with only a few notable exceptions.[43] Internal data are usually perceived as being more homogeneous than literature data but to date no systematic study has been published to address this question. Rather, it is assumed that all companies involved in safety evaluation, either using *in vitro* or *in vivo* methods, is operating under a standard operating procedure and that, particularly for *in vitro* data, the results are meant to be compared to results from other compounds. So while industrial scientists publish methods for data modeling,[44–49] seldom are internal data released and thus either the data modeled are already public or the underlying data are not given but only methods and results are given. This is a frustrating situation for both academic scientists who want to analyze industrial data in different ways and for industrial scientists who know that exposing internal data to outside analysis would possibly yield greater value from the data. This situation is compounded by the fact that each company has roughly the same types of data and even greater value could be gained from cross-industry merging of data.

There are now a few initiatives of note that are aiming to break down the traditional ways of thinking in this area. As mentioned above there is the model of outright release of data to the public as illustrated by the release by GSK of a large malaria dataset.[43] While not related to drug safety, this does set an important precedent regarding sharing of datasets in a 'pre-competitive' manner that will benefit everyone in a particular community. The second mechanism in current operation is bilateral or multilateral sharing of specific data between two pharmaceutical companies. This can be by direct exchange or by the use of a third party. Two good examples are of this kind of agreement are hosted by Lhasa, Ltd, one being the Genetox Impurities data sharing consortium (Intermediates Data Sharing Group) into which various partner companies can contribute data. The contribution of data then qualifies that particular company to access all data in the collection thereby facilitating SAR analysis of potential genotox impurities using a greatly expanded set of data. Similarly there is a consortium sharing data on *in vivo* data for excipients. Another interesting effort in this style is the Tox21 project in which pharmaceutical companies are encouraged to contribute both chemical substance and associated safety data to a central source.[50,51] One objective of Tox21 would be that the contributed data will be standardized and mined, but uniquely, Tox21 intends to also generate additional standardized data (primarily *in vitro*) using the compounds it is provided. This combination of existing safety data with data from modern *in vitro* methods intended to assess toxic liabilities or mechanisms is a unique step in safety evaluation. Finally, in the area of pre-competitive sharing of safety-related data specifically, the European Commission has taken the bold step of not only encouraging, but also resourcing initiatives aimed directly at sharing of pre-competitive data[52] under the umbrella of the Innovative Medicines Initiative (IMI). One of the efforts within IMI which promises to have an immediate impact on data sharing is the e-Tox project.[53] E-Tox is a framework in which safety-related *in vitro*, *in vivo* animal and ultimately clinical data from drug discovery and development are shared across industry with the ultimate goal of building computational models of the data. Despite the difficulties of legal release, lack of electronic versions of critical data and insufficient resources required to retrieve and organize internal data, the e-Tox project is unique in its ambition and represents an important step in more transparent and responsible use of safety data.

### 5.2.4 Limitations of Data Sources as Predictive Tools

Whilst there is a great deal of data available now in the public domain, using these sources to assess the likelihood of seeing a certain toxicity with a novel compound poses many difficulties which need to be considered by the assessor when using them to draw comparisons. Errors exist in every single public data source and these can be as simple as typographical errors or as complex as using the wrong term to describe an event. Indeed, even something as straightforward as the chemical being tested can be misrepresented in the data source either through the use of non-standardized names, incorrect or ambiguous CAS numbers, or errors in the chemical structure representation itself.[54] These errors can even be propagated from one source to another as they will often draw from each other rather than going to the original source. The simple problem is that no one source of data is free of errors and so can be considered a definitive source for information of a specified type.

Comparing biological data from different sources is a constant challenge when conducting data searches and comparisons. *In vitro* data can be easier to handle and combine but where data comes from more than one database but this too can have issues. It is well known that assays run using different protocols or conditions can give rise to very different responses in the assay for the same chemical. Common issues can be the reagents used in the assay, for example the source of the metabolic activation reagent commonly referred to as the S9 mix used in an Ames assay for detecting mutagenicity can result in whole classes of compounds registering as mutagens when they previously were thought to be inactive under different conditions.[55] Indeed, something as trivial as the temperature at which the assay is conducted can cause variation in the assay results. For example, temperature effects have been noted with assays that look at the ion flow in key ion channels such as the hERG potassium channel associated with an elongation of the interval between the onset of the Q wave and the end of the T wave, which represents the total time for ventricular depolarization and repolarization, (prolonged QT syndrome) which is thought to be linked to rare and often fatal arrhythmias in humans.[56]

A whole variety of issues exist when attempting to compare data from studies using preclinical species. The complex nature of *in vivo* studies often makes it difficult to compare across compounds. There are many variables to consider in comparing one experiment to another such as the species and strain used; the route of administration for treatment; the dosing frequency and formulation; the dose levels and the duration of the study *etc.* as all of these will influence the nature and type of outcomes observed in the experiment. These issues can be further compounded by circadian rhythm effects especially if one is considering expression levels of genes or even physiological responses.[57,58]

In addition, most reports pertaining to *in vivo* experiments only list those parameters which changed under treatment when compared to a control group but do not list everything that was measured during the course of the study. This creates a problem when trying to identify compounds that do not cause a specific phenotype so that they can be compared to those that do. The absence of evidence does not necessarily infer the absence of effect. The absence of an internationally accepted standard for the lexicon, taxonomy and ontology used in describing safety effects of compounds means that automated extraction of information from published literature using text mining becomes an almost insurmountable hurdle to creating data sets for comparison and so manual curation becomes the only alternative.[59–61]

Finally, and probably most importantly, *in vivo* experiments are often published where treatments administered are described in terms of the dose per unit of body weight on a daily intake. This presents multiple challenges when comparing one compound to another as the actual amount of active ingredient administered is dependent on the relative molecular weight of the compound in question, in that a dose of 10 mg $kg^{-1}$ of a compound that has a molecular weight of 100 is in fact six times that of a compound that has a molecular weight of 600 also administered at the same 10 mg $kg^{-1}$ dose. In addition, for compounds administered orally, the absorption of the compound into the bloodstream of the treated animal may vary by several orders of magnitude depending on the characteristics of the compound in question. A recent evaluation of bloodstream exposure *versus* administered dose shows that the exposure can vary across seven orders of magnitude for compounds administered at the same dose (Figure 5.1).

In summary, comparing data between different sources or compiling data sets from multiple sources can be time consuming as well as prone to errors and potential misunderstandings.

## 5.3 Use of Toxicology Data for Prediction

### 5.3.1 Capturing Structure–Activity Relationships in Toxicology Data

It was Galileo Galilei who set out the basic principles of SAR and QSAR with his assertion that we should observe the quantitative aspects of the world around us and to use these observations to deduce consequences from them. It was in fact a form of toxicology for which the first qualitative structure–activity relationships (QSAR) were produced in the mid-19$^{th}$ Century using what we now recognize as QSAR techniques.[62–64] As statistical methods and physical (quantum mechanical) description of the atomic environments of organic molecules improved later in the 20$^{th}$ Century,[65] those interested in modeling the effect of chemical variation on nearly any endpoint of interest were provided

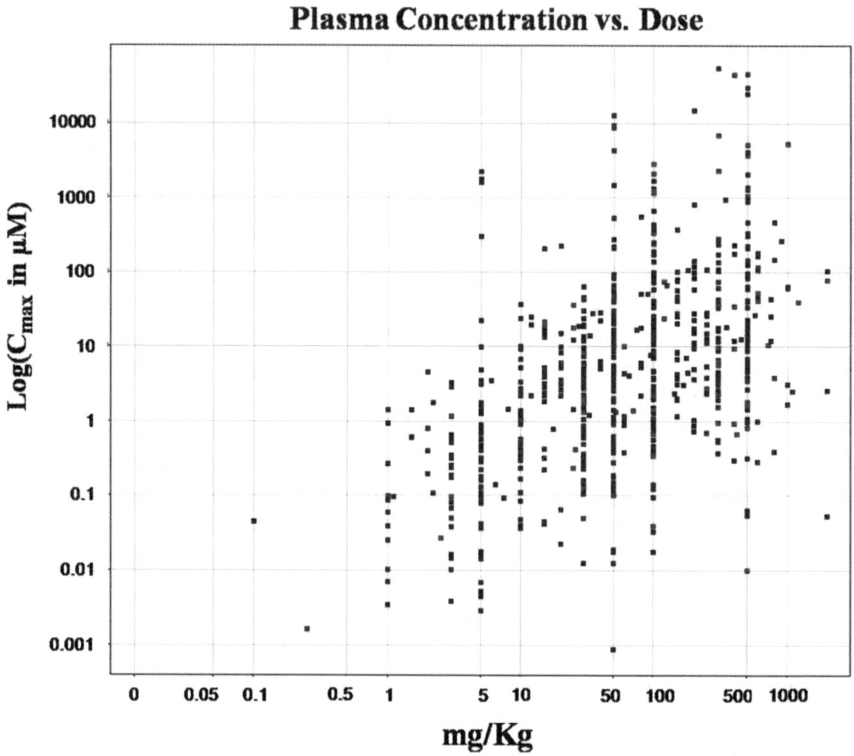


**Figure 5.1** Plot of $C_{max}$ plasma concentration in µM *versus* administered dose for compounds administered orally in rats and dogs in dose per unit body weight.

with a significantly enhanced set of tools with which to work. In addition, better understanding of the physics governing molecular structure and its effects on biological systems offered the possibility to interpret QSAR models and develop hypotheses regarding how modifications may alter the biological activity.

With respect to the application of these technologies to modern toxicological data, the most significant step forward was the production of higher quality toxicology datasets in the 1970s in the form of reverse mutation assay (Ames assay)[66] data which was produced under more controlled and consistent conditions thus making these data more amenable to QSAR modeling. Since the Ames mutagenicity data were primarily regarded as either 'Positive' or 'Negative', initial analyses of the data produced SAR 'rules' in which certain chemical structural features were regarded as ground for concern. These structural alerts were used to great effect in identification and risk mitigation of mutagenic compounds, particularly in the drug, industrial chemical and pesticide areas. These structural alerts are still used in combination with a number of other QSAR models to assess the overall risk of mutagenicity and many very useful and insightful treatments of this problem have been published over the years.[67–71] Availability of Ames data has also stimulated large collaborative efforts to assemble, mine and exploit these data in chemical design decisions[72,73] as well as promoting ongoing treatments of the problems of the accuracy of genetic toxicity prediction methods.[74] The methods in this area are advancing rapidly and the availability of relatively consistent datasets has facilitated work on the interpretation of complex QSAR models—a long-standing problem in the QSAR field.[75]

SAR and QSAR is currently used throughout the discipline of toxicology and several recent reviews have been published which cover the primary areas of drug discovery[76] environmental risk assessment[77,78] and drug and chemical regulation[79,80] and drug impurity assessment.[81,82] The specific area of regulatory use of QSARs will be discussed in more detail below. What is clear from most of the work in this area is that the data, and specifically the quality and quantity of the data, play a pivotal role in the overall quality, but also in the form of the final SAR or QSAR used.[83]

The proliferation of chemical structure analysis tools and methods, developed primarily to aid in drug discovery are now being regularly employed in the analysis of toxicity data. If one only looks at Ames mutagenicity data, one can find analyses that extend the structural alerts of Ashby and Tennant[69] and attempt to use these to predict new compounds, analyses using fixed substructural features to assess the statistical contribution to positive or negative activity,[73] and of course 'traditional' QSAR approaches using a variety of descriptors, some of which are more interpretable than others.[70,71] One can also find Ames QSAR analyses that include a direct interpretation of the relevant descriptors that contribute to the activity decision of just the particular molecule being predicted.[75] Finally, there is the more intuitive approach of read-across, in which structural analogs of the compound of interest are gathered, using a standard method of molecular description and similarity metric, and compared to the query compound.[84] For the activity of structurally similar compounds the activity of the query compound is then inferred. Read across methods, also known as k-nearest neighbor methods,[85] depend on a certain density of the compounds from which activity can be inferred. Lack of near neighbors, or if neighbors are of conflicting activities, results in uncertain conclusions in most cases. Almost universally, these methods have been used in isolation and if more than one method is used in a single report the tendency is to assess them in competition with each other. The future will demand that the various methods are used in concert and finding ways to use these methods in a way that they complement each other and contribute to a transparent and interpretable weight of evidence conclusion is an area in need of acute attention.

A more specific discussion of the areas in which predictive systems are being built will be presented in the final section of this chapter. Generally however, one can say that the effective use of toxicology data, with all of the issues regarding data quality outlined above, for predictions will require an enormous amount of research into what data mining and machine-learning methods are most appropriate for each data set and endpoint. Some examples of this type of research are given in the following sections.

### 5.3.2 Use of Biological Fingerprints in Assessing Toxicity

#### *5.3.2.1 What is a Biospectrum?*

New compounds in drug discovery are routinely screened in *in vitro* assay panels in order to predict potential off-targets and investigate the polypharmacology of compounds.[86–89] The panel usually consists of >80 targets spanning a wide range of protein families (*e.g.*, G protein-coupled receptors (GPCRs), enzymes, hormone receptors, transporters), and compounds are tested at a consistent, high dose (usually 10 μM). Activity is reported as percent inhibition and dose–response curves are usually subsequently generated for the identified off-targets to derive $IC_{50}$ or $K_i$ values. These matrices of target–protein interactions provide a rich source of data and can serve as a window into the interactome, and form the basis of the relatively new discipline of chemogenomics. In addition to the direct identification of off-targets, the ligand–target interactions can also be envisioned as a biospectrum or biological fingerprint, containing information not captured by common chemical similarity analysis, useful for *in silico* modeling. Here each ligand–target interaction populates a bin in the spectrum/fingerprint. These biospectra have mainly been used for three different types of tasks: retrieving neighbors in pharmacological space to identify potentially new targets and build *in silico* models to predict activity (either primary or off-targets); relating the binding profiles to *in vivo* effects such as predicting side-effects; searching for chemical features relating to promiscuity/selectivity.[90]

#### *5.3.2.2 Early Efforts*

Kauvar *et al.*[91] were among the first to utilize binding affinities to multiple targets as descriptors of chemical structure with their affinity fingerprint approach. As a proof-of-concept they create an information rich compound–target interaction matrix by determining the $IC_{50}$ values of a set of diverse compounds in a panel of eight targets, selected from a larger set of targets based on their low co-correlation. Employing stepwise linear regression fitting of the training compounds $IC_{50}$ values against the eight binding affinities to the experimental $IC_{50}$ value of the new target, models were derived to predict affinities for two unrelated targets with reasonable accuracy. The panel was subsequently expanded to 18 targets to ensure the generality of the surrogate proteins when applied to a larger set of chemicals. The models generated using 54 compounds were able to reasonably predict the activity of approximately 5000 compounds against four targets. Traditionally, the early stages of medicinal chemistry had been focused on optimizing the potency of the compounds and only screened for selectivity against a small set of related targets. With rising awareness of the safety concerns promiscuous compounds bring and advances in automated *in vitro* screening Poulain *et al.*[92,93] employed the pharmacological profiles of μ-opiate receptor modulators to prioritize which compound class to progress. From two different classes of actives they performed screening against not only opiate receptors but a broader panel of targets. The two classes differed in pharmacological profile with one being much more promiscuous, and therefore down-prioritized. They found that similar compounds exhibited a reasonable neighborhood behavior, and that early pharmacological profiling was useful to prioritize between series.

#### *5.3.2.3 Bioprint*

The BioPrint database[29] contains consistently measured binding data for ~1200 marketed drugs and additional relevant compounds in binding assays at Cerep, and a complete matrix of ligand–target interactions. In addition they also collected known records of adverse drug reactions (ADRs) providing links between chemicals, targets and *in vivo* effects. As a proof-of-concept they showed that it was possible to predict the ADRs for benperidol solely based on *in vitro* assay profile similarity. A set of 20 compounds was identified as similar, and by collecting ADRs of these compounds they were able to predict the majority of the important ADRs.

In a similar fashion, Fliri *et al.*[94] employed parts of this dataset to validate the biological spectra analysis as a biologically meaningful chemical similarity measure. By employing hierarchical clustering to the interaction matrix of 1567 compounds in 92 assays, they were able to show that clusters with a confidence in cluster score (CCS) >0.8 were likely to share similar biological activities and also a large structural similarity, as exemplified by an imidazole class of antifungals. In this dataset they observed 73 clusters containing 317 compounds with a CCS above 0.8, with all clusters having structurally and pharmacologically related compounds. Using the same dataset they inspected the use of biospectra as molecular descriptors to model agonism/antagonism of dopamine ligands.[95] Looking at a subset of 24 compounds related to dopamine they firstly investigated the effect of shortening the biospectra. As expected, compounds with high CCS continue to be close, whereas lower CCS pairs tend to diverge, leading to a refined CCS cut-off of 0.82. Secondly the functional activity of the 24 compounds was addressed. Interestingly, the functional activity of the studied compounds aligned well to the biospectral clustering of the compounds, implying the usefulness of biospectra as molecular descriptors beyond pure binding affinity predictions. Another unexpected finding was that this functional activity similarity could not be found when using $IC_{50}$ values as the base of clustering, since it, according to the authors, introduces a "pharmacophore bias" that do not reflect high and low-affinity interactions equally. Finally, a subset of 1045 marketed drugs, with associated clinical effects, was selected from the Bioprint database to investigate if the biospectra could be used to model side effects.[95,96] Side-effects were expressed as binary vectors based on the presence or absence of specific Coding Symbols for a Thesaurus of Adverse Reaction Terms (COSTART), and hierarchical clustering was then performed to find relations between specific side-effects. These side-effect profiles were also related to the biospectra using 872 compounds. Both the side-effect and biospectral profiles were analyzed using hierarchical clustering and the resulting clusters were inspected for overlap. Several similarities between the profiles were observed.

### 5.3.3 Predicting Pharmacology

In spite of the increased efforts of both industry and academia to fill the target–ligand matrix there are still a huge portion of this data missing,[97] and much work has gone into deriving i*n silico* methods that circumvent this problem.

One of the first *in silico* methods to predict a pharmacological profile was by Briem and Kuntz,[98] who used the docking program DOCK to generate an affinity profile similar to Kauvar *in silico*. Although their method performed consistently worse than regular 2D chemical structure similarity they observe that the "biologically similar" compounds found by docking differed from those identified using conventional chemical similarity. Given the limitations and approximations used in docking the inferior results were not surprising, still their finding hints at the potential of biological profiling to identify non-trivial chemical neighbors sharing biological activity.

Bender *et al.*[99] have built *in silico* models of target activity and ADRs using ECFP_4 fingerprints. These models were then correlated to each other to identify relationships between a specific ADR and target activity related *via* chemical features, extending the scope of applicability outside only explicitly tested compounds. Multi-category Bayes models for 70 targets and for 166 side-effects were generated and related based on their similarity in feature space. This methodology does therefore not require a full compound–target matrix, since it works with the structural features of molecules rather than complete compounds.[99] They show a good correlation between target activity and ADR, as exemplified by the μ-opiod receptor, M2 and COX2. Continuing on this method, Scheiber *et al.* address the question as to why often dissimilar chemotypes share side-effects. Instead of relating ADRs to specific targets, they relate a specific ADR to the known pathways the predicted targets are parts of.[100] To investigate the utility of this approach the activity of set of compounds against a panel of 2190 targets was predicted. Then all pathways containing at least one of the predicted targets for all compounds associated with a specific ADR was collected from MetaBase to retrieve the pathway likely to be responsible for the ADR. For instance, they identify cAMP signaling as an important pathway in the development of rhabdomyolysis.

Mestres and co-workers have in a series of publications described the development and validation of *in silico* receptome predictions, and from these predicted the side-effect profiles of compounds. In an early adaptation Mestres *et al.*[101] used the SHED[102] descriptors to build a ligand-guided nuclear hormone receptor (NHR) binding profile. Firstly they show that ligand information can be used to identify the NHR's phylogenetic relationships, and in addition highlight several less obvious connections. Secondly, they profile four targeted libraries (GPCR, protease, kinase and ion channels) and identify NHR hit rates between 4.4 and 9.7% indicating low false-positive rates of the models. Finally, a set of 2944 drugs were profiled, and several cases of off-target NHR activity were found some of which could be validated with literature data. In a similar fashion Vidal and Mestres[103] showed the potential of *in silico* approaches to predict a pharmacological profile using 13 antipsychotic drugs tested against 34 targets. The affinity of a drug to a target was calculated using an inverse distance weighting scheme. Each drug was represented by three different two-dimensional descriptors (PHRAG, FPD, SHED), and compared to a set of compounds with publically available target affinities. The method was evaluated for its scope of predictability, recall and accuracy. It was seen that the method works really well for high-affinity compounds, and has an overall scope of predictability of about 70%. Inspection of recall and precision indicates that the method usually is able to predict the affinity within 1 log unit of the known affinity. Campillos *et al.*[104] show how compounds can be related using their side-effect profiles, and also that primary activities of the related compounds can be transferred. Garcia-Serna and Mestres expand on this, and shows that the whole pharmacological profile instead of just primary targets of compounds,[105] is related by side-effect similarity. They also describe the predictions in the other direction, *i.e.*, from an *in silico* generated biospectra to adverse reactions. By identifying neighbors in biological space with known side-effect profiles and weighting the strength of their associations the query compound's side-effect profile is predicted. To exemplify they use ziprasidone, an antipsychotic. Three compounds were found to have a similar enough predicted biospectra, one antidepressant and two antipsychotics, and 83% of the predicted ADRs had strong literature evidence.

In an effort to understand which kinases are related to chromosomal damage Olaharski *et al.*[106] looked at inhibition profiles derived from a 290 kinase panel. A set of 113 compounds were used as the training set and by using several statistical techniques they derived a support vector machine model that was predictive for genotoxicity. The model building also resulted in a subset of kinases of particular interest to genotox being identified, a subset that therefore constitutes a relevant panel of kinases to avoid. Recently Oprea *et al.*[107] reported on the construction of a platform associating drugs, targets and clinical outcomes. Using the DRUGS database, containing annotations between 3837 small molecules and 1750 proteins, and text mining of approved drug labels, adverse reactions were extracted for 988 unique drugs. Drugs and side-effects were then related using a ten-dimensional PCA, which afforded links between side-effects and targets *via* the interacting drugs. The drugs were then also used to link targets to the clinical outcome of a compound, resulting in a conceptual implementation of a computer-aided drug repurposing tool.

## 5.4 Applications of Data-Driven Toxicity Assessments

### 5.4.1 Drivers for Higher Throughput Methods for Toxicity Assessments

Over the last few decades increased demand to ensure greater public and environmental safety from either accidental or deliberate exposure to chemicals has resulted in new legislation and with it increased pressure on both regulatory authorities and commercial organizations to conduct adequate risk assessments of novel chemicals. Current estimates are that in the European Union (EU) alone there are over 10 000 chemicals without adequate safety data available for conducting risk assessments and testing would require around 9 million laboratory animals at a cost of 1.3 billion Euros.[108,109] Naturally, this data gap has created a need for faster, cheaper and more accurate ways to assess the potential toxicity presented by a compound. With public pressure mounting to reduce the numbers of animals used in laboratory testing there is an increasing need for ways to assess and prioritize chemicals for further study and regulation based on prior knowledge or *in vitro* assays.

European regulations introduced in 2004 proposed to restrict and eliminate the use of animal testing for cosmetic ingredients by 2013 have spurred on the development of alternative methods including *in silico* models for toxicological endpoints such as skin sensitization.[110] There have been many efforts to develop data-driven models for this toxicological endpoint and these are now in common use across the personal product industries.[111–114]

In 2007, the European Community issued new regulations on chemicals and their safe use called REACH (Regulation, Evaluation, Authorization, and Restriction of Chemical substances).[115] This legislation places greater responsibility on industry to provide safety data on the substances they produce. The guidance does however provide general rules for the use of existing information as well as techniques such as (Q)SARs and read-across approaches to help in the evaluation process and so this also has spurred investment in these cheaper and faster alternatives to using animals.

The EU has also initiated several rounds of funding to explore and expand the use of *in silico* methods in order to meet these recent legislative changes. The previously mentioned Innovative Medicines Initiative[116] is focused primarily on the pharmaceutical industry but other projects such as OpenTox[117] have also been funded to help address the impact of REACH on industries in the EU. Similarly, The Joint Research Centre of the European Commission has commissioned the development of an open-source application for toxicological assessments called ToxTree.[118]

In the United States there have been similar efforts to consider alternatives to using animals, most notable of which is the recent Tox21 initiative.[119] This collaboration was catalyzed by a report from the National Research Council (NRC) entitled "Toxicity Testing in the 21$^{st}$ Century"[120] which prompted a five-year collaboration to assess and develop *in silico* and *in vitro* approaches for toxicity assessments. This collaboration was originally formed to capitalize on the experimental toxicology experience of the National Toxicology Program (NTP), headquartered at the NIH National Institute of Environmental Health Sciences (NIEHS); the high-throughput screening (HTS) technology of the NIH Chemical Genomics Center (NCGC), managed by the National Human Genome Research Institute (NHGRI); and the computational toxicology capabilities of the EPA's National Center for Computational Toxicology (NCCT). However, since its inception, the US Food and Drug Administration have also entered into the agreement. This effort also aligns with the US EPA ToxCast initiative[121] which set out to evaluate new ways to assess toxicity and aid in the prioritization of the thousands of chemicals that need to be tested for potential safety concerns.

Just how data-driven toxicity assessment approaches are used in practice is highly dependent on the context of when and where they are being used and by who, as often the questions being asked are context specific and the need for high sensitivity or specificity of the assessments may well be different.[122] Often in computational modeling there is a trade-off between sensitivity (*i.e.*, the ability of a model to identify all the actives in a set of molecules) and specificity (*i.e.*, the ability of a model to correctly identify inactive molecules in a set). Understanding how a model behaves for a test set of compounds will ultimately define how and where the model is applied.

For example, understanding the risks associated with environmental exposure or from low-level contaminants in food or drug products that are being consumed by the general public will require a more conservative approach with few false negatives as they need to address public safety concerns. Whereas, the application of SAR in the early stages of drug discovery faces a scenario where the models are used to filter out compounds that we are confident will have undesirable properties whilst not eliminating compounds that are believed to be good, *i.e.*, the models need to have high specificity. This is because any false negatives will be picked up by the subsequent screening cascades before there is any potential risk posed to human health. The thought here is to not restrict the chemical space available too early as it is a difficult enough task to find a pharmacologically active molecule to begin with.

Of course, there is the counter-argument here that we should perhaps only place our limited resources against developing those molecules we believe have the best chance of success. We should be prepared to accept that we may have a number of false predictions but we are confident that those molecules we are developing will not encounter safety issues as we progress through the development process. In this scenario, a high sensitivity is preferred so long as the specificity is not too low.

### 5.4.2 Applications in Drug Discovery and Development

Adverse safety issues are one of the leading causes for failure of new drug candidates either during the development process or post-launch when the drug is more readily available to the general public. The coupling of this fact with the relatively low productivity rate for new drugs, has meant an ever increasing interest in the early identification of potential toxicity and the avoidance of late-stage or post-launch failures which are most costly for the industry to bear. Toxicity assessments in the pharmaceutical industry are therefore used extensively throughout the drug discovery and development process.

Drug discovery can be viewed as a series of filters and experiments that help narrow the universe of possible chemistry down to the molecule or series of molecules that have all of the desired properties, *i.e.*, they interact with their primary pharmacology in the right way to provoke the right biological response to treat the intended disease for the appropriate duration whilst not having undesirable or unacceptable effects on the biological system in question. Much of the information that conveys these biological properties is encoded in the chemical structure and so the structure–activity relationship (SAR) concept is one of the fundamental tools used to differentiate chemicals and their effects on a biological system.[76]

It has been suggested that the adverse biological effects of a compound can be attributed to one of four primary causes:[123]

1) Toxicity linked directly to the primary pharmacology or mechanism of action of the compound;
2) Toxicity linked to a defined secondary pharmacology of the compound;
3) Toxicity linked to the presence of a structural fragment (toxicophore or structural alert);
4) Toxicity linked to the overall physicochemical properties of the molecule.

However, these primary drivers of *in vivo* toxicity are frequently observed simultaneously and so tend to correlate with one another making it difficult to tease apart which of them is the true primary cause.

One of the most famous cases where the adverse effects of a molecule were thought to result from its primary pharmacology is the case of the anti-obesity medication, Fen-phen. This medicine was shown to cause potentially fatal pulmonary hypertension and cardiac valvulopathy in some 30 percent of those patients examined. The adverse effects of Fen-phen have been attributed to its ability to act as a full or partial agonist of the 5-$HT_{2B}$ receptor.[124] Most drug companies now routinely screen compounds to ensure that they do not have this undesirable off-target activity and the development of models to predict this have also been developed and applied as part of a screening cascade.

### *5.4.2.1 Genotoxic Impurities in Drug Products*

The most common applications of data-driven toxicity assessments in drug discovery have been in the field of structural alerts, and as we have discussed previously, the application of structure–activity relationships for toxicology endpoints in the pharmaceutical industry really took a foothold with the development of the Ames assay. The development and acceptance of this *in vitro* assay resulted in large sets of compounds being screened thus enabling the application of SAR techniques to safety-related endpoints. The state-of-the-art in this field has now advanced to a point whereby these SAR methods are being proposed as part of a regulatory screening cascade for use in the identification and control of low-level impurities in drug products thus potentially removing the need to conduct actual testing of the chemicals in question. This screening cascade involves the use of both structural alerts and read-across assessments to bucket compounds into five categories of concern.[125] In this proposed scheme. Category 1 compounds are those that are known carcinogens and mutagens thus requiring control to low levels in the final product, whereas Category 5 compounds are those believed to have no structural alerts or evidence of carcinogenic potential and so of least concern for control as impurities. Dobo *et al.* went on to demonstrate that this proposed scheme would indeed yield high success rates in identifying those impurities of highest concern for human health with adequate high sensitivity and reasonable specificity.[81]

A recent survey of some pharmaceutical companies showed that most were using at least one SAR system for assessing the genotoxic potential of impurities as well as read-across comparisons to either public or proprietary databases (see Table 5.3).

Regulatory authorities such as the Food and Drug Administration (FDA) are also now embracing these data-driven approaches as part of their own formal review processes for potentially genotoxic impurities and other chemicals for which it is responsible for regulation and oversight.[82,126] The computational toxicology group within the FDA in particular has been proposing to use a consensus approach to applying the commercially available models since they believe this offers the maximum sensitivity and specificity when compared to using just one approach. The premise here is that if each model is trained to be highly specific that if just a single system predicts a compound to be positive then the overall call for the chemical is that it will most likely be Ames positive irrespective of the predictions made by the other models. Similarly, if no model identifies a cause for concern with the submitted structure then the thought is that this molecule will most likely be negative in the Ames assay. This approach

**Table 5.3** Survey of tools used by pharmaceutical companies when assessing impurities.

| *Tool used* | *AstraZeneca* | *GSK* | *Johnson & Johnson* | *Eli Lilly* | *Novartis* | *Pfizer* |
|---|---|---|---|---|---|---|
| DEREK | ✓ | ✓ | ✓ | ✓ | ✓ | ✓ |
| DEREK+[a] | | ✓ | | | ✓ | ✓ |
| MCASE | ✓ | | | | ✓ | |
| MCASE+[b] | | | | | ✓ | |
| Proprietary tool | ✓ | | | | ✓ | |
| Proprietary database search | ✓ | ✓ | | ✓ | | ✓ |
| Public database search | ✓ | ✓ | | ✓ | ✓ | ✓ |
| Compare to active pharm. ingredient | ✓ | ✓ | | ✓ | ✓ | ✓ |
| Chemist consult | ✓ | ✓ | | ✓ | ✓ | ✓ |

[a]DEREK+ is a modified version of DEREK based on company data.
[b]MCASE+ is a modified version of MCASE based on company data.

will work well provided that the compound in question is within the applicability domain of all the models being used and each negative prediction is thought to be reliable.

However, defining applicability domains for a model is not straightforward and is a topic of much debate within the scientific community.[127,128] Applicability domains are an expression of the scope and limitation of a model and as such it is assumed that predictions for compounds that lie within a model's applicability domain will be more accurate than those for molecules that are outside of the scope of the training set used. Most often these are defined by a similarity measure between the test compound and the training set and/or a check to ensure that the test article descriptors are within the range of those for the training set. Applicability domains work best when the training set of molecules all act by a single, common mechanism. The assumption is that if the test compound is similar enough to the training set and the values for its descriptors used in making the prediction are within the scope of those previously seen, then the chemical will have similar biological properties to those it is closest to in the training set.

However, for models that predict Ames mutagenicity, the training sets are often non-congeneric structures and so by their very nature encompass molecules that do not act by a common mechanism. As a consequence, those descriptors which describe the activity of one subset of molecules may well be inverse or orthogonal in nature to those that describe the activity of different subset. In addition, Ames mutagenicity often results from the presence of a small reactive functional group on a much larger molecular skeleton. Most similarity measures look at the whole molecule for comparison and as such are prone to be insensitive to small yet important substitutions that could infer biological activity or inactivity.

#### *5.4.2.2 Assessing Genotoxic Metabolites*

By natural extension, the concept of conducting risk assessments on metabolites formed uniquely by administration to humans, *i.e.*, these were not observed in preclinical species and so were not evaluated as part of the standard preclinical testing paradigm has been a topic of some debate between the pharmaceutical industry and the regulatory agencies.[129–131] Decision trees that incorporate the absolute abundance as well as consideration of the chemical structure including its similarity to the parent drug and presence of reactive functionalities have been proposed as a way to address concerns.[131] To date the regulatory guidance and incorporation of computational models is still an emerging field of science.

### 5.4.3 Expanding to Other Key Toxicological Endpoints

Over the last decade there has been a rapid expansion of the application of SAR techniques to other endpoints of toxicological concern. In the late 1990s there was a realization that certain drugs could induce cardiac arrhythmias that were both rare and unpredictable but potentially fatal. With this discovery came the observation that these compounds often caused prolonged QT syndrome which in turn was linked to a compounds ability to block or inhibit the human Ether-a-go-go Related Gene (hERG) which is a potassium ion channel.[76] The development of an *in vitro* assay capable of measuring a compounds effect on this important anti-target in the routine assessment of drug candidates has led to numerous *in silico* models that attempt to predict this interaction.[45]

More recent efforts have focused on other major causes of drug candidate failure. One such area of concern is hepatotoxicity or drug-induced liver injury (DILI). Types of DILI fall into two major classes, those classed as intrinsic where the effect is seen across species and will demonstrate a dose–response relationship and those classed as idiosyncratic where the incidence of injury is often rare but usually more severe. The idiosyncratic events are usually only within certain subset of the population and typically without any obvious dose–response relationship making these very difficult to predict.[132] Despite this being a complex biological area where numerous mechanisms can lead to DILI there have been some successes in predicting this severe and potentially fatal adverse event. Structural alerts have been identified that often occur in classes of molecules that would predispose them to causing DILI.[133] Other work has focused on the use of Bayesian modeling techniques,[134] k-nearest neighbor (Q)SAR approaches[135] or using a structural fragment-based QSAR method.[136–138]

Mitochondrial dysfunction has been implicated as one underlying mechanism of idiosyncratic DILI as well as a variety of other key attrition causes in drug development such cardiac toxicity, neuronal damage and muscle toxicity such as rhabdomyolysis.[139,140] There have been ongoing efforts to identify compounds that have mitochondrial effects using *in vitro* assays.[141,142] These assays have naturally led on to the development of structural alerts and other modeling strategies to predict mitochondrial dysfunction from the chemical structure.[143,144]

There has also been limited work done in exploring structure–activity relationships for compounds that can lead to reproductive and developmental toxicity or cause teratogenicity.[145] Finally, access to *in vivo* data in structured databases has led to the observation of trends in the physicochemical properties of compounds that lead to an increased incidence at low exposure thresholds.[146,147] With increasing access to preclinical safety data in formats that are amenable to data mining through initiatives like the eTox project within IMI, new relationships will no doubt be discovered and advance the state-of-the-art in relating the observed toxicity to the chemical properties of the compounds being studied.

## 5.5 Conclusions

This review has provided an overview of the various data sources and the methods commonly employed to analyze them. This is an enormously promising area for improving risk assessment. However, it should be recognized that the data are generated with very different purposes in mind and therefore the 'quality' varies widely. Familiarity with the data sources, their original purpose and their history is critical in effectively using the multitude of toxicology data sources available. Comparison of various compounds with each other using similarity-based methods should be one of the first things an investigator should attempt, keeping in mind that chemical representations also vary across the various data sources and that ionization states and tautomer forms can cause errors even in the most basic chemical similarity searches. Another very central aspect of comparison of compounds to each other in relation to their toxicology is exposure. Without exposure information one can erroneously extrapolate very high dose effects and overstate the risk. Thus while it is absolutely necessary to use all available toxicological data to assess risk, it is equally necessary to know the context in which the data were generated, relative exposures and limitations of the data gathered in that particular experiment. Without this, significant under- and over-estimation of toxicological risk will be very probable.

## References

1. P. Wexler, *Am. Fam. Physician*, 1995, **52**(6), 1677–1678.
2. G. C. Fonger, D. Stroup, P. L. Thomas and P. Wexler, *Toxicol. Ind. Health*, 2000, **16**, 4–6.
3. P. Wexler, *Toxicology*, 2001, **157**, 3–10.
4. P. Tomasulo, *Med. Ref. Serv. Q.*, 2002, **21**, 53–59.
5. A. M. Richard, L. S. Gold and M. C. Nicklaus, *Curr. Opin. Drug Discovery Dev.*, 2006, **9**, 314–325.
6. R. Judson, A. Richard, D. Dix, K. Houck, F. Elloumi, M. Martin, T. Cathey, T. R. Transue, R. Spencer and M. Wolf, *Toxicol. Appl. Pharmacol.*, 2008, **233**, 7–13.
7. O. Norager, W. G. Town and J. H. Petrie, *J. Chem. Inf. Comput. Sci.*, 1978, **18**, 134–140.
8. M. D. Waters and A. Auletta, *J. Chem. Inf. Comput. Sci.*, 1981, **21**, 35–38.
9. A. E. Auletta, M. Brown, J. S. Wassom and M. C. Cimino, *Environ. Health Perspect.*, 1991, **96**, 33–36.
10. Z. L. Ji, L. Y. Ha, C. W. Yap, L. Z. Sun, X. Chen and Y. Z. Chen, *Drug Saf.*, 2003, **26**, 685–690.
11. M. Kanehisa, *Science & Technology in Japan*, 1996, **59**, 34–38.
12. J.-X. Zhang, W.-J. Huan, J.-H. Zeng, W.-H. Huang, Y. Wang, R. Zhao, B.-C. Han, Q.-F. Liu, Y.-Z. Chen and Z.-L. Ji, *Bioinformatics*, 2007, **23**, 1710–1712.
13. E. Lim, A. Pon, Y. Djoumbou, C. Knox, S. Shrivastava, A. C. Guo, V. Neveu and D. S. Wishart, *Nucleic Acids Res.*, 2010, **38**, D781–D786.
14. C. J. Mattingly, G. T. Colby, J. N. Forrest and J. L. Boyer, *Environ. Health Perspect.*, 2003, **111**, 793–795.
15. C. J. Mattingly, M. C. Rosenstein, G. T. Colby, J. N. Forrest Jr. and J. L. Boyer, *J. Exp. Zool. Part A*, 2006, **305**, 689–692.
16. A. P. Davis, B. L. King, S. Mockus, C. G. Murphy, C. Saraceni-Richards, M. Rosenstein, T. Wiegers and C. T. Mattingly, *Nucleic Acids Res.*, 2011, **39**, D1067–D1072.
17. D. J. Dix, K. A. Houck, M. T. Martin, A. M. Richard, R. W. Setzer and R. J. Kavlock, *Toxicol. Sci.*, 2007, **95**, 5–12.

18. http://www.epa.gov/ncct/Tox21/
19. http://www.multicase.com/
20. http://www.leadscope.com/
21. https://www.lhasalimited.org/vitic/
22. http://www.cdc.gov/niosh/rtecs/default.html
23. http://www.gvkbio.com/database_pdf/Mechanism_Based_Toxicity.pdf
24. http://www.gvkbio.com/
25. E. E. Bolton, Y. Wang, P. A. Thiessen and S. H. Bryant, *Annu. Rep. Comput. Chem.*, 2008, **4**, 217–241.
26. Y. Wang, E. Bolton, S. Dracheva, K. Karapetyan, B. A. Shoemaker, T. O. Suzek, J. Wang, J. Xiao, J. Zhang and S. H. Bryant, *Nucleic Acids Res.*, 2010, **38**, D255–D266.
27. http://www.chemspider.com/
28. http://www.cerep.fr/Cerep/Users/pages/ProductsServices/bioprintservices.asp
29. C. M. Krejsa, D. Horvath, S. L. Rogalski, J. E. Penzotti, B. Mao, F. Barbosa and J. C. Migeon, *Curr. Opin. Drug Discovery Dev.*, 2003, **6**, 470–480.
30. http://www.aureus-sciences.com/aureus/web/guest/databases
31. http://www.sunsetmolecular.com/index.php
32. M. Olah, M. Mracec, L. Ostopovici, R. Rad, A. Bora, N. Hadaruga, I. Olah, M. Banda, Z. Simon, M. Mracec and T. I. Oprea, in *Chemoinformatics in Drug Discovery*, ed. T. I. Opreas, Wiley-VCH, New York, 2004, pp. 223–239.
33. C. Southan, P. Varkonyi and S. Muresan, *Curr. Top. Med. Chem.*, 2007, **7**, 1502–1508.
34. C. Southan, P. Varkonyi and S. Muresan, *J. Cheminform.*, 2009, **1**, 10.
35. http://www.ingenuity.com/products/pathways_analysis.html
36. http://www.genego.com/metacore.php
37. http://www.camcellnet.com/products.php?id=14&smenu=sub1
38. http://www.biowisdom.com/tag/sip/
39. http://www.ariadnegenomics.com/products/pathway-studio/
40. http://www.cas.org/products/scifindr/index.html
41. http://www.info.pharmapendium.com/
42. http://www.fda.gov/Drugs/GuidanceComplianceRegulatoryInformation/Surveillance/AdverseDrugEffects/default.htm
43. F.-J. Gamo, L. M. Sanz, J. Vidal, C. de Cozar, E. Alvarez, J.-L. Lavandera, D. E. Vanderwall, D. V. S. Green, V. Kumar, S. Hasan, J. R. Brown, C. E. Peishoff, L. R. Cardon and J. F. Garcia-Bustos, *Nature*, 2010, **465**, 305–310.
44. A. M. Aronov and B. B. Goldman, *Bioorg. Med. Chem.*, 2004, **12**, 2307–2315.
45. A. M. Aronov, *Drug Discovery Today*, 2005, **10**, 149–155.
46. C. L. Gavaghan, A. C. Hasselgren, N. Blomberg, G. Strandlund and S. Boyer, *J. Comput.-Aided Mol. Des.*, 2007, **21**, 189–206.
47. G. Papadatos, M. Alkarouri, V. J. Gillet, P. Willett, V. Kadirkamanathan, C. N. Luscombe, C. N. Luscombe, G. Bravi, N. J. Richmond,

S. D. Pickett, J. Hussain, J. M. Pritchard, A. W. J. Cooper and S. J. F. Macdonald, *J. Chem. Inf. Model.*, 2010, **50**, 1872–1886.
48. D. J. Pelletier, D. Gehlhaar, A. Tilloy-Ellul, T. O. Johnson and N. Greene, *J. Chem. Inf. Model.*, 2007, **47**, 1196–1205.
49. S. Glowienke and C. Hasselgren, in *Genotoxic impurities: Strategies for identification and control*, ed. A. Teasdale, John Wiley & Sons, Hoboken, New Jersey, 2010, pp. 97–120.
50. F. S. Collins, G. M. Gray and J. R. Bucher, *Science*, 2008, **319**, 906–907.
51. R. J. Kavlock, C. P. Austin and R. R. Tice, *Risk Anal.*, 2009, **29**, 485–487; discussion 492–497.
52. A. J. Hunter, *Drug Discovery Today*, 2008, **13**, 371–373.
53. T. Steger-Hartmann, F. Pognan, F. Sanz, C. Diaz, A. Sutter and M. Pastor, *Toxicol. Lett.*, 2010, **196**, S250–S251.
54. D. Fourches, E. Muratov and A. Tropsha, *J. Chem. Inf. Model.*, 2010, **50**, 1189–1204.
55. M. J. Prival, V. D. King and A. T. Sheldon Jr., *Environ. Mutagen.*, 1979, **1**, 95–104.
56. G. E. Kirsch, E. S. Trepakova, J. C. Brimecombe, S. S. Sidach, H. D. Erickson, M. C. Kochan, L. M. Shyjka, A. E. Lacerda and A. M. Brown, *J. Pharmacol. Toxicol. Methods*, 2004, **50**, 93–101.
57. S. Sukumaran, R. R. Almon, D. C. DuBois and W. J. Jusko, *Adv. Drug Deliv. Rev.*, 2010, **62**, 904–917.
58. S. Sukumaran, B. Xue, W. J. Jusko, D. C. Dubois and R. R. Almon, *Physiol. Genomics*, 2010, **42**, 141–152.
59. H. J. Ahr, N. Alepee, S. Breier, C. Brekelmans, I. Cotgreave, L. Gribaldo, G. Dal negro, O. De Silva, T. Hartung, A. Lacerda, B. Leblanc, C. Lecerf, J. P. Linge, S. Louhimies, I. Manou, G. Maxwell, K. K. Muller, W. Pape, K. Redhead, K. R. Schroder, D. Sladowski, K. van der Jagt and P. Vanparys, *Altern. Lab. Anim.*, 2008, **36**, 459–464.
60. R. A. Becker, C. J. Borgert, S. Webb, J. Ansell, S. Amundson, C. J. Portier, A. Goldberg, L. H. Bruner, A. Rowan, R. D. Curren and W. T. Stott, *Regul. Toxicol. Pharmacol.*, 2006, **46**, 18–22.
61. A. M. Goldberg and T. Hartung, *Sci. Am.*, 2006, **294**, 84–91.
62. A. Crum-Brown and T. R. Fraser, *Trans.–R. Soc. Edinburgh*, 1868, **25**, 151–203.
63. M. C. Richet, *Corps C. R. Soc. Biol.*, 1893, **45**, 775–776.
64. H. Kubinyi, *Quant. Struc.–Act. Relat.*, 2002, **21**, 348–356.
65. C. Hansch, *Acct. Chem. Res.*, 1969, **2**, 232–239.
66. B. N. Ames, E. G. Gurney, J. A. Miller and H. Bartsch, *Proc. Natl. Acad. Sci. U. S. A.*, 1972, **69**, 3128–3132.
67. J. Ashby, *Environ. Mutagen.*, 1985, **7**, 919–921.
68. J. Ashby and R. W. Tennant, *Mutat. Res.*, 1991, **257**, 229–306.
69. J. Kazius, R. McGuire and R. Bursi, *J. Med. Chem.*, 2005, **48**, 312–320.
70. R. Benigni, *Chem. Rev.*, 2005, **105**, 1767–1800.
71. F. T. Hatch, M. G. Knize and M. E. Colvin, *Environ. Mol. Mutagen.*, 2001, **38**, 268–291.

72. A. M. Richard and C. R. Williams, in *QSARs of Mutagens and Carcinogens*, CRC Press, New York, 2003.
73. C. Yang, C. H. Hasselgren, S. Boyer, K. Arvidson, S. Aveston, P. Dierkes, R. Benigni, R. D. Benz, J. Contrera, N. L. Kruhlak, E. J. Matthews, X. Han, J. Jaworska, R. A. Kemper, J. F. Rathman and A. M. Richard, *Toxicol. Mech. Meth.*, 2008, **18**, 277–295.
74. R. D. Snyder, *Environ. Mol. Mutagen.*, 2009, **50**, 435–450.
75. L. Carlsson, E. Ahlberg-Helgee and S. Boyer, *J. Chem. Inf. Model.*, 2009, **49**, 2551–2558.
76. S. Boyer, *Altern. Lab. Anim.*, 2009, **37**, 467–475.
77. J. C. Dearden, M. D. Barratt, R. Benigni, D. W. Bristol, R. D. Combes, M. T. D. Cronin, P. N. Judson, M. P. Payne, A. M. Richard, M. Tichy, A. P. Worth and J. J. Yourick, *Altern. Lab. Anim.*, 1997, **25**, 223–252.
78. M. Zeeman, C. M. Auer, R. G. Clements, J. V. Nabholz and R. S. Boethling, *SAR QSAR Environ. Res.*, 1995, **3**, 179–201.
79. C. Yang, L. G. Valerio Jr., and K. B. Arvidson, *Altern. Lab. Anim.*, 2009, **37**, 523–531.
80. M. T. D. Cronin, J. D. Walker, J. S. Jaworska, M. H. I. Comber, C. D. Watts and A. P. Worth, *Environ. Health Perspect.*, 2003, **111**, 1376–1390.
81. K. L. Dobo, N. Greene, M. O. Cyr, S. Caron and W. W. Ku, *Regul. Toxicol. Pharmacol.*, 2006, **44**, 282–293.
82. N. L. Kruhlak, J. F. Contrera, R. D. Benz and E. J. Matthews, *Adv. Drug Delivery Rev.*, 2007, **59**, 43–55.
83. J. J. Sutherland, L. A. O'Brien and D. F. Weaver, *J. Med. Chem.*, 2004, **47**, 5541–5554.
84. R. H. Hanway and P. F. Evans, *Toxicol. Lett.*, 2000, **116**, 61–68.
85. Y. C. Martin, J. L. Kofron and L. M. Traphagen, *J. Med. Chem.*, 2002, **45**, 4350–4358.
86. B. Faller, J. Wang, A. Zimmerlin, L. Bell, J. Hamon, S. Whitebread, K. Azzaoui, D. Bojanic and L. Urban, *Expert Opin. Drug Metab. Toxicol.*, 2006, **2**, 823–833.
87. S. Whitebread, J. Hamon, D. Bojanic and L. Urban, *Drug Discovery Today*, 2005, **10**, 1421–1433.
88. J. U. Peters, P. Schnider, P. Mattei and M. Kansy, *ChemMedChem*, 2009, **4**, 680–686.
89. J. Bowes, M. G. Rolf, J.-P. Valentin, V. Hamon, M. Crawford and T. Jean, in *The Process of New Drug Discovery and Development*, ed. C. G. Smith and J. T. O'Donnell, Informa Healthcare, New York, 2nd edn, 2006, pp. 103–134.
90. A. Steffen, T. Kogej, C. Tyrchan and O. Engkvist, *J. Chem. Inf. Model.*, 2009, **49**, 338–347.
91. L. M. Kauvar, D. L. Higgins, H. O. Villar, J. R. Sportsman, A. Engqvist-Goldstein, R. Bukar, K. E. Bauer, H. Dilley and D. M. Rocke, *Chem. Biol.*, 1995, **2**, 107–118.
92. R. Poulain, D. Horvath, B. Bonnet, C. Eckhoff, B. Chapelain, M. C. Bodinier and B. Déprez, *J. Med. Chem.*, 2001, **44**, 3391–3401.

93. R. Poulain, D. Horvath, B. Bonnet, C. Eckhoff, B. Chapelain, M. C. Bodinier and B. Déprez, *J. Med. Chem.*, 2001, **44**, 3378–3390.
94. A. F. Fliri, W. T. Loging, P. F. Thadeio and R. A. Volkmann, *Proc. Natl. Acad. Sci. U. S. A.*, 2005, **102**, 261–266.
95. A. F. Fliri, W. T. Loging, P. F. Thadeio and R. A. Volkmann, *J. Med. Chem.*, 2005, **48**, 6918–6925.
96. A. F. Fliri, W. T. Loging, P. F. Thadeio and R. A. Volkmann, *Nat. Chem. Biol.*, 2005, **1**, 389–397.
97. J. Mestres, E. Gregori-Puigjane, S. Valverde and R. V. Sole, *Nat. Biotechnol.*, 2008, **26**, 983–984.
98. H. Briem and I. D. Kuntz, *J. Med. Chem.*, 1996, **39**, 3401–3408.
99. A. Bender, J. Scheiber, M. Glick, J. W. Davies, K. Azzaoui, J. Hamon, J. Hamon, L. Urban, S. Whitebread and J. L. Jenkins, *ChemMedChem*, 2007, **2**, 861–873.
100. J. Scheiber, B. Chen, M. Milik, S. C. Sukuru, A. Bender, D. Mikhailov, S. Whitebread, J. Hamon, K. Azzaoui, L. Urban, M. Glick, J. W. Davies and J. L. Jenkins, *J. Chem. Inf. Model.*, 2009, **49**, 308–317.
101. J. Mestres, L. Martin-Couce, E. Gregori-Puigjane, M. Cases and S. Boyer, *J. Chem. Inf. Model.*, 2006, **46**, 2725–2736.
102. E. Gregori-Puigjane and J. Mestres, *J. Chem. Inf. Model.*, 2006, **46**, 1615–1622.
103. D. Vidal and J. Mestres, *J. Mol. Inf.*, 2010, **29**, 543–551.
104. M. Campillos, M. Kuhn, A. C. Gavin, L. J. Jensen and P. Bork, *Science*, 2008, **321**, 263–266.
105. R. Garcia-Serna and J. Mestres, *Expert Opin. Drug Metab. Toxicol.*, 2010, **6**, 1253–1263.
106. A. J. Olaharski, N. Gonzaludo, H. Bitter, D. Goldstein, S. Kirchner, H. Uppal and K. Kolaja, *PLoS Comput. Biol.*, 2009, **5**, e1000446.
107. T. I. Oprea, S. K. Nielsen, O. Ursu, J. J. Yang, O. Taboureau, S. L. Mathias, I. Kouskoumvekaki, L. A. Sklar and C. G. Bologa, *Mol. Inf.*, 2011, **30**, 100–111.
108. New study inaccurate on the number of test animals for REACH, available at: http://echa.europa.eu/doc/press/pr_09_11_animal_testing_20090828.pdf
109. T. Höfer, I. Gerner, U. Gundert-Remy, M. Liebsch, A. Schulte, H. Spielmann, R. Vogel and K. Wettig, *Arch. Toxicol.*, 2004, **78**, 549–564.
110. J. Fentem, M. Chamberlain and B. Sangster, *Altern. Lab. Anim.*, 2004, **32**, 617–623.
111. G. Maxwell, P. Aeby, T. Ashikaga, S. Bessou-Touya, W. Diembeck, F. Gerberick, P. Kern, M. Marrec-Fairley, J. M. Ovigne, H. Sakaguchi, K. Schroeder, M. Tailhardat, S. Teissier and P. Winkler, *ALTEX*, 2011, **28**, 50–55.
112. G. Patlewicz, D. W. Roberts and E. Uriarte, *Chem. Res. Toxicol.*, 2008, **21**, 521–541.
113. G. Patlewicz, A. O. Aptula, E. Uriarte, D. W. Roberts, P. S. Kern, G. F. Gerberick, I. Kimber, R. J. Dearman, C. A. Ryan and D. A. Basketter, *SAR QSAR Environ. Res.*, 2007, **18**, 515–541.

114. D. W. Roberts, A. O. Aptula, M. T. D. Cronin, E. Hulzebos and G. Patlewicz, *SAR QSAR Environ. Res.*, 2007, **18**, 343–365.
115. http://ec.europa.eu/environment/chemicals/reach/reach_intro.htm
116. http://www.imi.europa.eu/
117. http://www.opentox.org/
118. http://ecb.jrc.ec.europa.eu/qsar/qsar-tools/index.php?c = TOXTREE.
119. http://www.alttox.org/ttrc/overarching-challenges/way-forward/austin-kavlock-tice/
120. Committee on Toxicity Testing and Assessment of Environmental Agents, National Research Council, *Toxicity Testing in the 21st Century: a Vision and a Strategy*, The National Academies Press, Washington, DC, 2007.
121. Available at: http://www.epa.gov/ncct/toxcast/
122. L. G. Valerio Jr, *Toxicol. Appl. Pharmacol.*, 2009, **241**, 356–370.
123. J. Blagg, *Annu. Rep. Med. Chem.*, 2006, **41**, 353–368.
124. R. B. Rothman, M. H. Baumann, J. E. Savage, L. Rauser, A. McBride, S. J. Hufeisen and B. L. Roth, *Circulation*, 2000, **102**, 2836–2841.
125. L. Müller, R. J. Mauthe, C. M. Riley, M. M. Andino, D. De Antonis, C. Beels, J. DeGeorge, A. G. M. De Knaep, D. Ellison, J. A. Fagerland, R. Frank, B. Fritschel, S. Galloway, E. Harpur, C. D. N. Humfrey, A. S. Jacks, N. Jagota, J. Mackinnon, G. Mohan, D. K. Ness, M. R. O'Donovan, M. D. Smith, G. Vudathala and Larry Yotti, *Regul. Toxicol. Pharmacol.*, 2006, **44**, 198–211.
126. R. D. Benz, *Expert Opin. Drug. Metab. Toxicol.*, 2007, **3**, 9–124.
127. T. I. Netzeva, A. Worth, T. Aldenberg, R. Benigni, M. T. D. Cronin, P. Gramatica, J. S. Jaworska, S. Kahn, G. Klopman, C. A. Marchant, G. Myatt, N. Nikolova-Jeliazkova, G. Y. Patlewicz, R. Perkins, D. W. Roberts, T. W. Schultz, D. T. Stanton, J. J. M. van de Sandt, W. Tong, G. Veith and C. Yang, *Altern. Lab. Anim.*, 2005, **33**, 155–173.
128. I. Sushko, S. Novotarskyi, R. Korner, A. K. Pandey, A. Cherkasov, Li J, P. Gramatica, K. Hansen, T. Schroeter, K.-R. Müller, L. Xi, H. Liu, X. Yao, T. Öberg, F. Hormozdiari, P. Dao, C. Sahinalp, R. Todeschini, P. Polishchuk, A. Artemenko, V. Kuz'min, T. M. Martin, D. M. Young, D. Fourches, E. Muratov, A. Tropsha, I. Baskin, D. Horvath, G. Marcou, C. Muller, A. Varnek, V. V. Prokopenko and I. V. Tetko, *J. Chem. Inf. Model.*, 2010, **50**, 2094–2111.
129. T. A. Baillie, M. N. Cayen, H. Fouda, R. J. Gerson, J. D. Green, S. J. Grossman, L. J. Klunk, B. LeBlanc, D. G. Perkins and L. A. Shipley, *Toxicol. Appl. Pharmacol.*, 2002, **182**, 188–196.
130. D. A. Smith and R. S. Obach, *Chem. Res. Toxicol.*, 2009, **22**, 267–279.
131. D. A. Smith, R. S. Obach, D. P. Williams and B. K. Park, *Chem.–Biol. Interact.*, 2009, **179**, 60–67.
132. H. J. Zimmermann, *Hepatotoxicity: The adverse effects of drugs and other chemicals on the liver*, Lippincott Williams & Wilkins, Philadelphia, 1999.
133. N. Greene, L. Fisk, R. T. Naven, R. R. Note, M. L. Patel and D. J. Pelletier, *Chem. Res. Toxicol.*, 2010, **23**, 1215–1222.

134. S. Ekins, A. J. Williams and J. J. Xu, *Drug Metab. Dispos.*, 2010, **38**, 2302–2308.
135. A. D. Rodgers, H. Zhu, D. Fourches, I. Rusyn and A. Tropsha, *Chem. Res. Toxicol.*, 2010, **23**, 724–732.
136. E. J. Matthews, N. L. Kruhlak, D. R. Benz, D. A. Sabaté, C. A. Marchant and F. J. Contrera, *Regul. Toxicol. Pharmacol.*, 2009, **54**, 43–65.
137. E. J. Matthews, C. J. Ursem, N. L. Kruhlak, R. D. Benz, D. A. Sabaté, C. Yang, C. Yang, G. Klopman and J. F. Contrera, *Regul. Toxicol. Pharmacol.*, 2009, **54**, 23–42.
138. C. J. Ursem, N. L. Kruhlak, J. F. Contrera, P. M. MacLaughlin, R. D. Benz and E. J. Matthews, *Regul. Toxicol. Pharmacol.*, 2009, **54**, 1–22.
139. J. A. Dykens and Y. Will, *Drug Discovery Today*, 2007, **12**, 777–785.
140. K. Chan, D. Truong, N. Shangari and P. J. O'Brien, *Expert Opin. Drug Metab. Toxicol.*, 2005, **1**, 655–669.
141. J. A. Dykens, J. D. Jamieson, L. D. Marroquin, S. Nadanaciva, J. J. Xu, M. C. Dunn, A. R. Smith and Y. Will, *Toxicol. Sci.*, 2008, **103**, 335–345.
142. C. V. Pereira, A. C. Moreira, S. P. Pereira, N. G. Machado, F. S. Carvalho, V. A. Sardao and P. J. Oliveira, *Curr. Drug Saf.*, 2009, **4**, 34–54.
143. P. Kovacic, R. S. Pozos, R. Somanathan, N. Shangari and P. J. O'Brien, *Curr. Med. Chem.*, 2005, **12**, 2601–2623.
144. R. Mehta, K. Chan, O. Lee, S. Tafazoli and P. J. O'Brien, in *Drug-induced mitochondrial dysfunction*, ed. J. A. Dykens and Y. Will, Wiley-Blackwell, Oxford, 2008.
145. E. J. Matthews, N. L. Kruhlak, R. D. Benz and J. F. Contrera, *Regul. Toxicol. Pharmacol.*, 2007, **47**, 115–135.
146. J. D. Hughes, J. Blagg, D. A. Price, S. Bailey, G. A. Decrescenzo, R. V. Devraj, E. Ellsworth, Y. M. Fobian, M. E. Gibbs, R. W. Gilles, N. Greene, E. Huang, T. Krieger-Burke, J. Loesel, T. Wager, L. Whiteley and Y. Zhang, *Bioorg. Med. Chem. Lett.*, 2008, **18**, 4872–4875.
147. D. A. Price, J. Blagg, L. Jones, N. Greene and T. Wager, *Expert Opin. Drug Metab. Toxicol.*, 2009, **5**, 921–931.

CHAPTER 6

# *Cellular Stress and* In Vitro *Predictive Toxicology*

XUEMEI LIU,*[a] JEFFREY A. KRAMER[a] AND ALAN G. E. WILSON[b]

[a] Alcon Research Ltd, Preclinical Safety, 6201 South Freeway, Fort Worth, TX 76134, USA; [b] Lexicon Pharmaceuticals Inc., Drug Metabolism, Pharmacokinetics, Toxicology and Pathology, 8800 Technology Forest Place, The Woodlands, TX 77381-1160, USA

## 6.1 Introduction

The number of new chemical entities gaining regulatory approval has fallen in recent years, although it has been argued that this trend is not due to a decrease in innovative practices within the industry.[1,2] The lack of appropriate animal models for novel human disease targets undoubtedly plays a role, emphasizing the importance of rapid progression to clinical trials for proof-of-concept in man.[2,3] In the area of preclinical toxicology, the relatively high incidence of drug candidates that demonstrate unacceptable toxicity profiles in animals, and therefore never advance to human trials, highlights the critical importance of safety assessment in pharmaceutical research and development and the need for improved predictive capabilities in support of drug candidate selection.[4] Classical toxicity testing relies primarily on observing adverse biological responses in homogeneous groups of animals exposed to high doses of a test agent.[5,6] However, these tests provide little information on modes and mechanisms of action, information which is critical for understanding inter-species differences in toxicity, and the translation of preclinical data to humans.

RSC Drug Discovery Series No. 12
New Horizons in Predictive Toxicology: Current Status and Application
Edited by Alan G. E. Wilson

Published by the Royal Society of Chemistry, www.rsc.org

Moreover, these preclinical studies are expensive, time-consuming, and require large numbers of animals. The current focus and urgency in the pharmaceutical industry is to shorten the timelines for all aspects of drug discovery and to improve the ability to filter out early potential safety issues.

The predictive toxicology screening for compound-mediated toxicity relies on a few *in vitro* assays conducted primarily with cells or cell lines, optimally from humans, and on acute to chronic studies with animal models.[7] The use of a mammalian cell system is preferable due to substantial differences in cellular outer surfaces and the fact that chemical interactions *via* transcription factors can be monitored only in mammalian cells.[8] Despite their frequent use, the reliability, relevance, and effectiveness of the *in vitro* methodologies are continuously questioned. Powerful technologies for functional genomics may provide new, mechanism-based, assays with a high predictive value for toxic risks in humans. Some examples of toxicity pathways have the potential to predict various toxicities and could be evaluated with high-throughput methods.

## 6.2 ER Stress and Heat-Shock Response

The endoplasmic reticulum (ER) is the major signal transducing organelle in eukaryotic cells for lipid synthesis, protein folding, and protein maturation.[9,10] The lumen of the ER provides an environment that is specifically for the production of secretory and membrane proteins. It has been estimated that ~30% of newly synthesized proteins are rapidly degraded, possibly as a result of improper protein folding.[11,12] Continuous production of proteins and selective degradation of defective or excessive proteins are essential processes for the maintenance of cellular homeostasis and for the regulation of cell function.[13] Thus an acute increase in the translation of secretory proteins may impose a major problem for the cell due to a potential build up of misfolded proteins.[13] The ER contains several chaperones to facilitate proper protein folding, including binding Ig protein (BiP). Also known as glucose-regulated protein 78 (Grp78), BiP is a member of the heat-shock 70 protein family that binds transiently to newly synthesized proteins.[14,15] Heat-shock proteins (HSPs) are molecular chaperones that appear to be necessary in the critical step of three-dimensional folding of some newly formed proteins within the cell.[16–18] They ensure that newly formed polypeptides proceed correctly through folding and unfolding to achieve their functional shape. The HSPs also assist in the repair of denatured proteins or promote their degradation after stress or injury.[17,18] Even though many of the HSPs are present in cells under normal conditions, they all have been shown to be increasingly expressed in response to stress.[19]

ER stress can be induced by an accumulation of unfolded protein aggregates (unfolded protein response, UPR).[9,10,20] The situation becomes even more critical if perturbations in the ER environment occur, such as alterations in redox state, calcium levels, or failure to post-translationally modify secretory proteins.[9,10] There is a UPR system that senses the ER environment, elicits appropriate responses to various perturbations that restore ER homeostasis, and provides other physiological functions in various cell types.[12] The UPR consists of three main signaling systems initiated by three prototypical ER localized stress sensors: PERK (protein kinase-like endoplasmic reticulum kinase), IRE1 (inositol-requiring enzyme-1), and ATF6 (Activating transcription factor 6).[21,22] Under homoeostatic conditions, BiP binds to the IRE1 lumenal domain rendering IRE1 monomeric and inactive. Under stress conditions, BiP is released from PERK, IRE1, or ATF6 to bind to the misfolded proteins and assist in ATP-mediated chaperone refolding.[14,15] The PERK kinase (or eIF2 kinase) phosphorylates the subunit of the eIF2 that leads to reduction of general protein synthesis.[23,24] Mammalian IRE-1 is a type-1 ER transmembrane bifunctional glycoprotein and two isoforms, $\alpha$ and $\beta$, have been identified in mammals.[25,26] Both IRE1$\alpha$ and $\beta$ are activated in response to PERK-mediated eIF2 activation, in mammals this initiates gene expression changes by processing the mRNA of the transcription factor XBP1.[27] The transcribed XBP1 then translocates to the nucleus and induces a wide range of ER-localized chaperones, including the Grp78 and Grp94 families.[27] These chaperones most likely play a role in protecting the cell by preventing protein aggregation (keeping the unfolded proteins in a folding-competent state) and keeping $Ca^{2+}$ in the ER lumen.[28] Besides PERK and IRE1, the third ER-stress sensor molecule ATF6 is a transcription factor that is essential for XBP1 mRNA expression and chaperone induction upon ER stress.[27,29,30]

In summary, UPR stress signals lead to decreased rates of protein translation to prevent further accumulation of unfolded proteins. Simultaneously, ER-resident chaperones are induced to deal with accumulated protein aggregates and then the ER degrading apparatus becomes activated to eliminate denatured proteins.[28] This co-ordinated response prevents accumulation of unfolded proteins, allows time for the elimination of unfolded proteins, and re-establishes cellular homeostasis. However, if the misfolded proteins are not refolded or cleared from the ER, the cell may be targeted for apoptosis.[31] Although the exact signaling mechanism underlying ER stress-induced apoptosis is poorly understood, two main pathways, a transcription-factor-mediated cascade and a caspase-dependent pathway, are activated. In the former, IRE1 is thought to serve a pro-apoptotic function possibly through up-regulation of the transcription factor, GADD153/CHOP, which may in turn amplify the pro-apoptotic signal by altering the balance between Bcl-2 and Bax.[32,33] ER stress can also initiate cell death through activation of caspases in a pathway that is independent from mitochondria and death receptors, and thought to be mediated by caspase-12.[34] ER stress has been associated with a wide range of diseases, including neurodegeneration, stroke, bipolar disorder, cardiac disease, cancer, diabetes, muscle degeneration, and others.[35] Utilization of the ER stress response pathway-based assays as indicators of toxic interactions of chemicals with basic cellular machinery will potentially permit the clustering of chemicals based on biological response profiles of common mode of action (MOA) and also the inference of the specific MOA of a toxicant.

## 6.3 Oxidative Stress and Mitochondrial Toxicity

All organisms must continuously confront and control the presence of both pro-oxidants and antioxidants. The balance between these is tightly regulated and extremely important for maintaining vital cellular and biochemical functions.[36–38] This balance is often referred to as the redox potential, and any interference in the balance in any direction may be deleterious for the cell and for the organism. Changing the balance toward an increase in the pro-oxidant level over the capacity of the antioxidant is defined as oxidative stress.[36–38] The pro-oxidants can cause damage to biological targets such as lipids, DNA, and proteins; and on the defensive systems of the cell, which are composed of enzymes and reducing equivalents, or antioxidants. In general, these pro-oxidants are referred to as reactive oxygen species (ROS) which can be classified into either free radicals, reactive anions containing oxygen atoms, or molecules containing oxygen atoms that can either produce free radicals or are chemically activated by them. Although the exposure of the organism to ROS is extremely high from exogenous sources, the exposure to endogenous sources is much more important and extensive, because it is a continuous process during the life span of every cell in the organism.[39]

The mitochondrion is a unique organelle developed from endocytosed bacteria. Most of the original bacterial genes translocated into the host cell nucleus over evolutionary time, and thus the host cell nucleus controls the biosynthesis of the present day mitochondrion. Only 37 genes remain as maternally-inherited mitochondrial DNA.[40] A few of these genes code for the lipophillic, proton-pumping subunits of Complexes I, III, and IV of the electron transport chain, which establish the mitochondrial transmembrane potential that powers the synthesis of ATP.[40] In specialized tissues, mitochondria perform a number of diverse functions, but the common function of all mitochondria is the generation of ATP, the chemical energy required for a cell's metabolism.[40] Each step of the mitochondrial energy conversion system must function efficiently for cell survival. The mitochondria serve as the major organelle responsible for ROS production and many processes throughout the cell cycle.[41] Complex I in the brain and complex III in the heart and lungs seem to be the primary sources of mitochondrial superoxide production under normal conditions.[42,43] In many cases there is a leakage of ROS from the mitochondria into the intracellular environment.[44] The massive production of mitochondrial ROS is increased further in the aging cell where the function of the mitochondrion is impaired and its membrane integrity increasingly compromised.[45] Another important free radical species produced by cells is NO, whose formation from arginine and oxygen is catalyzed by a family of NO synthases (NOSs).[46,47] Although its presence, localization, and physiological role are debated, a mitochondrial NOS isoform (mtNOS), possibly associated with the mitochondrial inner membrane, has recently been described.[48,49] Nitric oxide can bind to heme groups of hemoproteins, including cytochrome oxidase. In the latter case, the important consequence is inhibition of respiration.[50] At low concentrations, reactive oxygen/nitrogen Species (ROS/RNS) play an important role in immune-mediated defense against invading microorganisms and serve as cell-signaling molecules. However, at high concentrations, ROS/RNS are capable of damaging host tissues.

The mitochondrial death pathway induced by oxidative stress has lately drawn considerable attention.[51–53] However, specific mechanisms of enhanced ROS generation in mitochondria and their translation into apoptotic signals are not well understood. Mitochondrial DNA has a much higher mutation rate than nuclear DNA. This is because the mitochondrial DNA repair system is limited and it lacks histones. When the amount of mtDNA with a mutation or deletion in a cell reaches a tissue-dependent threshold, the cellular metabolism becomes critical and the cell undergoes necrosis.[54] Mutations in mtDNA, whether inborn or acquired, accelerate mitochondrial dysfunction that induces further damage, causing additional mutations and deletions.[55] ROS-induced deletion of fragments of mtDNA promotes premature aging, and migration of the deleted fragments into the nuclear genome has been linked to carcinogenesis.[56] Since a significant number of ROS is generated during mitochondrial oxidative phosphorylation, several studies have suggested that mtDNA may accumulate more oxidative DNA damage relative to nuclear DNA.[57] Thus persistent mitochondrial DNA damage may serve as a useful biomarker for ROS-associated diseases over time.[57]

## 6.4 Apoptosis and Cell Cycle

Cell injury, as a result of physical, biochemical, or biological insults, induces expression of adaptive stress response genes. These cellular responses are usually cytoprotective but can participate in apoptosis which is necessary for normal development and homeostasis of multicellular organisms and the removal of transformed cells.[58,59] The cell cycle is a complex series of events which must be finely regulated if a cell is going to proliferate, differentiate, or enter apoptosis. This cycle is subdivided into four successive phases: G1 (growth phase I, previously called gap1), S (DNA synthesis), G2 (growth phase 2, previously called gap 2), and M (mitosis). In addition, the G0 phase was introduced to describe non-cycling cells.[60,61] In eukaryotic cells, the activation of cell cycle checkpoints is a key aspect of the cellular stress response.[62] Cell cycle checkpoints monitor macromolecular integrity and the successful completion of cellular processes prior to initiating the next phase in the cell cycle.[63] There are two principal check-points which regulate the cell cycle in the late G1 phase and immediately prior to entry into the M phase, respectively.[60,61] Although a cell can enter apoptosis in any phase of the cell cycle, the G1 check-point is especially important for the onset of apoptosis. When a cell reaches the G1 check-point, it can either enter S phase or initiate the apoptotic process if there is cell damage.[64] The proper sequence of cell cycle events is regulated principally by two protein families: the cyclin-dependent serine/threonine kinases (CDKs) and their regulator subunits, the cyclins.[64]

It is clear that apoptosis has to be tightly regulated since too little or too much cell death may lead to pathology, including developmental defects, autoimmune disease, neurodegeneration, and cancer.[65] During the earlier phase of apoptosis, cells lose the cell-to-cell adhesion and separate from neighboring cells.[66] As apoptosis progresses, cells will fragment into apoptotic bodies with intact cell membranes and will contain cytoplasmic organelles with or without nuclear fragments.[59] Apoptosis can be executed *via* extrinsic and intrinsic pathways depending on the stimulus leading to apoptosis. The extrinsic signaling pathways that initiate apoptosis involve transmembrane receptor [such as tumor necrosis factor (TNF)] mediated interactions.[67,68] Extrinsic signals bind to their receptors and trigger intracellular signaling leading to caspase-8 activation.[59,68] The TNF and Fas ligand pathways can induce both apoptosis or cell survival depending on the intracellular signaling pathways that are induced by them, and the balance seems to be related to activation of nuclear factor-κB.[68] The intrinsic signaling pathways that initiate apoptosis involve a diverse array of non-receptor-mediated stimuli that produce intracellular signals that act directly on targets within the cell and are mitochondrial-initiated events.[59,69,70] Both extrinsic and intrinsic pathways end at the point of the execution phase considered the final pathway of apoptosis.[71] Execution caspases activate cytoplasmic endonuclease, which degrades nuclear material, and proteases that degrade the nuclear and cytoskeletal proteins.[72,73] Caspase-3, caspase-6, and caspase-7 function as effector caspases, cleaving various substrates that ultimately cause the morphological and biochemical changes seen in apoptotic cells.[71] Among these, caspase-3 is considered to be the most important execution caspases, and is activated by many of the initiator caspases (caspase-8, caspase-9, and caspase-10).[72,73] Different initiator caspases can be activated by diverse stimuli, but nonetheless at some point of the enzymatic cascade, these events overlap and the same effector caspases are activated. This may serve to explain why different apoptotic stimuli all result in the same morphological alterations.[72,74]

Since apoptosis occurs *via* a complex signaling cascade, there are many opportunities to evaluate the activity of the proteins involved.[59,75,76] More than 13 known caspases can be detected using various types of caspase activity assays.[77] Some methods of caspase detection require cell lysis in order to release the enzymes into the solution. The major disadvantage is that the integrity of the sample is destroyed thereby eliminating the possibility of localizing the apoptotic event within the tissue or determining the type of cell that is undergoing apoptosis.[59] In cases with low numbers of apoptotic cells, DNA fragmentation is not recommended. DNA fragmentation occurs in the later phase of apoptosis, and thus the absence of a DNA ladder does not eliminate the possibility that cells are undergoing early apoptosis.[59] Cytochrome *c* release from the mitochondria can also be measured, however cytochrome *c* becomes unstable once it is released into the cytoplasm.[78] Therefore a non-apoptotic control is required to ensure that the staining conditions used are able to detect any available cytochrome *c*.[59,78,79] Finally, there is an issue of distinguishing apoptosis from necrosis, two processes that can occur independently, sequentially, or simultaneously.[80,81] In some cases, the type of stimuli and/or the degree of stimuli determines if cells die by apoptosis or necrosis. At low doses, a variety of injurious stimuli such as heat, radiation, hypoxia, and cytotoxicity can induce apoptosis, but these same stimuli can result in necrosis at higher doses. Since many features of apoptosis and necrosis overlap, it is crucial to employ two or more distinct assays to confirm that cell death is occurring *via* apoptosis. One assay may detect early (initiation) apoptotic events and a different assay may target a later (execution) event. The second assay, used to confirm apoptosis, is generally based on a different principle.[59]

## 6.5 DNA Damage and Repair

Damage to DNA induces several cellular responses that enable the cell either to eliminate or cope with the damage, or to activate a programmed cell death process, presumably to eliminate cells with potentially catastrophic mutations.[82] The DNA damage response reactions include: 1) the repair of damage and restoration of the DNA duplex; 2) activation of a cell-cycle checkpoint to allow for repair and to prevent transmission of damaged chromosomes; 3) a transcriptional response, which may be beneficial to the cell; and 4) apoptosis, which eliminates seriously deregulated cells.[83–85] Unrepaired damage increases the risk of mutation during cell division and thereby increases the risk of cancer.[84,86] DNA damage occurs in numerous ways, ranging from specific base modifications, *e.g.*, 8-oxoguanine (8-oxo-7,8-dihydroguanine) formation, to more stressor-specific mechanisms, *e.g.*, pyrimidine dimer formation due to UV irradiation. Despite numerous types of DNA adducts and base modifications, DNA damage can be grouped into a few major types, including DNA double-strand breaks (dsb), DNA nucleotide adduct formation and base modification, DNA basepairing mismatches, and DNA single-strand breaks (ssb).[87,88] Accordingly, the major classes of DNA repair are homologous recombination (HR) or nonhomologous end-joining (NHEJ), nucleotide excision repair (NER), and nucleotide mismatch repair (NMR).

DNA damage sensors probably recognize common intermediates of the major types of DNA damage. Candidate intermediates are DNA ssb that occur during all types of DNA damage and recognition motifs that are common to different base mismatches and modifications.[89,90] Much of the cellular machinery involved in DNA damage sensing is highly conserved in both eukaryotes and prokaryotes.[91–93] In *E. coli*, the ssDNA binding protein RecA is an important DNA damage sensor. It plays a central role in the repair of stalled replication forks, double-strand break repair, general recombination, induction of the SOS response, and SOS mutagenesis.[94] The eukaryotic homolog of RecA is Rad51, which catalyzes the central step of homologous recombination and is the key protein for DNA dsb. The most stable and deleterious base modification caused by ROS is the formation of 8-oxoguanine (8-oxo-7,8-dihydroguanine; 8-oxoG). MutT/MTH protects cells from the mutagenic effects of 8-oxoG by degrading 8-oxo-dGTP to 8-oxo-dGMP.[95] Another potential DNA damage biomarker is topoisomerase, which alters DNA topology by introducing transient ssb into DNA during replication and NER. Since DNA ssb might represent a common intermediate recognized by DNA damage sensors,[96] topoisomerase may be a critical element of DNA damage sensing. Indeed, topoisomerase I is involved in NER during the bacterial SOS response to stress induced DNA damage,[97,98] and the homologous mammalian topoisomerase III is a sensor for the S phase DNA damage checkpoint.[99]

Much work during the past decade has focused on DNA damage response proteins.[100] However, it is still nearly impossible to distinguish primary sensors from secondary transducers of DNA damage. The problem lies in complex circuits of feedback regulation of proteins involved in sensing DNA damage. For example, many candidate proteins are part of multiprotein complexes that, when activated, become targets of further modification by their own substrates.[101] Most studies on DNA damage proteins have focused on responses of cells to damage induced by ionizing radiation or highly reactive chemicals.[102] However, recent work has demonstrated that during other types of stress, including osmotic stress and heat-shock, DNA damage occurs and key mechanisms involved in eukaryotic DNA damage sensing, transduction, and repair are activated.[103–105] These findings, in combination with extensive prior knowledge about the effects of many types of stress on protein folding and stability, led to the hypothesis that cellular stress response represents a universal reaction to macromolecular damage.[106]

The development of a broad range of short-term assays for genetic toxicology served to identify many mutagens and address the relationship between mutagens and carcinogens. Currently, screening of DNA damaging agents is achieved with a battery of standardized genetic toxicity assays that have the ability to monitor both cytotoxic and genotoxic effects.[107] These assays provide high precision and predictivity of potential mechanisms of genetic toxicity. Negative findings in these assays are a strong indication that the risk of carcinogenicity is likely to be minimal. In contrast, indications with multiple assays that a test article or treatment can produce DNA damage or subcellular damage may be a strong indication that the risks of carcinogenicity may be high and additional testing may be required. These regulatory approaches provide reliable prediction of human carcinogenic hazard, but time and cost factors limit the number of chemicals that can be evaluated in these systems, and most screens are still applied late in preclinical drug development. A variety of high-throughput tests, almost all of which are involved in direct or indirect assays of mutagenicity, have now been developed and are used to aid in the identification of potential carcinogens.[108–110]

## 6.6 Nuclear Receptors

Over the last 10 years data has been generated to support the concept that a large fraction of carcinogens are not mutagenic and do not directly damage DNA.[111] Those carcinogens that are not mutagenic are often called "nongenotoxic carcinogens" or "epigenetic carcinogens".[111] Development of reliable assays for the prediction of nongenotoxic (NGTX) rodent carcinogens is a key challenge in preclinical toxicology.[112–114] The modes of action for NGTX are numerous and diverse, including the modulation of metabolizing enzymes, the induction of peroxisome proliferation, the stimulation of oxidative stress, the alteration of intercellular communication, the suppression of apoptosis, and the stimulation of regenerative cell growth following cytotoxic effects.[115–118] Even more complicating is the fact that many NGTX carcinogens frequently affect several of these pathways.[115–118] A number of NGTX carcinogens can recognize specific intracellular proteins including members of the nuclear receptor family. Nuclear receptors are one of the most abundant classes of transcriptional regulators. They modulate diverse functions such as homeostasis, reproduction, development, and metabolism.[119] The nuclear receptor superfamily includes nuclear hormone receptors (NHRs) and orphan nuclear receptors. The NHRs are receptors for which hormonal ligands have been identified, whereas orphan receptors are isolated on the basis of their sequence similarity and conserved domain organization to other NHRs without prior knowledge of their endogenous ligand(s).[119] All of the nuclear receptors have common structural features, which include a central DNA binding domain (DBD) responsible for targeting the receptor to highly specific DNA sequences comprising a response element. A ligand binding domain (LBD) is contained in the C-terminal half of the receptor and recognizes specific hormonal and nonhormonal ligands directing specificity to the biological response.[120,121]

Some NGTX carcinogens appear to mimic the action of hormones and growth factors and perturb signal transduction pathways.[122] Steroid hormone receptors act directly on DNA, regulate the synthesis of their target genes, and are usually activated by ligand binding. Interfering endogenous hormonal pathways can influence and disrupt the hormonal regulation and hormonal imprinting (in the fetus) of normal cell differentiation, growth, development, metabolism, and reproduction throughout life.[123] Their carcinogenic activity may therefore result from the persistent stimulation of such pathways, promoting the growth of initiated cells.[122] These effects can occur at levels far lower than those of traditional concern to toxicologists. Sometimes high doses shut off effects that occur at low levels, and sometimes low and intermediate doses produce greater effects than those observed at high doses.[124]

Many exogenous compounds alter gene expression through the orphan nuclear receptors, such as the aryl hydrocarbon receptor (AhR), constitutive androstane receptor (CAR), peroxisome proliferator activated receptor alpha (PPARα), and pregnane X receptor (PXR).[125,126] The ligand-binding pocket of orphan receptors is larger than those of classic receptors, and they bind a large diversity of molecules with lower affinity.[127] To distinguish them from the classic high affinity receptors such as steroid or thyroid hormone receptors, these receptors are now referred to as sensors because their function is probably to monitor a given physiological status of the organism and to finely tune homeostasis.[128] PPARs are activated by fatty acids and their derivatives.

Elevation of fatty acids in the cardiac myocyte or hepatocyte instructs the PPARs to activate pathways involved in the burning of fat.[129] PXR regulates induction of several drug-metabolizing enzymes (*e.g.*, CYP3A, CYP2B6, CYP2C8/9) and transporters (P-gp, multi-drug resistance protein-1 and multi-drug resistance protein-2), which are responsible for eliminating conjugates of toxic molecules and biliary efflux of endogenous molecules, respectively.[130] The liver X receptors (LXRs) are nuclear receptors that regulate an integrated network of genes which control whole body cholesterol and lipid homoeostasis.[131–133] The FXR acts as a bile acid sensor, and plays an important role in overall sterol metabolism by regulating transcription of genes involved in bile acid metabolism. The function of LXR and FXR is highly integrated, creating a complex but complementary physiologic network for controlling various facets of cholesterol and sterol metabolism across different tissues.[134,135]

In summary, assessing the potential carcinogenicity of chemicals for humans represents an ongoing challenge. Regulatory toxicologists in the pharmaceutical area are faced with many chemical entities to be classified as rodent carcinogens, in most cases on the basis of a nongenotoxic mechanism. The increasing attention being given to epigenetic carcinogenesis points at the need for a thorough evaluation during the toxicological program for safety assessment. It had been suggested that modulation of the underlying gene expression patterns is profoundly distinct between GTX and NGTX carcinogens, and thus the gene expression profiling might be applicable for classification of chemical carcinogens as GTX or NGTX.[136]

## 6.7 Metabolite-Mediated Toxicity

Drug-induced toxicity represents a major impediment to the development of new drugs and is a leading cause of drug withdrawal.[137] Even though activation of xenobiotic metabolizing pathways might reduce circulating levels of the active xenobiotics by eliminating them from the body as metabolites, it may also increase the toxicity of some xenobiotics by transforming them into more toxic forms.[138] Therefore, in addition to potency and selectivity, drug candidates are now selected on the basis of acceptable metabolism/toxicology profiles in preclinical species. By using *in vitro* approaches, many compounds that might have serious adverse reactions associated with them are effectively eliminated before reaching clinical trials, however, idiosyncratic adverse drug reactions (IADRs) cannot be detected in regulatory animal toxicity studies, and given their low frequency of occurrence in humans (1 in 10 000 to 1 in 100 000), they are often not detected until the drug has gained broad exposure in a large patient population.[139] Idiosyncratic reactions can affect many different organ systems, either as an isolated event (*e.g.*, hepatitis) or as part of a syndrome (*e.g.*, drug hypersensitivity syndrome).[140] One of the proposed mechanisms for the development of idiosyncratic drug toxicity is the bioactivation of relatively inert functional groups (toxicophores) to reactive metabolites as an obligatory step in the pathogenesis of certain IADRs.[139,141–143] While it is now relatively straightforward to identify the short-lived electrophilic species through *in vitro* "trapping" assays, our current understanding of mechanistic aspects of drug-induced toxicities is such that we cannot predict which reactive intermediates are likely to cause a toxic insult and which are not.[144,145] For example, several hepatic proteins can be modified by reactive metabolites, but this in general equates poorly with the extent of toxicity.[146] In addition, little is known about the identities of the macromolecular targets (primarily proteins) of these electrophiles or the functional consequences of their covalent modification by reactive drug metabolites. Furthermore, the toxicity of reactive metabolites may be mediated by noncovalent binding mechanisms, which may also have profound effects on normal liver physiology.[147–150] Finally, the reactive free radicals derived from oxygen could be produced *in vivo* in significant quantities.[151] Research leading to a deeper insight into mechanistic aspects of toxicities caused by reactive drug metabolites will aid greatly in the rational design of drug candidates with superior safety profiles and represents a challenging and exciting opportunity for chemical toxicology.[147,152] Procedures have been implemented to evaluate bioactivation potential of new drug candidates with the goal of eliminating or minimizing reactive metabolite formation by rational structural modification of the lead chemical class.[153,154] In addition, it is important to identify species differences in metabolism that may lead to toxic metabolites that are unique either to humans or one of the common preclinical species. However, mirroring the metabolism of the whole animal by *in silico* and *in vitro* systems is a continuing and difficult challenge.[155] New approaches have been developed, which include extensive *in vitro* methods using human and animal hepatic cellular and subcellular systems, recombinant human drug metabolizing enzymes, increased automation for higher throughput screens, sensitive analytical technologies, and *in silico* computational models to assess the metabolism aspects of the new chemical entities.[156]

## 6.8 hERG (*Human Ether-a-go-go Related Gene*) Channel Interaction

In a small percentage of individuals, subsequent prolongation of a part of the cardiac action potential termed the 'QT interval' results in potentially life-threatening ventricular arrhythmia.[157] The hERG gene encodes the α-subunit of a channel that mediates the rapid delayed rectifier $K^+$ current, which plays a vital role in depolarizing the ventricles of the heart.[158] Several drugs, including cisapride, terfenadine, astemizole, sertindole, and grepafloxacin have been withdrawn from the market in recent years, partly as a result of cardiovascular toxicity associated with undesirable blockage of potassium channel.[159] Since most QTcI-prolonging drugs can inhibit the function of recombinant hERG $K^+$ channels, *in vitro* hERG assays are used widely as front-line screens in cardiac safety testing for novel chemical entities.[158–160] To date, the *in vitro* assessment of the drug-mediated interaction with these channels uses cell systems that express the hERG channel and uses methods that include patch clamping, fluorescent probes, and rubidium flux studies. A further approach that determines the probability of interaction of a drug with hERG uses the inhibition of [$^3$H]-dofetilide binding, which is a higher throughput method compared with the "gold standard" patch clamping. These methods produce data of varying quality and reliability that can be computationally modeled. Computational approaches, such as 3D-QSAR, which is a ligand-based approach, have been used to evaluate potential hERG inhibitors.[161–164] A pharmacophore derived from a comparative molecular field analysis (CoMFA) model for 31 inhibitors found that three aromatic (hydrophobic) functions and a central nitrogen were key for binding to hERG.[164]

## 6.9 Conclusions

Regulatory agencies are providing leadership in the improvement of toxicity prediction approaches. In 2007, the NIH Chemical Genomics Center (NCGC) of the National Human Genome Research Institute (NHGRI), the National Institute of Environmental Health Sciences (NIEHS) National Toxicology Program (NTP), and the Environmental Protection Agency (EPA), collaborated on a new high-throughput toxicity screening initiative. The goal was to develop automated, high-throughput molecular and cell-based approaches for determining the potential human toxicity of the thousands of chemicals currently in use in the US. These early high-throughput screening approaches, which can also be used in the early drug discovery, will gain increasing importance in the coming years to allow early identification of potential toxicity issue. This chapter has provided a conceptual description of the current strategies for the prediction of cellular stress, and how this might be applied to high-throughput toxicity testing.

Cells sense and respond to stress in various ways ranging from the activation of survival pathways to the initiation of cell death that eventually eliminates damaged cells. This represents a defense reaction of cells to damage that environmental forces inflict on macromolecules.[165,166] Many aspects of the cellular stress response are not stressor specific because cells monitor stress based on macromolecular damage without regard to the type of stress that causes such damage. Whether or not cellular stress eventually selects for cell survival or cell death also depends on the type and intensity of the stress stimulus as well as the cell type.[165,166] In general, *in vitro* cellular stress screens should be evaluated using at least two test systems, one with an earlier direct response and another with a later common cell death response. The nature of the desired predictive accuracy should be considered with respect to the "false positive rate", which could eliminate compounds that might turn out to be negative in regulatory assays,[167] *versus* the "false negative rate", which could increase the probability of a compound passing into development that would ultimately turn out to be positive in a required regulatory toxicity assay.[167,168] According to the current understanding, the early higher throughput screens might be expected to have less predictive accuracy than later, lower throughput screens. Improving the sensitivity of *in vitro* tests through improved understanding of the basic cellular processes and alterations that can affect the integrity of the genetic material will require new mechanistic insights and better cell and tissue culture models. However, it cannot be stressed strongly enough that for any predictive technology to add value by reducing cycle time and attrition rate, it will be critical that the relevance of these technologies and translatability to humans is fully understood. While no preclinical approach is expected to be totally predictive, the strategic application of a variety and combination of early *in silico*, *in vitro*, and *in vivo* assays heralds the possibility and opportunity for transforming the drug discovery and development process and, most importantly, in reducing human risk and safety concerns.

## References

1. E. F. Schmid and D. A. Smith, *Drug Discovery Today*, 2005, **10**, 1031–1039.
2. T. A. Baillie, *Chem. Res. Toxicol.*, 2006, **19**, 889–893.
3. H. Olson, G. Betton, D. Robinson, K. Thomas, A. Monro, G. Kolaja, P. Lilly, J. Sanders, G. Sipes, W. Bracken, M. Dorato, K. Van Deun, P. Smith, B. Berger and A. Heller, *Regul. Toxicol. Pharmacol.*, 2000, **32**, 56–67.
4. H. Olson, G. Betton, J. Stritar and D. Robinson, *Toxicol. Lett.*, 1998, **102–103**, 535–538.
5. R. D. Bruce, *Fundam. Appl. Toxicol.*, 1985, **5**, 151–157.
6. E. Walum, *Environ. Health Perspect.*, 1998, **106**, 497–503.
7. J. C. Davila, R. J. Rodriguez, R. B. Melchert and D. Acosta Jr., *Annu. Rev. Pharmacol. Toxicol.*, 1998, **38**, 63–96.
8. T. Criswell, K. Leskov, S. Miyamoto, G. Luo and D. A. Boothman, *Oncogene*, 2003, **22**, 5813–5827.
9. M. Schröder, *Cell Mol. Life Sci.*, 2008, **65**, 862–894.
10. S. J. Marciniak and D. Ron, *Physiol. Rev.*, 2006, **86**, 1133–1149.
11. U. Schubert, L. C. Anton, J. Gibbs, C. C. Norbury, J. W. Yewdell and J. R. Bennink, *Nature*, 2000, **404**, 770–774.
12. E. Lai, T. Teodoro and A. Volchuk, *Physiology*, 2007, **22**, 193–201.
13. R. J. Kaufman, *J. Clin. Invest.*, 2002, **110**, 1389–1398.
14. K. Zhang and R. J. Kaufman, *J. Biol. Chem.*, 2004, **279**, 25935–25938.
15. M. Calfon, H. Zeng, F. Urano, J. H. Till, S. R. Hubbard, H. P. Harding, S. G. Clark and D Ron, *Nature*, 2002, **415**, 92–96.
16. U. Zugel and S. H. Kaufmann, *Clin. Microbiol. Rev.*, 1999, **12**, 19–39.
17. F. U. Hartl, *Nature*, 1996, **381**, 571–579.
18. J. Buchner, *Trends Biochem. Sci.*, 1999, **24**, 136–141.
19. R. H. Burdon, *Biochem. J.*, 1986, **240**, 313–324.
20. C. Xu, B. Bailly-Maitre and J. C. Reed, *J. Clin, Invest.*, 2005, **115**, 2656–2664.

21. K. Mori, W. Ma, M. J. Gething and J. Sambrook, *Cell*, 1993, **74**, 743–756.
22. J. S. Cox, C. E. Shamu and P. Walter, *Cell*, 1993, **73**, 1197–1206.
23. Y. Shi, K. M. Vattem, R. Sood, J. An, J. Liang, L. Stramm and R. C. Wek, *Mol. Cell Biol.*, 1998, **18**, 7499–7509.
24. H. P. Harding, Y. Zhang and D. Ron, *Nature*, 1999, **397**, 271–274.
25. W. Tirasophon, A. A. Welihinda and R. J. Kaufman, *Genes Dev.*, 1998, **12**, 1812–1824.
26. S. G. Hussain and K. V. Ramaiah, *Biochem. Biophys. Res. Commun.*, 2007, **355**, 365–370.
27. M. Schröder and R. J. Kaufman, *Annu. Rev. Biochem.*, 2005, **74**, 739–789.
28. D. Ron and P. Walter, *Nat. Rev. Mol. Cell Biol.*, 2007, **8**, 519–529.
29. A. H. Lee, N. N. Iwakoshi and L. H. Glimcher, *Mol. Cell Biol.*, 2003, **23**, 7448–7459.
30. T. Okada, H. Yoshida, R. Akazawa, M. Negishi and K. Mori, *Biochem. J.*, 2002, **366**, 585–594.
31. K. Zhang and R. J. Kaufman, *Methods Enzymol.*, 2008, **442**, 395–419.
32. B. He, *Cell Death Differ.*, 2006, **13**, 393–403.
33. R. Jordan, L. Wang, T. M. Graczyk, T. M. Block and P. R. Romano, *J. Virol.*, 2002, **76**, 9588–9599.
34. N. Morishima, K. Nakanishi, H. Takenouchi, T. Shibata and Y. Yasuhiko, *J. Biol. Chem.*, 2002, **277**, 34287–34294.
35. S. Oyadomari and M. Mori, *Cell Death Differ.*, 2004, **11**, 381–389.
36. R. Kohen, E. Vellaichamy, J. Hrbac, I. Gati and O. Tirosh, *Free Radic. Biol. Med.*, 2000, **28**, 871–879.
37. D. P. Jones, J. L. Carlson, V. C. Mody, J. Cai, M. J. Lynn and P. Sternberg, *Free Radic. Biol. Med.*, 2000, **28**, 625–635.
38. F. Q. Schafer and G. R. Buettner, *Free Radic. Biol. Med.*, 2001, **30**, 1191–1212.
39. R. Kohen, *Biomed. Pharmacother.*, 1999, **53**, 181–192.
40. E. Fosslien, *Ann. Clin. Lab Sci.*, 2001, **31**, 25–67.
41. C. Richter, V. Gogvadze, R. Laffranchi, R. Schlapbach, M. Schweizer, M. Suter, P. Walter and M. Yaffee, *Biochim. Biophys. Acta.*, 1995, **1271**, 67–74.
42. A. H. Schapira, J. M. Cooper, L. Manneschi, C. Vital, J. A. Morgan-Hughes and J. B. Clark, *Brain*, 1990, **113**, 419–432.
43. A. H. Schapira, J. M. Cooper, D. Dexter, J. B. Clark, P. Jenner and C. D. Marsden, *J. Neurochem.*, 1990, **54**, 823–827.
44. B. N. Ames, M. K. Shigenaga and T. M. Hagen, *Biochim. Biophys. Acta*, 1995, **1271**, 165–170.
45. U. T. Brunk and A. Terman, *Eur J. Biochem.*, 2002, **269**, 1996–2002.
46. J. S. Beckman and W. H. Koppenol, *Am. J. Physiol.*, 1996, **271**, C1424–C1437.
47. G. Czapski and S. Goldstein, *Free Radic. Biol. Med.*, 1995, **19**, 785–794.
48. P. Ghafourifar and C. Richter, *FEBS Lett.*, 1997, **418**, 291–296.
49. C. Giulivi, *Biochem. J.*, 1998, **332**, 673–679.

50. J. J. Poderoso, M. C. Carreras, C. Lisdero, N. Riobo, F. Schopfer and A. Boveris, *Arch. Biochem. Biophys.*, 1996, **328**, 85–92.
51. R. Kohen and A. Nyska, *Toxicol. Pathol.*, 2002, **30**, 620–650.
52. K. Apel and H. Hirt, *Annu. Rev. Plant Biol.*, 2004, **55**, 373–399.
53. A. Spector, *J. Ocul. Pharmacol. Ther.*, 2000, **16**, 193–201.
54. J. Miquel, *Arch. Gerontol. Geriatr.*, 1991, **12**, 99–117.
55. M. Hayakawa, K. Hattori, S. Sugiyama and T. Ozawa, *Biochem. Biophys. Res. Commun.*, 1992, **189**, 979–985.
56. M. Berneburg, Y. Kamenisch and J. Krutmann, *Photochem. Photobiol. Sci.*, 2006, **5**, 190–198.
57. F. M. Yakes and B. Van Houten, *Proc. Natl. Acad. Sci. U. S. A.*, 1997, **94**, 514–519.
58. C. J. Norbury and I. D. Hickson, *Annu. Rev. Pharmacol. Toxicol.*, 2001, **41**, 367–401.
59. S. Elmore, *Toxicol. Pathol.*, 2007, **35**, 495–516.
60. G. I. Evan, L. Brown, M. Whyte and E. Harrington, *Curr. Opin. Cell Biol.*, 1995, **7**, 825–834.
61. I. F. Tannock, *Lung Cancer*, 1994, **10**, S29–S51.
62. M. L. Smith and A. J. Fornace Jr, *Mutat. Res.*, 1996, **340**, 109–124.
63. L. H. Hartwell and T. A. Weinert, *Science*, 1989, **246**, 629–634.
64. S. Herwig and M. Strauss, *Eur. J. Biochem.*, 1997, **246**, 581–601.
65. S. W. Lowe and A. W. Lin, *Carcinogenesis*, 2000, **21**, 485–495.
66. P. R. Bar, *Life Sci.*, 1996, **59**, 369–378.
67. F. H. Igney and P. H. Krammer, *Nat. Rev. Cancer*, 2002, **2**, 277–288.
68. R. M. Locksley, N. Killeen and M. J. Lenardo, *Cell*, 2001, **104**, 487–501.
69. X. Saelens, N. Festjens, L. Vande Walle, M. van Gurp, G. van Loo and P. Vandenabeele, *Oncogene*, 2004, **23**, 2861–2874.
70. C. Du, M. Fang, Y. Li, L. Li and X. Wang, *Cell*, 2000, **102**, 33–42.
71. E. A. Slee, C. Adrain and S. J. Martin, *J. Biol. Chem.*, 2001, **276**, 7320–7326.
72. N. A. Thornberry and Y. Lazebnik, *Science*, 1998, **281**, 1312–1316.
73. M. T. Santini, G. Rainaldi and P. L. Indovina, *Crit. Rev. Oncol. Hematol.*, 2000, **36**, 75–87.
74. N. A. Thornberry, *Chem. Biol.*, 1998, **5**, R97–R103.
75. M. Watanabe, K. Suzuki and S. Kodama, *Nippon Igaku Hoshasen Gakkai Zasshi*, 2002, **62**, 540–544.
76. Y. Otsuki, Z. Li and M. A. Shibata, *Prog. Histochem. Cytochem.*, 2003, **38**, 275–339.
77. V. Gurtu, S. R. Kain and G. Zhang, *Anal. Biochem.*, 1997, **251**, 98–102.
78. J. C. Goldstein, N. J. Waterhouse, P. Juin, G. I. Evan and D. R. Green, *Nat. Cell Biol.*, 2000, **2**, 156–162.
79. L. Scorrano, M. Ashiya, K. Buttle, S. Weiler, S. A. Oakes, C. A. Mannella and S. J. Korsmeyer, *Dev. Cell*, 2002, **2**, 55–67.
80. T. Hirsch, P. Marchetti, S. A. Susin, B. Dallaporta, N. Zamzami, I. Marzo, M. Geuskens and G. Kroemer, *Oncogene*, 1997, **15**, 1573–1581.

81. C. J. Zeiss, *Vet. Pathol.*, 2003, **40**, 481–495.
82. W. K. Kaufmann and R. S. Paules, *FASEB J.*, 1996, **10**, 238–247.
83. K. Hiom, *Curr. Biol.*, 2009, **19**, R331–333.
84. M. A. Cohn and A. D. D'Andrea, *Mol. Cell*, 2008, **32**, 306–312.
85. F. Altieri, C. Grillo, M. Maceroni and S. Chichiarelli, *Antioxid. Redox. Signal.*, 2008, **10**, 891–937.
86. M. S. Sheikh, M. C. Hollander and A. J. Fornance Jr, *Biochem. Pharmacol.*, 2000, **59**, 43–45.
87. M. R. Volkert, *Environ. Mol. Mutagen.*, 1988, **11**, 241–255.
88. T. E. Wilson, U. Grawunder and M. R. Lieber, *Nature*, 1997, **388**, 495–498.
89. J. K. Moore and J. E. Haber, *Mol. Cell Biol.*, 1996, **16**, 2164–2173.
90. S. J. Boulton and S. P. Jackson, *EMBO J.*, 1996, **15**, 5093–5103.
91. G. Gill, *Curr. Opin. Genet. Dev.*, 2003, **13**, 108–113.
92. M. Markstein and M. Levine, *Curr. Opin. Genet. Dev.*, 2002, **12**, 601–606.
93. M. S. Cyert, *J. Biol. Chem.*, 2001, **276**, 20805–20808.
94. J. W. Beaber, B. Hochhut and M. K. Waldor, *Nature*, 2004, **427**, 72–74.
95. M. Sekiguchi and T. Tsuzuki, *Oncogene*, 2002, **21**, 8895–8904.
96. N. Liu, J. E. Lamerdin, R. S. Tebbs, D. Schild, J. D. Tucker, M. R. Shen, K. W. Brookman, M. J. Siciliano, C. A. Walter, W. Fan, L. S. Narayana, Z. Q. Zhou, A. W. Adamson, K. J. Sorensen, D. J. Chen, N. J. Jones and L. H. Thompson, *Mol. Cell*, 1998, **1**, 783–793.
97. Y. Mao and M. T. Muller, *DNA Repair*, 2003, **2**, 1115–1126.
98. O. I. Kovalsky, L. Grossman and B. Ahn, *J. Biol. Chem.*, 1996, **271**, 33236–33241.
99. R. K. Chakraverty, J. M. Kearsey, T. J. Oakley, M. Grenon, M. A. de La Torre Ruiz, N. F. Lowndes and I. D. Hickson, *Mol. Cell Biol.*, 2001, **21**, 7150–7162.
100. G. Fritz, K. Tano, S. Mitra and B. Kaina, *Mol Cell Biol.*, 1991, **11**, 4660–4668.
101. D. Kultz, *Annu. Rev. Physiol.*, 2005, **67**, 225–257.
102. A. J. Fornace Jr, D. W. Nebert, M. C. Hollander, J. D. Luethy, M. Papathanasiou, J. Fargnoli and N. J. Holbrook, *Mol. Cell Biol.*, 1989, **9**, 4196–4203.
103. A. J. Fornace Jr, I. Alamo Jr, M. C. Hollander and E. Lamoreaux, *Nucleic Acids Res.*, 1989, **17**, 1215–1230.
104. D. Kultz and D. Chakravarty, *Proc. Natl. Acad. Sci. U. S. A.*, 2001, **98**, 1999–2004.
105. D. Kultz, S. Madhany and M. B. Burg, *J. Biol. Chem.*, 1998, **273**, 13645–13651.
106. C. C. Harris, *Science*, 1993, **262**, 1980–1981.
107. D. Kirkland, M. Aardema, L. Muller and H. Makoto, *Mutat. Res.*, 2006, **608**, 29–42.
108. X. Liu, J. A. Kramer, J. C. Swaffield, Y. Hu, G. Chai and A. G. Wilson, *Mutat. Res.*, 2008, **653**, 63–69.

109. R. M. Walmsley, *Expert Opin. Drug Metab. Toxicol.*, 2008, **4**, 827–835.
110. N. Billinton, P. W. Hastwell, D. Beerens, L. Birrell, P. Ellis, S. Maskell, T. W. Webster, S. Windebank, F. Woestenborghs, A. M. Lynch, A. D. Scott, D. J. Tweats, J. van Gompel, R. W. Rees and R. M. Walmsley, *Mutat. Res.*, 2008, **653**, 23–33.
111. Y. Hayashi, *Exp. Toxicol. Pathol.*, 1992, **44**, 465–471.
112. D. G. Hoel, J. K. Haseman, M. D. Hogan, J. Huff and E. E. McConnell, *Carcinogenesis*, 1988, **9**, 2045–2052.
113. R. W. Tennant, M. R. Elwell, J. W. Spalding and R. A. Griesemer, *Mol. Carcinog.*, 1991, **4**, 420–440.
114. C. R. Elcombe, J. Odum, J. R. Foster, S. Stone, S. Hasmall, A. R. Soames, I. Kimber and J. Ashby, *Environ. Health Perspect.*, 2002, **110**, 363–375.
115. J. Ashby, *IARC Sci. Publ.*, 1992, **116**, 135–164.
116. B. Silva Lima and J. W. Van der Laan, *Regul. Toxicol. Pharmacol.*, 2000, **32**, 135–143.
117. G. Nguyen-Ba and P. Vasseur, *Oncol. Rep.*, 1999, **6**, 925–932.
118. G. M. Williams and J. Whysner, *Exp. Toxicol. Pathol.*, 1996, **48**, 189–195.
119. M. Robinson-Rechavi, H. Escriva Garcia and V. Laudet, *J. Cell Sci.*, 2003, **116**, 585–586.
120. V. Giguere, N. Yang, P. Segui and R. M. Evans, *Nature*, 1988, **331**, 91–94.
121. G. Benoit, A. Cooney, V. Giguere, H. Ingraham, M. Lazar, G. Muscat, T. Perlmann, J. P. Renaud, J. Schwabe, F. Sladek, M. J. Tsai and V. Laudet, *Pharmacol. Rev.*, 2006, **58**, 798–836.
122. S. Green, *Trends Pharmacol. Sci.*, 1992, **13**, 251–255.
123. A. Aranda and A. Pascual, *Physiol. Rev.*, 2001, **81**, 1269–1304.
124. M. N. Jacobs and D. F. Lewis, *Proc. Nutr. Soc.*, 2002, **61**, 105–122.
125. V. Giguere, *Endocr. Rev.*, 1999, **20**, 689–725.
126. S. A. Kliewer and T. M. Willson, *J. Lipid Res.*, 2002, **43**, 359–364.
127. G. Benoit, M. Malewicz and T. Perlmann, *Trends Cell Biol.*, 2004, **14**, 369–376.
128. A. J. Watt, W. D. Garrison and S. A. Duncan, *Hepatology*, 2003, **37**, 1249–1253.
129. P. Honkakoski, R. Moore, J. Gynther and M. Negishi, *J. Biol. Chem.*, 1996, **271**, 9746–9753.
130. S. A. Kliewer, J. T. Moore, L. Wade, J. L. Staudinger, M. A. Watson, S. A. Jones, D. D. McKee, B. B. Oliver, T. M. Willson, R. H. Zetterstrom, T. Perlmann and J. M. Lehmann, *Cell*, 1998, **92**, 73–82.
131. P. J. Willy, K. Umesono, E. S. Ong, R. M. Evans, R. A. Heyman and D. J. Mangelsdorf, *Genes Dev.*, 1995, **9**, 1033–1045.
132. B. A. Laffitte, J. J. Repa, S. B. Joseph, D. C. Wilpitz, H. R. Kast, D. J. Mangelsdorf and P. Tontonoz, *Proc. Natl. Acad. Sci. U. S. A.*, 2001, **98**, 507–512.
133. C. L. Cummins and D. J. Mangelsdorf, *Biochem. Soc. Trans.*, 2006, **34**, 1110–1113.

134. M. Ananthanarayanan, N. Balasubramanian, M. Makishima, D. J. Mangelsdorf and F. J. Suchy, *J. Biol. Chem.*, 2001, **276**, 28857–28865.
135. B. Blumberg and R. M. Evans, *Genes Dev.*, 1998, **12**, 3149–3155.
136. K. Mathijs, K. J. Brauers, D. G. Jennen, A. Boorsma, M. H. van Herwijnen, R. W. Gottschalk, J. C. Kleinjans and J. H. van Delft, *Toxicol. Sci.*, 2009, **112**, 374–384.
137. C. Prakash, R. Sharma, M. Gleave and A. Nedderman, *Curr. Drug Metab.*, 2008, **9**, 952–964.
138. D. W. Nebert, *Biochem. Pharmacol.*, 1994, **47**, 25–37.
139. A. S. Kalgutkar and M. T. Didiuk, *Chem Biodivers.*, 2009, **6**, 2115–2137.
140. S. R. Knowles, L. E. Shapiro and N. H. Shear, *Clin. Rev. Allergy Immunol.*, 2003, **24**, 229–238.
141. B. K. Park, M. Pirmohamed and N. R. Kitteringham, *Chem. Res. Toxicol.*, 1998, **11**, 969–988.
142. J. P. Uetrecht, *Chem. Res. Toxicol.*, 1999, **12**, 387–395.
143. D. J. Naisbitt, S. F. Gordon, M. Pirmohamed and B. K. Park, *Drug Saf.*, 2000, **23**, 483–507.
144. D. C. Liebler, M. J. Meredith and F. P. Guengerich, *Cancer Res.*, 1985, **45**, 186–193.
145. B. Wen, L. Ma, S. D. Nelson and M. Zhu, *Anal. Chem.*, 2008, **80**, 1788–1799.
146. Y. Qiu, L. Z. Benet and A. L. Burlingame, *J. Biol. Chem.*, 1998, **273**, 17940–17953.
147. J. Uetrecht, *Drug Metab. Rev.*, 2006, **38**, 745–753.
148. J. Uetrecht, *Annu. Rev. Pharmacol. Toxicol.*, 2007, **47**, 513–539.
149. J. M. Shenton, M. Teranishi, M. S. Abu-Asab, J. A. Yager and J. P. Uetrecht, *Chem. Res. Toxicol.*, 2003, **16**, 1078–1089.
150. J. Gan, Q. Ruan, B. He, M. Zhu, W. C. Shyu and W. G. Humphreys, *Chem. Res. Toxicol.*, 2009, **22**, 690–698.
151. M. M. Tarpey, D. A. Wink and M. B. Grisham, *Am. J. Physiol. Regul. Integr. Comp. Physiol.*, 2004, **286**, R431–R444.
152. T. Usui, M. Mise, T. Hashizume, M. Yabuki and S. Komuro, *Drug Metab. Dispos.*, 2009, **37**, 2383–2392.
153. N. Masubuchi, C. Makino and N. Murayama, *Chem. Res. Toxicol.*, 2007, **20**, 455–464.
154. D. C. Evans, A. P. Watt, D. A. Nicoll-Griffith and T. A. Baillie, *Chem. Res. Toxicol.*, 2004, **17**, 3–16.
155. S. Coecke, H. Ahr, B. J. Blaauboer, S. Bremer, S. Casati, J. Castell, R. Combes, R. Corvi, C. L. Crespi, M. L. Cunningham, G. Elaut, B. Eletti, A. Freidig, A. Gennari, J. F. Ghersi-Egea, A. Guillouzo, T. Hartung, P. Hoet, M. Ingelman-Sundberg, S. Munn, W. Janssens, B. Ladstetter, D. Leahy, A. Long, A. Meneguz, M. Monshouwer, S. Morath, F. Nagelkerke, O. Pelkonen, J. Ponti, P. Prieto, L. Richert, E. Sabbioni, B. Schaack, W. Steiling, E. Testai, J. A. Vericat and A. Worth, *Altern. Lab. Anim.*, 2006, **34**, 49–84.

156. H. van de Waterbeemd and E. Gifford, *Nat. Rev. Drug Discovery*, 2003, **2**, 192–204.
157. K. Finlayson, H. J. Witchel, J. McCulloch and J. Sharkey, *Eur. J. Pharmacol.*, 2004, **500**, 129–142.
158. B. T. Priest, I. M. Bell and M. L. Garcia, *Channels*, 2008, **2**(2), 87–93.
159. B. A. Wible, P. Hawryluk, E. Ficker, Y. A. Kuryshev, G. Kirsch and A. M. Brown, *J. Pharmacol. Toxicol. Methods.*, 2005, **52**, 136–145.
160. X. Yao, D. L. Anderson, S. A. Ross, D. G. Lang, B. Z. Desai, D. C. Cooper, P. Wheelan, M. S. McIntyre, M. L. Bergquist, K. I. MacKenzie, J. D. Becherer and M. A. Hashim, *Br. J. Pharmacol.*, 2008, **154**, 1446–1456.
161. S. Ekins, W. J. Crumb, R. D. Sarazan, J. H. Wikel and S. A. Wrighton, *J. Pharmacol. Exp. Ther.*, 2002, **301**, 427–434.
162. G. Ermondi, S. Visentin and G. Caron, *Eur. J. Med. Chem.*, 2009, **44**, 1926–1932.
163. K. Yoshida and T. Niwa, *J. Chem. Inf. Model.*, 2006, **46**, 1371–1378.
164. R. A. Pearlstein, R. J. Vaz, J. Kang, X. L. Chen, M. Preobrazhenskaya, A. E. Shchekotikhin, A. M. Korolev, L. N. Lysenkova, O. V. Miroshnikova, J. Hendrix and D. Rampe, *Bioorg. Med. Chem. Lett.*, 2003, **13**, 1829–1835.
165. S. Fulda, A. Gorman, O. Hori, and A. Samali, *Int. J. Cell Biol.*, 2010, 214074.
166. S. Fulda, *Int. J. Cell Biol.*, 2010, 370835.
167. D. Kirkland, S. Pfuhler, D. Tweats, M. Aardema, R. Corvi, F. Darroudi, A. Elhajouji, H. Glatt, P. Hastwell, M. Hayashi, P. Kasper, S. Kirchner, A. Lynch, D. Marzin, D. Maurici, J. Meunier, L. Müller, G. Nohynek, J. Parry, E. Parry, V. Thybaud, R. Tice, J. Benthem, P. Vanparys and P. White, *Mutat. Res.*, 2007. **628**(1), 31–55.
168. D. Kirkland, M. Aardema, L. Henderson and L. Müller, *Mutat. Res.*, 2005, **584**(1-2), 1–256.

CHAPTER 7

# In Vitro *Genotoxicity*

JOHN J. NICOLETTE,[a] SUNDAR VENKATACHALAM,[b] BRINDA MAHADEVAN[a] AND PATRICIA A. ESCOBAR*[c]

[a] Abbott Laboratories, Abbott Park, IL 60064-6112, USA; [b] Biochemistry & Cellular Molecular Biology Department, University of Tennessee, Knoxville, TN 37996, USA; [c] Boehringer Ingelheim Pharmaceuticals, Ridgefield, CT 06877-0368, USA

## 7.1 Introduction

Genetic toxicology is a subspecialty of toxicology that encompasses the study of genetic damage, the agents that induce such damage, and the biological response to genetic that damage.[1] Modification of the DNA or genetic damage includes structural chromosome distortions or breaks (clastogenicity) which interfere with replication and transcription, and at the DNA level, point mutations resulting in heritable changes in DNA sequence.[2] Unlike other toxicities, traditionally, genetic toxicity has been viewed as having a linear dose–response relationship with no safety threshold; that is, one insult or "hit" from a genotoxic material could result in one mutation which could lead to heritable changes in somatic or germ cells. Genetic toxicity or 'genotoxicity' falls into a unique class of toxicants where any exposure might be concerning. There are certain types of damage, however, where the mechanism of damage has a threshold, that is, a certain exposure level must be achieved in order to see the damage. This is more often seen *in situ*ations where a chemical induces chromosome number changes, either loss or gain, also called aneuploidy. In such a case, the chemical disrupts the mechanisms for chromosomal segregation or nuclear division. Understanding when one has a clastogen that directly

RSC Drug Discovery Series No. 12
New Horizons in Predictive Toxicology: Current Status and Application
Edited by Alan G. E. Wilson

Published by the Royal Society of Chemistry, www.rsc.org

interacts with the DNA or an aneugen where the "DNA damage" is secondary to other effects becomes extremely important when trying to identify the true risk of exposure to agents that cause such damage. A chemical that can be shown to have a threshold for genotoxic endpoints may have safe daily or lifetime exposures associated with it, where exposure below an identified practical threshold would mean a reduction in the potential for carcinogenesis. However, establishing a threshold requires mechanistic evidence, not merely negative results from certain dose levels from several genetic toxicology tests.[3] Some of these mechanistic tests will be described.

Chemical carcinogens can form DNA adducts, or promote other modifications to DNA, such as oxidative damage, alterations to the ultrastructure (DNA-strand crosslinking, strand breakage, chromosomal rearrangements and deletions) and alter repair mechanisms leading to mutations. Although cells possess mechanisms to repair virtually all types of DNA damage, these are not always completely effective, and residual un-repaired or mis-repaired DNA damage can lead to the insertion of an incorrect base during DNA replication. Mutation fixation followed by transcription and translation ultimately leads to the synthesis of altered proteins that can affect the survival of the species if the genetic changes affect the germ line or induce pre-carcinogenic events in somatic cells.[4,5] While the process of carcinogenesis is a multi-step, complex process, DNA damage can be an important first step; the role of genetic toxicology is to predict this first step. More significantly, genetic toxicology tests, while detecting the adverse effects of chemicals relating to DNA stability, tend to be highly sensitive for predicting carcinogenic potential. Individual tests range from about 60 to 80% sensitivity, and when multiple tests are used (a 'battery' approach) the sensitivity can increase to almost 87% accuracy for predicting rodent carcinogenicity.[6]

Genetic toxicology as such plays an indispensable role in determining the safety profile of industrial chemicals, pharmaceuticals and environmental pollutants. The high degree of sensitivity of these tests for identifying potential genotoxic hazards requires testing highly pure test materials (typically $>98\%$ purity). For example, a test material less than 95% pure may be shown to be positive in a bacterial mutagenicity test due to the presence of a genotoxic impurity.[7]

Genotoxicity testing is used as an early surrogate for carcinogenicity testing, and is required for initiation of drug clinical trials and as a minimum initial safety assessment for most industrial chemicals.[8] These tests are usually conducted in a battery approach, using multiple tests to characterize any potential hazard.[9] As a minimum, *in vitro* testing is typically required, usually consisting of a gene mutation assay conducted in bacteria and a mammalian chromosome damage test. Some industries such as the pharmaceutical industry are required to conduct *in vivo* tests as well, such as the *in vivo* micronucleus test.

In addition, *in vitro* genotoxicity testing is especially important given legislation worldwide such as those to reduce, refine or replace animal testing (3Rs), Registration, Evaluation, Authorisation and Restriction of Chemical substances (REACH), the Cosmetic Directive, and the Canadian Dangerous Substances

List.[10–13] Despite the high degree of predictivity for carcinogenic potential seen in the *in vitro* genetox battery, efforts are constantly being made to identify tests that are higher in throughput, require less test material or provide more mechanistic data than the traditional genetox assays. It is important to note that "higher throughput" modifications/alternative tests should not be confused with "high-throughput" testing that is often seen in early drug-discovery efforts, for example, where thousands of compounds can be assayed in one test. At best, most modifications to improve the efficiency of genetox evaluations can be described as "medium throughput" with some tests achieving up to about 100 compounds per assay. Still, it is critical to note that there are tests which offer the researcher a reliable understanding of genotoxic liability on many more compounds than can be evaluated by the "standard" tests

In the following sections the various standard (or regulatory acceptable) *in vitro* genotoxicity assays, their predictive capabilities and limitations, application-based variations, complementary/mechanistic assays that address issues relating to equivocal results in the standard tests and recent developments that are applicable to predictive toxicology are described. *In vivo* genotoxicity assays are beyond the scope of this chapter and will be discussed elsewhere in this book.

## 7.2 Standard *In Vitro* Assays for Genotoxicity

Described in this section are the basic genotoxicity tests, traditionally referred to as standard or regulatory assays for genotoxicity. These tests all have commonly agreed upon methods in the form of guidelines established by the Organization of Economic Cooperation and Development (OECD) and are often the suggested or required tests in batteries or testing schemes to assess the genotoxicity of chemicals prior to or in lieu of animal testing or human testing in clinical trials.[9,14–20] As will be described later in this chapter, there are variations of these standard tests which offer higher throughput or other advantages over the standard design at the cost of some level of accuracy.

### 7.2.1 Ames Test

One of the earliest tests that is still widely used in genotoxicity testing was developed by Ames and colleagues in the mid 1970s and serves as an important initial assay to determine the mutagenic potential of chemicals and is widely known as the bacterial reverse mutation or Ames assay.[21,22] Briefly, this assay is based on the ability of chemicals to induce mutations in bacteria that require the exogenous supply (auxotrophy) of amino acids (either histidine or tryptophan) due to the presence of distinct mutations in the operon necessary for the biosynthesis of either of these amino acids. Chemicals that are mutagenic lead to the reversion of the mutation(s) in the bacterial strain (prototrophy), allowing the reverted bacteria to grow independently as the exogenously supplied amino acids are exhausted. The numbers of revertant colonies are enumerated by counting the resulting colony formation on the agar Petri dish.

In the presence of a mutagenic agent, more bacteria will revert to prototrophy, and an increase in revertant colonies will be observed. The mutagenic potential will be indicated by the increase number if revertant colonies when compared to the spontaneous reversion rate seen in vehicle or untreated controls. The bacteria (various strains of *S. typhimurium* or *E. coli*) are further engineered to allow a variety of mutagens the opportunity to attack the DNA with a lack of bacterial repair capability and a deep rough mutation in the cell wall allowing larger molecules access to the cell. This assay also has the ability to differentiate the type of mutations by employing a number of tester strains with different type of mutations. *Salmonella* strains TA98, TA1537 and TA97a are proficient at identifying frameshift mutagens, strains TA100 and TA1535 primarily identify mutations that involve basepair substitutions. *Salmonella* TA102 or *E. coli* WP2 strains are generally used to detect mutagens that can cause DNA crosslinking, oxidative damage and hydrazine-like chemicals.[23] For chemicals that need to be metabolized to the ultimate mutagenic form, a variety of exogenous metabolic activation sources can be built in to the standard design of the test (for example, rat or hamster liver Aroclor-induced S9). Ames assay results are typically obtained two to three days after plating. The test has been shown to be about 65% concordant with rodent carcinogenicity or *in vivo* genotoxicity.[6] Thus, in a typical predictive paradigm, without further investigation into the mode of action, a chemical is often considered potentially carcinogenic when a positive Ames assay (mutagenic) result is seen. These features make the Ames test the gold standard *in vitro* mutation assay used globally to assay for a chemical's genotoxic capabilities.

To investigate mechanisms of mutagenesis, specialized strains of bacteria have been further engineered in the years since the original Ames strains were established. For example, there are several strains deficient in nitroreductase (*e.g.*, TA98NR) or those that contain elevated nitroreductase or acetyl-CoA:*N*-hydroxylamine *O*-acetyltransferase levels that can help elucidate the metabolic pathways promutagens may need to go through to be transformed to the ultimate mutagen. Such information may be critical in ascertaining if a bacterial mutation result has relevance in an intact mammalian system.[24,25]

The Ames test has been instrumental in determining the mutagenic potential of thousands of compounds and generating data sets for various computational modeling efforts.[26] The wealth of data has lead to the association of a number of chemical classes and structural moieties with mutagenicity.[27] By employing such structure–activity relationships, chemicals can be grouped amongst similar structures for the purposes of drug development, safety handling, work-related or environmental exposure concerns, in lieu of actual mutation data.

Among the salient technical features of the Ames test, that make it one of the most widely used for early prediction of potential carcinogenicity, are its simplified format, short assay times, the need for lower quantities of test compound, the availability of multiple bacterial strains with distinct mutations, and the adaptability of the test to assay metabolites from S9 liver factions. It should be noted that, the Ames test identifies only about 65% of genotoxic carcinogens. For this reason a battery of *in vitro* tests is typically required to identify the additional genotoxic carcinogens that may be missed by the Ames test.[9,28]

### 7.2.2 Mouse Lymphoma Test

The mouse lymphoma test utilizes a forward mutation assay in the heterozygous thymidine kinase (tk+/–) locus in L5178Y mouse lymphoma cells to determine the mutagenicity of chemicals. In this assay, L5178Y cells that acquire inactivating mutations of the wild-type tk allele become resistant to triflurothymidine- (TFT) induced toxicity and this is measured by determining cloning efficiency on soft agar. The increased mutant frequency from exposure to chemicals can be directly proportional to the mutagenic potential. Exposure periods consist of short exposures with and without metabolic activation and a continuous exposure arm without activation. Expression of mutant cells in the form of colonies typically takes two days.[16] Recently, a microwell version was developed as an alternate format for testing.[29]

This assay is able to detect mutagenicity (point and frameshift mutations evidenced by large colonies) and small deletions (small colonies) that involve the tk locus, either directly or through metabolism from S9 liver microsomes. Thus, the assay may be used to detect both mutation and chromosome damage. It is typically included in an *in vitro* battery to identify chromosome breakage (clastogenicity). Care needs to be taken when interpreting data from exposures that cause extreme changes in pH, osmolarity or extreme reduction in relative cell growth.[16] Such conditions especially in assays designed to evaluate chromosome damage have been shown to increase the incidence of DNA damage by non-direct means, leading to positive results in the assays that are not the result of genotoxicity.[30,31] Where earlier results were called into question regarding the assay's ability to distinguish inherent genotoxicity from toxicity-induced damage, changes to the evaluation criteria and re-evaluation of questionable data indicate the mouse lymphoma test has a high degree of sensitivity for rodent carcinogens that act through a genotoxic mechanism.[32] However, the mouse lymphoma test has not been shown to reliably detect chromosome number changes (aneuploidy) on a consistent basis which may hinder early mechanistic understanding of the risk of the genotoxicity seen.[28]

### 7.2.3 *In Vitro* Chromosome Aberration Test

The chromosome aberration test is performed usually either in human peripheral blood lymphocytes (HPBL) or Chinese hamster cells in culture. Chromosome aberrations are visualized in metaphase spreads of chemically treated cells. The assay can incorporate metabolic activation systems such as rat liver S9 to help detect damaging agents that require metabolism to be active. The assay usually incorporates a short duration exposure (three to six hours) of cells to the test agent with a recovery period (1.5–2 cell cycles), as well as a continuous exposure arm that is usually 2–2.5 cell cycles in duration. In the final hours of testing (either in the recovery period or the continuous exposure), cells are arrested in metaphase by the addition of colcemid. Slides are then prepared, fixed and stained. Using microscopy, typically at least 100 metaphases from each culture are evaluated for the cells containing chromosomes which possess rearrangements or contain multiple aberrations.[15] Thus the assay reports on direct DNA damage as measured by breaks or rearrangements. Metaphase analysis can also give insight into possible indirect modes of genotoxic damage by scoring the number of cells that display polyploidy (extra complete sets chromosomes per metaphase) or endoreduplication (aberrant separation of replicated chromosomes). The chromosome aberration assay is a frequently employed first-tier *in vitro* test to compliment the bacterial mutation assay to provide additional coverage in assessing chemicals for the possibility of inducing DNA damage.[9]

The *in vitro* chromosome aberration test, like other cytogenetic assays, is considered a very sensitive test to identify possible genotoxicants, owing to the capability of exposing cells to large concentrations of test material.[6] This same aspect though has led to concerns about the specificity of the assay for predicting *in vivo* geneotoxic agents or rodent carcinogens. Chromosome aberrations can be induced not only by test materials through genotoxic mechanisms, but by extreme culture conditions such as low acidity or high osmolarity.[15] Under conditions where there is a high degree of cytotoxicity, metaphase spreads can also show a high incidence of aberrations.[30,31] Typically, the level of cytotoxicity evaluated should not exceed 50–55%; however, there are various methods to measure cytotoxicity, which can lead to differences in limit concentration evaluation.[33] Some major drawbacks of this assay are the technical complexity, longer time periods for analysis and limited automation capability that limit the potential for metaphase analysis as a high-throughput tool for genotoxicity.

### 7.2.4 *In Vitro* Micronucleus Assay

Similar to the *in vitro* chromosome aberration assay, the *in vitro* micronucleus (MNvit) assay examines a chemical's ability to cause chromosome damage as evidenced by the presence of small, DNA staining bodies (a micronucleus or MN) in a cell whose nucleus has gone through replication. The exposure procedures are very much the same as those used in the chromosome aberration test, only cells in interphase are examined, and nuclear division can be estimated by the addition of a cytokinesis-blocking agent such as cytochalasin B.[34] In addition to providing information on chromosomal breakage, this assay can also provide some limited information on the loss or gain of whole chromosomes and chromatids, usually when special staining techniques such as fluorescent *in situ* hybridization (FISH) are used (see Section 7.4.2.1). Furthermore, the technical simplicity of the assay, adaptability for most cell types and the ability to score a large number of cells even by microscopy make it a powerful analytical tool for *in vitro* genotoxicity testing. Like other cytogenetic assays, caution must be used when interpreting data from cultures exposed to extremes of pH, osmolarity or cytotoxicity.[17] If the assay is conducted without cytochalasin B, the analyst must score twice as many cells since, after division, one daughter cell will contain the micronucleus and one will not. Platforms such as flow cytometry or image analysis can positively impact throughput and content as will be described later in this chapter.[35,36]

More detail on the specific assays in the standard genetox battery can be found elsewhere.[19,20]

## 7.3 Improving Throughput of Genetic Toxicity Tests

The previously mentioned assays were described in reference to fully regulatory compliant protocols and procedures to support hazard identification, aid in assessment of risk of exposure and/or support clinical trials of investigational new drugs. These *in vitro* tests are rapid when compared to *in vivo* studies for genotoxicity or carcinogenicity, use less test material, are cost effective, do not involve animal usage, and have extensive historical data sets on various chemicals, drugs and natural genotoxicants. Despite these advantages, the standard tests as described could not be considered 'higher throughput' by any stretch of the definition. For example, for a full standard Ames test, using five bacterial strains, under conditions with and without metabolic activation and in pre-incubation and plate incorporation mode, nearly 500 Petri plates would need to be utilized. Because of holding temperature differences of the components (cold S9, hot overlay agar, room temperature bacterial culture), automation of the assay is nearly impossible. While the chromosome aberration test can show direct consequence of exposure to the chemical on the chromosome, manually scoring up to four concentrations in each of the three required exposure conditions for chromosome aberrations can take several weeks, is laborious and requires special training to accurately distinguish true chromosome damage from gaps.

When faced with the task of evaluating many chemicals for worker safety assessments, impact on biological systems from environmental exposure or for potential genotoxicity in a drug-discovery setting, higher throughput methods may be needed. Key factors to consider for a higher throughput assay are low compound requirements for testing (milligrams instead of grams), more compounds tested per assay, rapid turnaround, ease and clarity of evaluation. The assays should have reasonable sensitivity and specificity when compared with those seen in the standard tests as well. In fact, it is important to understand that these modified tests are actually trying to predict genotoxicity that their full-scale counterparts would reveal. In subsequent sections, methods employed to increase throughput and add value in identifying mechanisms of genotoxicity will be discussed.

### 7.3.1 Modifications of Standard Mutation Assays

The simplest forms of higher throughput *in vitro* genetox assays are those that are simply scaled-down (miniaturized) modifications of the standard tests.

To increase throughput, reduce turnaround and compound needs, standard assays can be conducted with only a portion of the regulatory requirements met, such as testing on two of the three exposure times/conditions in the cytogenetics assay or reducing the number of strains employed in the Ames assay. The performance of these modified assays is often quite comparable to the standard test they are based on, although obviously would not be 100% correlative.

Further gains can be made by proportionally scaling the tests down, often leading to "mini" or "micro" versions of the tests. These versions offer comparable, though somewhat reduced, performance to the standard test and can typically be performed with far less material than the standard tests they are based upon. In 2000, Diehl *et al.* introduced a MiniScreen Ames assay which is conducted with the same standard design, but is scaled back in reagents to 20% of the original recipe and uses a six-well plate format.[37] The assay shows a high fidelity with the standard Ames assay, and requires only 42 mg of compound (this allowing for two replicates per treatment dose/condition). Similar efforts have been made to reduce the assay further into 24-well plates, where the same proportion of reagents are used but reduced in quantity even further. These reductions allow more compounds to be evaluated per assay as less material and less plating is done for each compound. By analyzing the chemical space being interrogated (through historical experience or by employing structure–activity models), it can be possible to reduce the number of strains to increase the throughput but not reduce the integrity of the identification of the hazards. Typically, a screening strategy that includes reduction in strains used will include use of *Salmonella* TA98 and TA100, which are proficient in detecting frameshift mutagens and base-pair substitution mutagens, respectively.[38] This offers the user an opportunity to evaluate a set of chemicals and have coverage over the wide range of genotoxin induced mutations typically seen. However, many reduced sized or alternate method tests incorporate other standard strains and could be employed if needed.

Other modifications have also been used to increase the throughput of the Ames-type mutation test. The Spiral plating assay took advantage of the limited diffusion of Ames test components through agar and, using a specially designed plater and stylus delivery system, applied identical quantities of bacteria and S9 to the plate, while adding a gradient of the formulated test compound over the same parts of the plate.[39] As little as one tenth of the mass of the standard Ames test requirements could be plated for multiple strains and multiple concentrations to obtain mutagenicity results against increasing dosage after incubation, using the companion plate reader and software. Aubrecht and colleagues introduced the lux (CDABE) operon from *Xenorhabdus luminescens* into the standard Ames *Salmonella* and scaled the test down to the 24-well plate level.[40] Bioluminescence is used as a reporter of active metabolism, as seen in a revertant colony on the plate. Using the fluorescence from the colonies, a photon-counting CCD camera can be employed to identify the colonies per well.[40] Finally, a liquid-based Ames II assay utilizes TA98 and a mix of other strains in a simple assay that determines mutagenicity by colorimetric evaluation of changes to an indicator medium in the presence of revertant bacteria that have been exposed to mutagens. After the exposure period, each well of a 24-well plate containing bacteria and indicator medium is dispersed onto 48 wells in a 384 well plate. The proportion of wells that exhibit color change (purple to yellow) after two days of incubation are compared in the exposed wells to those of the controls.[41,42] These assays employ a simple approach to answer the questions the larger standard Ames test does and use reagents and procedures familiar to most Ames laboratories. As the scale goes down, though, care must be made in deciding the criteria employed for a positive response. For example, reducing the number of bacteria employed in an Ames test will reduce the number of spontaneous revertants. As the test gets smaller, the criteria for a positive response in the small assay may need to be modified from the standard test to be meaningful.

### 7.3.2 Cytogenetics Tests

Like the mutation assays, scaled-down versions of the cytogenetics tests can increase throughput by cutting down evaluation time, which is often the rate-limiting aspect of these tests. Strategies include reduced numbers of cells per culture scored or reduced treatment conditions to get a quick assessment of a chemical's clastogenic or aneugenic ability, depending on the assay being employed. Assessment tools such as flow cytometry or image analysis can also greatly impact turnaround time. For example, flow-based procedures have advantages over manual microscopy evaluations, such as increasing the number of cells that can be evaluated in a culture without scorer fatigue. Along with automation of analysis, there are frequently opportunities to reduce the overall testing platform size from large culture flasks or tubes to as small as 96-well plates.[43,44] These reductions can come at a cost in numbers of cells or growth characteristics of the cells, so it is important to establish these parameters prior to implementing a reduced-sized testing scheme. As with any new laboratory technique, rigorous validation allows for more confidence in the final result with minimal intervention by the researcher. In addition to improving throughput, modifications of the platforms in the *in vitro* micronucleus assay may help gain more than just a "damage *vs.* no damage" answer; these tests can become rapid, high-content assays as will be described later.

### 7.3.3 Chromosome Aberration: RadarScreen

RadarScreen measures DNA damage to yeast through the promoter of the RAD54 (recombinatorial repair) gene with a β-galactosidase readout. The expression of this β-galactosidase can easily be quantified by use of the substrate D-luciferin-*O*-β galactopyranoside, which is converted into galactose and luciferin that can be measured luminometrically. This is a much higher throughput ($\sim$100 compounds/day) assay than a conventional chromosome aberration test, with the requirement of a low amount of compound ($<$5 mg). The RadarScreen assay has been demonstrated to show a good predictivity of chromosomal damage with a low number of false positive results.[45] This makes the assay a useful tool to understand the potential hazard of many chemicals before the need to create or obtain more test material for the more rigorous regulatory aberration assay.

### 7.3.4 GreenScreen HC Assay

The GreenScreen HC (HC = human cells) assay is a high-throughput microplate-based reporter assay. The assay is performed in the p53 competent human TK6 lymphoblastoid cell line that has been transfected with a stable replicating plasmid that has the GADD45α promoter sequence and a gene encoding green fluorescence protein (GFP).[46] The human GADD45a (Growth Arrest and DNA Damage) gene family is regulated by p53 and it is involved in the DNA damage and repair process. In addition to p53-dependent induction, it is regulated by, amongst others, BRCA1, c-MYC, and NF-κB.

The GADD45a gene has been considered a DNA damage stress biomarker, because it is up-regulated (3- to 14-fold) as a consequence of cellular response to DNA insult. In addition, the GADD45a gene has been linked to apoptosis, cell cycle delay, DNA replication delay to allow time for repair and induction of DNA repair genes.[47,48] Green fluorescence protein (GFP) is a very stable protein isolated from the jellyfish *Aequorea victoria*. Its fluorescence is readily measured, and is widely used in reporter assays. The detection of GFP in the assay requires an excitation wavelength of 488 nm and emitted light is measured at around 520 nm.

In order to detect all classes of genotoxins, cells must progress through a full cell cycle, so data are collected at 24- and 48-h time points so as to account for possible cell cycle delay (increased cell doubling time). Increased transcription of GADD45a over the constitutive level and significant induction in cellular fluorescence is indicative of genotoxicity, while the measurement of the reduction in optical absorbance, proportional to the inhibition of cell proliferation, is used to quantify general cytotoxicity compared to that achieved in the vehicle-treated controls, both with reference to statistically defined thresholds explain by Hastwell *et al.*[46] Fluorescence induction in the test strain is corrected for both cell density and background of the control strain.

Intrinsic fluorescence has limited the use of the assay with strongly fluorescent compounds because it might bias the results. However, by incorporating flow cytometric analyses, strongly colored/fluorescent compounds are more accurately evaluated in the assay.

In summary, the main advantage of the GreenScreen HC assay is that it evaluates the cellular response to overall genome damage, and is not limited to measure of a particular type of DNA damage.[49]

### 7.3.5 Vitotox Assay

Vitotox is a medium-/higher throughput bioluminescent assay. It is an *S. typhimurium* test that uses the light emission of bacteria to detect the genotoxicity, cytotoxicity and mutagenic potential of compounds. The main principle of the assay is based on a reporter gene system where luciferase activity is used as a measure of the genotoxicity. Luciferase expression is activated *via* a cascade of reactions known as the SOS response. The general principle of SOS induction involves the de-repression of the RecN gene that is achieved by placing a Lux reporter system under transcriptional control of the RecN promoter.[50] The important benefit of this assay is that the entire genome of the cell functions as a target for the genotoxin to display its effect. Most often a cytotoxicity assay is also performed together with each sample to define the functional dose range for each compound. The assay can be conducted using a very low amount of the compound (2.5–5 mg) and has been demonstrated to have a good correlation and excellent predictivity to the Ames assay thus reducing positive Ames scores later in development.[51] However, for this assay, highly pure compounds may be an essential element to reduce the false positive results induced by impurities. Taken together, screening with the Vitotox and subsequently deselecting/ranking compounds has proven useful to predict Ames results.[51]

## 7.4 Other Approaches for *In Vitro* Genotoxicity Testing

As mentioned earlier, the main rationale for conducting gentotoxicity assays is to understand the potential of a chemical compound to induce damage in DNA that can manifest as mutations which could range from single or double strand breaks, adducts, DNA-strand crosslinks, and chromosomal damage (chromosomal rearrangements and deletions). Earlier in this chapter, standard assays used for mutation and chromosomal damage hazard identification in the regulatory arena were explained (*i.e.*, Ames, MLA, chromosomal aberration assay and micronucleus). However, the scope of DNA damage induced by chemicals is so diverse that such damage or a combination of DNA damage-related cellular processes (*e.g.*, oxidative DNA damage) has a high potential to induce pre-carcinogenic lesions. Below we expand our discussion of genotoxicity into other ancillary *in vitro* assays that can be used to help elucidate the genotoxic potential of a compound. Furthermore, drugs may elicit a positive genotoxic response in one or more *in vitro* assays, despite having no obvious structural features predictive of covalent drug–DNA interactive potential or known mechanistic basis. Something other than direct covalent drug–DNA interaction can be involved that may trigger a chromosome aberration positive. For example, clastogenicity may arise from other mechanisms that exhibit a threshold phenomenon. Chemicals that bind non-covalently to DNA (such as Topo II inhibitors) can result in irreparable DNA double-strand breaks, chromosomal aberration/micronuclei.[52–54] Therefore, assessing for genotoxicity to detect chromosome breakage related to Topo II inhibition using specific centromeric or topoisomerase probes or spindle tubule staining may be of predictive value in cases where a chromosome aberration positive, but an Ames negative finding is observed.

As industries (such as the cosmetic industry) and governmental committees drive the 3Rs (reduce, replace, refine) to lower the number of animal tests being conducted, *in vitro* screening testing strategies have been pressured to evolve from more than just hazard identification tools into specialized fields/disciplines that can be used to identify mechanisms of DNA damage and help add to the body of knowledge to create better risk assessments for a variety of exposure situations. Some approaches use higher level cellular organisms that can provide more relevant data on a chemical's ability to mutate such a system. Assay systems that can elucidate the mode of action of the genotoxicant can inform and guide the risk assessment process. For example, a positive result in an *in vitro* MN assay may be shown to be less concerning if aneuploidy and a threshold can be established. DNA damage can occur by a variety of mechanisms; tests that measure oxidative stress may show that anti-oxidants can mitigate the genotoxicity. Newer assays may function to identify hazards or risks that standard assays may not. For example, the H2AX assay may provide information on risk of exposure to a dose of genotoxicant, and track the time course where that damage may be seen. Some of these assays are described briefly below.

## 7.4.1 Assays to Detect Mutations

### *7.4.1.1 HGPRT Assays*

The hypoxanthine-guanine phosphoribosyl transferase (HGPRT) mutation assay is similar to the MLA assay and is based on the X-linked HGPRT gene in Chinese hamster ovary (CHO) cells.[55,56] In this assay, untreated and treated cells are grown in the presence of purine analogs (*e.g.*, 6-thioguanine or 8-azaguanine) that are converted to toxic intermediates by the purine salvaging enzyme HGPRT. The mutation frequency is measured by analyzing the clonogenic potential of CHO cells in the presence of 6-thioguanine or 8-azaguanine. By conducting the cloning aspect, one can see how many mutations are viable and by sequencing the new clones, the actual mutations can be revealed.[57] Unfortunately, the cloning step takes two weeks to complete; thus this assay is not suitable for rapid, high-throughput testing.

### *7.4.1.2 Yeast DEL Assay*

The yeast DEL assay is a simple assay that has been shown to detect primarily the clastogenic activity of chemicals.[58] This assay primarily detects intrachromosomal recombination between two genetically engineered mutant *his3* alleles within the endogenous HIS3 gene in yeast. In addition to disrupting the endogenous HIS3 gene, the yeast DEL system also incorporates a LEU2 gene sequence that allows for the measurement of leucine auxotrophy in addition to measuring histidine prototrophy in cells that undergo recombination in response to chemical treatment.[59,60] To address the need for greater screening efficiency, a high-throughput, 384-well plate version of the assay has been developed. Since the yeast cell wall limits uptake of particularly large lipophilic chemicals, a strain with a permeable cell wall has recently been developed and could enhance the utility of the yeast DEL assay for evaluating a broader spectrum of chemicals.[61] This assay is useful in detecting clastogenic agents that lead to double-strand breaks, leading to inappropriate recombination. The advantages of the assay included technical simplicity and its ability to detect both genotoxic and nongenotoxic carcinogens, while having a 70–80% concordance with the *in vitro* micronucleus assay.[62,63]

### 7.4.2 Assays to Detect Aneuploidy

Several assays can be used to achieve the goal of assessing the potential of aneuploidy prior to conducting an *in vivo* rodent micronucleus test, which is often done after clinical trials are in progress.[64] This concept is important, as aneuploidy represents a class of genotoxicity that may have a threshold. Such damage can arise by a variety of mechanisms such as disruption of cell division, disruption of chromosome segregation, inhibition of DNA synthesis, inhibition of topoisomerases, nucleotide pool imbalance, overloading of oxidative defense mechanisms, metabolic overload (Phase II enzymes *etc.*), ion chelation, disturbance of metal homeostasis, extremes of pH/osmolarity and cytotoxicity.[31] Historically these assays have not been high throughput, (such as the anti-kinetochore assay described below). However, since early detection of genotoxicity may lead to deprioritization of a chemical or drug candidate for development, more and more early detection of thresholded genotoxicity has become a priority. Several assays are described below.

#### 7.4.2.1 *Anti-Kinetochore Staining/Fluorescent In Situ Hybridization*

Utilizing special staining techniques in combination with an *in vitro* micronucleus assay by cytokinesis block, it is possible to distinguish damage that occurs from clastogenic compounds and chromosome loss from exposure to aneugenic compounds. This mechanistic assay can be used as additional testing to support weight of evidence and is not higher throughput. The objective of anti-kinetochore staining is to determine if micronuclei (MN) are due to a clastogenic or an aneugenic mode of action. The staining allows for visualization of centromeres (indicative of whole chromosomes). This is achieved using anti-kinetochore antibodies derived from CREST (Calcinosis, Raynaud's phenomenon, Esophageal dysfunction, Sclerodactyly, Telangiectasia) patients and are directed against the kinetochore protein coat of the centromeric region of chromosomes. These antibodies are non-species specific and may be tagged with fluorochromes to allow the visualization of the presence/absence of centromeres and thereby whole chromosomes. A shift in the proportion of centromere-negative MN to centromere-positive MN is considered to indicate aneugenicity.[65]

#### *7.4.2.2 Mnvit—Flow Cytometer (MN/High-Content Screening)*

The standard Mnvit assay is widely used to assess genotoxic potential of test substances by measuring the frequency of MN in cultured mammalian cells. Traditionally, MN events have been evaluated by microscopy. *In vitro* flow cytometric methods of enumeration of micronuclei significantly shorten analysis time and can enhance assay throughput.[35] However, to successfully adapt such methods, the following elements have to be rigorously established. The assay needs to measure true MN rather than other cellular or subcellular components, be reproducible and proprietary substance validation/sensitivity is required when part of a screening strategy. Current application of testing in human TK6 cells, or Chinese hamster V79 or ovary cells has proven to yield important information in assessment of genotoxicity of predevelopment compounds[66,67] but low throughput has hindered the ability to use this assay as a screen. Technological advances have made it feasible to use 96-well plates for screening pharmaceutical compounds, enhancing throughput.[44] An advantage of the flow MN method is the capability of identifying potentially aneugenic compounds with the Chinese hamster fibroblast cells within the same test to identify micronucleus formation, as well as obtaining information on cell cycle perturbations.[44,67] With proper gating set up, increases in hypodiploid nuclei, a marker of aneugenicity can be identified, as well as "sizing" of the MN by measuring the fluorescence signal of the MN, can discriminate cultures exposed to aneugens from those exposed to clastogens.[67–69] In short, this seems to be an adaptable methodology for laboratories with access to a flow cytometer. Utilizing such technology, a single screening evaluation can replace a number of *in vitro* assays, identifying compounds that have a genotoxic signal, may disrupt the cell cycle or cause aneuploidy.

Obtaining more than just a qualitative positive/negative response from a genotoxicity assay is becoming more important in predictive toxicology. As described above, a small sample of test material in an *in vitro* micronucleus assay can provide data on genotoxicity, aneuploidy *vs.* clastogenicity and cell cycle perturbations by flow cytometry. With only one or two milligrams of compound, an automated assessment of MN can be done on potentially hundreds of compounds in a week, which in the context of solubility and cytotoxicity determinations has nearly equivalent fidelity to the standard, low-throughput microscopy evaluation.[70] Indeed, genetic toxicologists are being asked to provide more than just hazard identification for early drug-discovery support, and these tools may provide routine high-content screening tests towards this effort.

### 7.4.3 Indicators of DNA Damage

Standard *in vitro* genotoxicity tests detect mutagenicity arising from unrepaired or mis-repaired DNA damage Given the fact that genotoxicity may arise from direct or indirect DNA damage resulting from exposure to chemicals, the measurement of DNA damage provides a correlation to the genotoxic potential of chemicals. However, it is important to note that the mutagenicity of a chemical is also dependent on additional factors that include the rate and fidelity of DNA and the proclivity of each DNA adduct type to yield mutations during DNA replication. There are various assays that have been developed to analyze DNA damage. We will focus here on the tests that have been utilized more frequently to evaluate damage after a positive result has been seen in a standard genetox assay.

#### *7.4.3.1 DNA Adducts*

The 32P-postlabeling assay has a well-established methodology that determines the propensity of chemicals to bind covalently to DNA. It has been used in analyzing the formation of DNA adducts by carcinogens and chemotherapeutic agents as well as naturally occurring environmental and biological entities.[71,72] Unlike other approaches that measure DNA damage indirectly, adduct detection provides valuable information on the spectrum of covalent DNA adducts. More importantly, this assay can detect a wide variety of structurally distinct chemical adducts from alkylations to bulky adducts formed by polycyclic hydrocarbons at very high sensitivity in the range of 1 adduct per $10^9$–$10^{10}$ nucleotides. In brief, this technique involves the enzymatic digestion of potentially adducted DNA to deoxynucleoside 3′-monophosphates, enrichment of modified nucleotides *via* the removal of unmodified bases, labeling of the 5′-hydroxyl group of modified bases to generate 3′,5′-biphosphate, separation of modified bases using thin layer chromatography (TLC) and detection of DNA adducts by autoradiography.[73] While this assay provides no information on the mutagenicity, it serves as a confirmatory test to determine if the chemical does or does not have DNA adducting activity.

#### *7.4.3.2 8-OH-DG Measurements*

Many chemicals can induce DNA damage *via* an oxidative mechanism, and induction of oxidative lesions can be an important etiological factor in carcinogenesis. Oxidative DNA damage can occur through the formation of reactive oxygen species during the metabolism/detoxification of the compound and can be analyzed by monitoring the levels of oxidized nucleotides in the urine of treated individuals by high-performance liquid chromatography (HPLC) or liquid chromatography-tandem mass spectrometry (LC-MS/MS).[74,75] The analysis of oxidized nucleotides provides an indirect measurement for the potential for mutagenesis and subsequent carcinogenesis. While a major advantage of this method is the non-invasive *in vivo* approach, it does not provide unequivocal evidence for the genotoxicity of chemicals.

#### *7.4.3.3 Comet Assay*

The Comet Assay, also known as Single Cell Gel Electrophoresis (SCGE), provides the simplest platform and a sensitive methodology to measure DNA strand-breaks at the level of a single mammalian cell. Cells embedded in agarose, on a microslide, are subjected to electrophoresis under alkaline conditions. DNA damage is observed as an increase in the number of DNA fragments that have migrated out of the cell nucleus, forming a streak, upon DNA staining, similar to the tail of a comet.[76] The degree of fragmentation in the comet tail, relative to that in the head, is directly proportional to the extent of DNA damage. The alkaline (pH 13) version of the comet assay enables the detection of single- and double-strand breaks, and single-strand breaks arising due to repair or to formation of alkali-labile sites. DNA double-strand breaks may specifically be detected by running the assay under neutral rather than alkaline conditions.

The *in vitro* comet assay has not yet been frequently applied to regulatory submissions, but it is useful for helping understand compound-related DNA damage mechanisms, that is, to determine if a compound induces direct DNA damage, DNA crosslinks or effects on DNA repair. The major advantages of the *in vitro* comet assay are: a higher throughput, short experiment times, ease of analysis and its use as a general screening assay for DNA damage; any cell line in suspension, monolayer (primary cell cultures or cell line) or 3D organ cultures can be used as a small cell number is required; allows the investigation of damage to single cells rather than providing an indication of DNA damage in the cell population as a whole; and requires reduced amounts of test material.[77,78] In addition, it can be modified for testing DNA repair capacity by treating cells with a damaging agent and monitoring the remaining damage at specific time intervals. For the *in vitro* comet assay, as for any other genetox assay, cytotoxicity has to be taken into account in study interpretation, and a large presence of highly damaged cells can be used as an intrinsic indicator of cytotoxicity.[79]

By combining the comet assay with fluorescent *in situ* hybridization (FISH), using labeled probes to particular DNA sequences, we can examine DNA damage and repair at the level of chromosome, single genes or DNA sequences.[80,81] Thus, the combination of both techniques has been applied in particular for detection of site-specific breaks in DNA regions which are relevant for the development of different diseases, understanding genotoxicity potential, DNA repair, cytogenetic biomonitoring, cancer, *etc.*[79,82–84]

#### *7.4.3.4 H2AX*

Recent data indicate that DNA damage induces a variety of post-translational modifications on specific core histones and histone variants.[85] Among the various chromatin modifications that occur after DNA damage, the phosphorylation of the histone variant, H2AX at Serine 139 (also known as γ-H2AX), after double-strand break (DSB), has been thoroughly studied. These studies have helped to elucidate that DSBs, whether alone or as one type of a spectrum of DNA lesions, are involved in many cellular processes.[86] The phosphorylation of H2AX is induced by the DNA damage signaling kinase,

ATM (ataxia telangiectasia mutated).[87] H2AX phosphorylation then leads to the aggregation of a variety of DNA damage response proteins in the vicinity of the DNA damage leading to downstream events that include repair of damage and signal transduction events that ultimately lead to cell cycle arrest or programmed cell death.[85,88]

γ-H2AX molecules accumulate in the chromatin flanking the DSB and antibodies developed against this γ-H2AX focus, allow the visualization of the DSB site. These antibodies can be used as biomarkers in genetic toxicology testing, a biodosimeter for drug development, radiation exposure, and for clinical trials for cancer chemo- and radiotherapy.[89,90]

### 7.4.4 DNA Repair

DNA repair maintains the balance between DNA damage and permanent mutations. Changes in DNA repair activity can allow the mutation burden to increase and ultimately fix the mutation in the DNA, so impediment in the DNA repair process has been considered a gentotoxic endpoint. By necessity, DNA repair systems are extremely active and accurate because they need to keep the cell mutation rate at a level that maintains the species but allows variation. This has been estimated (in pseudogenes) to be $2.5 \times 10^{-8}$ mutations per nucleotide site, or 175 mutations per diploid genome per generation.[2]

DNA repair is a vast research field, which encompasses a huge range of cellular and biological events. Due to the complex process in each of the DNA repair mechanism (*i.e.*, base excision repair, nucleotide excision repair, non-homologous end joining, *etc.*) finding DNA repair assays that can be reliably used in the regulatory arena has been difficult. The DNA repair assays traditionally used in genetic toxicology had the objective of measuring DNA damage potential by inducing DNA repair. Two classic examples are the *in vitro* unscheduled DNA synthesis (UDS) assay performed with rat hepatocytes, and the BrdU (bromodeoxyuridine) incorporation method.[91,92] These *in vitro* assays are similar to their *in vivo* counterparts and will be described in more detail in the chapter on *in vivo* genetic toxicology.

However, new approaches like the comet assay, comet-FISH, and antibodies for γ-H2AX, among others, could be used in the future to understand DNA repair in the context of gentotoxicity testing.[80,82,93,94]

## 7.5 Future Areas for Consideration

The need for early safety data has led to a drive to improve the throughput of many safety assays including genotoxicity tests. The assays described previously in this chapter have been a good start to meeting this need. However, these improvements have not kept pace with technological improvements in other arenas. For pharmaceuticals in particular, in comparison to the tremendous advances in combinatorial chemistry and molecular biology that have lead to an exponential increase of potential drug candidates as well as drugable cellular targets, advances in highly predictive genetic toxicology tests have only been incremental. However, it is important to note that under the current regulatory environment, new, high-throughput tests are expected to mimic their regulatory counterparts, assessing similar endpoints with similar predictivity. A concerted effort has been made in developing computer models and knowledge-based systems for assessing the structure–activity relationship for genotoxicity. These efforts are discussed elsewhere in a dedicated topic on computational modeling approaches. The need for developing predictive *in vitro* genotoxicity screens that are less time consuming, more cost effective and mechanism-based is tremendous both for the regulatory agencies and industry. However, improving the mechanistic understanding of genotoxicity using the same tried and tested platforms (bacterial mutation tests, classical cytogenetics) has proven to be elusive; assays are being employed to be more than just the hazard identification tools they were designed to be. Clearly, new approaches are needed to gain better understanding of the meaning of genotoxicity seen in hazard ID tests and the risk such damage poses. In the following section, advances in less "traditional" methodologies as well as initiatives that have the potential to accelerate analysis, improve predictive power, provide greater mechanistic information and perhaps transform the field of *in vitro* genetic toxicology are discussed.

### 7.5.1 Toxicogenomics

One of the most promising developments expected to revolutionize the field of predictive *in vitro* and *in vivo* toxicology is toxicogenomics. It can be defined as the study of the structure and function of the genome as it responds to adverse xenobiotic exposure. It is a field that combines toxicology with genomics or other high-throughput molecular profiling technologies such as transcriptomics (mRNA expression), proteomics (cell and tissue-wide protein expression) and metabolomics (metabolic profiling). In pharmaceutical drug discovery and development, toxicogenomics is used to study adverse (toxic) effects of drugs in defined model systems in order to draw conclusions on the risk to patients. The application of toxicogenomics is broad, ranging from chemical hazard identification and characterization, to risk assessment. In this regard it is emerging as a science that can provide tools for improving the understanding of mechanisms of toxicity, identifying biomarkers of toxicity and exposure, reducing uncertainty in grouping of chemicals for risk assessments and providing alternative methods for chemical screening and predicting toxicological outcomes. In brief, toxicogenomics refers to the transcriptional profiling of genes in response to toxic stimuli at the cellular and tissue levels. Unlike other genetic toxicology methods that provide data on a single endpoint (mutation, chromosome aberration, other forms of DNA damage), this approach is truly a high-content methodology that allows the researcher to analyze the effect of chemicals on global gene expression patterns on a cell-type or tissue-specific manner. Systematic evaluation of toxicogenomic data can provide valuable and early information on potential toxicity and genotoxicity of chemicals. Toxicogenomics provides important information on the mode of action of chemicals in addition to details on the carcinogenic potential of chemicals.[95,96] Toxicogenomics also holds promise to solve important issues relating to genetic toxicology that include the use of alternative *in vitro* methods, early prediction to decrease drug attrition and the need for assays that provide global readouts on the effects of drugs and chemicals. Compounds with similar modes of genotoxic action may induce specific gene expression changes. Thus the genotoxicity of unknown compounds may be predicted after comparison of their profiles with the gene expression profiles of known genotoxicants.[97] Ironically, some of the strengths of toxicogenomics such as the large amount of data relating to gene expression patterns as well as the need for complex multidisciplinary analyses (bioinformatics, mechanistic toxicology and molecular biology) have limited its wider use. However, efforts by consortia of academics, government and industry partnerships (*e.g.*, ILSI HESI Genomics committee; the Critical Path Initiative) have been initiated to further streamline the use of toxicogenomics and possibly validate its use in predictive toxicology.[98] The success of such efforts and the tremendous analytical advances in genomics can be expected to drive the field of applied toxicogenomics within the realm of predictive genetic toxicology.

### 7.5.2 Epigenetics

Epigenetics refers to inherited changes in gene expression patterns that do not involve changes in DNA sequence information. The epigenetic regulation of gene expression during normal physiological development and the importance of abnormal epigenetic changes during cancer progression are beginning to be understood.[99–101] While a majority of the studies have focused on direct changes in the DNA methylation patterns of specific genes during cancer formation, recent studies have shown the important role of histone modification in DNA damage responses as well as tumor progression.[102,103] Epigenetic change is important in various disease conditions; as such, modulation of epigenetic mechanisms that can in turn be used to reverse aberrant gene expression patterns has become an important avenue for therapeutic approaches. Interestingly, several new candidate drugs that inhibit DNA methyl transferases and histone deacetylases (*e.g.*, suberoylanilide hydroxamic acid, 5-azacytidine, depsipeptide) have shown promising clinical results and approved for the treatment of specific cancers.[104] Despite these advances and prospects, there is limited information on the effectiveness, adverse effects and risks of epigenetic modulators. This new area of research that is changing our thinking of normal development, disease progression and disease therapy has immense implications for predictive genotoxicity at multiple levels. First and foremost, our understanding of epigenetics can provide important clues to the late-stage failure of drugs that have initially passed *in vitro* genotoxicity testing. Secondly, the development of epigenetic therapies provides an important challenge for the field of predictive toxicology (and genetic toxicology) as the current battery of *in vitro* genotoxicity analyses (that are based on DNA stability and mutations) will be inadequate for determining potential adverse effects. Finally, further elucidation of epigenetic pathways will provide possible mechanistic explanation of non-genotoxic carcinogenicity of chemicals and drugs.

### 7.5.3 High-Throughput Screening (HTS)—Tox21 Community

The collaborative efforts between the US National Toxicology Program (NTP), the National Institutes of Health Chemical Genomics Center (NCGC), and the US Environmental Protection Agency (US EPA) (commonly known as the Tox21 Community) have established research, development, validation, and translation of new and innovative test methods that characterize key steps in toxicity pathways. A key focus has been on the use of quantitative high-throughput screens (qHTS) used at the NCGC in 1536-well format to identify genotoxic compounds, including an approach based on increased cytotoxicity in DNA-repair-deficient chicken DT40 cell lines *versus* the corresponding wild-type cell line. The US EPA (National Center for Computational Toxicology) introduced ToxCast™, a research program to address chemical screening and prioritization needs by using a comprehensive battery of high-throughput and high- content screens to generate biological fingerprints and predictive signatures. The resulting data is released *via* a web site called ACToR (Aggregated Computational Toxicology Resource). In Phase I, 320 compounds (predominantly data-rich pesticides) were tested in over 500 different assays. The next phase of qHTS at the NCGC will include the screening of a library of ~10 000 compounds with known structures as part of the Tox21 project. This library is being developed in collaboration with the EPA NCCT and the NCGC, and will include the full EPA ToxCast™ chemical library (approx 1000 chemicals), for which a broader spectrum of commercial and research qHTS assay technologies are being employed through the affiliated ToxCast™ project.

High-throughput technologies available to identify genome-wide epigenetic alterations will help understand their role in health, disease and toxicant-induced biological outcomes. These tools provide the potential to help understand the risk associated with various chemical agents. In addition, emerging areas such as toxicogenomics, epigenomics and other global approaches may help routinely distinguish direct DNA interaction from damage as a consequence of cytotoxicity or non-covalent DNA binding DNA damage secondary to mechanism (Topo II inhibition, DNA polymerase inhibition, *etc.*). Toxicogenomics and HTS testing strategies are giving researchers, for the first time, the ability to broadly probe biological targets, pathways, and mechanisms in relation to toxicity endpoints, including genetic toxicity, for large numbers of chemicals. The use of toxicogenomics in the 21st century can serve as a bridge between genotoxicity and carcinogenicity. The coordinated approaches and efforts by ToxCast/Tox21, highlight the expectations for the future, supporting a new paradigm for predictive toxicology.[105]

## 7.6 Conclusions

The benefit of early *in vitro* genotoxicity screening is that it improves the safety profile of compounds that are selected in the early research phase and also contributes to the risk assessment process. It also helps by reducing costly late drug attrition. Limited amounts of pharmaceutical or environmental samples demand conservation of sample and reduce the available approaches one can take to assess their safety. Therefore, one has to be prudent in choosing the assays with medium-/high-throughput screening capacity and sufficient predictive power to make informed decisions based on less information than would be ideal. With a well-considered early screening strategy, the information from performing several of these assays upfront in the discovery process allows us to prioritize compounds not only on the basis of structure "activity" but also provides structure "toxicity" relationship insights. The information obtained then facilitates further development and enables us to make informed choices as to which compounds should be moved forward in drug development using *in vivo* animal studies. The information gained on many compounds can then be fed into other tools, such as computational models that could now better predict potential genotoxicity from chemical structures, obviating the need to test every compound in a laboratory test, and improving the performance of these *in silico* tools. Likewise, large sets of genetox data can enhance the understanding gleaned from toxicogenomics, leading to the development of mutation or clastogenesis profiles that could further enhance our understanding of mechanisms and the decision- making process.

In view of the complexities of the cellular and molecular processes that affect the genotoxic characteristics of chemicals, the costs associated with *in vivo* carcinogenicity assays and the need to expedite the analysis of potential therapeutic candidates, *in vitro* genotoxicity testing provides a rational choice that balances the aforementioned needs with the practical requisite to develop effective drugs with minimal side-effects. Furthermore, the robustness of standard *in vitro* genotoxicity testing assays is well suited to a variety of applications that involve the testing of chemicals (with potential human exposure), pharmaceutical candidates, and environmental pollutants. More importantly, the inter-laboratory reliability and the availability of an extensive experience-/evidence-based knowledge base for these assays make them methods of choice that are accepted by regulatory agencies around the world and indicate their potential to predict chemical-induced carcinogenesis.

Assessing genotoxicity is an important aspect of both drug development and chemical safety testing (including the REACH program). The *in vitro* testing battery has been designed to be a highly sensitive hazard identification battery to increase the potential to predict chemical carcinogenicity. However, the design of tests that provide extremely high sensitivity leads to low specificity when multiple tests are employed. For instance, 50% of non-carcinogens among pharmaceuticals have some DNA damage signal in genotoxicity assays.[106,107] Furthermore, the current testing paradigm is incapable of detecting a variety of non-genotoxic carcinogens, such as hormone-type agents, which may impose a considerable human health risk.

*In vitro* genetic toxicology under the current design can only attempt to reproduce a portion of the immensely complex process of tumorigenesis. Advances such as toxicogenomics and in the area of epigenetics have provided researchers with opportunities to learn more about chemical genotoxicants and their relationship with the tumorigenic process that were unavailable when the current battery was designed. Our ability to better screen for genotoxicity and predict carcinogenicity is expected to vastly improve with the advent of robust genomic tools that are being evaluated for genotoxicity testing. Such improvements will be vital, as more and more, society expects safe products without the need for animal testing. Currently the only way to assure a compound is truly non-carcinogenic is to conduct an expensive animal bioassay. While we may never be able to eliminate the need for animal testing in all situations, improvement in predictive *in vitro* genetic toxicology testing, along with the further development of assays to understand the pathways and mechanisms that lead to tumor formation, and improved systems such as computer-based modeling, testing paradigms and mechanistic evaluations will help reduce the number of bioassays required.

In the future, it will be important to consider what role genetic toxicology can play in a new HTS *in vitro* toxicity testing paradigm, and what the implications of the new HTS testing programs, such as Tox21 and ToxCast, for the genetic toxicology community and predictive toxicology are.

## Acknowledgements

The authors would like to thank Dr Ronald Snyder for his diligent review of this chapter.

## References

1. D. Brusick, *Principles of Genetic Toxicology*, Plenum Press, New York, 1987, p. 284.
2. E. C. Friedberg, *Cell Res.*, 2008, **18**, 3–7.
3. M. Kirsch-Volders, L. Gonzalez, P. Carmichael and D. Kirkland, *Mutat. Res.*, 2009, **678**, 72–75.
4. J. H. Hoeijmakers, *Nature*, 2001, **411**, 366–374.
5. M. C. Poirier, *Nat. Rev. Cancer*, 2004, **4**, 630–607.
6. D. Kirkland, M. Aardema, L. Henderson and L. Müller, *Mutat. Res.*, 2005, **584**, 1–256.
7. M. O. Kenyon, J. R. Cheung, K. L. Dobo and W. W. Ku, *Regul. Toxicol. Pharmacol.*, 2007, **48**, 75–86.

8. A. Jacobs and K. D. Jacobson, *Toxicol. Sci.*, 2004, **81**, 260–262.
9. *S2B: Genotoxicity: a standard battery for genotoxicity testing of pharmaceuticals*, International Organization for Harmonisation, Geneva, Switzerland, 1997.
10. Commission of the European Communities, *Directive 2003/15/EC of the European Parliament and of the Council of 27 February 2003 amending Council Directive 76/768/EEC on the approximation of the laws of the Member states relating to cosmetic products*, Brussels, 2003.
11. Commission of the European Communities, *Regulation (EC) No. 1907/2006 of the European Parliament and of the Council of 18 December 2006 concerning the Registration, Evaluation, Authorisation and Restriction of Chemicals (REACH), establishing a European Chemicals Agency, amending Directive 1999/45/EC and repealing Council Regulation (EEC) No. 793/93 and Commission Regulation (EC) No. 1488/94; Council Directive 76/769/EEC; Commission Directives 91/155/EEC, 93/67/EEC, 93/105/EC and 2000/21/EC*, Brussels, 2006.
12. Commission of the European Communities, *REACH Technical Guidelines*, Brussels, 2007, available from: http://ecb.jrc.it/reach/rip/.
13. European Chemicals Agency, *Guidance on information requirements and chemical safety assessment*, Helsinki, Finland, 2008, ch. R6, available from: http://guidance.echa.europa.eu/docs/guidance_document/information_requirements_r6_en.pdf?ver=20_08_08.
14. Organization for Economic Cooperation and Development, *Guideline 471: Bacterial Reverse Mutation Test*, Paris, France, 1997.
15. Organization for Economic Cooperation and Development, *Guideline 473: In vitro Mammalian Chromosome Aberration Test*, Paris, France, 1997.
16. Organization for Economic Cooperation and Development, *Guideline 476: In vitro Mammalian Cell Gene Mutation Test*, Paris, France, 1997.
17. Organization for Economic Cooperation and Development, *Guideline 487: In vitro Mammalian Cell Micronucleus Test*, Paris, France, 2010.
18. *S2A: Guidance on specific aspects of regulatory genotoxicity tests for pharmaceuticals*, International Conference on Harmonisation, Geneva, Switzerland, 1995.
19. D. Putman, J. Clarke, P. Escobar, R. Gudi, L. Krsmanovic, K. Pant, V. Wagner III and R. San, in *Toxicological Testing Handbook: Principles, Applications and Data Interpretaion*, ed. D. Jacobson-Kram and K. Keller, Informa Healthcare, New York, 2006, pp. 185–248.
20. P. Guzzie-Peck, J. Sakaki and S. Weiner, in: *Pharmaceutical Toxicology in Practice – A Guide to Non-Clinical Development*, ed. A. Lodola and J. Stadler, John Wiley & Sons, Hoboken, New Jersey, 2011.
21. B. Ames, J. McCann and E. Yamasaki, *Mutat. Res.*, 1975, **31**, 347–364.
22. D. Maron and B. Ames, *Mutat. Res.*, 1983, **113**, 173–215.
23. D. Gatehouse, S. Haworth, T. Cebula, E. Gocke, L. Kier, T. Matsushima, C. Melcion, T. Nohmi, T. Ohta, S. Venitt and E. Zeiger, *Mutat. Res.*, 1994, **312**, 217–233.

24. P. Einisto, M. Watanabe, M. Ishidate Jr and T. Nohmi, *Mutat. Res.*, 1991, **259**, 95–102.
25. Y. C. Ni, R. H. Heflich, F. F. Kadlubar and P. P. Fu, *Mutat. Res.*, 1987, **192**, 15–22.
26. R. D. Snyder, G. S. Pearl, G. Mandakas, W. N. Choy, F. Goodsaid and I. Y. Rosenblum, *Environ. Mol. Mutagen.*, 2004, **43**, 143–58.
27. J. Ashby and R. W. Tennant, *Mutat. Res.*, 1991, **257**, 229–306.
28. Committee on Mutagenicity of Chemicals in Food Consumer Products and the Environment, *Guidance on a strategy for testing of chemicals for mutagenicity*, Department of Health, London, 2000.
29. M. Honma, M. Hayashi, H. Shimada, N. Tanaka, S. Wakuri, T. Awogi, K. I. Yamamoto, N.-U. Kodani, Y. Nishi, M. Nakadate and T. Sofuni, *Mutagenesis*, 1999, **14**, 5–22.
30. T. Morita, T. Nagaki, I. Fukuda and K. Okumura, *Mutat. Res.*, 1992, **268**, 297–305.
31. D. Scott, S. M. Galloway, R. R. Marshall, M. Ishidate Jr., D. Brusick, J. Ashby and B. C. Myhr, *Mutat. Res.*, 1991, **257**, 147–205.
32. M. M. Moore, M. Honma, J. Clements, G. Bolcsfoldi, B. Burlinson, M. Cifone, J. Clarke, R. Delongchamp, R. Durward, M. Fellows, B. Gollapudi, S. Hou, P. Jenkinson, M. Lloyd, J. Majeska, B. Myhr, M. O'Donovan, T. Omori, C. Riach, R. San, L. F. Stankowski Jr, A. K. Thakur, F. Van Goethem, S. Wakuri and I. Yoshimura, *Environ. Mol. Mutagen.*, 2006, **47**, 1–5.
33. D. Kirkland, *Mutat. Res.*, 2010, **702**, 135–138.
34. M. Fenech, *Mutat. Res.*, 2000, **455**, 81–95.
35. S. M. Bryce, J. C. Bemis, S. L. Avlasevich and S. D. Dertinger, *Mutat. Res.*, 2007, **630**, 78–91.
36. I. Decordier, A. Papine, G. Plas, S. Roesems, K. Vande Loock, J. Moreno-Palomo, E. Cemeli, D. Anderson, A. Fucic, R. Marcos, F. Soussaline and M. Kirsch-Volders, *Mutagenesis*, 2009, **24**, 85–93.
37. M. S. Diehl, S. L. Willaby and R. D. Snyder, *Environ. Mol. Mutagen.*, 2000, **36**, 72–77.
38. D. M. Maron and B. N. Ames, *Mutat. Res.*, 1983, **113**, 173–215.
39. L. D. Claxton, V. S. Houk and S. Warren, *Mutat. Res.*, 2001, **488**, 241–257.
40. J. Aubrecht, J. J. Osowski, P. Persaud, J. R. Cheung, J. Ackerman, S. H. Lopes and W. W. Ku, *Mutagenesis*, 2007, **22**, 335–342.
41. S. Fluckiger-Isler, M. Baumeister, K. Braun, V. Gervais, N. Hasler-Nguyen, R. Reimann, J. Van Gompel, H. G. Wunderlich and G. Engelhardt, *Mutat. Res.*, 2004, **558**, 181–197.
42. P. Gee, D. M. Maron and B. N. Ames, *Proc. Natl. Acad. Sci. U. S. A.*, 1994, **91**, 11606–11610.
43. S. M. Bryce, J. Shi, J. Nicolette, M. Diehl, P. Sonders, S. Avlasevich, S. Raja, J. C. Bemis and S. D. Dertinger, *Environ. Mol. Mutagen.*, 2010, **51**, 260–266.
44. S. M. Bryce, S. L. Avlasevich, J. C. Bemis, S. Phonethepswath and S. D. Dertinger, *Mutat. Res.*, 2010, **703**, 191–199.

45. D. Kirkland, P. Kasper, L. Müller, R. Corvi and G. Speit, *Mutat. Res.*, 2008, **653**, 99–108.
46. P. W. Hastwell, L. L. Chai, K. J. Roberts, T. W. Webster, J. S. Harvey, R. W. Rees and R. M. Walmsley, *Mutat. Res.*, 2006, **607**, 160–175.
47. D. Liebermann and B. Hoffman, *Blood Cells, Mol., Dis.*, 2007, **39**, 329–335.
48. S. Jin, H. Zhao, F. Fan, P. Blanck, W. Fan, A. Colchagie, A. J. Fornace and Q. Zhan, *Oncogene*, 2000, **19**, 4050–4057.
49. R. M. Walmsley, *Expert Opin. Drug Metab. Toxicol.*, 2008, **4**, 827–835.
50. D. van der Lelie, L. Regniers, B. Borremans, A. Provoost and L. Verschaeve, *Mutat. Res.*, 1997, **389**, 279–290.
51. W. M. Westerink, J. C. Stevenson, A. Lauwers, G. Griffioen, G. J. Horbach and W. G. Schoonen, *Mutat. Res.*, 2009, **676**, 113–130.
52. R. Snyder and P. J. Gilles, *Environ. Mol. Mutagen.*, 2002, **40**, 266–276.
53. R. Snyder and M. R. Amone, *Mutat. Res.*, 2002, **503**, 21–35.
54. R. Snyder, D. E. Ewing and L. B. Hendry, *Environ. Mol. Mutagen.*, 2005, **45**, 100–105.
55. D. Clive and J. F. Spector, *Mutat. Res.*, 1975, **31**, 17–29.
56. J. P. O'Neill, P. A. Brimer, R. Machanoff, G. P. Hirsch and A. W. Hsie, *Mutat. Res.*, 1977, **45**, 91–101.
57. P. Keohavong, L. Xi and S. G. Grant, *Methods Mol. Biol.*, 2005, **291**, 161–170.
58. A. Galli and R. H. Schiestl, *Biotherapy*, 1998, **11**, 129–133.
59. R. H. Schiestl, *Nature*, 1989, **337**, 285–288.
60. R. H. Schiestl, R. D. Gietz, R. D. Mehta and P. J. Hastings, *Carcinogenesis*, 1989, **10**, 1445–1455.
61. W. W. Ku, J. Aubrecht, R. J. Mauthe, R. H. Schiestl and A. J. Fornace, *Toxicol. Sci.*, 2007, **99**, 20–25.
62. Z. Kirpnick, M. L. Homiski, E. Rubitski, M. Repnevskaya, N. Howlett, J. Aubrecht and R. H. Schiestl, *Mutat. Res.*, 2005, **582**, 116–134.
63. R. J. Brennan and R. H. Schiestl, *Methods. Mol. Biol.*, 2004, **262**, 111–124.
64. H. F. P. Joosten, F. A. A. van Acker, D. J. van den Dobbelsteen, G. J. M. J. Horbach and E. I. Krajnć, *Toxicol. Lett.*, 2004, **151**, 113–134.
65. D. A. Eastmond and J. D. Tucker, *Mutat. Res.*, 1989, **224**, 517–525.
66. S. M. Bryce, J. C. Bemis, S. Avlasevich and S. D. Dertinger, *Mutat. Res.*, 2007, **630**, 78–91.
67. J. Nicolette, M. Diehl, P. Sonders, S. Bryce and E. Blomme, *Environ. Mol. Mutagen.*, 2011, **52**, 355–362.
68. S. M. Bryce, J. Shi, J. Nicolette, M. Diehl, P. Sonders, S. Avlasevich, S. Raja, J. C. Bemis and S. D. Dertinger, *Environ. Mol. Mutagen.*, 2010, **51**, 260–266.
69. J. Shi, R. Bezabhie and A. Szkudlinska, *Mutagenesis*, 2010, **25**, 33–40.
70. M. S. Mondal, J. Gabriels, C. McGinnis, M. Magnifico, T. H. Marsilje, L. Urban, A. Collis, D. Bojanic, S. A. Biller, W. Frieauff, H. J. Martus, W. Suter and P. Bentley, *Toxicol. Sci.*, 2010, **118**, 71–85.

71. R. C. Gupta, M. L. Sopori and C. G. Gairola, *Cancer Res.*, 1989, **49**, 1916–1920.
72. S. Kato, K. Yamashita, T. Kim, T. Tajiri, M. Onda and S. Sato, *Mutat. Res.*, 1988, **202**, 85–91.
73. A. C. Beach and R. C. Gupta, *Carcinogenesis*, 1992, **13**, 1053–1074.
74. C. W. Hu, C. J. Wang, L. W. Chang and M. R. Chao, *Clin. Chem.*, 2006, **52**, 1381–1388.
75. M. T. Wu, C. H. Pan, Y. L. Huang, P. J. Tsai, C. J. Chen and T. N. Wu, *Environ. Mol. Mutagen.*, 2003, **42**, 98–105.
76. J. P. Banath, M. Fushiki and P. L. Olive, *Int. J. Radiat. Biol.*, 1998, **73**, 649–660.
77. R. R. Tice, E. Agurell, D. Anderson, B. Burlinson, A. Hartmann, H. Kobayashi, Y. Miyamae, E. Rojas, J. C. Ryu and Y. F. Sasaki, *Environ. Mol. Mutagen.*, 2000, **35**, 206–221.
78. R. Ghaoui, B. C. Sallustio, P. C. Burcham and F. R. Fontaine, *Chem.–Biol. Interact.*, 2003, **145**, 201–211.
79. W. Shi, Z. Feng, J. Zhang, I. Gonzalez-Suarez, R. P. Vanderwaal, X. Wu, S. N. Powell, J. L. Roti Roti and S. Gonzalo, *Carcinogenesis*, 2010, **31**, 994–1002.
80. S. Shaposhnikov, P. Thomsen and A. Collins, *Methods Mol. Biol.*, 2011, **682**, 115–132.
81. P. A. Escobar, M. T. Smith, A. Vasishta, A. E. Hubbard and L. Zhang, *Mutagenesis*, 2007, **22**, 321–327.
82. G. Hovhannisyan, *Mol. Cytogenet.*, 2010, **3**, 17.
83. G. Spivak, R. A. Cox and P. C. Hanawalt, *Mutat. Res.*, 2009, **681**, 44–50.
84. A. C. Guimaraes, L. M. Antunes, H. F. Ribeiro, A. K. dos Santos, P. C. Cardoso, P. L. de Lima, A. D. Seabra, T. B. Pontes, C. Pessoa, M. O. de Moraes, B. C. Cavalcanti, C. M. Sombra, O. Bahia Mde and R. R. Burbano, *Cell Biol. Toxicol.*, 2010, **26**, 403–419.
85. W. M. Bonner, C. E. Redon, J. S. Dickey, A. J. Nakamura, O. A. Sedelnikova, S. Solier and Y. Pommier, *Nat. Rev. Cancer*, 2008, **8**, 957–967.
86. J. Dickey, C. Redon, A. Nakamura, B. Baird, O. Sedelnikova and W. Bonner, *Chromosoma*, 2009, **118**, 683–692.
87. K. J. McManus and M. J. Hendzel, *Mol. Biol. Cell*, 2005, **16**, 5013–5025.
88. S. Nowsheen, R. Wukovich, K. Aziz, P. Kalogerinis, C. Richardson, M. Panayiotidis, W. Bonner, O. Sedelnikova and A. Georgakilas, *Mutat. Res.*, 2009, **674**, 131–136.
89. C. E. Redon, A. J. Nakamura, O. A. Martin, P. R. Parekh, U. S. Weyemi and W. M. Bonner, *Aging*, 2011, **3**, 168–174.
90. C. E. Redon, A. J. Nakamura, O. Sordet, J. S. Dickey, K. Gouliaeva, B. Tabb, S. Lawrence, R. J. Kinders, W. M. Bonner and O. A. Sedelnikova, *Methods Mol. Biol.*, 2011, **682**, 249–70.
91. Organization for Economic Cooperation and Development, *Guideline 482: Genetic Toxicology: DNA Damage and Repair/Unscheduled DNA Synthesis in Mammalian Cells In Vitro*, OECD, Paris, France, 1986.

92. C. Smith and P. Hanawalt, *Biochim. Biophys. Acta*, 1976, **447**, 121–132.
93. A. Nakamura, V. Rao, Y. Pommier and W. Bonner, *Cell Cycle*, 2010, **9**, 389–397.
94. G. Spivak, *Methods Mol. Biol.*, 2010, **659**, 129–145.
95. H. Ellinger-Ziegelbauer, J. Aubrecht, J. C. Kleinjans and H.-J. Ahr, *Toxicol. Lett.*, 2009, **186**, 36–44.
96. M. D. Waters, M. Jackson and I. Lea, *Mutat. Res.*, 2010, **705**, 184–200.
97. A. Lynch, J. Sasaki, R. Elespuru, D. Jacobson-Kram, V. Thybaud, M. De Boeck, M. J. Aardema, J. Aubrecht, R. D. Benz, S. Dertinger, G. Douglas, P. White, P. Escobar, A. J. Fornace, M. Honma, R. Naven, J. Rusling, R. Schiestl, R. Walmsley, E. Yamamura, J. van Benthem and J. Kim, *Environ. Mol. Mutagen.*, 2010, **52**, 205–223.
98. W. B. Mattes, *Methods Mol. Biol.*, 2008, **460**, 221–238.
99. M. Verma and S. Srivastava, *Lancet Oncol.*, 2002, **3**, 755–763.
100. A. P. Feinberg, *Semin. Cancer Biol.*, 2004, **14**, 427–432.
101. M. Lohrum, H. G. Stunnenberg and C. Logie, *Int. J. Biochem. Cell Biol.*, 2007, **39**, 1450–1461.
102. G. G. Wang, C. D. Allis and P. Chi, *Trends Mol. Med.*, 2007, **13**, 363–372.
103. G. G. Wang, C. D. Allis and P. Chi, *Trends Mol. Med.*, 2007, **13**, 373–380.
104. C. Mund and F. Lyko, *Bioessays*, 2010, **32**, 949–957.
105. B. Mahadevan, R. Snyder, M. D. Waters, R. D. Benz, R. A. Kemper, R. R. Tice and A. M. Richard, *Environ. Mol. Mutagen.*, 2011, **52**, 339–354.
106. S. Hoffmann and T. Hartung, *Hum. Exp. Toxicol.*, 2006, **25**, 497–513.
107. R. Snyder and J. Green, *Mutat. Res.*, 2001, **488**, 151–169.

CHAPTER 8

# *Cardiac Toxicity Prediction: To Simplify, or to Integrate, that is the Question*

VIVEK J. KADAMBI*, COLLEEN SYNAN AND KATHERINE BREWER

Millennium: The Takeda Oncology Company, Drug Safety Evaluation, 35 Landsdowne Street, Cambridge, MA 02139, USA

## 8.1 Introduction

The goal of nonclinical toxicology studies is to identify potential adverse effects associated with administration of a drug candidate. Safety pharmacology studies, which aim to detect functional effects on critical organ systems, are an essential part of the nonclinical evaluation of a drug candidate. Included in the safety pharmacology core battery, as outlined in International Conference on Harmonisation S7A (ICH S7A)[1] are studies to thoroughly explore effects on the central nervous, cardiovascular and respiratory systems. Non-rodent *in vivo* studies have traditionally been the "gold standard" for evaluating effects on cardiovascular function. *In vitro* studies represent an important tool in safety pharmacology investigations, as evidenced by the ICH S7B guidelines on the use of *in vitro* assays to determine the potential effects of pharmaceuticals on ventricular repolarization.[2] More recently, because cardiovascular function and structure can be altered in ways not easily recognized in *in vivo* cardiovascular toxicology studies, *in vitro* studies have found favor as tools for performing mechanistic cardiotoxicity studies. While the predictivity of *in vitro* assays is

RSC Drug Discovery Series No. 12
New Horizons in Predictive Toxicology: Current Status and Application
Edited by Alan G. E. Wilson

Published by the Royal Society of Chemistry, www.rsc.org

commonly questioned, these assays offer certain advantages which make them invaluable to the field of drug development.

*In vitro* assays, such as ion channel binding assays, electrophysiology assays using single cells or freshly isolated preparations, Langendorff preparations, and cardiomyocyte toxicity assays represent a relatively inexpensive option for investigating potential cardiovascular liabilities. These assays require only a small amount of test article and can generally be conducted rapidly; qualities which make them attractive options for first-tier assays employed early in the drug development process. Although these *in vitro* systems are tremendously helpful, they represent only a fraction of a complex *in vivo* system and are not infallible in predicting cardiovascular effects in humans. Therefore, when evaluating results of an *in vitro* assay, it is important to consider that *in vivo* additional interactions may be at play, and to carefully weigh the potential risks and benefits associated with administration of a drug candidate.

In this chapter, many of the *in vitro* assays used today to evaluate cardiotoxic potential of drug candidates will be discussed in detail, including an explanation of how these assays differ and how each can be used to answer specific questions.

## 8.2 Ion Channel Binding Assays

Ion channels serve as the molecular work-horses of the cardiovascular system, conducting the flow of ionic charges and thus regulating the electrical activity of the heart. Changes in the electrochemical gradient across the cardiomyocyte cell membrane, generated by the flow of ions through the protienaceous pores in ion channels, form the basis for the cardiac action potential (Figure 8.1). Given the precision required for proper synchronization and conduction of the action potential through each cardiomyocyte, it is not difficult to believe that dysregulation of this process can occur. A variety of factors can contribute to ion channel dysfunction, including drug administration, with the end result being cardiac arrhythmias. The possibility is perhaps best illustrated by the

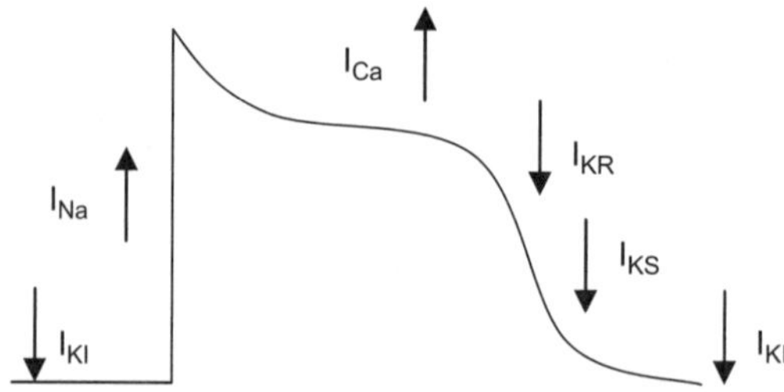


**Figure 8.1** Ion channel currents contributing to the cardiac action potential. Reproduced with permission from T. J. Jentsch, C. A. Hübner and J. C. Fuhrmann, *Nat. Cell Biology*, 2004, **6**, 1039–1047. Copyright Nature Publishing Group, 2004.

withdrawal of several commercially successful pharmaceuticals [Seldane® (terfenadine; Hoechst Marion Roussel, Kansas City, Missouri), Propulsid® (cisapride; Janssen Pharmaceutica, Titusville, New Jersey), Hismanal® (astemizole; Janssen Pharmaceutica, Titusville, New Jersey)], in the 1990s due to reports of QT interval prolongation and an associated ventricular tachycardia known as Torsades de Pointes (TdP) which resulted in an increased risk for sudden cardiac deaths in patients receiving these pharmaceuticals. Blocking of the hERG channel, a voltage-gated potassium channel responsible for the current ($I_{Kr}$) which produces the rapid phase of ventricular repolarization, was ultimately found to be the mechanism by which these pharmaceuticals induced QT interval prolongation. Binding of a small molecule to the hERG channel can impede the efflux of potassium ions, resulting in delayed ventricular repolarization. Ventricular repolarization is represented by the QT interval on a surface electrocardiogram; therefore, delayed ventricular repolarization results in prolongation of the QT interval. Delayed ventricular repolarization leaves ventricular myocytes vulnerable to early after-depolarizations (EADs), which can lead to TdP, a rapid, polymorphic ventricular tachycardia visualized on an ECG as a twisting of the QRS complex around the isoelectric baseline (Figure 8.2). Untreated, TdP may spontaneously revert to normal sinus rhythm or degenerate into ventricular fibrillation.

Interaction with the hERG channel is not, in and of itself, sufficient to cause TdP but is a useful surrogate which affords for an accessible endpoint in early screening of drug candidates. These screening assays assess a test compound's affinity for the hERG channel heterologously expressed in whole cells or cell membranes isolates. These assays can be performed using radioactivity or fluorescence polarization to measure displacement of a labeled ligand with known affinity for the hERG channel by the test compound. Multiple concentrations of the test compound are evaluated in order to generate a dose–response curve and calculate an $IC_{50}$ value, the concentration at which 50% of the bound known ligand is displaced. The $IC_{50}$ is then used to calculate an absolute inhibition constant, or $K_i$, for the test compound using the Cheng–Prusoff equation [eqn (8.1)].[3] Calculation of a $K_i$ value is necessary to correct for assay-to-assay differences in membrane concentration and ligand-membrane affinity.

$$K_i = \frac{IC_{50}}{1 + [S]/K_m} \tag{8.1}$$

Where [S] is the concentration of hERG membranes in the reaction and $K_m$ is the concentration of membranes at which known ligand activity is at half maximal.

The displacement assay format described here for the hERG channel assay is a staple of general pharmacology testing and has been used for ion channel, enzyme and receptor testing. This assay format is amenable to use for any cardiac ion channel of interest simply by substituting a cell line (or membrane homogenate) expressing the appropriate ion channel and a labeled ligand whose affinity for that channel is known. Due to the low material requirement,

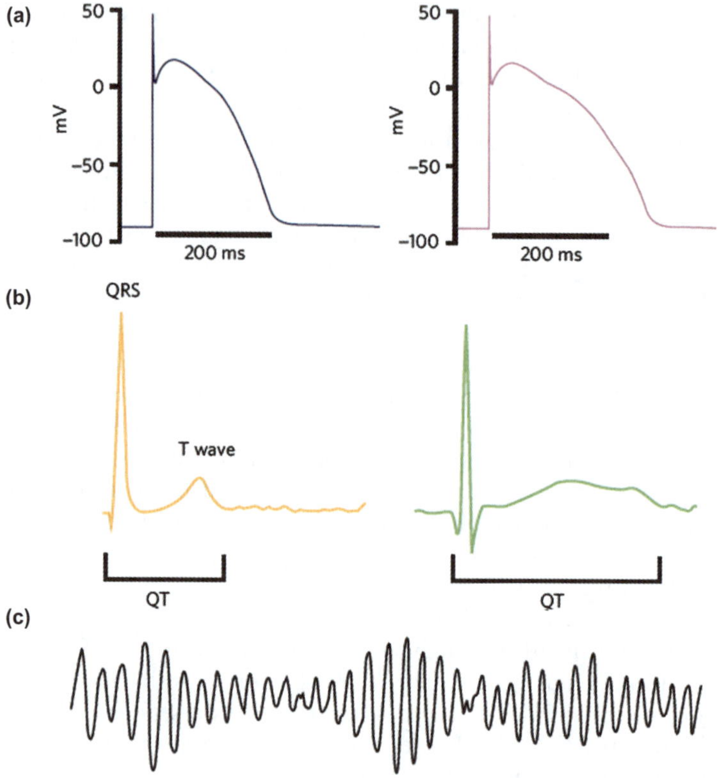


**Figure 8.2** Reduced hERG current delays ventricular repolarization and can induce arrhythmia. (a) Normal human ventricular myocyte action potential (left) and a prolonged action potential simulated[4] by reducing hERG current by 80% (right). (b) Normal ECG trace for a single cardiac cycle (left) and abnormal ECG trace with prolonged QT interval (right). The QRS complex represents depolarization, and the T-wave indicates repolarization of the ventricles. The QT interval represents the time between initial depolarization and final repolarization of the ventricles. (c) Diagram of an ECG tracing showing a TdP arrhythmia. Reproduced with permission from M. C. Sanguinetti and M. Tristani-Firouzi, *Nature,* 2006, **440**, 463–469. Copyright Nature Publishing Group, 2006.

compatibility with automation platforms and rapid turnaround time, these ion channel binding assays can be employed in a high-throughout manner to screen candidate compounds early in the drug development process. Pairing these assays with early pharmacology assays (*i.e.*, target enzyme activity) can be useful for understanding structure–activity relationships and supporting rational design to decrease undesired ion channel activity, while retaining or even enhancing the desired target activity of drug candidates. Additionally, these assays can be employed later in the development process to aid in mechanistic understanding of a cardiovascular effect observed *in vivo*.

## 8.3 Patch Clamp Assay

Methods for recording action potentials in cells capable of conducting electrical impulses date back to the experiments of Hodgkins and Huxley on the giant squid axon.[5] Further technical refinement, most notably the patch clamp method developed by Bert Sakmann and Erwin Neher,[6] allowed for measurement of the current through individual ion channels. For investigation of cardiac ion channel function, patch clamp electrophysiology studies can be conducted using freshly isolated myocytes or Purkinje fibers, *Xenopus laevis* oocytes expressing the ion channel of interest or the same stable heterologous expressing cell lines employed in binding assays. Methods for investigating interactions with a single ion channel type will be discussed in this section. Freshly isolated myocytes and Purkinje fibers, which contain the myriad of ion channels required for proper function *in vivo*, represent an additional level of complication and will be discussed further in the subsequent section.

Patch clamp electrophysiology is considered to be the "gold standard" *in vitro* format for assessing the potential for a drug candidate to interact with an ion channel. As with binding assays, multiple concentrations of a test compound are tested in order to calculate an $IC_{50}$ value. The advantage of patch clamp electrophysiology assay data is the functional endpoint. While data from a binding assay will only indicate that a candidate drug interacts with an ion channel, patch clamp electrophysiology data offers information about alterations to the ion channel current resulting from that interaction. In terms of understanding the potential for a drug candidate to prolong the QT interval, patch clamp electrophysiology is described in ICH S7B as an acceptable method from a regulatory perspective. Additionally, retrospective analysis has shown that data from patch clamp electrophysiology studies and an

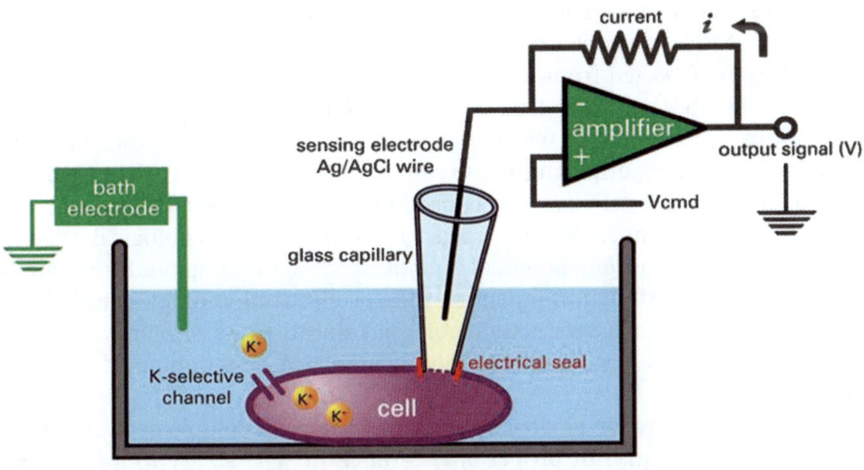


**Figure 8.3** Patch clamp assay schematic reproduced from http://www.discoverymedicine.com/Jeffrey-J-Clare/2010/03/24/targeting-ion-channels-for-drug-discovery/ (with permission from Discovery Medicine).

understanding of therapeutic plasma concentration are sufficient to predict for drug-induced QT prolongation and TdP in humans.[7]

Patch clamp assays have traditionally required a skill, trained operator. To perform the assay, negative pressure vacuum is applied to a portion of the cell membrane (the "patch") using a micropipette (Figure 8.3). Once a high-resistance seal, referred to as a gigaseal, is formed between the micropipette and the membrane, an electrode is placed inside the micropipette to record the current generated across the membrane patch. In order to determine the effects of a drug candidate on the ion channel current, the test compounds can be added to the buffer solution and alterations to the current recorded. The time-consuming and labor-intensive nature of this format has prevented its wide-spread use in early drug development and prompted the use of the high-throughput binding assays as described above. More recently, advances in engineering and robotics have resulted in the development of instruments which allow for the automation of patch clamp assays. Initial uptake of the automated platform was limited by the high capital cost for equipment and low assay success rates due to difficulties encountered with automated generation of an effective gigaseal. Second-generation automation instruments have increased both the throughput and the success rate using this platform by enabling the formation of multiple gigaseals per well on a multiwell plate.[8]

## 8.4 *Ex Vivo* Preparation Assays

Electrophysiological techniques can also be employed to investigate drug candidate effects on the entire concert of cardiac ion channels. Action potential duration (APD) is commonly assessed in isolated Purkinje fibers or ventricular wedge preparations. Studies validating these assay with known proarrhythmic drugs have found a strong correlation between the *in vitro* data and *in vivo* effects.[9–11] APD assays can be performed using Purkinje fibers isolated from hearts freshly dissected from rabbits, pigs, or dogs. Fibers are placed in buffer inside a chamber with electrodes at either end. The fibers themselves are attached to microelectrodes which measure the net voltage across each fiber. An illustration of the experimental set-up can be seen in Figure 8.4.[12] The fibers are placed in solutions with various concentrations of the test compound, and voltage across the fibers are recorded to assess electrophysiological changes such as resting membrane potential, amplitude of action potential rise, rate of rise, and duration of action potential. Similar electrophysiological techniques can be employed to assess action potential duration *ex vivo* in ventricular wedge preparations, *e.g.*, in a transmural sample of tissue obtained from the ventricle wall.

APD assays allow for *in vitro* assessment of the full complement of cardiac ion channels necessary for proper *in vivo* function. The ability to monitor the effect of a drug candidate on the action potential duration, representing the integrated output of cardiac sodium, calcium and potassium channels, is a distinct advantage of using an *ex vivo* assay format. Due to the use of freshly

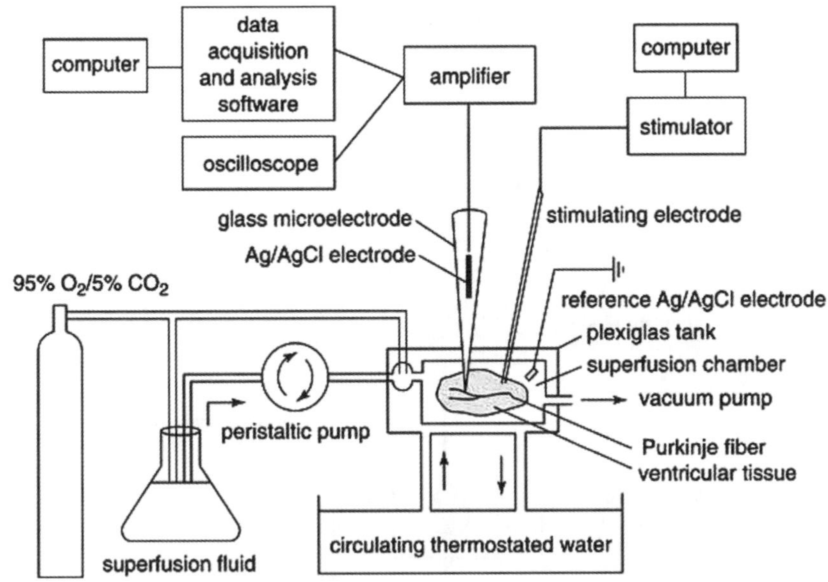


**Figure 8.4** Purkinje Fiber assay schematic. Reproduced from ref. 9 with permission. Copyright John Wiley & Sons, 2006.

isolated tissue and the time-consuming, labor-intensive manual electrophysiology recordings required, the APD assay is generally positioned as a second-tier assay when employed in drug development. Binding to an ion channel or changes in ion channel current observed in a first-tier assay may necessitate further investigation in an *ex vivo* preparation assay in order to determine if the earlier observations translate to alterations to the integrated action potential.

## 8.5 Langendorff Preparation

The isolated perfused heart, or Langendorff preparation, utilizes the entire heart (usually rabbit, guinea pig, or mouse), which, once isolated from the body of the animal, will continue to function for several hours. In addition to electrophysiologic data, the Langendorff heart model provides information about cardiac rhythm, mechanical parameters including contractility of the myocardium, and coronary pressure.[13] This assay was developed by Oskar Langendorff, a German physiologist, in the late 1800s and has been a valuable model in drug development for over a century.

This *ex vivo* preparation consists of an intact heart, blood vessels severed, attached to a stand with perfusion tubes attached. Oxygenated buffer is perfused into the heart through a cannula in the aorta (Figure 8.5).[14] After a calibration period that allows the heart to pump and flush the buffer through,

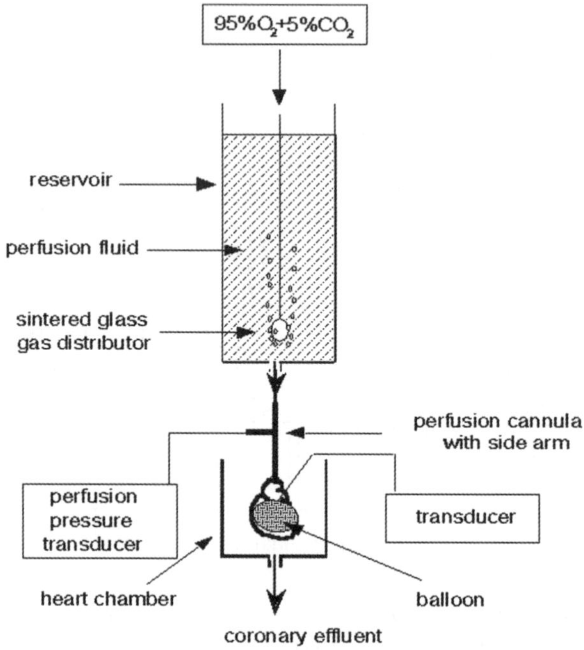


**Figure 8.5** Langendorff perfused heart model schematic. Reproduced from ref. 14 with permission. Copyright Elsevier, 2000.

increasing concentrations of the test compound are introduced into the buffer for 30–45 minutes each, and ECG tracings, contractility, coronary flow, and voltage data are recorded while the heart continues to beat. This assay is a comprehensive way of examining how a test article may acutely affect the function of the heart.

However, effects of chronic exposure cannot be assessed with this model due to the limited viability of the *ex vivo* preparation. Additionally, the model lacks the innervation and hormonal complication present in an intact animal model.

## 8.6 Isolated Cardiomyocyte Assays

Just as the black box warnings and drug withdrawals due to QT prolongation, TdP and sudden death drove development and use of ion channel assays, the need for a format amenable to performing studies to investigate drug-induced cardiotoxicity was demonstrated, in particular, by cardiotoxicity observed with agents targeting tyrosine kinase receptors.[15] Left ventricular dysfunction and congestive heart failure observed following clinical administration of drugs from this class prompted investigative studies which revealed a direct cytotoxic effect on cardiomyocytes. As cardiomyocytes have limited capacity for cell division and, therefore, limited ability for tissue repair, direct toxicity to cardiomyocytes has severe downstream consequences. Apoptotic or necrotic cardiomyocytes are replaced by fibrosis and leave the cardiac muscle with reduced contractility, the consequence of which is reduced cardiac output. Following these clinical observations and mechanistic studies, assays utilizing freshly isolated cardiomyocytes have been employed in drug development to investigate potential direct cardiotoxic effects of drug candidates.[16]

Freshly isolated rat neonatal cardiomyocytes have been employed to examine direct toxic effects through quantification of lactate dehydrogenase (LDH) activity levels in cardiomyocytes following exposure to a drug candidate. Incorporating investigations of caspase activity or mitochondrial membrane potential in *in vitro* cardiomyocyte assays may offer additional mechanistic information.

To examine electrophysiological effects in cardiomyocytes, the cells are patched into a patch clamp assay and treated as described above to investigate changes action potential duration (APD) across the cells. Researchers also use cardiomyocytes to predict for occurrence of EADs in response to treatment with test articles, which would predict for the potential of TdP *in vivo*.[17,18]

## 8.7 Conclusions

*In vitro* cardiac assays are essential in predicting cardiotoxicity liability and understanding the mechanism of observed cardiotoxicity of drug candidates. Researchers can employ ion channel binding assays, electrophysiology assays on single ion channels or *ex vivo* tissue preparations, Langendorff preparations and cardiomyocyte assays alone or in tandem to assess electrophysiological changes, direct cytotoxic effects and changes in contractility or cardiac output. Many studies have examined the correlation between *in vitro* and *in vivo* cardiovascular assay results and have found high concordance between *in vivo* assay data and *in vivo* observations;[19] these assays are important tools in drug safety evaluation. The *in vitro* assays discussed in this chapter are a great starting point for any cardiac investigation and can reveal important cardiotoxicities that should be investigated further and monitored closely as development proceeds.

## Acknowledgements

The authors would like to thank Dr. Craig Fisher for his assistance in obtaining reprint permissions for the figures used in this chapter.

## References

1. *S7A: Safety pharmacology studies for human pharmaceuticals*, International Conference on Harmonisation, Geneva, Switzerland, 2001.

2. *S7B: The non-clinical evaluation of the potential for delayed ventricular repolarization (QT interval prolongation) by human pharmaceuticals*, International Conference on Harmonisation, Geneva, Switzerland, 2005.
3. Y. Cheng and W. H. Prusoff, *Biochem. Pharmacol.*, 1973, **22**, 3099–3108.
4. L. Priebe and D. J. Beuckelmann, *Circ. Res.*, 1998, **82**, 1206–1223.
5. A. Hodgkin and A. Huxley, *J. Physiol.*, 1952, **117**, 500–544.
6. E. Neher, B. Sakmann and J. H. Steinbach, *European J. Physiol.*, 1978, **375**, 219–228.
7. W. S. Redfern, L. Carlsson, A. S. Davis, W. G. Lynch, I. MacKenzie, S. Palethorpe, P. K. Siegl, I. Strang, A. T. Sullivan, R. Wallis, A. J. Camm and T. G. Hammond, *Cardiol. Res.*, 2003, **58**, 32–45.
8. C. Möller and M. Slack, *Drug Discov. Today*, 2010, **15**, 334–390.
9. M. Aubert, R. Sterwalder, B. Wagner, I. Parrilla, I. Cavero, L. Doessegger and E. A. Ertel, *Drug Safety*, 2006, **29**(3), 237–254.
10. T. Liu, B. S. Brown, Y. Wu, C. Antzelevitch, P. R. Kowey and G. X. Yan, *Heart Rhythm*, 2006, **3**(8), 948–956.
11. G. A. Gintant, J. T. Limberis, J. S. McDermott, C. D. Wegner and B. F. Cox, *J. Cardiovasc. Pharmacol.*, 2001, **37**, 607–618.
12. S. Picard, S. Goineau and R. Rouet, *Current Protocols in Pharmacology*, John Wiley & Sons, Hoboken, NJ, 2006.
13. H. J. Döring, *Physiol. Bohemoslov.*, 1990, **39**, 481–504.
14. F. Sutherland and D. J. Hearse, *Pharmacol. Res.*, 2000, **41**, 613–627.
15. T. Force, D. S. Krause and R. A. Van Etten, *Nat. Rev. Cancer*, 2007, **7**, 332–344.
16. T. Inoue, K. Tanaka, M. Mishima and K. Watanabe, *AATEX*, 2007, **14**, 457–462.
17. J. Q. He, Y. Ma, Y. Lee, J. A. Thomson and T. J. Kamp, *Circ. Res.*, 2003, **93**, 32–39.
18. Y. M. Zhang, C. Hartzell, M. Narlow and S. C. Dudley, *Circulation*, 2002, **106**, 1294–1299.
19. T. Meyer, P. Sartipy, F. Blind, C. Leisgen and E. Guenther, *Expert Opin. Drug Metab. Toxicol.*, 2007, **3**, 507–517.

CHAPTER 9

# In Vitro *Approaches for Determining Liver-Specific Toxicity of New Drug Candidates*

JAMES M. McKIM JR

CeeTox Inc., 4717 Campus Drive, Kalamazoo, MI 49008, USA

## 9.1 Introduction

It is now generally accepted among pharmaceutical scientists that early drug-discovery research efforts should not only identify and optimize new chemical entities for the desired or druggable properties, but should also identify toxicity. The assessment of compound liabilities includes those related to the intended target and adverse effects related to the unique chemistry of the molecule (off-target). Early efforts to identify compound toxicity typically focus on the relative cytotoxicity of chemical hits in animal-derived immortalized cell lines. Data from these screening models can provide information on relative toxicity between molecules. More importantly, the data obtained can provide a means of relating the *in vitro* exposure concentrations that cause adverse effects to the maximum plasma concentrations required *in vivo* for efficacy. In addition, information on the mechanisms underlying the adverse effects can also be obtained. Although this type of information is useful for determining the toxic liability of a scaffold, rank-ordering hits, determining an *in vitro* margin of safety and guiding structure–activity relationships (SARs), it does not provide information on organ-specific toxicity in humans. Promising new drug candidates are often dropped from development due to kidney, heart, or liver specific

RSC Drug Discovery Series No. 12
New Horizons in Predictive Toxicology: Current Status and Application
Edited by Alan G. E. Wilson

Published by the Royal Society of Chemistry, www.rsc.org

toxicity. Many drugs that have made it to market have been withdrawn due to unanticipated organ specific toxicity. Identifying overt toxicity is not nearly as challenging as identifying risk profiles that will result in severe organ specific toxicity in a small patient population. *In vitro* systems that can accurately identify organ specific toxicity would be of great value. Models capable of predicting human organ specific toxicity are complex to build and cannot be achieved by simply adding a test drug to liver, kidney, or heart cells and measuring viability. In order for an *in vitro* cell model to be organ specific it must possess the anatomical, physiological, and biochemical properties that characterize the organ of interest. At least some of the endpoints measured *in vitro* must be specific to the organ of interest. After more than a decade of trying to predict *in vivo* risk with *in vitro* data it is clear that *in vitro* models add the most predictive power when several types of *in vitro* data are linked in a tiered approach to toxicity screening. This integrative approach should include an *in vivo* anchor, such as the maximum therapeutic plasma concentration (whether measured or estimated) to be sure that the data obtained with *in vitro* models was done within the boundaries of expected clinical use. This chapter will focus on *in vitro* systems that can provide a true indication of human liver specific toxicity.

## 9.2 Understanding Liver Structure, Cell Types, and Function

A prerequisite to the development of an *in vitro* model capable of assessing liver specific toxicity is to understand the normal structure, function, and biochemistry of this organ as it is *in vivo*. In other words, it is important to know and understand the unique properties that make a liver, a liver. The liver is the largest gland in the body and is located below the diaphragm and anterior to the stomach. It receives blood from the gastrointestinal system *via* the portal vein and blood from systemic circulation by the hepatic artery. Orally administered drugs are absorbed into the portal system and delivered to the liver before they enter general circulation (Figure 9.1). The liver consists of functional units known as the liver lobules. This multifunctional organ is responsible for many essential biochemical processes and is a primary target organ of toxicity for many orally administered drugs.

### 9.2.1 Structure

Structurally, the human liver consists of two wedge-shaped lobes with the right lobe being slightly larger than the left lobe. As mentioned above, blood enters the liver by two vessels, the hepatic portal vein, which carries dissolved nutrients derived from digestion of food in the gut, and the hepatic artery, which brings oxygenated blood from the lungs. Blood flows from the hepatic artery and portal vein to the hepatic central vein through sinusoids. Blood collected in the hepatic central vein then enters general circulation. Two ducts originate in

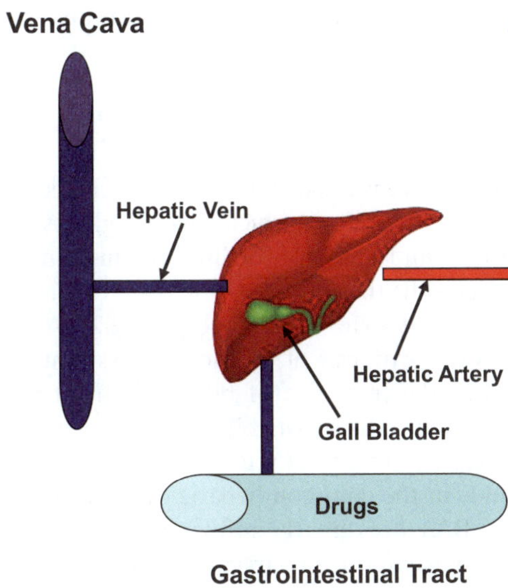


**Figure 9.1** Anatomical location of liver and blood flow.

the liver and these come together to form the common hepatic duct, which empties into the duodenum of the small intestine. Bile is formed by liver cells and stored in the gall bladder located under the liver. Each lobe of the liver is divided into many lobules about the size of a pin head. Each lobule contains several types of cells, connected with bile and blood channels. The entire liver is permeated with a network of blood, bile, and lymph capillaries.

### 9.2.2 Cell Types and their Roles

There are five main types of cells found in the liver; parenchymal (hepatocytes) and non-parenchymal, which include sinusoidal endothelial cells (SECs), kupffer cells, and stellate cells. The non-parenchymal cells are all found in the sinusoidal compartment. In addition, there are intrahepatic lymphocytes (IHL) also known as liver-specific natural killer cells or pit cells which can be found in the sinusoidal lumen. Hepatocytes comprise about 80% of the liver volume and perform nearly all of the biochemical functions associated with this organ. The non-parenchymal cells only comprise about 6.5% of the liver's volume, but represent 40% of the total number of cells. It is now well known that under both normal, as well as pathological conditions the substances released from non-parenchymal cells can impact many hepatic functions carried out in neighboring parenchymal cells. This means that non-parenchymal cells in the liver also have a pronounced impact on the development of liver toxicity following exposure to endogenous and exogenous compounds. Therefore, before discussing the various *in vitro* models for evaluating the effects of drugs and chemicals on the liver, it is important to have a general understanding of liver anatomy and function.

### 9.2.3 Liver Parenchymal Cells (Hepatocytes)

The parenchymal cell of the liver is the hepatocyte; this cell performs nearly all of the biochemical functions of the liver, which include glucose regulation, cholesterol synthesis, synthesis and secretion of lipoproteins, and fat metabolism. Hepatocytes are polygonal cells that join to form borders that face the sinusoid (basolateral) or adjacent hepatocytes (apical) (Figure 9.2). An important function of the hepatocyte is the synthesis of bile acids (BAs) and the formation of bile. Bile flow begins with the transport of bile acids from the cytosol of the hepatocyte into the bile canaliculus by the bile salt export pump (BSEP) or the multidrug resistant associated protein 2 (MRP2). Bile movement continues into the bile ductules and ends in the common hepatic duct outside of the liver.

Influx and efflux of BAs are greatly influenced by transporter proteins located on either the basolateral or apical surfaces (Figure 9.3). These

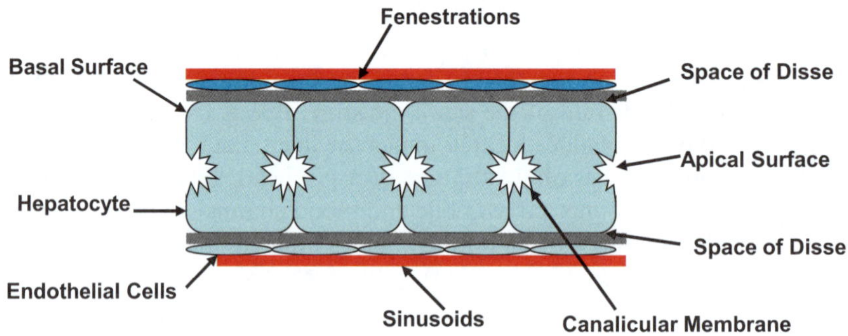


**Figure 9.2** Orientation of liver cells.

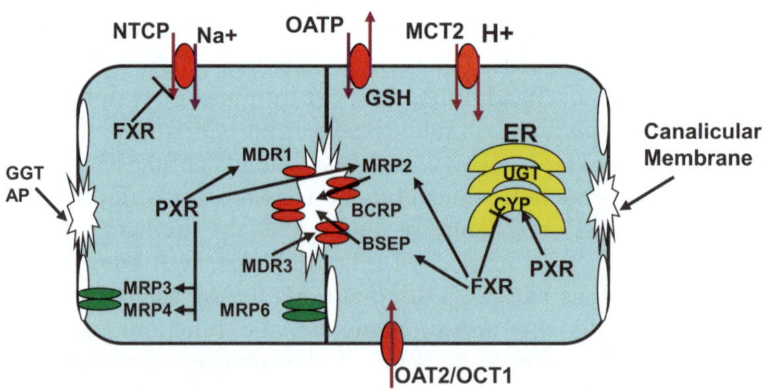


**Figure 9.3** Diagrammatic representation of hepatic transporter location, effects of FXR, and PXR activation.

transporters as well as cytochrome P450 (CYP) metabolizing enzymes (*e.g.*, CYP7A1 and CYP3A4) in the hepatocyte control BA synthesis, metabolism, and uptake from blood (NTCP), and movement into bile (BSEP, MRP) (Figure 9.3).

Maintaining the balance of BA concentration in the hepatocyte is critical for the formation of bile, and for the protection of the liver from toxicity. There are two primary bile acids formed in the hepatocyte, cholic acid (CA) and chenodeoxycholic acid (CDCA), as well as two derivatives [deoxycholic acid (DCA) and lithocholic acid (LCA)] known as secondary bile acids. The toxicity of BAs is inversely related to the number of hydroxyl groups (Figure 9.4).

Under normal conditions, BAs synthesized in the liver are metabolized by cytochrome P450 enzymes, conjugated by UDP-glucuronosyl transferases (UGT1A1) with glucuronic acid and pumped across the canalicular membrane by BSEP or MRP2. If the elimination of bile acids from the liver is inhibited by drugs, toxic BAs, such as LCA, can accumulate and cause liver toxicity. Stress induced by disease, drugs, or chemicals can cause changes in the relative abundance or activity of these important proteins, which then disrupts hepatic BA homeostasis.

When bile acid concentration increases in the liver, the BAs bind and activate the FXR, which can then mediate the expression of several transporter proteins and enzymes. FXR activation downregulates CYP7A1 and NTCP and upregulates BSEP and MRP2 (Figure 9.3). The consequence of this is that hepatic accumulation of BAs *via* CYP7A1-mediated biosynthesis from cholesterol and uptake of BAs from sinusoidal blood by NTCP are reduced. Bile acids can also increase the expression and activation of pregnane-X receptor (PXR).

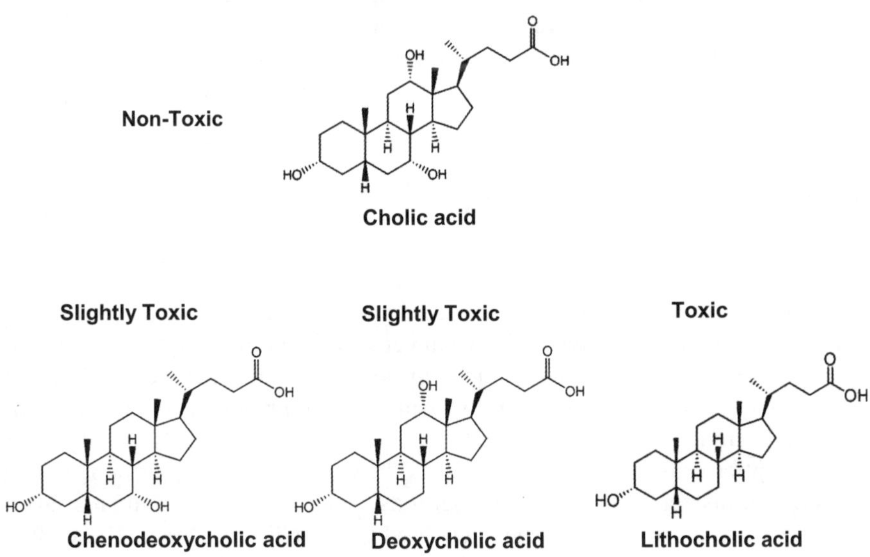


**Figure 9.4** Molecular structures of bile acids.

Activation of PXR causes an increase in CYP3A4 expression and activity, an increase in MRP2, MRP3, and MRP4 expression, and an increase in MDR1. CYP3A metabolizes BAs, while MRP transporters move BAs out of the hepatocyte.

The hepatic toxicity of drugs and chemicals can be greatly affected by the effects they exert on bile flow. Exogenous drugs or chemicals that inhibit efflux transporters or UGT1A1-mediated conjugation of BAs can cause cholestasis, resulting in an increase in the intracellular concentration of BAs and liver toxicity. In this example, toxicity is not directly caused by the drug or chemical, but by its affect on endogenous homeostatic systems. Some drugs are substrates for efflux pumps and are eliminated from the hepatocyte in bile. Drugs that are eliminated in bile enter the gut where they can be eliminated from the body in feces or de-conjugated by alkaline pH or bacterial glucuronidases. De-conjugation leads to reuptake of parent drug and to enterohepatic circulation. When the administration of a drug alters the pharmacokinetics or toxicity of a drug already in the system the effect is called a drug–drug interaction (DDI). Drug-induced changes in transporter activity or relative abundance is the cause of many DDIs.

Drugs or chemicals can be removed from the liver by transport into the biliary tree and subsequent elimination in bile, or by transport into blood for elimination in urine. Transporters that move compounds from the hepatocyte into the canaliculi include BSEP, MRP2, and the multidrug-resistance proteins MDR1, MDR2, and MDR3. Exposure to exogenous compounds can induce the expression of these transporters, which is mediated through the nuclear transcription factor PXR.[1]

Hepatocytes are in close proximity to blood circulation due to a complex network of microvesicles known as the sinusoids, which carry blood from the hepatic artery and portal vein to the central vein. This provides an ideal mechanism by which the liver can regulate blood glucose, fatty acids, lipoproteins, cholesterol, and the metabolism of endogenous and exogenous chemicals.

## 9.2.4 Non-Parenchymal Cells

### *9.2.4.1 Kupffer Cells*

Kupffer cells are macrophages that are located within the sinusoidal lumen anchored on or between the endothelial cells. Morphologically, these cells are characterized by an irregular shape, intracytoplasmic vacuoles, lysosomes, phagosomes, a well-developed endoplasmic reticulum, Golgi complexes, and vesicles all indicating that these cells possess endocytotic and secretory functions. Kupffer cells can be identified and differentiated from other hepatic cells by endogenous peroxidase staining methods.[2,3] They respond to inflammatory stimuli by proliferating, and when activated these cells secrete cytokines which can have significant effects on the liver hepatocyte and hence on total liver health and function.[4]

Alcohol toxicity is a good example of how kupffer cells can mediate overall liver toxicity. Chronic exposure to alcohol leads to the formation of acetaldehyde and an increase in fatty acids. There is also an increase in CYP2E1 expression and activity, leading to the hypothesis that CYP2E1 was responsible for the observed toxic responses. Gadolinium chloride ($GdCl_2$) transiently kills hepatic kupffer cells. When rats were exposed to $GdCl_2$ prior to alcohol there was still the expected increase in CYP2E1, but the liver toxicity associated with alcohol exposure was not observed when kupffer cells were not present.[5] These findings clearly separated the induction of CYP2E1 from at least part of the alcohol-induced liver toxicity and demonstrated the important role that kupffer cells can have on liver health.

The administration of some drugs and biologics can also alter kupffer cell function and affect liver health. In clinical trials the recombinant immunotoxin LMB-2, developed for the treatment of leukemia, caused significant liver toxicity. Investigations into the mechanism revealed that LMB-2 was concentrated in kupffer cells, which responded by producing high levels of the cytokine TNF-α. When induction of TNF-α was blocked, liver toxicity was reduced.[6]

Some drugs exhibit low toxicity under normal conditions, but become more toxic when the body is under stress. For example, in the presence of inflammation many drugs have more pronounced cytotoxicity. Activated kupffer cells can induce this inflammatory response. Drugs associated with gastrointestinal issues or those that were withdrawn because of liver toxicity (*e.g.*, troglitazone, phenylbutazone, diclofenac, and tolcapone) were considerably more toxic in the presence of inflammation, while the toxicity of drugs not associated with these issues was not affected.[7]

### *9.2.4.2 Endothelial Cells*

SECs possess fenestrations, or pores, with an average diameter of 150–175 nm. Endothelial cells have three primary functions: 1) filtration of particles, 2) endocytosis, and 3) secretion of bioactive factors. The fenestrations found in endothelial cells function like a sieve that enables transport and exchange of materials between the blood and the hepatocyte, while preventing larger molecules from passing. As a result, only particles that are smaller than 0.2 μm, such as chylomicron remnants, can pass through this sieve system. These small chylomicron particles are rich in cholesterol and pass into the space of Disse where they can be absorbed by the hepatocytes. Endothelial cells are also actively involved in three types of endocytotic processes: fluid phase pinocytosis, adsorptive non-receptor mediated pinocytosis, and adsorptive receptor mediated pinocytosis. Endothelial cells secrete bioactive molecules, such as prostaglandin E2, prostacyclin, and cytokines, and participate in the synthesis of the extracellular matrix.[4,8,9]

Acute liver failure resulting from normally therapeutic doses of acetaminophen (APAP) has been observed clinically in chronic alcoholics.

The observed hepatic toxicity consists of hemorrhagic centrilobular necrosis and large increases in serum transaminases, which is preceded by centrilobular microvascular injury. Liver sinusoidal endothelial cells are important mediators of hepatic toxicity resulting from APAP exposure. SECs have been shown to be an early and sensitive target for APAP-mediated toxicity. This effect is enhanced *in situ*ations of pre-exposure to alcohol. As early as 30 min post APAP exposure, the SECs become swollen and lose their ability to endocytose. Within 2 h post treatment and prior to damage in the hepatocytes, there is damage to the fenestrae and disruption of the sieve properties of the SECs. This can lead to a collapse of the sinusoid and a reduction in blood flow. Similar events are observed in early stages of hepatic venooclusive disease.[10] When eNOS was inhibited the toxicity increased, but when iNOS was inhibited the amount of injury was reduced. These data indicate a protective role for constitutive nitric oxide (NO) produced by SECs.

Hepatic venooclusive disease (HVOD) can occur in patients on long-term immunosuppressive therapy following a kidney or liver transplant. The immunosuppressive drug azathioprine has been associated with HVOD, sinusoidal dilation, sinusoidal fibrosis, and hyperplasia. All of these lesions may be linked to SEC damage resulting in disruption of hepatic circulation in the sinusoids. Azathioprine undergoes extensive metabolism in the intestine and liver by glutathione-*S*-transferase to 6-mercaptopurine, resulting in a dramatic decrease in liver glutathione (GSH) levels.[11] *In vitro*, azathioprine appears more toxic to SECs than to hepatocytes. Toxicity in both SECs and hepatocytes is related to cellular GSH levels (Figure 9.5). This was demonstrated by first depleting the cells of GSH with buthionine sulphoximine (BSO) exposure and then treating with drug. Under these conditions the drug was considerably more toxic. Protection of SECs to azathioprine exposure is conferred by GSH. Therefore, a key cytoprotective mechanism for SECs is their GSH-defense system.[12] These findings are in agreement with those observed following APAP exposure. APAP is metabolized to a reactive intermediate which can then be conjugated to GSH (Figure 9.6). SECs are sensitive to APAP and APAP can cause a sequence of events leading to HVOD.

#### *9.2.4.3 Stellate or Fat-Storing Cells*

Hepatic stellate cells (HSCs) also called Ito cells are located in the space of Disse between the sinusoids and the hepatocyte. In normal liver these cells represent about 5–8% of the total number of liver cells. HSCs have long protrusions that wrap around the sinusoids and are characterized by the storage of fat, which contains vitamin A (Figure 9.7). In their inactive state, these cells are believed to function as lipid antigen presenting cells, which stimulate the proliferation of natural killer cells.[13] Histologically, HSCs can be identified by the presence of fat droplets, gold chloride staining, or the expression of reelin.[14,15]

Damage to the liver can result in the activation of stellate cells. This is characterized by proliferation, loss of vitamin A, chemotaxis, and the secretion

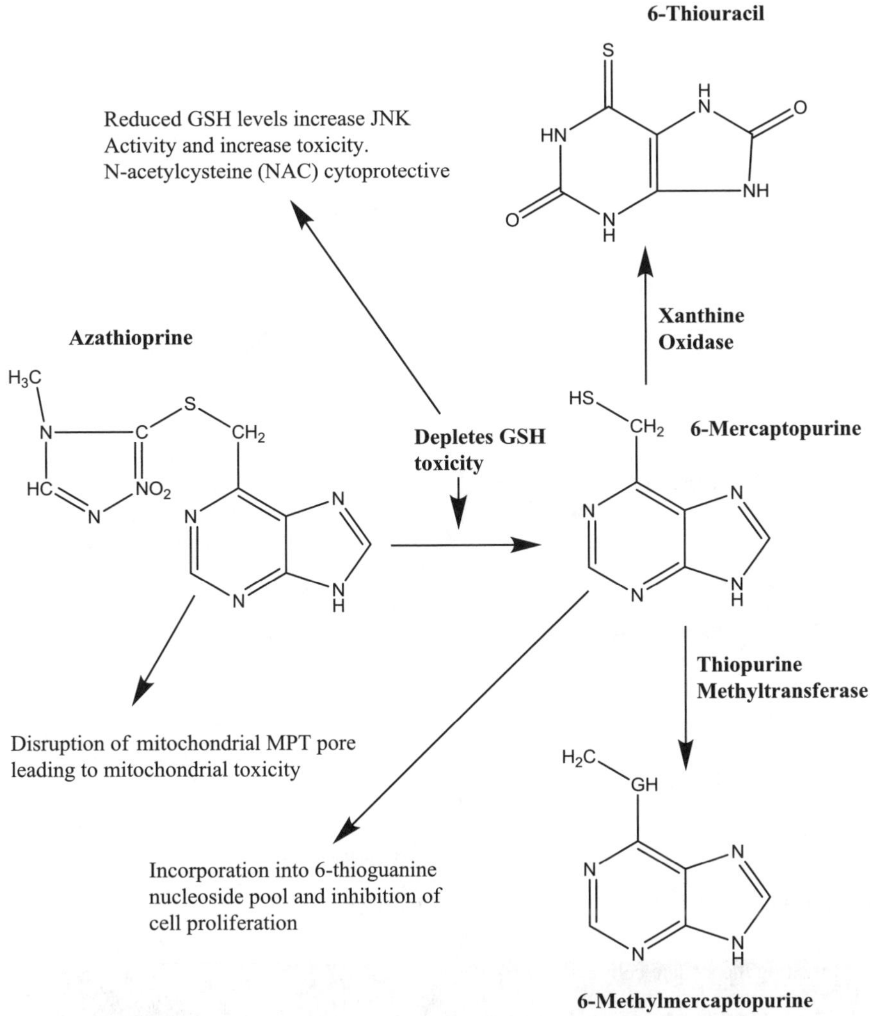


**Figure 9.5** Metabolic activation and cytotoxicity of azathioprine.

of collagen scar tissue (fibrosis) leading to the more chronic end-stage situation of liver cirrhosis.

Although several of the liver cell types discussed participate in the development of liver fibrosis, HSCs are especially important in this process because of their ability to secrete collagen, regulate vascular tone, and secrete inflammatory mediators such as transforming growth factor beta (TGF-β) and platelet-derived growth factor (PDGF). At some point in the fibrogenic process the stellate cells become regulated by an autocrine loop and as such begin to function independently of the other liver cells.[16] The crucial role that HSCs play in the development of liver fibrosis makes them important targets for new drugs designed to treat fibrotic liver disease.[17]

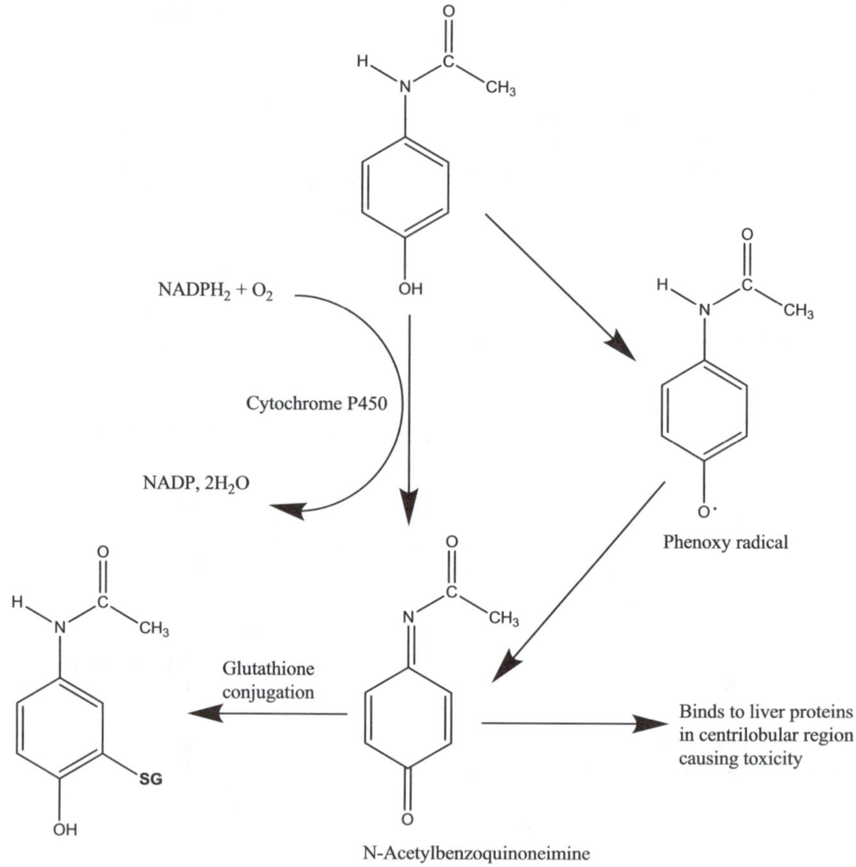


**Figure 9.6** Metabolic activation of acetaminophen.

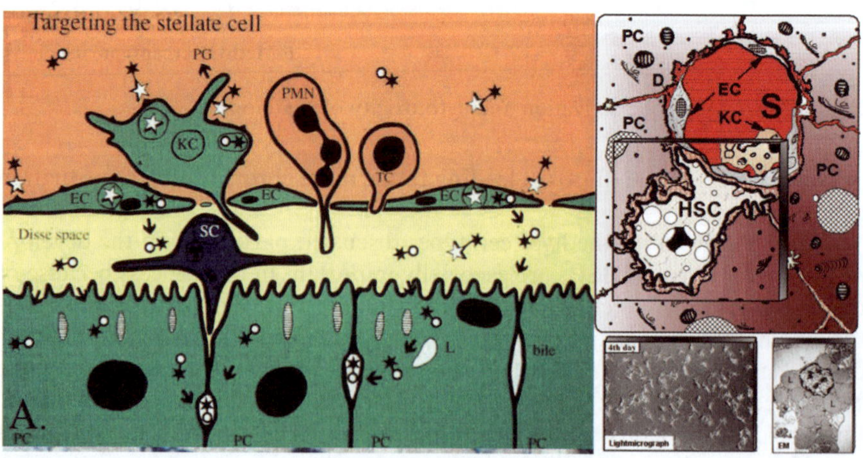


**Figure 9.7** Cell-to-cell communication in liver. Reproduced from ref. 16 with permission. Copyright Frontiers in Bioscience, 2002.

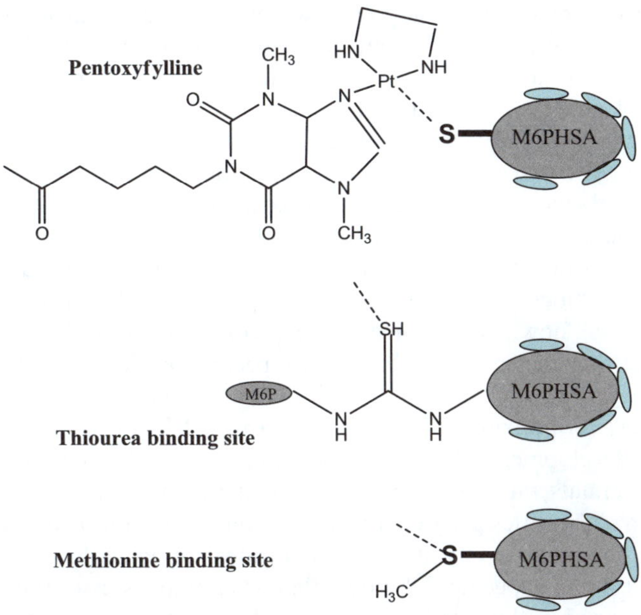


**Figure 9.8** Interaction of pentoxyfylline with M6PHSA. Reproduced from ref. 17 with permission. Copyright Elsevier Science Inc., 2006.

Activated HSCs are characterized by a high rate of proliferation and synthesis of extracellular matrix materials. Therefore, one strategy for the treatment of liver fibrosis is to deliver antiproliferative drugs to the stellate cells.[16] However, the location of HSCs in the liver has made it difficult to achieve efficacious drug concentrations in these target cells. To address this issue new anti-fibrotic drugs are being designed in a manner that specifically directs the drug to the HSC. Activated HSCs contain high levels of neoglycoprotein mannose-6-phosphate-albumin (M6PHSA). HSCs bind and take in M6PHSA *via* insulin-like growth factor II/mannose 6-phosphate receptor located in high abundance on activated HSCs. Thus, one approach to delivering more drug to HSCs involves linking the drug to M6PHSA, which then binds to the receptors on HSCs and is taken up by the cells.[17,18]

The anti-proliferative agent known as pentoxyfylline (PTX) inhibits HSC proliferation and activation *in vitro*. In order to improve efficacy *in vivo* the drug was linked to M6PHSA (Figure 9.8). Intracellular release of PTX is believed to be by competitive thiol displacement and not enzymatic activity.[17,19–21]

## 9.3 *In Vitro* Models That Predict Liver Specific Toxicity

Most *in vitro* models that use hepatocytes- or hepatoma-derived cell lines monitor cell viability, cell proliferation, mitochondrial function, apoptosis, and oxidative stress. These endpoints can provide important information on relative toxicity between drugs, but they are not specific to the liver and may not provide information on more subtle toxicity. In order for cell models to be predictive of adverse effects in a primary tissue or organ type, the endpoints monitored must be unique to that organ. Simply measuring membrane integrity with a leakage enzyme or mitochondrial function by ATP levels in a liver cell will not provide data that predicts liver specific toxicity. Organ-specific *in vitro* systems should mimic as closely as possible the cell type and functional structure of the intact organ. The liver is an important organ that carries out many different biochemical processes that impact the health of the entire body. This section will now discuss some of the *in vitro* models available and how to use the data they generate to predict liver specific toxicity.

Early drug-discovery programs rely heavily on standard safety studies done in rats, dogs, or monkeys. Therefore, *in vitro* models incorporated into early phases of development should provide predictive information on general toxicity in animals with less emphasis on predicting human toxicity. However, as new chemical entities progress to the candidate selection phase, just prior to beginning the animal safety studies, it is prudent to evaluate these lead compounds in a human specific cell model that accurately assesses the candidate's potential to produce human liver toxicity. These test systems should focus on mechanistic endpoints and more chronic effects, some of which may be mediated through mechanisms not present in the animal models.

Inter-species differences in metabolism are a major mechanism that describes why a compound that produces toxicity in a rodent safety study may not cause toxicity in humans. Conversely, this can also explain why compounds deemed safe based on animal testing may turn out to produce unacceptable toxicity in humans.

### 9.3.1 Dose and Systemic Exposure

An important consideration in the development of an *in vitro* screening strategy is the relationship between oral dose and systemic exposure, which can also be greatly affected by inter-species differences in metabolism. During the drug-development process, the risk associated with exposing humans to a new drug candidate is based on extrapolation of pre-clinical safety data obtained in rodents to humans. To be effective, this method relies on the assumption that the exposure–effect relationship across species remains constant. Exposing humans to doses that result in plasma concentrations not achieved in animal safety studies is unlikely, or is done with extreme caution. Therefore, in situations where rodent metabolism is much higher than human metabolism, basing human doses on multiples of animal data for clinical trials could result in much higher plasma concentrations in humans, which could result in toxicity. Species differences in metabolism and therefore differences in metabolite formation are common and must be considered when developing an *in vitro* approach. If one species metabolizes a drug or chemical *via* a pathway that results in a higher concentration of a reactive intermediate the result could be species-specific toxicity. It is therefore important to understand how a new drug or chemical is metabolized in commonly used test species (*e.g.*, rat, dog, and monkey) as well as humans.

### 9.3.2 Determining Species-Specific Metabolic Stability and Metabolic Activation

When a new drug is being evaluated for potential liver toxicity it is important to understand as early as possible how the drug is metabolized by rats, dogs, and humans. A comparison of the metabolic profiles obtained in each of these species can provide valuable information that can be used to guide subsequent experiments. The rate of metabolism determined with microsomes can provide an estimate of hepatic clearance and differences in metabolic rates can give hints into possible issues between species. In Figure 9.9, verapamil metabolism is compared in hepatic microsomes from mouse and human. Verapamil is metabolized more rapidly in the mouse than in humans. In this situation, if human doses were based on mouse kinetic data, plasma concentrations could reach levels that would produce toxicity. The narrower the therapeutic window the more important these data are for safety. Midazolam is also metabolized more rapidly in the mouse than in human microsomes. Metabolic stability data collected over several time points allow the determination of a half-life ($T_{1/2}$) *in vitro* and an estimate of hepatic clearance. Both values can be used to compare compounds in a therapeutic area. Metabolic profiles that are significantly different between species may indicate that one species may be more susceptible to liver toxicity than another.

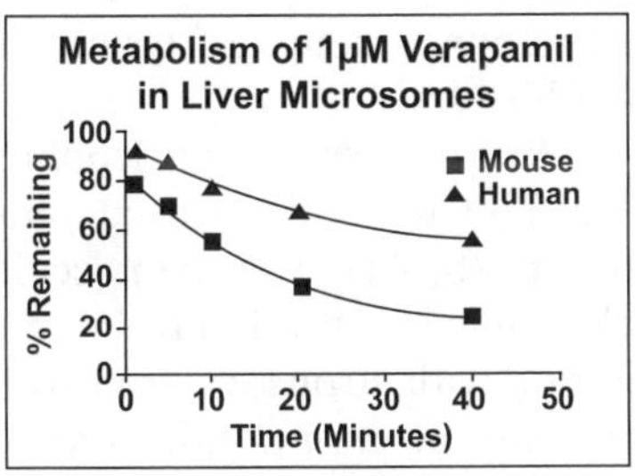


| | | $Cl_H$(ml/min/kg) | |
|---|---|---|---|
| | $T_{1/2}$(min) | Pred | Lit |
| Mouse | 22 | 73 | |
| Human | 52 | 15 | 19 |

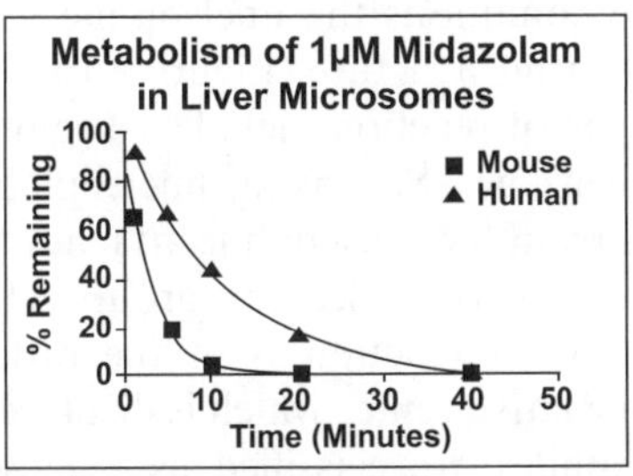


| | | $Cl_H$(ml/min/kg) | |
|---|---|---|---|
| | $T_{1/2}$(min) | Pred | Lit |
| Mouse | 3.1 | 87 | |
| Human | 6.8 | 20 | 8.7 |

**Figure 9.9** Determining hepatic half-life and clearance. Data provided by CeeTox, Inc. Kalamazoo, MI, USA. Pred = predicted value, Lit = reported value in the literature.

If either of these situations is detected it is important to determine whether any of the metabolites are reactive electrophiles.

### 9.3.3 Metabolic Activation Pathways

Drugs are eliminated from the body either as the unchanged parent molecule or as metabolites of the parent molecule. In most instances the metabolism of drugs and chemicals renders the molecule less reactive (*e.g.*, less toxic) and more water soluble. There are however many examples of drugs and chemicals that undergo metabolic conversion to electrophilic and highly reactive metabolites that have been linked to liver toxicity. A major concern with these reactive metabolites is that they are capable of binding to and forming covalent bonds with cellular nucleophiles, such as proteins, nucleic acids, and lipids. Irreversible covalent binding to proteins and DNA can lead to significant adverse effects.

Electrophiles are characterized as being electron-deficient chemicals capable of binding to nucleophiles (electron donors) by accepting electrons. Electrophiles and nucleophiles can be further defined as being either "hard" or "soft" depending on the polarizability of the electrophilc or nucleophilic center. In general, soft electrophiles are highly polarizable and bind to soft nucleophiles, while hard electrophiles have poorly polarizable centers and bind to hard nucleophiles. There is an abundance of nucleophilic sites in biological systems. These include nucleic acid polymers that contain S, N, and O atoms. Protein-based sites are soft electrophiles, while nucleic acid sites are defined as hard.[22,23] Examples of nucleophilic sites in cells and tissues with which soft electrophiles may react include the following in order of increasing hardness: 1) thiol of cysteine, 2) S atoms in methionine, 3) primary amino groups of lysine and arginine, and 4) the secondary amino groups of histidine.[23]

There are several types of reactions between electrophiles and nucleophiles and these reactions can span the continuum of soft to hard. Two common reactions are nucleophile aromatic substitution ($S_NAr$) and bimolecular nucleophilic substitution ($S_N2$). $S_NAr$ is a nucleophilic substitution reaction in which the electrophile consists of an aromatic ring with strong electron-withdrawing groups, such as nitro groups, in the *ortho*- or *para*-positions and a leaving group, such as a halide. Under these conditions the nucleophile displaces the leaving group and replaces it on the ring structure (Figure 9.10).

Examples of chemicals that undergo this type of reaction include 1-bromo-2,4-dinitrobenzene and 1-chloro-2,4-dinitrobenzene. $S_N2$ is a nucleophilic substitution reaction where a pair of electrons from the nucleophile attaches to an electron-deficient electrophilic center and displaces a leaving group. The most common chemical structure for this type of reaction is of the order $CH_2$–X, where "X" is a halide with an electronegative center which is displaced following a nucleophilic attack. Soft electrophiles are classified as reactive toxicants and bind with the greatest efficiency with strong soft-nucleophiles like GSH. Soft electrophiles are strongly polarizable and readily react with GSH. However, hard electrophiles have less affinity for GSH.[22,24]

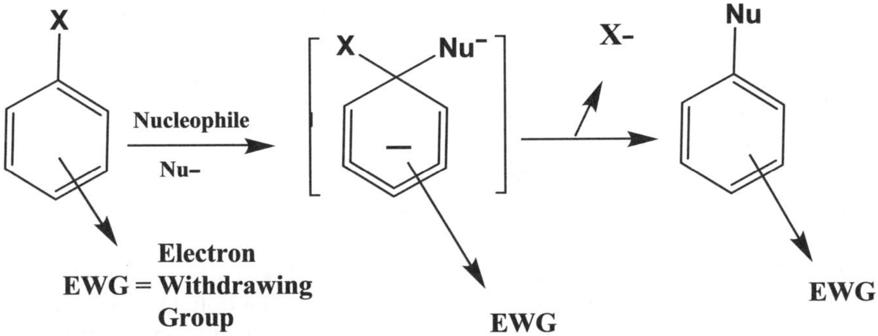


**Figure 9.10** Nucleophilic aromatic substitution.

The production of metabolites that are soft electrophiles is considered to be the most relevant to the development of adverse effects. Clearly, reactive molecules capable of binding to cellular macromolecules, such as DNA and proteins can lead to toxicity, but it is often unclear exactly which protein(s) is/are relevant to the observed toxicity. The importance of GSH conjugation in the detoxification of reactive molecules is based on the amount of type of electrophile formed. Metabolism of *N*,*N*-dimethyl-1,4-aminoazobenzene (DAB) yields a large quantity of soft electrophile which can directly bind to GSH. Because conjugation with GSH does not require enzymatic activity by glutathione *S*-transferase (GST), the amount of electrophile and the tissue concentrations of GSH would be expected to have a significant effect on toxicity.[24] Metabolism of acetaminophen yields a soft electrophile and therefore the GSH-conjugate 3-glutathione *S*-yl acetaminophen is an important detoxification step. The formation of strong soft electrophiles *via* metabolism in the liver results in a high amount of GSH conjugation. Conjugation can occur non-enzymatically or enzymatically when the electrophile is recognized as a substrate for GST. An important consideration is that when both enzymic and non-enzymic conjugation is occurring, there can be a significant depletion of cellular GSH. Although GSH levels in the hepatocyte can be as high as 10 mM, drugs or chemicals that deplete intracellular GSH by conjugation may increase the cells susceptibility to toxic insult if the GSH levels cannot be maintained. When GSH levels fall below a critical level, intracellular oxidative stress is likely to occur *via* an increase in reactive oxygen species such as superoxide anion, hydroxyl radicals, and lipid radicals.

## 9.4 *In Vitro* Models for Identifying Reactive Metabolites

Identifying whether a new drug candidate undergoes metabolic conversion to reactive intermediates is important for assessing potential human toxicity. Moreover, whenever possible the species of electrophile should be identified.

Because strong soft electrophiles react quickly and efficiently with GSH, a simple method of assessing bioactivation is by measuring GSH depletion in the presence and absence of metabolizing enzymes. The ratio of GSH depletion in the absence of enzymes relative to GSH depletion in the presence of human or rat liver microsomes (HLM/RLM) provides an indication of reactivity associated with parent *versus* metabolite. This assay provides information on inherent reactivity of the parent molecule and determines if the parent can be metabolized to a reactive intermediate that binds GSH.[25–27]

*In vitro* cell models that use primary hepatocytes or hepatic cell lines should evaluate intracellular GSH levels. If a significant depletion in GSH occurs independently of cell death or reduced cell proliferation the mechanisms of depletion should be investigated. There are four primary mechanisms by which GSH may be depleted and these include: 1) non-enzymatic conjugation, 2) enzymatic conjugation, 3) inhibition of GSH synthesis, and 4) increased oxidative stress and oxidation to glutathione disulfide (GSSG). The determination of non-enzymatic conjugation of GSH to a new drug can be done in a cell-free buffer that includes known amounts of GSH and test compound. Following an incubation period, the amount of unbound (free) GSH remaining may be determined by standard methods.[25,28] The enzymatic formation of GSH–drug conjugates can be determined using HLM or RLM preparations or primary hepatocytes. In this context enzymatic applies to the Phase I activation of the parent molecule, which may increase its reactivity and hence its binding to GSH, and Phase II reactions with GST, which enhances the rate of GSH conjugation either to the parent molecule or its metabolites.

The parent drug and its metabolites are then analyzed by LC-MS/MS or LC-MS to identify GS–drug Metabolites. This approach was used to understand the metabolic activation of diclofenac.[29] Diclofenac is a non-steroidal anti-inflammatory (NSAID) drug and is one of the most prescribed NSAIDS in the world. The drug has been linked to more than 200 cases of hepatocellular damage. About 10% of these cases progressed to more severe liver toxicity ending with acute liver failure and death.[30–32] Hepatoxicity resulting from diclofenac is multifaceted and includes disruption of the mitochondrial membrane potential, depletion of NADPH, metabolic activation, and protein adduct formation. Diclofenac undergoes redox cycling between 5-hydroxydiclofenac and *N*,5-dihydroxydiclofenac, which further depletes the NADPH pool.[33]

Diclofenac is extensively metabolized in rat and human liver, however, the metabolites formed and the cytochrome P450 enzymes responsible vary between species. In rats, CYP2C11 converts diclofenac to a highly reactive metabolite, which covalently binds to CYP2C11. In humans, CYP2C9 metabolism of diclofenac represents the major route of metabolism forming 4-hydroxydeclofenac *via* a reactive quinone imine intermediate at low concentrations ($K_m = 4–6\ \mu M$). However, this pathway does not appear to produce a measurable increase in protein adduct formation because when inhibited there is no change in adduct formation. At high concentrations, diclofenac is metabolized by human CYP3A4 to form 5-hydroxydiclofenac and a reactive quinone imine with $K_m > 80\ \mu M$. If CYP3A4 is inhibited, protein adduct formation is prevented. It is believed that cellular decomposition of 5-hydroxydiclofenac by a metal-catalyzed oxidation produces *p*-benzoquinone imine, which is highly reactive and is ultimately responsible for increased adduct formation (Figure 9.11). Individuals who have compromised cellular defense mechanisms, such as low levels of NADPH, or GSH are more susceptible to diclofenac toxicity.[34]

Glutathione is a small tripeptide consisting of glutamate, cysteine, and glycine. It is present in most tissues at high concentrations and is essential for maintaining the redox balance of cells.[35] The reduced form of GSH is capable of binding to soft electrophiles and is the primary antioxidant defense mechanism of the liver, lung, and many other tissues and organs. Under normal conditions, the liver as well as other tissues, synthesize GSH in a two step enzymatic reaction (Figure 9.12). The first and rate-limiting step is the

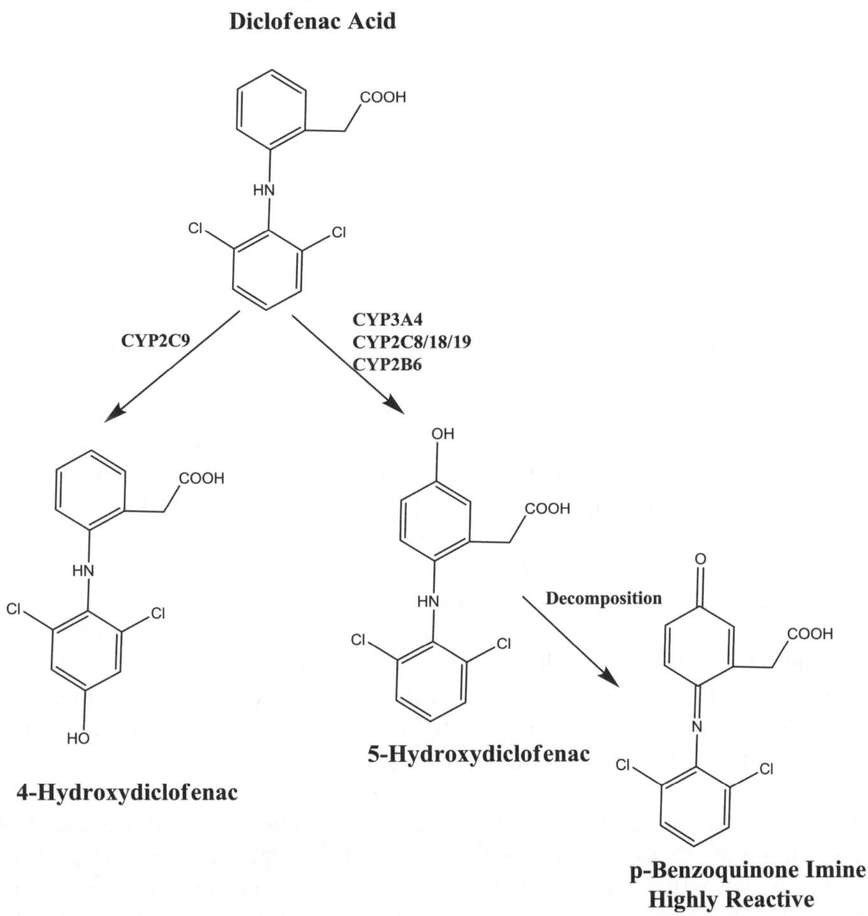


**Figure 9.11** Proposed metabolic pathways of diclofenac in humans.

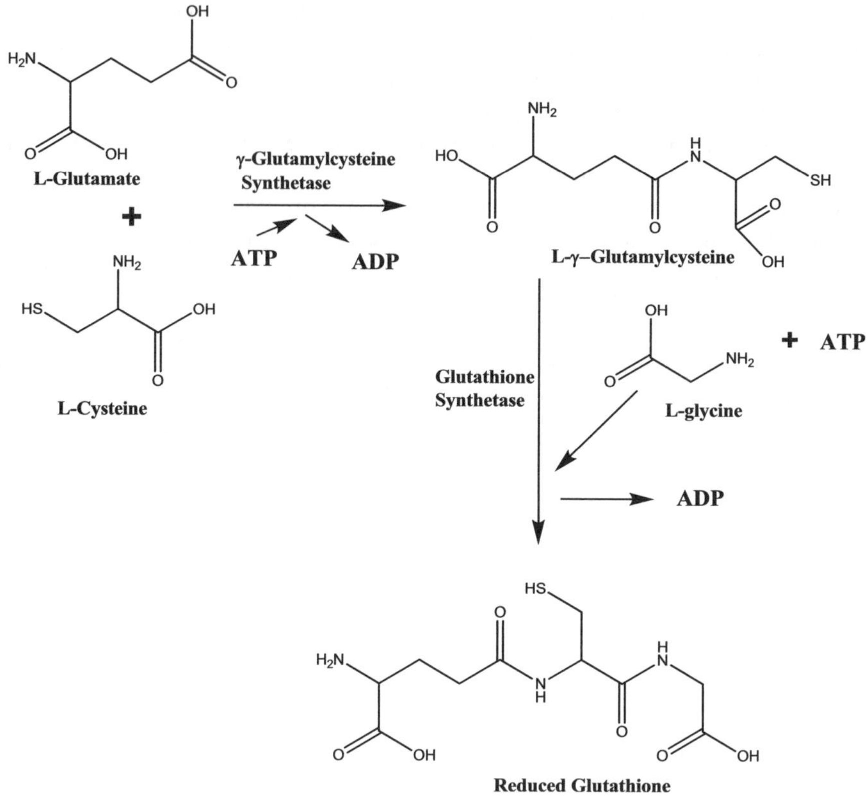


**Figure 9.12** Synthesis pathway for glutathione.

formation of the dipeptide glutamylcysteine which is catalyzed by γ-glutamylcysteine synthetase, also referred to as glutamate-cysteine ligase. In the second step, glycine is attached to form the tripeptide reduced glutathione (γ-L-glutamyl-L-cysteinylglycine), a reaction catalyzed by glutathione synthetase. Both reactions in the synthesis of GSH require ATP.

Under oxidative stress caused by the formation of reactive oxygen species, such as superoxide anion and hydrogen peroxide, GSH protects the cell by accepting electrons from these reactive species *via* the enzyme glutathione peroxidase forming the disulfide GSSG. Two molecules of reduced GSH can be returned to the cytosolic pool by glutathione reductase in the presence of NADPH (Figure 9.13). The ratio of GSH to GSSG is a primary indicator of the redox status of the cell or tissue.

The diagram in Figure 9.13 depicts the roll of GSH in the cell as an antioxidant defense mechanism. Under low-stress conditions the cell is capable of maintaining an excess of reduced GSH. Glutathione peroxidase ($GSH_{px}$) uses GSH to detoxify hydrogen peroxides forming GSSG. In the presence of NADPH, glutathione reductase ($GSH_{Red}$) converts GSSG back to GSH. The 'star bursts' in Figure 9.13 indicate points in the cycle where drugs could

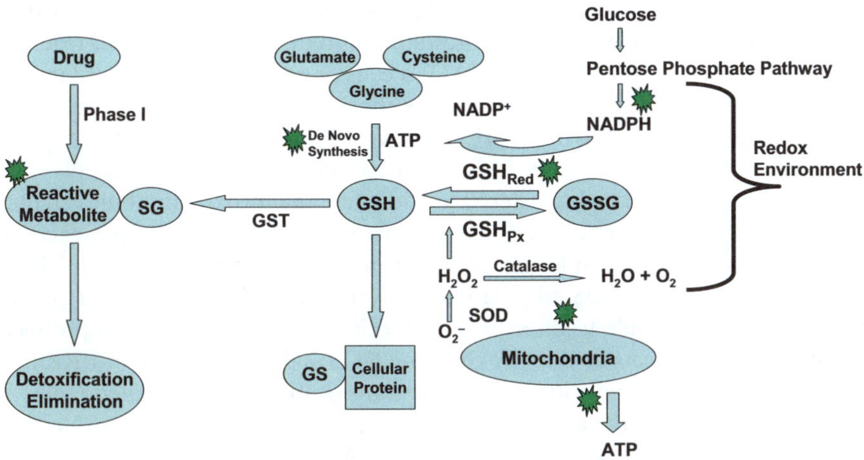


**Figure 9.13** Glutathione cycle and maintenance of cellular redox state. Diagram provided by CeeTox Inc., Kalamazoo, MI, USA.

interfere with GSH homeostasis. If the amount of GSH exceeds the amount being removed from the GSH cycle *via* direct binding to reactive metabolites or proteins or by inhibition of synthesis, the cell's ability to maintain homeostasis could be compromised and the redox state (GSH/GSSG) shifted to an oxidative and toxic state.

It should be evident from the discussion above that the introduction of drugs that are metabolized to reactive intermediates capable of binding GSH or drugs that inhibit the synthesis of GSH or reduce cellular ATP or NADPH or any combination of these could create an environment that overwhelms the GSH system and shifts the redox potential (GSH/GSSH) in favor of oxidation. Inhibition of GSH synthesis can be achieved by treating cells or animals with BSO. Depletion of GSH *via* direct chelation or binding can be achieved by the addition diethylmaleate (DEM). Addition of reduced glutathione does not work well as a means of supplementing cellular GSH because GSH does not cross cell membranes. A key component of the maintenance of cellular GSH concentrations is the availability of L-cysteine. N-acetyl cysteine (NAC) added to cells or given to animals causes a significant increase in GSH synthesis by increasing the pool of L-cysteine.

The synthesis of GSH is controlled by γ-glutamylcysteine synthetase (γ-GCS) and therefore drugs that induce its expression and activity would increase cellular GSH. Conversely, those agents that inhibit its synthesis would reduce cellular GSH and predispose or sensitize cells to oxidative mechanisms of toxicity. Oxidative stress activates mitogen-activated protein kinases (MAPKs) a family of kinases that respond to physiologic stimuli by mediating intracellular signaling pathways.[36] Three major MAPKs have been reported, JNK, ERK1/2, and p38. Inhibition of p38-MAPK inhibits γ-GCS and reduces cellular GSH, while induction or activation of p38-MAPK increases GSH synthesis.[37] Proteosome inhibitors have been shown to increase activated p38-MAPK prior to elevating GSH resulting in reduced toxicity from reactive oxygen species.[38] The addition of NAC to cells or animals can reduce damage caused by oxidative stress. It is commonly thought that this protective effect is due to increased synthesis of GSH. However, Zhang has demonstrated that NAC can directly reduce ROS toxicity independently of GSH synthesis.[39] In these studies, NAC was administered to a human renal proximal tubule cell line (HK-2) in combination with an inducer of oxidative stress. The presence of NAC provided considerable protection from ROS-mediated toxicity. There was a reduction in ROS-stimulated activation of p38-MAPK and JNK, however, NAC was able to directly activate ERK1/2. NAC appears to produce its cytoprotective effects by directly chelating ROS and by activation of ERK1/2. Proteosome inhibitors also induce nuclear translocation NF-E2 related factor 2 (Nrf2) a signaling pathway linked to the expression of many cytoprotective proteins *via* the antioxidant response element (ARE).

Many new anti-tumor drugs are designed to inhibit specific kinase signaling pathways. These new drug candidates should be evaluated for potential inhibition of GSH synthesis which may predispose tissues to toxicity.

Compounds tested in first-tier *in vitro* screens that cause a significant depletion in GSH, which is clearly independent of cell death or proliferation, should undergo additional studies designed to identify the mechanism of GSH depletion. Once this information is known, a realistic risk factor can be assigned to the new drug candidate.

### 9.4.1 *In Vitro* Assays that Identify Metabolic Activation

Depletion of reduced GSH in a microsomal system can be used as an indication that a reactive or electrophilic compound is present. There is a strong correlation between covalent protein binding and formation of GSH adducts *in vitro* ($R^2 = 0.93$) and this correlation exists whether human or rat microsomes are used as the test system.[40] Therefore, assays that measure covalent protein binding and GSH depletion or determine a rate of GSH conjugate formation can be useful tools for predicting risk for toxicity related to metabolic activation of parent drug. Unless the new drug is a prodrug that requires metabolism in order to become active, high susceptibility to metabolism or metabolic activation to a toxic intermediate are considered undesirable properties.

### 9.4.2 Determining *In Vitro* Covalent Binding of Drugs

If radiolabeled drug is available it is possible to measure GSH conjugate formation using HPLC and a radiometric detector. In this assay 10 μM (0.2 μCi per tube) of test drug is incubated at 37 °C with rat or human microsomes (1 mg $mL^{-1}$ per tube), in 100 mM potassium phosphate buffer (pH 7.4) containing 10 mM $MgCl_2$, and an NADPH-generating system (2 units/mL G-6-PDH, 25 mM G-6-P, and 2.5 mM β-$NADP^+$) in a total volume of 0.5 mL.

The reaction is carried out in the presence of 100 μM and 500 μM GSH. The reaction is initiated by the addition of β-NADP$^+$ and carried out for 30 min. At the end of the incubation time the reaction is stopped with the addition of 0.5 mL acetonitrile. Note that the linearity of this reaction, based on the amount of microsomal protein and a 30 min incubation time, should be confirmed with each lot of microsomes. The reaction tubes are then centrifuged at 1650 *g* for 5 min at 4 °C to collect precipitated protein. The protein pellet is washed two times with 80% (v/v) aqueous methanol containing 10% (w/v) trichloroacetic acid, then two times with 80% aqueous methanol. Following each wash the tubes are centrifuged at 1650 *g* for 5 min at 4 °C. After the final wash the radioactivity in the wash solution should be less than or equal to about three times background which is typically 100 dpms. The final protein pellet is then solubilized in 0.5 mL of 1 M NaOH at 55 °C for 12 h. The solution is then neutralized with 1 M HCL and the protein concentration determined. The amount of radioactivity in the solution represents the amount of covalent protein binding.[40]

### 9.4.3 Determining *In Vitro* GSH Conjugate Formation

When radiolabeled drug is not available, it is possible to measure the formation of GSH conjugates with the drug following incubation with liver microsomes. GSH binding has been shown to correlate well with covalent protein binding of drug. The reaction is as described above except that non-radiolabeled drug (10 μM) is used and $^{35}$S-GSH is included at 100 μM (0.25 μCi/tube). The reaction is performed as described above for covalent protein binding. Following the 30 min incubation, the reaction is stopped with the addition of acetonitrile. The reaction tube is then centrifuged at 1650 *g* for 5 min at 4 °C. A 50 μL aliquot is added to an HPLC column and the peak area of $^{35}$S-GSH conjugates to total radioactivity is determined.[41]

### 9.4.4 Determining *In Vitro* GSH Conjugate Formation without Radiolabeling

A quick and simple assay to determine GSH binding that does not require the use of radiolabeled material can also be employed. In this assay GSH depletion is taken as an indication of GSH conjugate formation in microsomes. The reaction mixture is as above, except that drug and GSH are unlabeled. At the end of the assay the loss of free GSH is determined by performing an assay to measure total GSH equivalents as described by Tietz and modified by Griffith (Figure 9.14).

In Figure 9.14, rat microsomes (0.5 mg mL$^{-1}$) isolated from phenobarbital and α-naphthoflavone-induced rats were incubated in a potassium phosphate buffer at pH 7.4 at room at 37 °C for 1 h. The general inhibitor of cytochrome P450, aminobenzotriazole (ABT), was included to demonstrate involvement of cytochrome P450 enzymes. Acetaminophen was included as a positive control.

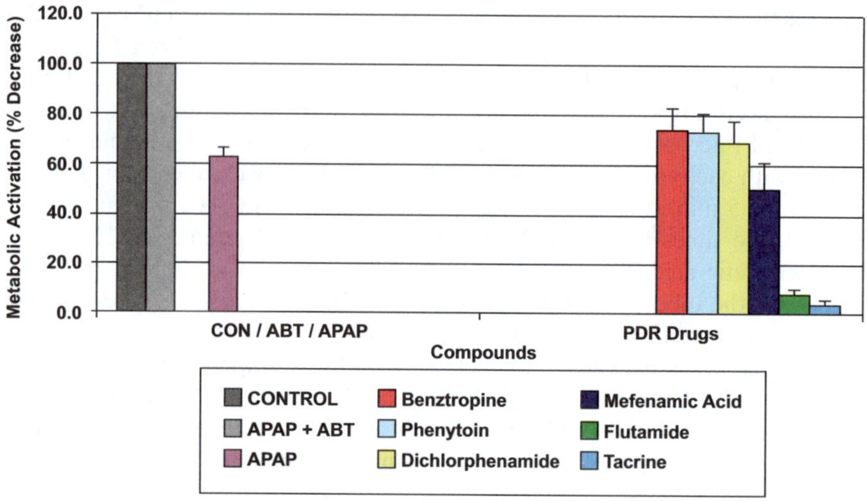


**Figure 9.14** Determining GSH conjugate formation as a measure of bioactivation. Data provided by CeeTox Inc. Kalamazoo, MI, USA.

It is important to include a complete reaction mix that does not contain drugs in order to control for peroxidase conversion of GSH to GSSG.

## 9.4.5 Species Differences in Metabolism

A classic example of liver toxicity related to species differences in metabolism is coumarin. Coumarin (1,2-benzopyrone) is naturally occurring in many foods and spices and is used as an ingredient in fragrances where it functions as a stabilizer and fragrance enhancer. Clinically, it has been administered to humans because of its chemo-preventive and anticoagulant properties.[42] Coumarin is hepatotoxic in rats and as a result its use has been restricted under FDA 21 CFR 189,130.

Although coumarin is hepatotoxic to rats, it is not toxic to humans, mice, hamsters, or gerbils. Differences in species susceptibility to coumarin liver toxicity are due to differences in metabolism (Figure 9.15).

In rats and mice the predominant pathway for coumarin metabolism is the formation of the 3,4-epoxide, which can bind to GSH or rearrange into the hepatotoxic intermediate *o*-hydroxyphenylacetaldehyde (*o*-HPA). The formation of *o*-HPA in rats and mice is nine to 38 times greater than in humans. In humans the major route of metabolism is the formation of 7-hydroxycoumarin, which is not hepatotoxic.[43,44] The detoxification of *o*-HPA to *o*-hydroxyphenylacetic acid (*o*-HPAA) has been identified as the major determinant of species differences in toxicity. Humans do form the *o*-HPAA product, and this is presumably *via* the toxic intermediate *o*-HPA, however the aldehyde dehydrogenase responsible for this conversion has higher activity in humans than in rats or mice. Thus, even though small amounts of the toxic form can be

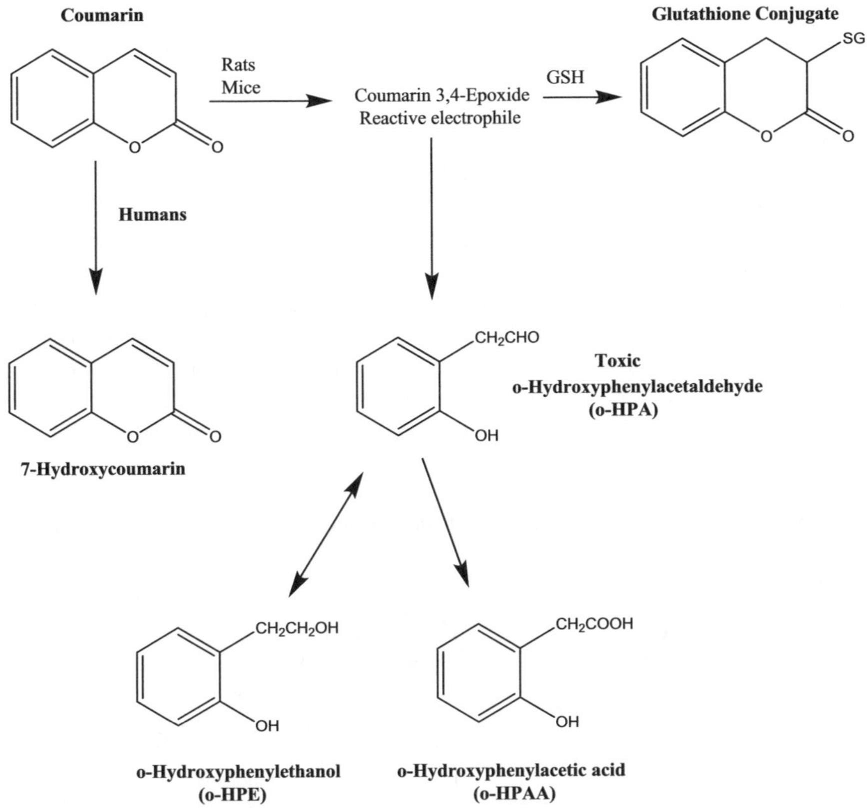


**Figure 9.15** Species-dependent metabolism of coumarin.

produced in human liver, the higher activity of the detoxification enzyme reduces accumulation of the toxic *o*-HPA intermediate and makes it unlikely that coumarin, at low clinically relevant doses, would produce liver toxicity.[44]

When precision-cut liver slices from rat, monkey, and human were used to compare the rate of diclofenac metabolism, clear species differences were observed with the rat > monkey ≫ human. When protein adduct formation in the same species was measured, the occurrence followed the same pattern with rat > monkey ≫ human.[45] The ability to identify species-specific differences in toxicity, as well as elucidate the mechanisms for these differences is essential for discovery teams who must make go-no-go decisions on data derived from animal models.

Tolbutamide is a sulfonylurea drug used to treat type 2 diabetes. The drug helps control blood sugar levels by inducing the pancreas to produce more insulin. The drug is orally absorbed and rapidly excreted in the urine. Metabolism in the liver follows two main pathways: 1) oxidation of the methyl group or 2) dealkylation of the sulfonyl group. Four primary metabolites are formed, hydroxymethyltolbutamide, carboxymethyltolbutamide, *p*-tolysulfonylurea, *p*-tolysulfonamide (Figure 9.16). Tolbutamide in humans is relatively safe; however, liver toxicity occurs in dogs.[46,47] It is now believed that the species differences observed in hepatic toxicity is due to the formation of the *p*-tolylsulfonamide and *p*-tolylsulfonylurea, which are found in dogs, but not in humans.

Early discovery teams faced with understanding animal pharmacokinetic, efficacy, and safety data must be able to identify species-specific mechanisms of toxicity. *In vitro* cell-based systems incorporated into early drug discovery must be able to identify the risk of species-specific toxicity. As discussed above, *in vitro* models such as precision-cut liver slices and primary hepatocytes from rat, dog, monkey and human have been useful models for identifying species differences in metabolism and toxicity.[45–47] In addition to primary hepatocytes and precision-cut liver slices, many investigators have used microsomes isolated from different species as a tool for identifying the CYP enzymes responsible for

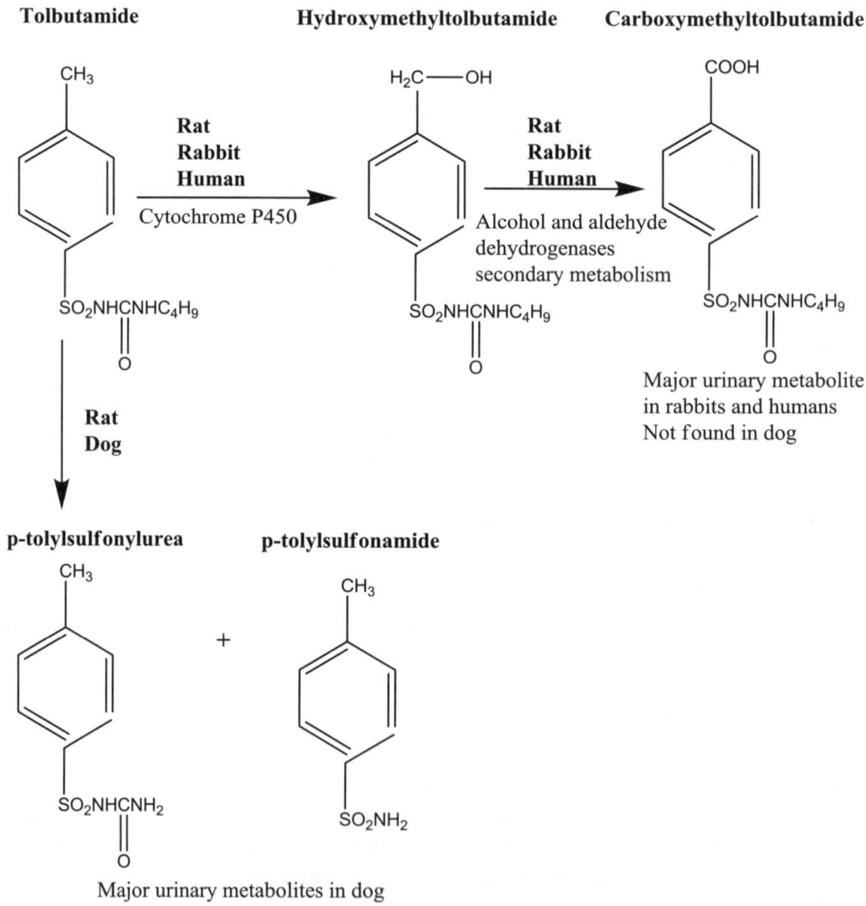


**Figure 9.16** Species-dependent metabolism of tolbutamide.

drug metabolism. Identifying metabolite profiles in multiple test species can provide insight into the species that may be most sensitive to toxicity.

Once it has been determined that the animal test systems produce metabolites that are different from those found in humans, it is necessary to understand the reactivity and toxicity of the metabolites in both species. To accomplish this, it is helpful to identify the specific CYP enzymes responsible for the metabolite formation.

## 9.5 Cytochrome P450 Reaction Phenotyping

The fraction of the dose metabolized by CYP enzymes is a major determinant of potential drug–drug interactions and is essential for understanding the impact of inter-individual differences in drug metabolism among humans.[39] Because metabolism plays a major role in both the elimination and toxicity of drugs, it is important to identify the primary metabolites and the enzymes responsible. Phenotyping is the process whereby hepatocytes, isolated microsomes, and recombinant CYP proteins are combined with enzyme specific inhibitors, substrate marker probes, and antibodies to determine the major metabolic pathways responsible for drug metabolism. Once obtained, these data can identify differences in metabolism between animals used in preclinical safety studies and humans. Reactive or toxic intermediates formed in one species, but not in another, can provide a mechanistic rationale for the level of risk expected in humans.

Reaction phenotyping is typically done using multiple approaches. The process combines a metabolism model, such as recombinant P450 enzymes or microsomes combined with antibody inhibition, chemical inhibition, and correlation analysis to provide conclusive evidence for the participation and relative contribution to metabolism and clearance of a drug.[39,48] Chemical substrates with a high specificity for a single CYP enzyme are of greatest value as a probe substrate. Probe or marker substrates can be used to determine the activity of a specific CYP enzyme *in vivo* or in an *in vitro* cell or microsome system. The specific activity of each CYP enzyme, once known, can be used to correlate metabolite formation with predetermined CYP activity.[49] Probe substrates can also be used to determine if an unknown compound has the potential to inhibit specific CYPs. For example, to evaluate the effect of a new drug as an inhibitor of CYP1A2 the probe substrate might be phenacetin, and phenacetin *O*-deethylation would be the activity assay used to determine inhibition. Phenacetin is incubated with microsomes with and without the test drug and with a known inhibitor (*e.g.*, α-naphthoflavone, a potent inhibitor of CYP1A2 with an $IC_{50}$ of 0.068 nM). The best chemical inhibitor is one that only reacts with a single target CYP.[49,50] Chemical inhibition experiments should be conducted over a wide concentration range in order to establish an accurate $IC_{50}$ (Table 9.1).

Chemical inhibition should be verified with antibody inhibition experiments. Highly specific monoclonal antibodies for most of the human P450s are now commercially available. Antibody inhibition experiments should be done at low

**Table 9.1** Human cytochrome P450 substrates, metabolites, inducers and inhibitors.[39,49,50]

| *Enzyme* | *Probe substrate* | *Activity assay* | *Inducer* | *Inhibitors* | *Inhibitor concentration (μM)* |
|---|---|---|---|---|---|
| CYP1A2 | Phenacetin | Phenacetic *O*-deethylation | 3-Methylchloanthrene | α-Naphthoflavone, furafylline | 10–30 |
| CYP2A6 | Coumarin | Coumarin 7-hydroxylation | Dexamethasone | Methoxsalen, tranylcypromine | 1 |
| CYP2B6 | Bupropion | Hydroxybupropion | Phenobarbital | Triethylenethiophosporamide (ThioTEPA) | 50 |
| CYP2C8 | Paclitaxel | Paclitaxel 6α-hydroxylation | Rifampin | Quercetin, montelukast | 0.1 |
| CYP2C9 | Diclofenac | Diclofenac 4′-hydroxylation | Phenobarbital, rifampin | Sulfaphenazole | 10 |
| CYP2C19 | (*S*)-Methenytoin | (*S*)-Mephenytoin 4′-hydroxylation | Rifampin | Ticlopidine | 1 |
| CYP2D6 | Dextramethorphan | Dextramethorpan O-demethylation | — | Quinidine | <2 |
| CYP2E1 | Chlorzoxazone | 6-Hydroxy chlorzoxazone | Ethanol | Diethyldithiocarbamate | 50 |
| CYP3A4/5 | Midazolam | Midazolam 1′-hydroxylation | Dexamethasone | Ketoconazole | 1 and 10 |
| CYP3A4/5 | Testosterone | Testosterone 6β-hydroxylation | — | Ketoconazole, troleandomycin | 50 |

and high concentrations of antibody in order to define the titration curve. If a single enzyme is responsible for a drugs metabolism the inhibition should be at least 90%. When more than one enzyme is suspected to be involved with a compounds metabolism, several antibodies should be employed and tested in at least 10, and preferably 20, microsomal preparations in order to clearly identify the relative contributions of each enzyme. This number of microsomal preparations isolated from different individuals is necessary due to large inter-individual variation in CYP activities and differences in microsomal isolations.

Correlation studies compare the activity of a known CYP enzyme (*x*-axis) with formation of a metabolite (*y*-axis). In the example shown in 10.17, the formation of metabolite M1 correlates well ($R^2 = 0.74$) with increasing activity of CYP3A4. This type of correlation analysis experiment is important for an unknown metabolite as a confirmation that the enzymes identified in the inhibition experiments are directly responsible for the metabolite formation[49,51–53] (Figure 9.17).

The relationship between the dose of a drug administered and systemic exposure can vary greatly between test animals and humans. This in turn can have a dramatic impact on the observed adverse effects and the assessment of human safety. Understanding the metabolism of new drug candidates and how both the parent molecules and their metabolites can affect toxicity is an essential piece of information that can be generated using *in vitro* models. The information obtained is directly applicable to predicting *in vivo* effects. It is important for pre-clinical discovery to identify and understand the major pathways of metabolism in order to anticipate potential drug–drug interactions and liver toxicity issues.[54]

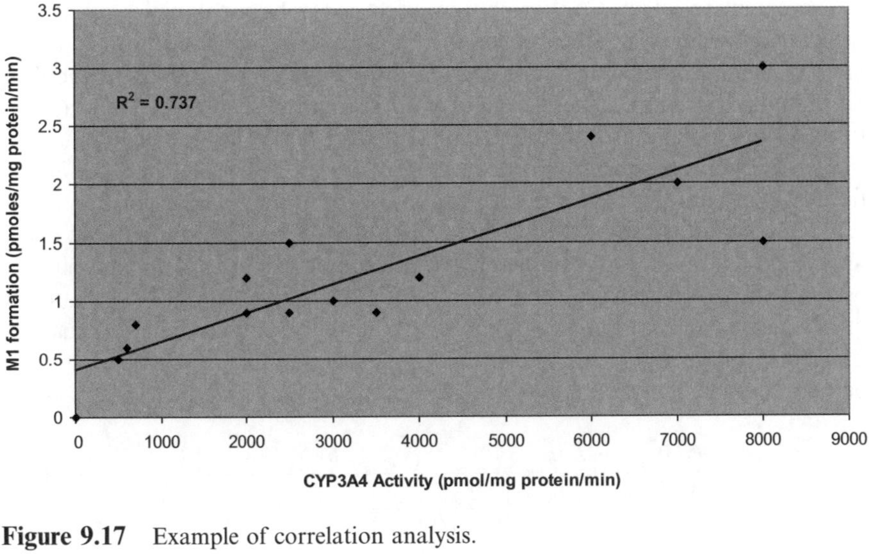


**Figure 9.17** Example of correlation analysis.

## 9.6 Identifying Potential Drug–Drug Interactions

Drug–drug interactions (DDI) between two or more co-administered drugs occurs when one drug affects the pharmacokinetics of another by either reducing its half-life and therefore its efficacy or inhibiting its elimination, resulting in higher than expected plasma concentrations and potential toxicity. In other words, if one drug changes the absorption, distribution, metabolism, or excretion of another, a DDI has occurred.[54,55] Inhibition and induction of drug-metabolizing enzymes can alter the rate of metabolic transformation and elimination and as such represent two major reasons for DDIs. When one drug changes the rate of metabolism of another drug the result can dramatically affect the safety or efficacy of a drug. The metabolism of most exogenous molecules that enter the body *via* ingestion occurs in the liver. The most important family of enzymes involved with the metabolism of drugs and chemicals is cytochrome P450.

Although CYP enzymes are ubiquitous; they are in high concentration in the liver. Therefore, the liver is an important site of CYP inhibition and induction. Because CYP enzymes can recognize many different molecules as substrates, it is highly likely that two drugs can be metabolized by the same enzyme. Therefore, if these drugs are administered together they can compete for the same metabolic site. In this situation, the relative concentration of drugs and the affinity of each drug for the same metabolic site on the enzyme will determine the extent of competitive inhibition. It is also possible for a drug to inhibit a CYP enzyme that is not involved with its metabolism. Finally, a molecule may enter a CYP binding site where it is transformed into a reactive intermediate which can than covalently bind to the active site and inactivate the protein. This type of inhibition is the most serious and is called irreversible inhibition. Therefore, compounds that inhibit CYPs can be classified as competitive, non-competitive, or irreversible inhibitors.

The extent to which CYP inhibition affects the pharmcokinetics of another drug is dependent on the number of CYP enzymes involved with a drug's metabolism, and the contribution that each CYP makes to a drug's metabolism and elimination. Thus, although important information such as reaction rate and turnover can be obtained from recombinant CYP (rCYP) systems containing a single enzyme, it is generally recognized that this model represents a configuration that does not represent the *in vivo* situation accurately. Therefore, in order to fully understand the impact of CYP inhibition as it pertains to potential drug–drug interactions it is recommended that complete reaction phenotyping be performed, which includes the use of rCYP systems, known substrates in microsomal systems, chemical and antibody inhibitors, and correlation analysis. The data obtained by this integrative approach can then be used (eqn (9.1) below) to model how an inhibitor will affect changes in a substrate drug's AUC.

$$\frac{\mathrm{AUC}_{\mathrm{po(I)}}}{\mathrm{AUC}_{\mathrm{po(C)}}} = \frac{f'_{\mathrm{g}}}{f_{\mathrm{g}}} \times \frac{1}{\left[\dfrac{f_{\mathrm{m}} f_{\mathrm{m,CYP}}}{\mathrm{CL}_{\mathrm{int,I}}/\mathrm{CL}'_{\mathrm{int,I}}}\right] + [1 - (f_{\mathrm{m}} f_{\mathrm{m,CYP}})]} \tag{9.1}$$

Eqn (9.1) describes how the presence of an inhibitor or inducer can alter another drug's AUC, where $AUC_{po(I)}$ and $AUC_{po(C)}$ represent the AUC in the presence and absence of the perpetrator molecule (inhibitor or inducer), respectively. The availability of drug to the intestinal wall in the presence ($f_g'$) and absence ($f_g$) of the perpetrator molecule. The fraction metabolized by all CYPs ($f_m$) and fraction of the total CYP-dependent metabolism catalyzed by the affected CYP ($f_{m,CYP}$) and intrinsic clearance defined as metabolite formation in the absence ($CL_{int,l}$) and presence ($CL_{int,l}'$) of the perpetrator molecule. This general equation has been used extensively, but it is based on several key assumptions which are as follows:

1) the inhibitor does not affect $f_g$;
2) the liver is the only organ for clearance;
3) a well-stirred kinetic model applies;
4) $[S] << K_m$.

In addition to the general equation, there are other models that help describe the effect of CYP inhibition. Eqn (9.2) compares the ratio of intrinsic clearance (absence of inhibitor) to the intrinsic clearance (presence of inhibitor). This equation describes reversible competitive or noncompetitive inhibition. In this equation [I] is the concentration of inhibitor, $K_i$ is the dissociation constant of the inhibitor–enzyme complex.

$$CL_{int,I}/CL'_{int,I} = 1 + \frac{[I]}{K_i} \tag{9.2}$$

Mechanism-based inhibition can be described by eqn (9.3) where $k_{inact}$ is the rate constant for CYP inactivation, $K_i$ is the half maximal rate of inactivation, [I] is the concentration of inhibitor, and $k_{deg}$ is rate constant of CYP degradation or turnover.

$$CL_{int,I}/CL'_{int,I} = 1 + \frac{k_{inact}}{K_i}\frac{[I]}{k_{deg}} \tag{9.3}$$

Although the inhibition of CYP enzymes is not in itself considered to be a toxic event in the liver, the effect can predispose the liver, and for that matter the entire body, to an adverse event produced by another drug, as direct result of the CYP inhibition. Therefore, CYP induction and inhibition should be considered as adverse events and incorporated into the pool of *in vitro* safety data that can be collected in early discovery. This information can assist chemists early in discovery during lead optimization by directing the SAR as they modify molecules to improve druggable attributes.[55]

### 9.6.1 Importance of Cytochrome P450 Inhibition

When one drug inhibits the enzyme responsible for the metabolism of another drug the result can an increase in plasma concentration and the development of adverse effects. A good example of this can be illustrated by reviewing the drug terfenadine. Terfenadine, a non-sedating H1 receptor antagonist, was used as an antihistamine in the treatment of allergies. Terfenadine is a prodrug rapidly absorbed from the gut where it undergoes significant first-pass metabolism by two routes: the first is an *N*-dealkylation to azacyclonol and the second is hydroxaylation of the *t*-butyl group to form hydroxyterfenadine.[56] Hydroxyterfenadine is further oxidized to the carboxylic acid which is the biologically active form of terfenadine (Figure 9.18). Therefore under normal circumstances the actual plasma concentrations of the parent molecule terfenadine are low.

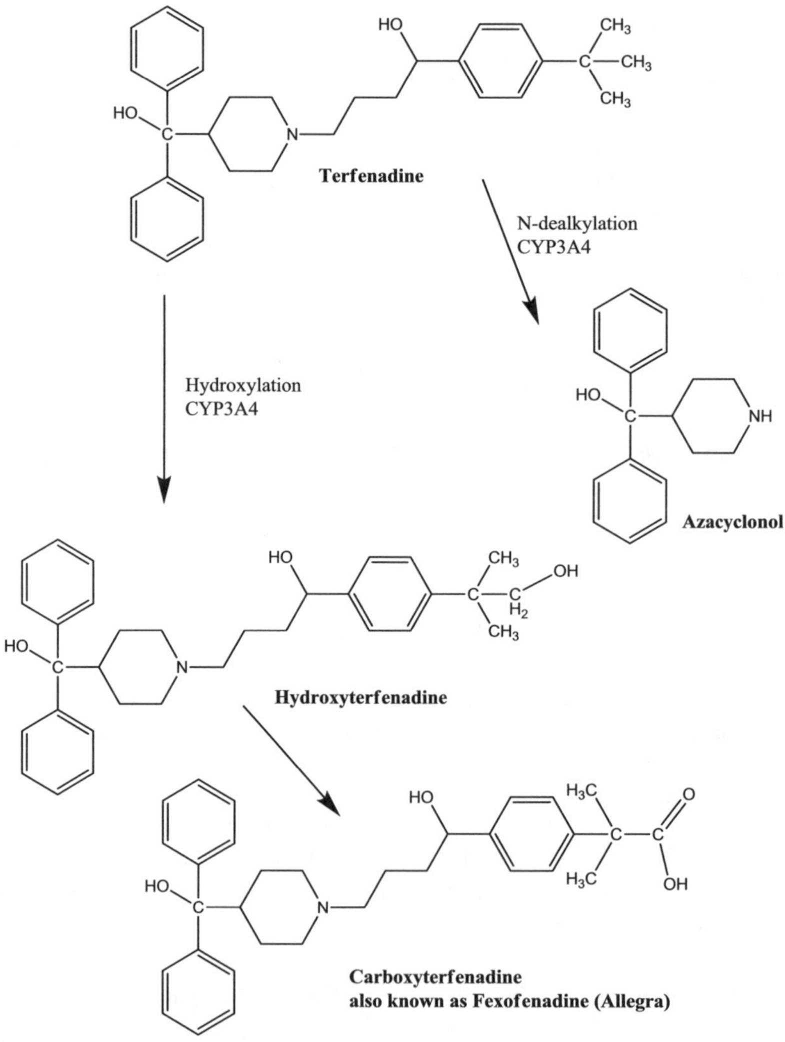


**Figure 9.18** Metabolic pathways for terfenadine.

CYP3A4 is the primary enzyme responsible for the metabolism of terfenadine to both azacyclonol and hydroxyterfenadine. The antifungal agent ketoconazole is a potent inhibitor of CYP3A4. The co-administration of terfenadine with ketoconazole to patients in clinical studies increases the half-life ($T_{1/2}$) of terfenadine, with a corresponding increase in the AUC that ranged from 13–59 fold above those measured in patients that did not receive ketoconazole.[57] The higher plasma concentrations and increased half-life caused a prolongation of the cardiac QT interval leading to a fatal arrhythmia known as TdP. As a result, terfenadine was withdrawn from the market. Later, the carboxylic acid metabolite (fexofenadine) of terfenadine was marketed as the antihistamine known as Allegra, which is not associated with cardiac toxicity.

There are three general categories of drug inhibition: 1) competitive, 2) quasi-competitive and 3) non-competitive (metabolism-dependent or suicide). Competitive inhibition occurs when two drugs compete as substrates for the same CYP enzyme. For example, omeprazole and diazepam are both metabolized by CYP2C19. When co-administered, omeprazole increases the half-life of diazepam. Quasi-competitive inhibition occurs when the inhibitor drug is not a substrate for the enzyme it is inhibiting. The primary pathway of dextromethorphan metabolism is CYP2D6. Quinidine significantly reduces the clearance of dextromethorphan because it is a potent inhibitor of CYP2D6, but is not a substrate for this enzyme. The third type of CYP inhibition is non-competitive, also called mechanism-based, or suicide inhibition, and is characterized by metabolism to a metabolite that can act as a competitive inhibitor or one that forms a tight, near-covalent, bond with the haem moiety of the CYP enzyme or with the CYP protein and inactivates the enzyme. The bond is so tight that the drug is not released and the enzyme is killed or permanently inactivated (suicide inhibition). Recovery from mechanism-based inhibition requires the synthesis of new protein. This type of inhibition is often characterized by an increasing potency of inhibition over time.[58] Time-dependent, mechanism-based inhibition of CYP metabolism generally has more profound clinical implications and therefore is important to identify early.[59]

The evaluation of new chemical entities for possible CYP inhibition can be done with *in vitro* screening methods. Two commonly used methods are the standard single substrate assays and the fluorescent probe method with recombinant CYPs. The standard method uses human liver microsomes as the enzyme system, combined with a probe substrate specific for the enzyme of interest. CYP1A1/2 inhibition can be assessed by monitoring the formation of ethoxyresorufin-*O*-deethylase in the presence of the test (inhibitor) compound. The fluorescent probe assay is done in a 96-well plate by adding the incubation buffer which contains the substrate at various concentrations and the cDNA expressed CYP of interest. The reaction is started by adding an NADPH-generating system. Activity is measured by the formation of a fluorescent metabolite from the starting substrate. In this assay, CYP1A2 inhibition is determined by adding 7-ethoxyresorufin as substrate and measuring the formation of the fluorescent metabolite resorufin in the presence of the test compound.[60]

The type and potency of CYP inhibition are important pieces of information to obtain early in the drug-discovery process because these data are normally included in the investigative new drug (IND) application.

### 9.6.2 Role of Cytochrome P450 Induction

It has been known for years that many drugs can induce cytochrome P450 enzymes. The increased levels of metabolizing enzymes can significantly reduce the plasma concentration of drugs that are metabolized by the induced enzymes. This can lead to a reduction or complete loss in drug efficacy or in some instances to increased toxicity due to formation of highly reactive intermediates. One example is the induction of CYP3A4 in human liver by rifampicin, which causes a decrease in the AUC of midazolam and simvastatin that can be as high as 90% compared to patients that were not treated with rifampicin. Induction requires a series of cellular processes that include transcription of the gene to form mRNA, followed by translation of the mRNA to functional protein. Thus, CYP induction requires several days of repeated exposure to see maximal enzyme effects and drug interactions.

Induction *per se* is not considered to be an adverse or toxic event in the liver, however, CYP induction in the liver is a major reason for changes in the half-life of a drug and can be responsible for the production of reactive metabolites that do cause liver toxicity. For this reason it is important to know if metabolism of a new chemical entity (NCE) results in a reactive intermediate. Metabolic activation can be determined from *in vitro* assays and the data obtained incorporated into the decision-making process of drug design.

The induction of these CYP enzymes is mediated by several nuclear transcriptions factors, such as the aryl hydrocarbon receptor (AhR), the *constitutive* androstane receptor (CAR), and the pregnane-X receptor (PXR). These transcription factors control the expression of CYP1A, CYP2B, and CYP3A enzymes respectively. Although many tissues contain CYP enzymes and are capable of responding to inducers, the organ where the induction of drug-metabolizing enzymes occurs to the greatest extent is the liver. Several *in vitro* models are currently used to obtain induction information. These include human primary hepatocytes, ligand binding assays, and cell-based reporter gene constructs.[39]

In late-lead optimization it is important to identify liver-specific issues in both the rat and human models. By collecting data that can be related to both test groups it may be possible to identify potential species-specific toxicities. All the putative new drug candidates still under consideration should have been tested for QT prolongation (hERG), and genotoxicity at this point in development. Potential drug–drug interactions can be assessed by determining the effect of the drug on the induction and inhibition of CYP enzymes. Because the liver CYP metabolizing system represents an important pathway by which drugs are cleared from the body, changes in their relative abundance or activity can have important clinical consequences. Induction can increase the clearance of co-administered drugs thereby reducing their effect. Induction can also increase the metabolism of prodrugs to their active form, which may change their efficacy and pharmacokinetics. Finally, induction may increase the bioactivation of drugs and in so doing, increase the concentration of reactive forms that can cause liver toxicity.[61]

## 9.7 Hepatocytes in Sandwich Culture

The hepatocyte model considered to be the gold standard for determining liver CYP induction is the primary hepatocyte in sandwich culture. Hepatocytes grown sandwiched between collagen or collagen and Matrigel have a morphology that more closely resembles hepatocytes (*e.g.*, cuboidal), and maintain metabolism and growth for longer periods of time. In addition, this type of culture allows the formation of canalicular membrane networks which provide a means of evaluating liver specific transporters (Figure 9.19).

Nearly all aspects of the culture system should be optimized for best results. Most parameters have been well defined and described previously.[61–63] The type of matrix used, the media, seeding density, and species have all been shown to impact induction results and interpretation of data (reviewed by Hewitt). When using human hepatocytes, similar induction data was obtained using either freshly isolated or cryopreserved hepatocytes.[61] The US FDA draft guidelines recommend that induction studies are performed with hepatocytes obtained from a minimum of three individuals in order to minimize inter-individual differences in responses.[64] Animal hepatocytes should not be used to predict human induction; however, animal induction profiles compared to human induction profiles may provide important information on potential

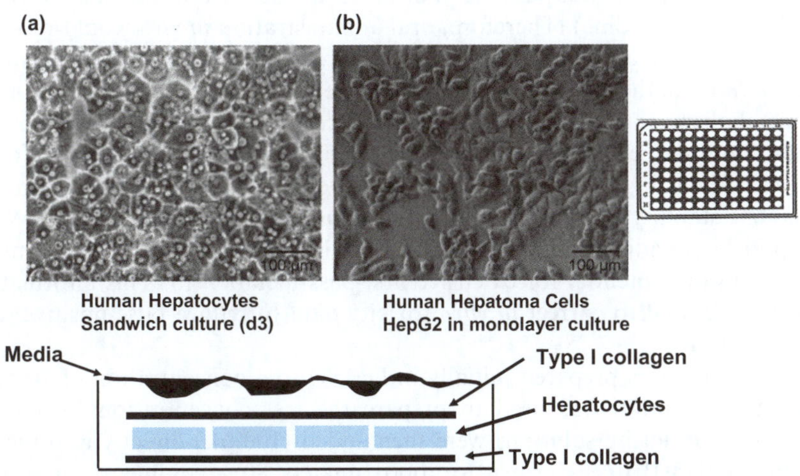


**Figure 9.19** Comparison of human primary hepatocytes in sandwich culture to HepG2 cells. Reproduced from ref. 131 with permission. Copyright American Society for Pharmacology and Experimental Therapeutics, 2003.

species-specific toxicity or confirm animal pharmacokinetic data. The confluency of the culture systems is important, as low-density human hepatocyte cultures have a lower induction response. A confluency of 70% is recommended for human cultures. For human hepatocytes common media include Dulbecco's minimal essential, Leibovitz L-15, modified Chee's medium, and Williams medium E. Most induction studies are carried out in serum-free media supplemented with insulin and submicromolar amounts of dexamethasone.[65,66] The equilibration and growth period (time of seeding to addition of test agents) is 24–48 h. The induction period following the addition of the test compound is three days for enzyme activities and two days for mRNA. The most relevant endpoint is enzyme activity expressed specific activity as this is the form that will determine whether there is a change in the metabolism of a drug. Following the induction period, CYP substrates may be added directly to the cell culture system or microsomes can be prepared from the cell monolayer.

### 9.7.1 Importance of Understanding Metabolic Stability

Determining the metabolic stability of a test compound is an important piece of information that greatly improves the predictive power of *in vitro* models. An example of this can be seen with terfenadine. *In vitro* assessment of cytotoxicity using multiple endpoints of cell health reveals a concentration–response curve consistent with compounds that would cause organ toxicity *in vivo* (Figure 9.20). This is interesting because terfenadine was tested in a full battery of preclinical and clinical safety studies and was approved by the FDA. The explanation for this apparent false positive result *in vitro* can be found by understanding the metabolism of the drug. As mentioned above, terfenadine undergoes extensive first-pass metabolism to the active and less toxic form of the drug (fexofenadine). Therefore, oral administration *in vivo* would result in very low a plasma concentrations of the parent drug due to first-pass metabolism. *In vitro*, the parent drug is applied directly to the cells. Due to low rates of metabolism *in vitro*, a much higher concentration of the drug comes in contact with the cells. The drug is known to affect ion channels, and therefore it is toxic at the higher concentrations achieved in culture. By incorporating metabolic stability into the interpretation of *in vitro* toxicity data (Figure 9.21) it is possible to adjust for low metabolic stability (high rates of metabolism) of NCEs and the potential for extensive first-pass metabolism. This information can then be used to correct *in vitro* toxicity data to reduce false-positive data interpretations.

Terfenadine was prepared initially in DMSO to a concentration of 20 mM. This stock solution was used to prepare the test concentrations in culture medium. The dosing solutions were then added (100 μL) directly into the rat hepatoma (H4IIE) cells grown to approximately 80% confluency in 96-well culture plates and incubated at 37 °C in 5% $CO_2$ for 6 and 24 h. Each plotted value represents the mean of six wells. The coefficient of variation was between 10 and 15%. Final DMSO concentrations did not exceed 0.5%. Metabolic

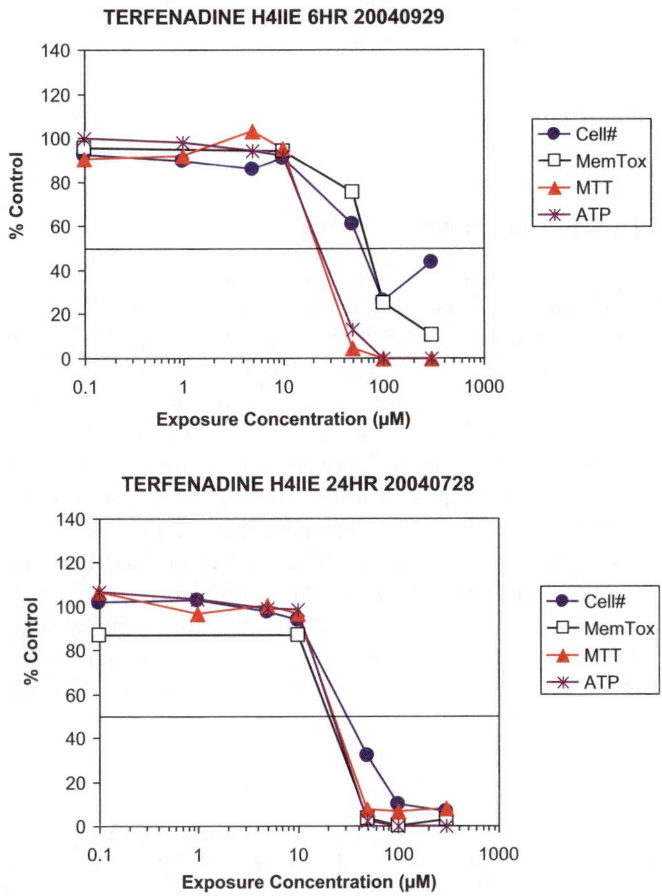


**Figure 9.20** *In vitro* cytotoxicity of terfenadine at two time points.

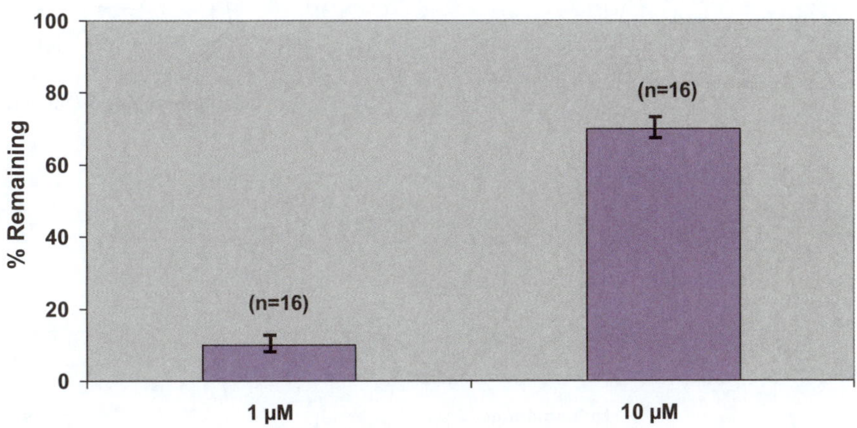


**Figure 9.21** Metabolic stability of terfenadine in rat microsomes.

stability was determined with rat microsomes (0.5 mg $mL^{-1}$) in pH 7.4 buffer. Terfenadine was added to final concentrations of 1 or 10 μM and incubated at room temperature for 30 min. The parent drug was analyzed by LC-MS and the data are reported as the mean ± SEM and expressed as a percent of parent remaining (%R).

### 9.7.2 Formation of Reactive Metabolites

The formation of reactive metabolites (bioactivation) has been associated with many approved drugs that have either been removed from the market due to liver toxicity or have received a black box warning. Examples of drugs known to undergo metabolic activation include troglitazone (diabetes), nefazodone (antidepressant), iproniazid (antidepressant), benoxaprofen (NSAID), tienilic acid (diuretic), trovafloxacin (antibacterial), diclofenac (NSAID), furosemide (diuretic), imiprimine (tricyclic antidepressant), indomethacin (NSAID), isoniazid (antibacterial), clozapine (antipsychotic), acetaminophen (NSAID), amodiaquine (antimalarial), and carbamazepine (antiseizure). All of these drugs can be metabolized to reactive intermediates and as such may produce toxicity *via* covalent binding to proteins. An example is provided in Figure 9.22 for carbamazepine.[67,68] In many instances, toxicity due to metabolic activation is missed during animal preclinical safety studies and this can result in adverse events in humans after the drug has been introduced into the market. It is

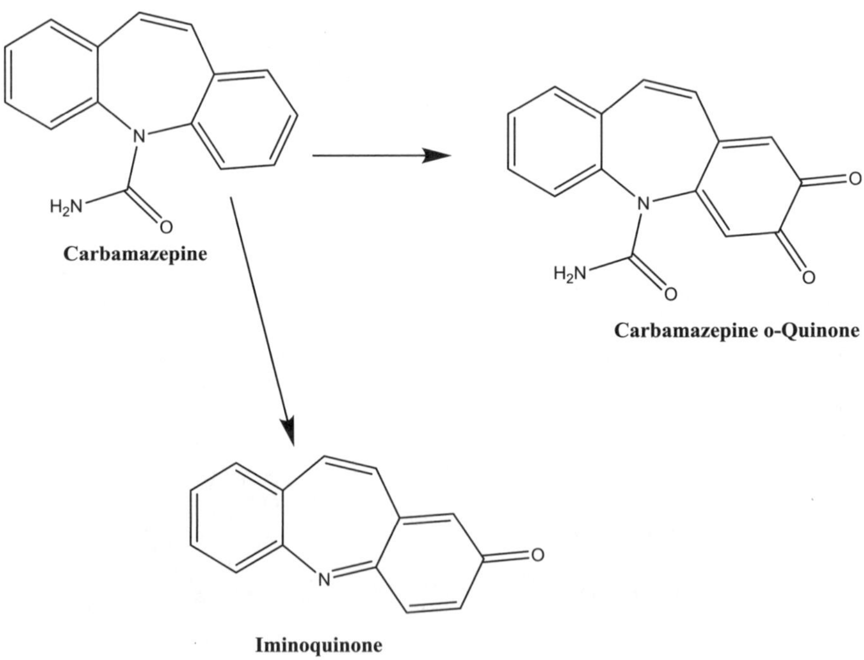


**Figure 9.22** Metabolic activation of carbamazepine.

generally recognized that risk for adverse effects in humans can be reduced by mitigating the formation of reactive metabolites.[40,69,70]

The potential to form reactive metabolites can be determined with *in vitro* systems. Most compounds susceptible to activation through metabolism form electrophilic sites which can bind to nucleophiles on proteins or other macromolecules in the cell. As a result the potential to form electrophilic compounds and their ability to bind covalently to proteins can be used to design *in vitro* assays to identify these intermediates. Moreover, it is well known that electrophiles can bind to and activate the Nrf2/keap1 nuclear transcription factor, which upon activation, releases keap 1 translocates to the nucleus, binds to the antioxidant response element (ARE) and induces the expression of several cytoprotective genes.[69] This pathway has been used as an indicator of reactivity, and is considered to be an intrinsic sensing system in cells for reactive intermediates.[71,72] Genes controlled by the Nrf2/keap1 activation of the ARE promoter include thioredoxin, aldoketoreductase, NADPH quinone reductase 1; UDP-glucuronosyltransferases, and γ-glutamylcysteine synthetase.[73]

### 9.7.3 The Importance of Bile Acid Homeostasis in the Liver

The liver is a complex organ with both apical (canalicular membrane) and basolateral (sinusoidal blood) orientation. An important function of the liver is the regulation of bile acid concentration in blood and the initiation of bile production. This process involves Phase I metabolism of bile acids by cytochrome P450 enzymes, Phase II conjugation enzymes such as UDP-glucuronosyl transferase (UGT1A1), and Phase III hepatobiliary transport systems, such as the bile salt export pump, BSEP. These processes are regulated by several nuclear receptors which include the constitutive androstane receptor (CAR), the farnesoid-X receptor (FXR) and the pregnane-X-receptor (PXR).[1,74] The liver maintains an intricate balance between *de novo* synthesis of bile acids from cholesterol in the hepatocyte, uptake of bile acids from blood into the hepatocyte, and elimination or efflux out of the hepatocyte (Figure 9.23).

The two primary bile acids chenodeoxycholic and cholic acid are synthesized by two pathways. The "classic" pathway involves hydroxylation at the 7′-position by cholesterol 7-α-hydroxylase or CYP7A to form 7-hydroxycholesterol. 7-Hydroxycholesterol can then be converted to chenodeoxycholic or cholic acid through a series of enzymatic reactions. The ratio of CDCA to CA is determined by the activity of sterol 12-α-hydroxylase (CYP8B1). Metabolism *via* this enzyme results in the formation of CA. Substrates that are not captured by this step become CDCA. CDCA represents about 45% of the bile acids while CA represents about 31%. The second pathway occurs in the mitochondria and is known as the "acidic" pathway of bile acid synthesis. In this pathway cholesterol is hydroxylated at the 27′-position by sterol 27-α-hydroxylase (CYP27A1) and the resulting product is hydroxylated at the 7′-position by oxysterol 7-α-hydroxylase (CYP7B1) resulting in the formation of CD*CA*. In rodents this pathway may represent as much as 25% of the bile acids

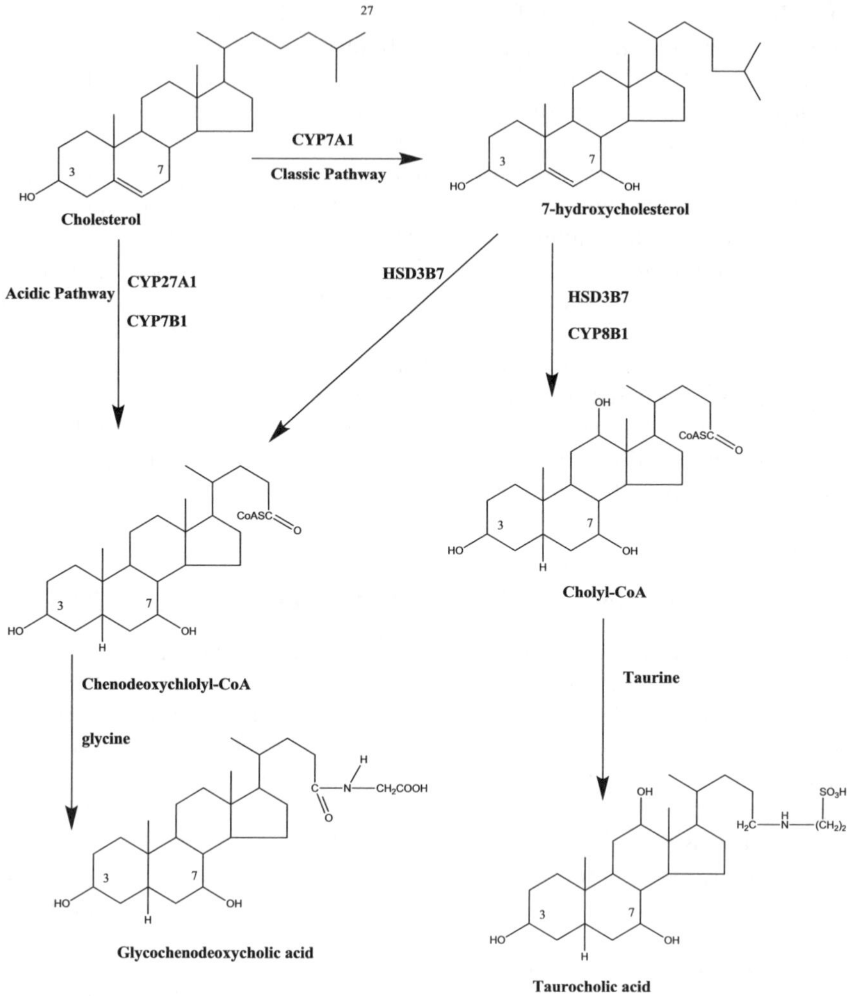


**Figure 9.23** Hepatic synthesis of bile acids.

synthesized, however in humans it is only 6%. Although the contribution of bile acid synthesis in humans by the acidic pathway is low, it appears critical for normal fetal development, as infants born with mutations in CYP7B1 develop cholestatic liver disease that can lead to cirrhosis.

In order to be transported across the canalicular membrane into the bile, the primary bile acids must be conjugated to either glycine or taurine. In the example shown in Figure 9.23, CDCA is conjugated to glycine yielding glycochenodeoxycholic acid, while CA is conjugated to taurine yielding taurocholic acid. Conjugation enhances their amphipathic properties, which improves secretion into the bile canaliculi and reduces toxicity. Conjugated primary bile acids represent the primary solutes in bile. Bile acids accumulate in the gall bladder and aid in the digestion of fatty foods. After a meal, bile release into the duodenum is stimulated by the hormone cholecystokinin (CCK) to help assimilate lipids into the body. The conjugated primary bile acids in the gut undergo de-conjugation reactions mediated by gut bacteria to yield the secondary bile acids deoxycholate (from CA) and lithocholate (from CDCA). Both the primary and secondary bile acids are reabsorbed into portal circulation and returned to the liver. As much as 95% of the bile acids released from the gall bladder into the gut are reabsorbed, a process known as enterohepatic circulation.

Bile acid homeostasis is complex and is controlled by multiple processes. Bile acids can regulate the expression of genes that control their synthesis and uptake into the hepatocyte. A key component to the activity of this important feedback loop is the nuclear transcription factor FXR. There are two forms of this transcription factor, FXR$\alpha$ and FXR$\beta$, and in humans there are four $\alpha$-isozymes. When bile acids bind to FXR$\alpha$ it is activated, translocates to the nucleus, forms a heterodimer with RXR, and binds to hormone response elements (FXE). A primary function of FXR is to repress the expression and activity of CYP7A1, the rate-limiting enzyme in bile acid synthesis. FXR does not interact directly with the promoter of CYP7A1, rather FXR activation induces the expression of small heterodimer protein (SHP). SHP binds to the promoter region of CYP7A1 and suppresses expression. Under normal conditions, SHP is ubiquitinated and rapidly degraded by proteosomes; however, when bile acid levels in the liver rise, there is an increase in the expression of bile-acid-induced intestinal fibroblast growth factor 19 (FGF19).[75] FGF19 increases the stability of SHP *via* inhibition of SHP proteosomal degradation. This prolongs the half-life of SHP and enhances its activity toward inhibition of CYP7A1. Bile acids also repress the expression of genes encoding CYP8B1 and CYP27, two enzymes involved in bile acid synthesis.[76] It has also been shown that induction of SHP by bile acids inhibits the function of a membrane transporter $Na^+$-taurocholate contransporting peptide (NTCP) located on the basolateral side of the hepatocyte. Organic anion transport protein (OATP1B1) is another uptake transporter that is $Na^+$-dependent and whose expression is repressed by high levels of bile acids. Bile acids in the hepatocyte are transported by efflux pumps located in the canalicular membrane into bile (Figure 9.24). Both NTCP and OATP1B1 transport bile acids from sinusoidal blood into the hepatocyte.[77]

FXR activation induces the expression genes whose products are responsible, either directly or indirectly, for transporting bile acids out of the hepatocyte. These include the bile salt export pump (BSEP), multi-drug resistance protein 3 (MDR3), and multi-drug resistance associated protein 2 (MRP2). MDR3 transports phospholipids into the bile and is therefore necessary for the formation of phospholipid, cholesterol, and bile acid micelles which protect the liver from bile acid toxicity.

Another important nuclear receptor in the liver is PXR. PXR activation induces CYP enzymes such as (CYP3A4) which hydroxylates bile acids and

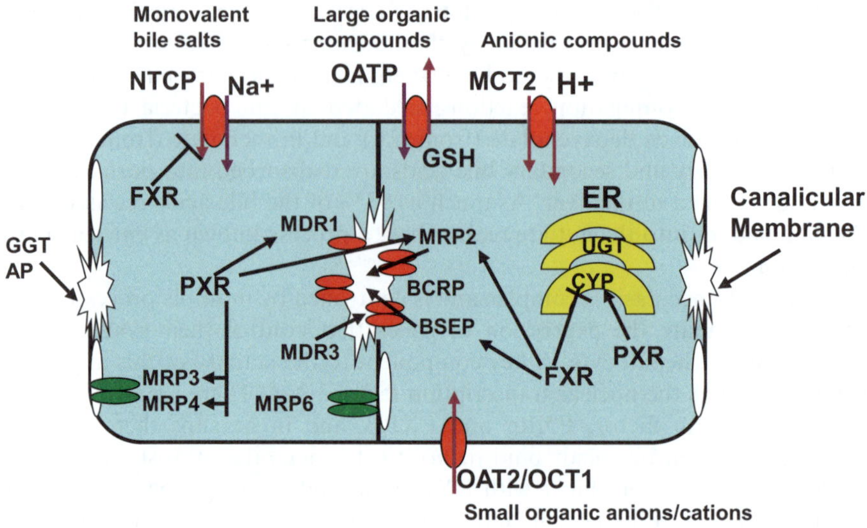


**Figure 9.24** Diagrammatic representation of hepatic transporter location and effects of FXR and PXR activation.

allows them to be transported out of the cell. PXR activation also controls the expression of several transporter proteins in the hepatocyte including BSEP, MDR1, MRP1, MRP2, MRP3, and OATP2.[1,78–80] PXR activation protects the liver from bile acid toxicity by increasing bile acid metabolism, and efflux.[81–83] MRP3 seems to play an important role in the mechanisms underlying the hepatoprotective effects of PXR activation against bile acid toxicity.[1]

From the preceding discussion it should be apparent that new chemical entities that disrupt bile acid homeostasis can indirectly increase liver toxicity *via* increased bile acids and may directly affect liver toxicity by changing the uptake, metabolism, and clearance of drugs that may be substrates for the CYP enzymes or efflux transporters. Disruption of these processes has clinical relevance. Genetic mutations resulting in the absence of BSEP and MDR3 have been linked to inherited cholestatic liver disorders. Mutations in MRP2 are linked to Dubin–Johnson syndrome or inherited hyperbilirubinemia.

New chemical entities that are FXR antagonists, inducers of CYP7A1, inducers of NCTP, or inhibitors of BSEP, MDR3, or MRP2 will cause an increase in bile acids in the hepatocyte. High concentrations of bile acids are toxic to the liver and can lead to chlolestatic liver disease, fibrosis, and eventual liver failure. Compounds that are PXR agonists can increase CYP expression, as well as transporter expression. These changes can lead to alterations in the pharmacokinetic properties of the drug resulting in drug–drug interactions (DDIs).

Therefore, it is important to understand how new chemical entities will affect these receptors, transporters, and CYPs in order to accurately predict direct liver toxicity and indirect toxicity related to DDIs.

## 9.8 *In Vitro* Methods for Evaluating PXR, FXR, and CAR Binding

Several methods are available for measuring nuclear receptor binding. Some examples include time-resolved fluorescence resonance energy transfer (TR-FRET), a microplate format for binding that uses time-resolved fluorescence, and a format based on ALPHAScreen technology.[84] Most methods are available in multi-wall formats and can be obtained from commercial sources.

Nuclear receptor binding can also be assessed in whole cell culture by exposing cells to known agonists and measuring the expression of genes known to be controlled by the nuclear receptor of interest by qRT-PCR. PXR controls the expression of CYP3A4, and exposure of human hepatocytes and some human immortalized cell lines to rifampicin or pregnenolone 16-α-carbonitrile (PCN), results in significant induction of CYP3A4. FXR can be activated with the addition of the synthetic ligands such as GW4064 which induces the expression of SHP, and CAR can be activated by phenobarbital as measured by the expression of CYP2B enzymes.[74,85]

### 9.8.1 Determining Transporter Inhibition

Inhibition of the bile salt export pump can be assessed using BSEP vesicles prepared from an insect cell system transfected with a baculovirus that expresses BSEP. Transport activity and the effect of the test compound on this activity can be determined by measuring the amount of radiolabeled substrate (*e.g.*, taurocholate) incorporated into the vesicles. Incubations in the presence of test compounds can provide information on inhibition and identify potential liver toxicity. BSEP vesicles for rat, dog, and human may be obtained from commercial sources.[86] An example of species-dependent inhibition of BSEP can be seen in Table 9.2 below.

In addition to BSEP vesicles, it is also possible to obtain vesicles that express several different MRPs and MDR1.

## 9.9 Developing Liver-Specific *In Vitro* Toxicity Screens

Un-anticipated liver toxicity observed in preclinical animal safety studies, in human clinical trials, or in patients after a drug as been approved and marketed

**Table 9.2** Comparison of BSEP inhibition between species.[86]

| *Inhibitor* | *Concentration tested (μM)* | *Rat BSEP % of control* | *Dog BSEP % of control* | *Human BSEP % of control* |
|---|---|---|---|---|
| Pravastatin | 500 | 88 | 48 | 42 |
| Rifampicin | 500 | 28 | 11 | 9 |
| Troglitazone | 100 | 30 | 17 | 1 |
| Vinblastin | 500 | 8 | 18 | 6 |

still represents a major reason for drug failure in the approval process and withdrawal from the market once approved. Therefore, it is prudent to incorporate a robust *in vitro* screening paradigm that can identify potential issues related to liver toxicity early in the discovery process. The liver is one of the most important organs to monitor because drugs dosed orally will enter the liver before entering systemic circulation. The liver is one of the most important organs in the metabolism, detoxification, and elimination of drugs. Many drugs are metabolized by cytochrome P450 enzymes in the liver, conjugated to glucuronide, sulfate, or glutathione and either returned to general circulation for elimination in the urine, or direct elimination *via* transport into bile. These factors can determine not only the concentration in plasma, but the half-life as well. Drugs may act directly on subcellular sites to cause adverse effects in the liver or they may act on pathways of normal liver function thereby causing toxicity *via* indirect mechanisms (*e.g.*, inhibition of bile flow). Early toxicity screening to identify acutely toxic agents requires a different model than later stage toxicity screening to examine species-specific toxicity issues, or chronic toxicity that may manifest as idiosyncratic toxicity in small patient populations after a drug has made it to market. *In vitro* toxicity screens designed to determine liver specific toxicity must incorporate multiple endpoints in an integrated systems biology approach to evaluating the potential toxicity of new drug candidates.[72] Wherever possible, the *in vitro* exposure concentrations should bracket the maximum therapeutic plasma concentrations expected during therapy. There should be an *in vivo* anchor, such as plasma concentration, that links the concentration–response profiles developed *in vitro* to something real *in vivo*. It is not enough to simply put test compound in a dish with cells and measure lactate dehydrogenase (LDH) leakage or an 3-(4 5-dimethylthiazol-2-yl)-2,5-diphenyltetrazolium bromide (MTT) assay. These endpoints alone often generate false negative or false positive results and are nearly impossible to interpret in isolation of other pertinent data. The cells used should mimic as closely as possible the complexities of the *in vivo* organ. To be successful, *in vitro* test systems must provide a value that can be used by others to make a decision about the molecule being tested. These individuals must be convinced that the *in vitro* data they are receiving can be translated to *in vivo* effects.

### 9.9.1 Different Models for Different Questions

The development and implementation of a useful *in vitro* screening strategy for identifying compounds that have a high probability of causing liver toxicity requires careful consideration. Clearly, a single cell model with one or two biochemical endpoints for cell viability will not be robust enough to define the more subtle mechanisms leading to hepatic toxicity in a small population of patients. Therefore, *in vitro* platforms with the greatest potential for providing meaningful data that can be used to predict *in vivo* effects, and make key decisions, will undoubtedly be comprised of a well-defined and understood test system. The successful screening platform should combine concentration response, and multiple endpoints in an integrated systems approach. Some of the endpoints selected should be specific for liver effects. In early discovery when it is important to understand all liabilities that a new molecule may possess, the use of immortalized cell lines can be very useful. The type of cell used and the number of endpoints measured is determined by where in the discovery funnel the assessment is to be placed. At this point predicting adverse effects in humans is not the issue. Discovering and understanding the underlying mechanisms of adverse effects relative to other compounds in the same chemical space should be the focus early at this toxicity screening stage. Speed, accuracy, and low cost are the primary requirements of early *in vitro* toxicity screening systems. Chemists must be able to identify and separate toxicophores from pharmacophores, target from off-target effects, and relative toxicity between molecules. As chemical modifications are made to the structure during efforts to improve potency or solubility, it is important to have at hand a rapid screening system that can assess how these changes may affect toxicity.

## 9.9.2 Early-Toxicity Screening Strategies

The FDA requires that all new chemical entities undergo safety testing in both rodent and non-rodent species. It is unlikely that NCEs that cause severe toxicity in rats will ever be approved for humans, unless the mechanism of the adverse effects can be identified as specific to rodents and therefore unlikely to occur in humans. Therefore, the use of rodent derived immortalized cell lines can provide excellent toxicity data, at low cost and reasonable turnaround times. Furthermore, because the primary effect being evaluated is acute toxicity, and because orally administered drugs will enter the liver before systemic circulation, the probability is high that any acute cytotoxicity measured is indeed predictive of liver toxicity. This of course is not the case for toxicity that is metabolism dependent, or that is more chronic in nature. These very specific types of toxicities require more sophisticated cell models.

There are many cell lines available for evaluating acute toxicity. The choice of a particular cell line should be based on laboratory understanding of its biochemical properties and experience with the model. One cell line that has many excellent and some unique properties that have been useful in our laboratories is the rat hepatoma (H4IIE) cell line. This cell line grows well in serum concentrations that range from 2.5–20%, making it possible to assess how protein binding affects toxicity. The cells do not revert to anaerobic metabolism (Crabtree effect) in culture, but remain oxidative, a trait much more similar to *in vivo* conditions. This property is important because many drug toxicities are linked to mitochondrial damage, and cells that revert to anaerobic metabolism for energy are less sensitive to mitochondrial effects. This is why the HepG2 cells when cultured in the presence of glucose cannot detect rotenone toxicity, a chemical that potently inhibits oxidative phosphorylation.[87,88] In comparison, rotenone-mediated mitochondrial toxicity is easily detected in H4IIE cells.[25,89] Finally, the H4IIE cells possess low constitutive cytochrome P450 activities and hence low metabolism. This property is fine for early screening work when the issue of toxicity must be simplified and the focus is on the parent molecule.

### 9.9.3 Importance of Multiple-Endpoint Analysis and Concentration Response

Over the years many biochemical assays have been developed to assess cytotoxicity in cells grown in culture. The use of *in vitro* cytotoxicity assays has provided important information on relative toxicity between chemicals as well as information on the mechanisms of toxicity. However, the ability to extrapolate *in vitro* toxicity to predict *in vivo* effects has been less successful. One reason for this apparent disconnect is the use of a single endpoint and exposure concentrations that would not be expected *in vivo*. Ideally, *in vitro* exposure concentrations should bracket those expected *in vivo*. The interpretation of *in vitro* data can change dramatically as the number of endpoints increases. Figure 9.25 illustrates how the interpretation of the data changes with different

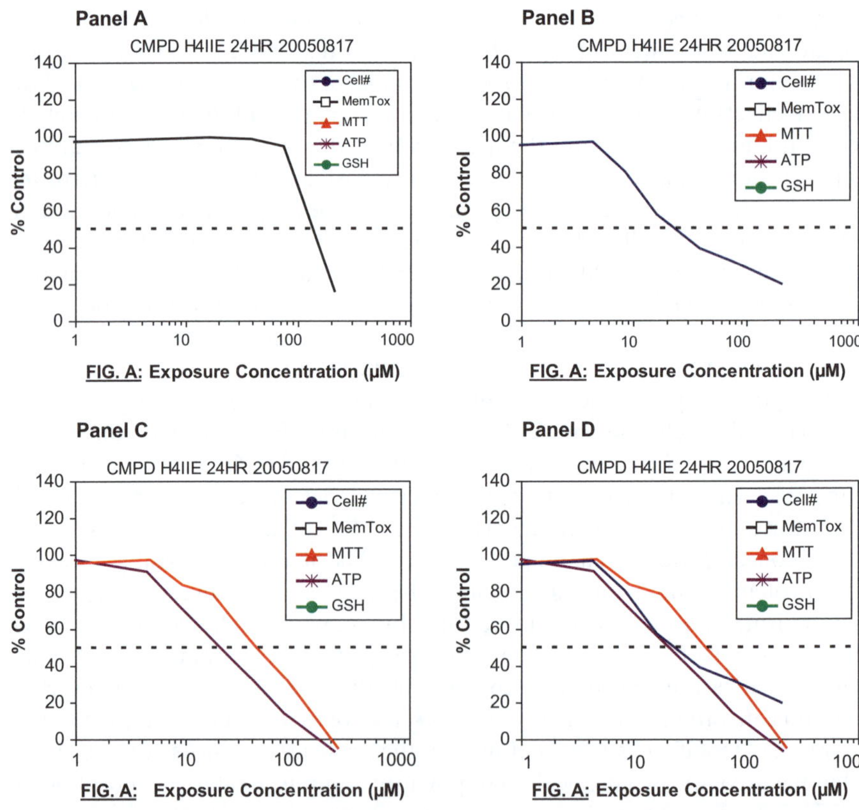


**Figure 9.25** Interpretation of *in vitro* data requires multiple endpoints.

endpoints. In Panel A, a typical membrane leakage marker is analyzed in the culture medium as a measure of viability. Based on this endpoint toxicity is low with no cell death detected until concentrations exceeding 100 μM are achieved.

In Panel B changes in cell mass are reported. Now it appears that the compound is considerably more toxic, but is the loss in cell mass due to cell death or changes in proliferation? Clearly, the interpretation of effect is considerably different when viewing each panel alone without the benefit of the other. However, by combining Panels A and B it is clear that the compound is altering cell proliferation prior to cell death. Let's continue with this compound a bit more. In Panel C two common markers (MTT and ATP) of cell health are shown. If Panel C data were all that was available it would not be clear whether the loss in MTT and ATP was due to cell death, a reduction in cell number, or a direct effect on mitochondria. However, when these data are plotted with cell mass (Panel D) it becomes much clearer. The reduction of MTT activity and ATP levels are due to a loss in cell mass that is the result of an inhibition in cell proliferation. Thus, the correct interpretation of the data is that the test compound's primary effect was on cell proliferation, and not on cell viability.

From the example above it should be clear that it is important to analyze *in vitro* responses relative to cell mass, protein, or DNA/RNA. This is especially true if the cell model being used is proliferating.

Bortezomib (Velcade®) is a potent and selective inhibitor of the 26S proteosome, a ubiquitous enzyme that controls many cellular signaling pathways. The drug has been effective in the treatment of several hematologic malignances and was approved in 2003 for the treatment of relapsed refractory multiple myeloma.[90–92] The drug was evaluated in the H4IIE model using four endpoints for cell viability and health (membrane leakage, ATP, MTT, and cell mass). Following a 24 h exposure to the drug (Figure 9.26, Panel A) all of the cell-based markers showed a maximal response of about 50% and were unchanged with increasing concentration of drug. The H4IIE cells have a doubling time of 22–24 h, therefore, in a 22–24 h exposure scenario if cell proliferation were inhibited, the maximum effect could only be 50% relative to controls. Note that the response curve for the media-based marker for membrane integrity was separate from the cell-based assays.

The approved drug bortezomib was evaluated in the *in vitro* cytotoxicity model by exposing H4IIE cells to concentrations ranging from 0.001 to 300 μM. The cells were seeded at a density of 10 000 per well in 100 μL of medium. The cells were allowed to grow and equilibrate for 48 h prior to applying the test material. Following the application of the test compound and a 24 h exposure time, cell health was assessed by assays that measure cell mass (circle), membrane integrity (square), incorporation of bromodeoxyuridine (BrdU) (diamonds), MTT (triangles), and ATP (asterisk). Each point on the concentration response curves represents the mean of 4–6 replicate wells. In Panel A, a concentration range of 1 to 300 μM resulted in all of the cell-based markers responding at the low exposure concentration and then not responding as exposures were increased, suggesting a potent and maximal effect at the lowest exposure tested. In order to define the concentration–response curve, the drug

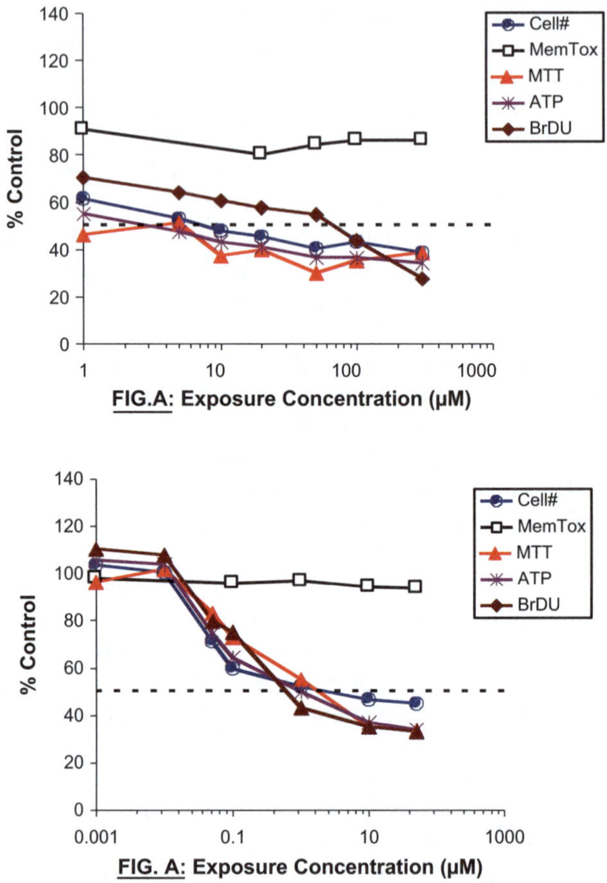


**Figure 9.26** *In vitro* toxicity testing of Velcade® using an H4IIIE cell line. Data provided by CeeTox Inc. Kalamazoo, MI.

was tested again at lower concentrations (Panel B). Under these conditions a full response profile was observed.

Note, when a response profile like the one in Panel A is obtained, it is necessary to adjust the exposure concentrations in order to define a concentration–response profile. Therefore, in Panel B the exposure concentrations were reduced and the result was a well-defined concentration–response profile. It is important to point out that the only parameter affected by the drug was cell proliferation. MTT activity and ATP levels tracked with loss in cell mass, and hence cannot be considered as independent events. There was no cell death as determined by membrane integrity, so this conclusion is valid under the experimental conditions presented. In this case the *in vitro* effects measured represent efficacy, the desired effect of the drug, and not toxicity.

The assay approach described above is rapid, low cost, and provides useful data sets that can be used by project teams to evaluate how changes in chemistry affect toxicity, to identify target from off-target effects, and understand mechanisms of adverse effects. As new drug candidates move through the lead optimization phase of discovery it is important to employ cell-based models that are more complex and varied in order to identify potential issues specific to the liver that may arise in the animal safety studies, in clinical trials, or in the market.

### 9.9.4 Liver-Specific Assay Systems

The evaluation of liver-specific liability should include metabolic stability, bioactivation, CYP induction/inhibition, PXR, CAR, AhR, and LXR binding, BSEP inhibition, UGT1A1 inhibition, and cytotoxicity parameters measured in primary hepatocytes grown in sandwich culture. All of these data should be combined and reviewed prior to making a final assessment of the hazard/risk profile.

To assess liver toxicity *in vitro*, primary hepatocytes are grown in sandwich culture and several biochemical endpoints are measured following exposure to a broad range of concentrations. Endpoints should include for acute toxicity, membrane integrity, mitochondrial function, cell mass, extrinsic and intrinsic apoptosis, redox status (GSH/GSSG), oxidative stress, and canalicular toxicity markers such as γ-glutamyl transferase (GGT) or alkaline phosphatase (AP), both specific to the canalicular membrane. Steatosis and phospholipidosis can be determined with simple assays. Changes in Nrf2/ARE controlled gene expression (HMOX1, TXN, NQO1, CYP1A1/2, ALDH3) can provide a good indication of cellular stress.

### 9.9.5 Membrane Integrity

There is a difference between biochemical events that may lead to cell death and cell death itself. This distinction is important in order to correctly interpret *in vitro* data sets as previously discussed in this chapter. When a cell loses the integrity of its plasma membrane, there is no possible way for survival. Osmotic balance is lost, redox potential is lost, and the internal environment mixes with the external. Therefore, true cell viability should be based on this parameter. There are several enzyme leakage markers routinely used to assess viability. Lactate dehydrogenase (LDH), GST, and ALT/AST are a few common examples. It is important to include controls for compound interference on the endpoints being measured and this is especially true in high-throughput laboratories where test compounds can represent a large chemical space. Activity-based assays are more susceptible to interference than assays that measure protein by ELISA. A prudent approach is to conduct initial evaluations by monitoring LDH activity, and if the results are equivocal, a follow up assay such as the α-GST ELISA (Argutus Medical, Dublin Ireland) can be included to verify the results. Membrane integrity is a vital anchor needed to interpret *in vitro* data.

### 9.9.6 Cell Proliferation

It is important to measure changes in cell number as a function of proliferation or cell death. This is most important when using an immortalized cell line where proliferation is active. Methods for determining cell proliferation include incorporation of BrdU, which is specific for S-phase, or methods that measure changes in total cellular DNA/RNA pools. Cell proliferation and membrane integrity serve as key reference points for interpreting all other endpoints. Effects observed on other cell functions that occur independently of cell death or changes in cell number can be identified as specific to the test compound.

### 9.9.7 Mitochondrial Function

Many drugs can produce adverse effects on mitochondrial function. This organelle is essential to the survival of cells in all tissues. Mitochondria are composed of two membranes that separate the inter-membrane compartment and the inner compartment, which holds the mitochondrial matrix. The inner membrane separates the mitochondrial matrix on the inside from the inter-membrane space on the outside (Figure 9.27). This organelle provides quantitatively the highest amount of energy (ATP) for the cell. Mitochondrial generation of ATP is by aerobic metabolism and is accomplished by oxidative phosphorylation (OXPHOS). The mitochondria contain many enzymes and functions that include β-oxidation of fatty acids, citric acid cycle, and OXPHOS. Two of the most relevant functions to toxicology are OXPHOS and

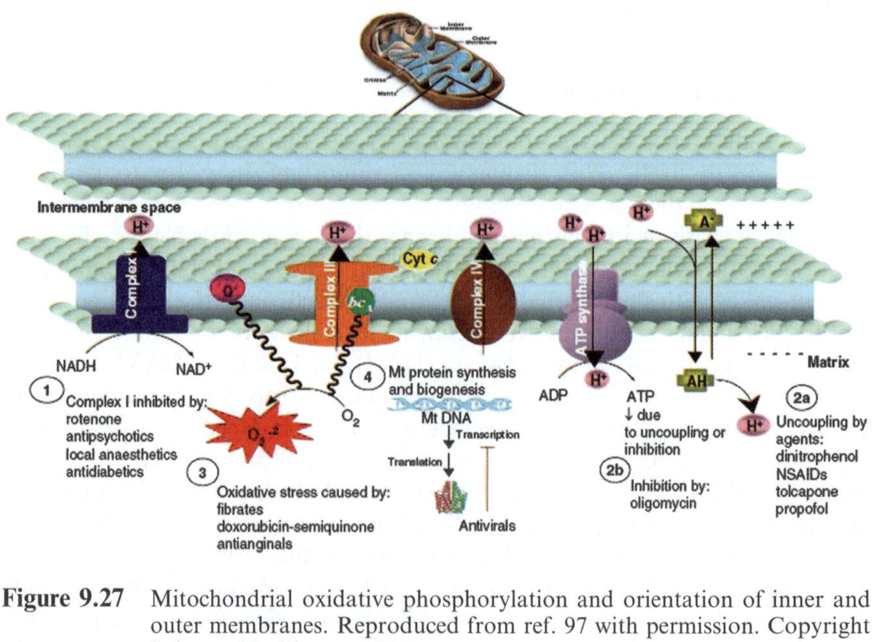


**Figure 9.27** Mitochondrial oxidative phosphorylation and orientation of inner and outer membranes. Reproduced from ref. 97 with permission. Copyright Informa Healthcare, 2005.

integrity of the dual-membrane system. The respiratory chain catalyzes electron transfer from reduced donors like NADPH and FADH2 with the generation of 10 $H^+$ protons for each pair of electrons used to form molecular oxygen. This creates an unequal movement of $H^+$ protons, which accumulate on the outside of the inner membrane and as a result an electrochemical gradient between the inside of the inner mitochondrial membranes and the outside ($\Delta\Psi$) is established. Maintenance of this proton gradient is essential to the health of the mitochondria and ultimately to the cell.

Drugs or chemicals can induce a mitochondrial permeability transition (MPT) which is the result of the opening of the MPT pore. The MPT pore is a protein pore formed in the mitochondrial membrane under stress. These pores are believed to be formed through the actions of pro-apoptotic proteins of the bcl-2 family (*e.g.*, Bad, Bax or Bid), which can be activated by stress, such as reactive oxygen, NO, and depletion of growth factors. Proteins in the bcl-2 family include bcl-2 and bcl-XL, which are anti-apoptotic and Bad, Bax or Bid, which are pro-apoptotic proteins. Bax is localized primarily in the cytosol, but translocates to the mitochondria when activated by stress stimuli where it binds to bcl-2 and forms PT-pores.[93] The relative abundance of pro- *versus* anti-apoptotic proteins determines how sensitive a cell is to apoptosis. Activation of the MPT-pore can destabilize the proton gradient and disrupt the membrane potential resulting in the leakage of cytochrome *c* and other pro-apoptotic

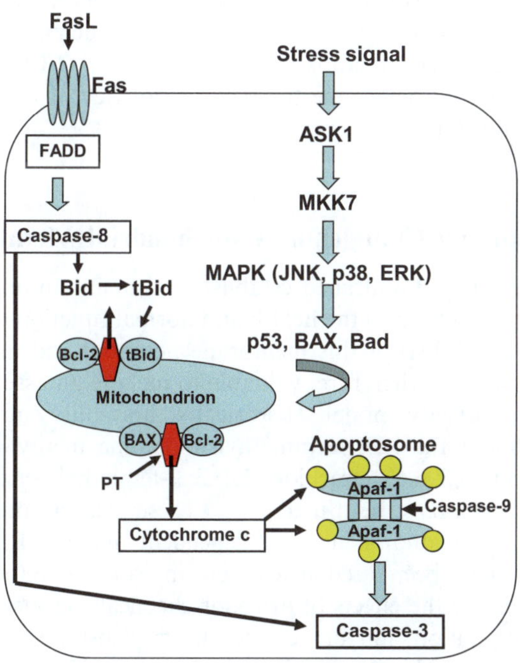


**Figure 9.28** Intracellular signaling pathways leading to apoptosis.

proteins into the cytosol of the cell. Cytochrome *c* binds to Apaf-1 to form an apoptosome, which then recruits the inactive pro-form of caspase 9 into the complex and activates it (Figure 9.28). The activation of caspase-9 begins a cascade that eventually results in the activation of caspase-3 or caspase-6, which represents the committed steps in programmed cell death characterized by DNA fragmentation.[94,95]

Drugs that inhibit the complexes I, III, and IV can cause an increase in ROS as the result of auto-oxidation of reduced complexes.[96] Examples of compounds that inhibit specific complexes are rotenone, formaldehyde, and chloramphenical (complex I), antimycin A (complex III), and cyanide (complex IV). Inhibition of these complexes causes an increase in ROS, which in turn activates mitochondrial PT leading to disruption in membrane potential and induction of apoptosis. Uncoupling agents are characterized as protonorphic. They shunt protons across the inner membrane thereby disrupting the proton gradient, effectively shutting down OXPHOS, reducing the amount of superoxide anion formed and reducing the production of cellular ATP.[96–98] Uncouplers reduce the formation of superoxide anion.[99]

Drug-induced damage to the mitochondria is a key event in the initiation of cellular toxicity and therefore assays designed to monitor mitochondrial health are essential. Therefore, *in vitro* toxicity screening for liver toxicity should include an extensive panel of assays designed to identify mitochondrial toxicity. Endpoints should include MTT, ATP levels, BAX/bcl-2 ratios, activation of caspases-3, 6, 8, and 9, changes in the REDOX state of the cell, and changes in $\Delta\Psi$. The inclusion of positive controls such as rotenone and antimycin, as inhibitors of OXPHOS, as well as uncoupling agents such as dinitrophenol and carbonylcyanide-*p*-trifluoromethoxy phenylhydrazone (FCCP), can improve data interpretation and determine the relative potency of the test drug *versus* known mitochondrial toxins.

### 9.9.8 Determining Changes in Mitochondrial Membranes ($\Delta\Psi$)

The ability of the mitochondria to establish and maintain an electrochemical proton gradient is essential to the health and normal function of this important organelle. Drugs can disrupt this membrane potential and disrupt OXPHOS and ATP synthesis. It is therefore, valuable to include an assessment of $\Delta\Psi$ in the *in vitro* liver toxicity model. Historically, lipophilic cationic fluorescent dyes such as rhodamine-123, tetramethylrhodamine methyl ester (TMRM), rhodamine-800, and 5,5′,6,6′-tetrachloro-1,1′,3,3′-tetraethyl-benzimidazolylcarbocyanine iodide (JC-1), have been used.[100–103] These dyes are preferentially taken up into healthy mitochondria in a $\Delta\Psi$-dependent manner. Rhodamine-123 or its methyl ester have been used extensively in isolated mitochondria and in intact cells to monitor the effects of drugs or chemicals on membrane potential, mitochondrial respiration, ion or volume effects, substrate transport, or ATP synthesis. Rhodamine-123 is taken up into viable mitochondria in a manner directly proportional to the $\Delta\Psi$. During this process the dye forms J-aggregates and stacks in

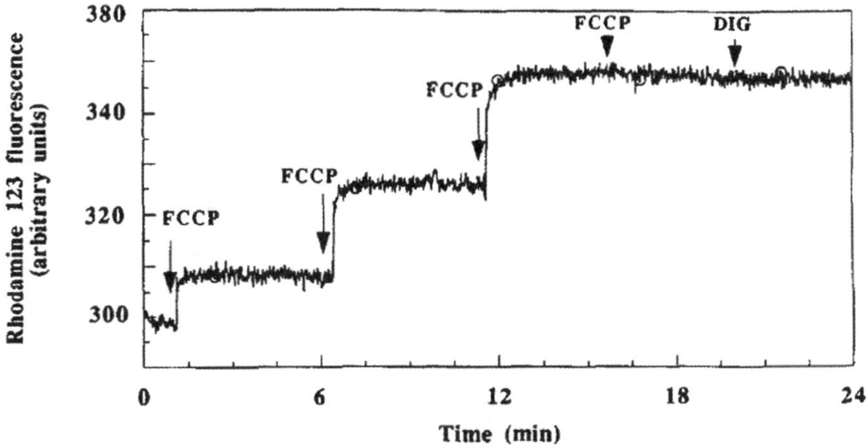


**Figure 9.29** Measuring disruption in mitochondrial membrane potential. Reproduced from ref. 104 with permission. Copyright Elsevier Science Inc., 1996.

a manner that quenches more than 70% of the fluorescent signal. As a result, treatment with drugs that disrupt the ΔΨ, cause an increase in the fluorescent signal as the dye is released back into the cytosol. In the example shown in Figure 9.29, hepatocytes isolated from rats were loaded with rhodamine-123 and then incubated in the presence of varying concentrations of the uncoupler FCCP for 10 min at 30 °C. A clear concentration-dependent increase in fluorescence was observed, at an excitation wavelength of 505 nm and an emission wavelength of 525 nm, indicating a disruption of ΔΨ and subsequent release of the fluorphore.[104]

At high concentrations rhodamine-123 has been shown to be cytotoxic. This is most likely due to inhibition of key mitochondrial proteins, such as ATPase, and inhibition of state-3 respiration at concentrations $>100$ μM. Concentrations as low as 10 μM have caused rapid swelling of mictochondria.[101] Therefore, when using this dye care should be taken to ensure that the dye is not cytotoxic to the cells. Optimization of the dye-loading concentrations should be determined for each cell type.

Another commonly used dye to measure ΔΨ is JC-1. In its monomer state the dye fluoresces green with an emission peak at 535 nm, which corresponds to a low ΔΨ. As the potential gradient increases (*e.g.*, healthy mitochondria) the dye forms aggregates and the emission peak shifts to red, with an emission peak at 595 nm. To determine the state of membrane polarization the ratio of $I_{595}/I_{535}$ is calculated. A higher ratio indicates healthy membranes while a lower ratio indicates a loss of membrane polarization and ΔΨ.[100] This assay was used in combination with mouse hepatocyte cell line (AML-12) to measure the effects of the drug clofibrate on mitochondria. These experiments revealed that the drug causes a concentration-dependent loss in ΔΨ and increases cellular ROS, both of which occurred prior to cell death (Figure 9.30).

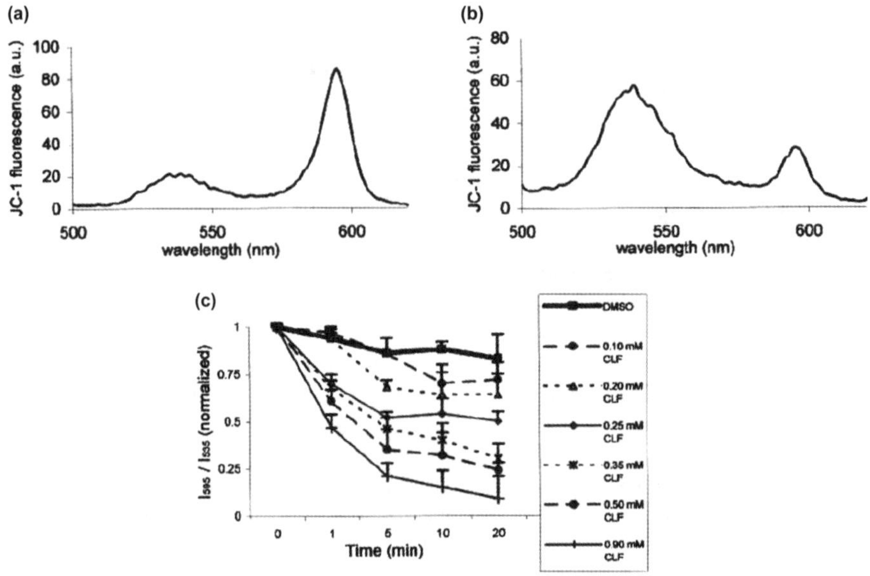


**Figure 9.30** Measuring mitochondrial $\Psi\Delta$ with JC-1 in the presence of clofibrate (CLF). Reproduced from ref. 100 with permission. Copyright Elsevier Science Inc., 1996.

## 9.9.9 Measuring Effects on Glutathione

Glutathione is the cells primary defense against oxidative injury and reactive electrophiles. GSH is a strong soft nucleophile that binds soft electrophiles in substitution-type reactions. Cellular GSH levels can be monitored by taking advantage of the highly specific reaction between monochlorobimane (mBCl) and GSH. Unbound mBCl is non-fluorescent, but in the presence of GSH and the enzyme GST a stable fluorescent adduct is formed.[105] The assay is simple and does not require the disruption of cells in culture. Changes in total cellular GSH (GSH + GSSG) can be determined by a modified Tietz assay as described by Jaeschke and Mitchell.[106] This method has the advantage of accounting for both reduced and oxidized GSH equivalents. This assay provides an indication of GSH lost from the cellular pool, which can occur when GSH binds to reactive drugs or their metabolites, is lost following cell death, or when there is direct inhibition of GSH synthesis. When total cellular GSH pools are depleted it is important to understand which mechanism is involved. Determining whether a test compound inhibits the rate limiting (γ-glutamylcysteine synthetase) enzyme in GSH synthesis is an important piece of information.[107–110]

## 9.9.10 Measuring Reactive Oxygen Species

Increased production and release of ROS, such as superoxide anion, hydrogen peroxide, hydroxyl radical, and lipid hydroperoxides can lead to significant liver toxicity. This effect is significantly enhanced when there is a concomitant loss in GSH, the primary antioxidant of the liver. ROS can be generated by the upregulation of CYP2E1, by inhibition of OXPHOs, or disruption of the mitochondrial membrane potential. Identifying compounds that increase cellular oxidative stress is important for predicting chronic liver toxicity. Activation of the Nrf2/ARE signaling pathway induces the expression of cytoprotective proteins under control of the antioxidant response element (ARE). Therefore, monitoring the expression of ARE controlled genes, such as glutamate cysteine ligase (GCL), heme oxygenase (HO-1), and thioredoxin (TXN) can serve as an indicator of oxidative stress.[28,72]

Increases in cellular hydroperoxides can be measured using the probe 2′,7′-dichlorofluorescein diacetate (DCFDA). DCFDA is non-fluorescent and able to diffuse across cell membranes. Once inside the cell the acetate moieties are cleaved by endogenous esterases to form the polar non-fluorescent 2′,7′-dichlorofluorescein, trapped inside the cell, which can react with reactive oxygen species to form the fluorescent form 2′,7′-dichlorofluorescin. The rate of change in fluorescence is determined at an excitation wavelength of 490 nm and an emission wavelength of 525 nm by determining the fluorescence intensity (FI) at time $t=0$ and after each exposure time ($t$). The DCF assay should be conducted over a short time course of exposure that ranges from 20 min to 12 h.[100,111–114]

### 9.9.11 Importance of Cell-to-Cell Communication

At the beginning of this chapter the cellular heterogeneity of the liver and its unique physiology and location in the body were discussed. Although most of the key biochemical functions normally associated with liver function can be found in the parenchymal cells (hepatocytes), it is important to remember how the effects of drugs on the other liver cells can influence toxicity. Compounds that elicit their primary effects on non-parenchymal cells *in vivo* may exhibit less toxicity when evaluated in a primary hepatocyte cell culture model. Therefore, it is important to evaluate the effects of new drug candidates on non-parenchymal cells.

The hepatic sinusoids contain four different cell types:

1) Endothelial cells, which form the lining of the sinusoid (capillary). These cells are unique in that they possess fenestrations that enable them to filter small molecules between the blood, cells in the sinusoids, and the parenchymal cells through the space of Disse.[4,8] Co-cultures of liver endothelial cells and hepatocytes have been used to study the role of IGF-II/M6P in the activation of latent TGF-β.[115]
2) Kupffer cells which are the macrophages of the liver and accumulate in periportal areas where their primary function is the endocytosis of bacterial endotoxin. When kupffer cells are exposed to endotoxins they become activated and release the proinflammatory cytokines IL-1, IL-6, TNF, and various eicosanoids. These cells can also take up and kill

tumor cells. The release of these bioactive cytokines can induce toxicity in nearby parenchymal cells and is the underlying mechanism of endotoxin induced liver injury.[116–118] Although these cells reside in the sinusoid they can have direct cell-to-cell contact with hepatocytes *via* cytoplasmic extensions. Several studies have been carried out using isolated hepatocytes in co-culture with kupffer cells. Work by Hoebe demonstrated that direct cell-to-cell contact between kupffer cells and hepatocytes is necessary in the development of a hepatic inflammatory response.[116] Drugs that activate macrophages can therefore initiate processes that lead to liver injury.

3) Stellate cells (SCs) are characterized by fat droplets and large amounts of vitamin A. The extracellular matrix (ECM) is composed of collagens, fibronectin, laminin, and proteoglycans. Under normal conditions stellate cells provide the primary source of these important materials. However, when the liver is injured or under chemical stress, these cells are stimulated to differentiate into myofibroblasts, which is characterized by a loss of vitamin A and of their fat droplets, and the production of α-actin. These cells play an important role in the development of hepatic fibrosis. When a stellate cell line (CFSC-2G) was co-cultured with hepatocytes the system behaved in a manner consistent with the pathogenesis of fibrosis as characterized by impaired adenylate charge and succinate dehydrogenase activity, and increased collagen.[119]
4) Pit cells are the natural killer cells of the liver. These cells can be activated by exogenous chemicals can enhance their activity and proliferation. Kupffer cells appear to control pit cell motility, adherence, viability, and cytotoxicity.[8] Examples of co-cultures with hepatocytes and pit cells could not be found, but this may be an important area for future research.

## 9.10 Precision-Cut Liver Slices

Precision-cut liver slices (PCTS) in dynamic organ culture provide a well studied and accepted method of evaluating drug metabolism and toxicity.[120–123] PCTS has several advantages over standard monolayer culture models. The slices maintain normal cell architecture, cell heterogeneity, relative abundance of cell types, and cell-to-cell interactions. In addition this method can also be used to study other tissues (*e.g.*, kidney, lung, and heart) obtained from the same source. To prepare slices, liver tissue from the species of choice is obtained and cored using a biopsy punch. The core is then placed into a tissue slice instrument, such as the Krumdieck Tissue Slicer and sliced into discs that have a thickness of 200–250 nm (Figures 9.31 and 9.32). The slices can then be placed into multi-well cell culture plates for study.[124,130]

Recent advances in the ability to cryopreserve human and rat tissue slices has made this method more attractive for routine screening work.[125,126] Cytochrome P450 (CYP) induction has been well studied and shown to be similar to primary hepatocytes. CYP2B induction by phenobarbital and CYP2E1 by

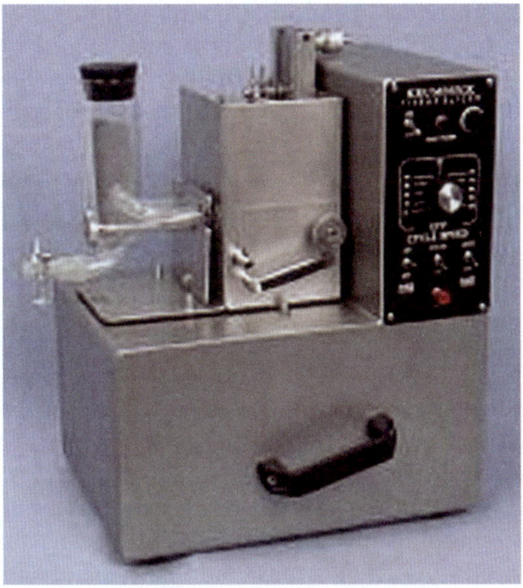

**Figure 9.31** Photograph of the Krumdieck tissue slicer.

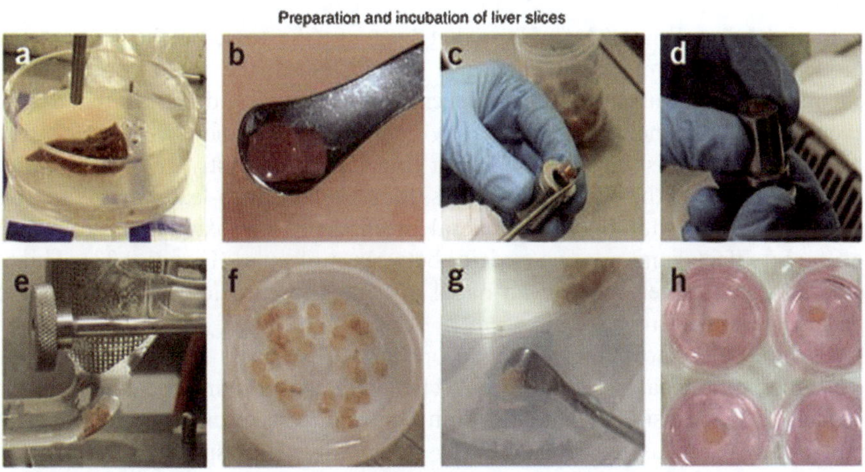


**Figure 9.32** Preparation of precision-cut liver slices. Reproduced from ref. 130 with permission. Copyright Nature America, Inc., 2010.

isoniazid has been recently reported.[123] This model has also been used to study the regional cytochrome P450 activities.[127]

PCTS is also useful for evaluating metabolism and toxicity of several drugs in the same class. An example is the work reported by Onderwater which compared several *N*-substituted *N*′-(4-imidazole-ethyl) thiourea compounds, which undergo Phase I and II metabolism in the liver.[128] The model provided data that could be used to relate chemical structure with toxicity and metabolism and provided a means of rank ordering these compounds.

Slices prepared from livers undergoing fibrosis were shown to provide a functional model for studying the antifibrotic properties of new drug candidates.[129]

This model provides an excellent alternative to primary culture and cell lines for the study of drug metabolism and toxicity.

## 9.11 Conclusions

Drug-induced liver injury is a major reason for the failure of promising new drugs in preclinical safety studies and in small patient populations after it enters the market. The liver is a complex organ that serves many important functions essential for survival. All drugs administered orally must enter the liver prior to entering systemic circulation. This means that the liver may achieve high concentrations of drugs and their metabolites. A systematic approach (Table 9.3) to the generation of *in vitro* safety data combined with a gated Boolean logic pattern for making decisions can ensure that the best science is applied in a way that optimizes the probability of success for new drugs.

In order for *in vitro* data to predict liver specific toxicity, the *in vitro* cell model should mimic key functional properties of the intact organ. Biochemical or molecular endpoints specific to the liver and linked to adverse events should be included in the assay panel. The placement of assays in the discovery funnel is important. Labor-intensive and costly models are not required early in the discovery process during the hit-to-lead phase. In this phase the focus should be on general mechanisms of toxicity, target *versus* off-target effects, and relative toxicity between molecules (Figure 9.33). This is where the use of cell lines and a panel of general cytotoxicity markers would be most useful (Table 9.3).

As molecules move into the lead-optimization phase, ADME and drug–drug interaction data should be collected with the primary focus on human models. The inclusion of models from common test species, such as the rat and dog, can be useful in identifying potential species specific effects or to provide a mechanistic explanation for effects observed in preclinical safety studies. The addition of more complex human-cell-based models should be used at this stage. Finally, all *in vitro* information collected should be analyzed in order to make a final assessment of risk going forward. An estimate of maximum plasma concentration expected in therapy, therapeutic endpoint, and length of dosing are only a few of the important parameters needed to make an intelligent go-no-go decision. The probability of drug-induced liver injury in either animals or humans can be greatly reduced by implementing an *in vitro* toxicity screening program that focuses on cell models with liver-specific properties combined with intelligent selection of multiple parameters

**Table 9.3** Suggested *in vitro* screening strategy for identifying liver toxicity.

| *In Vitro model* | *Timing* | *Species* | *Cellular function* | *Assay* | *Interpretation* |
|---|---|---|---|---|---|
| CL | HL | R, H | Membrane integrity | GST, LDH, ALT | Cell viability live/dead[a] |
| CL | HL | R, H | Mitochondrial function | ΔΨ, ATP, MTT | Mitochondrial toxicity |
| CL | HL | R, H | Oxidative stress (redox) | GSH, DCFDA | Reactivity and redox, oxidative stress |
| CL | HL | R, H | Cell proliferation | BrdU caspase activation | Determines test compound's affect on cell division |
| CL | HL | R, H | Apoptosis | DNA fragmentation | Determines programmed cell death |
| MIC | HL | R, H | Metabolism loss of parent | LC-MS %R | Provides metabolic stability and intrinsic clearance |
| MIC | LO | H, R, D | GSH depletion and conjugation | GSH-binding | Determines parent reactivity and formation of reactive metabolites and species differences |
| | LO | H | Nuclear receptor binding | PXR, LXR, CAR binding | |
| PHSC | LO | H, R, D | Bile flow | BSEP inhibition | Determines cholestatic potential and species differences |
| IV | LO | H, R, D | Bile flow | BSEP inhibition | Determines cholestatic potential and species differences |
| PHSC | LO | H, R, D | CYP induction | CYP activity | Determines induction of major CYPs |
| MIC | LO | H | CYP inhibition | CYP inhibition | Determines test compound's ability to inhibit key CYPs |
| PE | LO | H | CYP inhibition | CYP inhibition | Determines test compound's ability to inhibit key CYPs |
| PHSC | LO | H, R, D | Membrane integrity | GST, LDH, ALT | Provides toxicity data in normal tissue, species differences |
| PHSC | LO | H, R, D | Cannalicular toxicity | GGT, AP | Identifies toxicity specific to cannalicular membrane and species differences |
| PHSC | LO | H, R, D | Mitochondrial function | ΔΨ, ATP, MTT | Mitochondrial health |
| PHSC | LO | H, R, D | Gene panel toxicity | Array with 10 toxicity target pathways | Identifies signaling pathways related to toxicity |
| PCLS | LO | H | Membrane integrity, mitochondrial function | GST, LDH, ALT ΔΨ, ATP, MTT | Evaluates toxicity in a liver model with all cell types present, assesses direct and indirect toxicity |
| | | | Apoptosis | Caspase activation, DNA fragmentation | Determines programmed cell death |

[a]Panel provides estimate of plasma concentration where general toxicity would be expected to occur. Determine *in vitro* therapeutic index. Rank order compounds. CL = cell lines, MIC = microsomes, PHSC - primary hepatocytes sandwich culture, IV - isolated vesicles, PE = purified enzymes, PCLS - precision-cut liver slices, HL - Hit-to-Lead, LO - lead optimization.

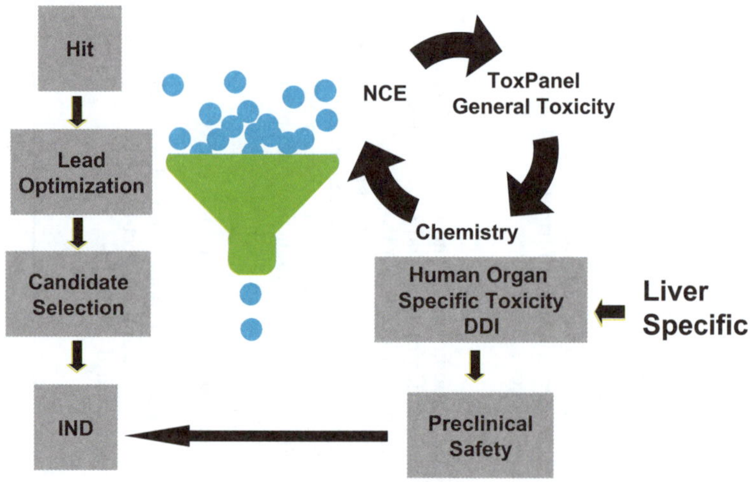


**Figure 9.33** Incorporating *in vitro* liver toxicity screening into drug discovery.

that provide clear information on cell health over an exposure concentration range that is relevant to expected *in vivo* plasma concentrations.

## Acknowledgements

I would like to thank the scientific staff at CeeTox, Inc (Kalamazoo, MI) for their dedication to the development and validation of *in vitro* models that predict *in vivo* toxicity and to Ms. Muriel Reva for her outstanding technical support. I would also like to thank Mr. Paul Wilga for his critical review of this manuscript and for his excellent comments and suggestions. I would like to thank my wife Lindsay P. South who gave me the space to write this and to my father the late Dr. James M. McKim III, who is always with me.

## References

1. S. Teng and M. Piquette-Miller, *Br. J. Pharmacol.*, 2007, **151**, 367–376.
2. J. M. McKim Jr, J. Liu, Y. P. Liu and C. D. Klaassen, *Toxicol. Appl. Pharmacol.*, 1992, **112**, 324–330.
3. S. Angermuller, M. Schunk and K. Kusterer, *Hepatology*, 1995, **21**, 1594–1601.
4. L. Bouwens, L. P. De Bleser, K. Vanderkerken, B. Geerts and E. Wisse, *Enzyme*, 1992, **46**, 155–168.
5. D. R. Koop, B. Klopfenstein, Y. Iimuro and R. G. Thurman, *Mol. Pharmacol.*, 1997, **51**, 944–950.
6. M. Onda, M. Willingham, Q. C. Wang, R. J. Kreitman, Y. Tsutsumi, S. Nagata and I. Pastan, *J. Immunol.*, 2000, **165**, 7150–7156.

7. S. Tafazoli, D. D. Spehar and P. J. O'Brien, *Drug Metab. Rev.*, 2005, **37**, 311–325.
8. E. Wisse, F. Braet, D. Luo, R. De Zanger, D. Crabbé and A. Vermoesen, *Toxicol. Pathol.*, 1996, **24**, 100–111.
9. A. M. De Leeuw, A. Brouwer and D. L. Knook, *J. Electron Microsc. Technol.*, 1990, **14**, 218–236.
10. R. S. McCuskey, *Clin. Hemorheol. Microcirc.*, 2006, **34**, 5–10.
11. C. Menor, M. D. Fernández-Moreno, J. A. Fueyo, O. Escribano, T. Olleros, E. Arriaza, C. Cara, M. Lorusso, M. Di Paola, I. D. Román and L. G. Guijarro, *J. Pharmacol. Exp. Ther.*, 2004, **311**, 668–676.
12. L. D. DeLeve, X. Wang, J. F. Kuhlenkamp and N. Kaplowitz, *Hepatology*, 1996, **23**, 589–599.
13. M. Emoto and S. H. Kaufmann, *Trends Immunol.*, 2003, **24**, 364–369.
14. A. Stanciu, C. Cotuţiu and C. Amălinei, *Rev. Med. Chir. Soc. Med. Nat. Iasi.*, 2002, **107**, 235–239.
15. D. Kobold, A. Grundmann, F. Piscaglia, C. Eisenbach, K. Neubauer, J. Steffgen, G. Ramadon and T. Knittel, *J. Hepatol.*, 2002, **36**, 607–613.
16. L. Beljaars, D. K. Meijer and K. Poelstra, *Front. Biosci.*, 2002, **7**, e214–e222.
17. T. Gonzalo, E. G. Talman, A. van de Ven, K. Temming, R. Greupink, L. Beljaars, C. Reker-Smit, D. K. Meijer, G. Molema, K. Poelstra and R. J. Kok, *J. Control. Release*, 2006, **111**, 193–203.
18. R. Greupink, H. I. Bakker, W. Bouma, C. Reker-Smit, D. K. Meijer, L. Beljaars and K. Poelstra, *J. Pharmacol. Exp. Ther.*, 2006, **317**, 514–521.
19. L. Beljaars, G. Molema, B. Weert, H. Bonnema, P. Olinga, G. M. Groothuis, D. K. Meijer and K. Poelstra, *Hepatology*, 1999, **29**, 1486–1493.
20. L. Beljaars, G. Molema, D. Schuppan, A. Geerts, P. De Bleser, B. Weert, D. K. Meijer and K. Poelstra, *J. Biol. Chem.*, 2000, **275**, 12743–12751.
21. L. Beljaars, P. Olinga, G. Molema, P. De Bleser, A. Geerts, G. M. Groothuis, D. K. Meijer and K. Poelstra, *Liver*, 2001, **21**, 320–328.
22. E. M. Gagan, M. W. Hull, T. W. Schultz, G. Pöch and D. A. Dawson, *Arch. Environ. Contam. Toxicol.*, 2007, **52**, 283–293.
23. D. A. Dawson, J. L. Allen, T. W. Schultz and G. Pöch, *J. Environ. Sci. Health, Part A: Toxic/Hazard. Subst. Environ. Eng.*, 2008, **43**, 43–52.
24. B. Ketterer, B. Coles and D. J. Meyer, *Environ. Health Perspect.*, 1983, **49**, 59–69.
25. J. M. McKim Jr, D. J. Keller III and J. R. Gorski, *J. Toxicol., Cutan. Ocul. Toxicol.*, 2010, **29**, 171–192.
26. T. W. Schultz, J. W. Yarbrough and E. L. Johnson, *SAR QSAR Environ. Res.*, 2005, **16**, 313–322.
27. T. W. Schultz, J. W. Yarbrough and S. K. Koss, *Cell Biol. Toxicol.*, 2006, **22**, 339–349.
28. A. Natsch, H. Gfeller, M. Rothaupt and G. Ellis, *Toxicol. in Vitro*, 2007, **21**, 1220–1226.

29. K. G. Madsen, C. Skonberg, U. Jurva, C. Cornett, S. H. Hansen, T. N. Johansen and J. Olsen, *Chem. Res. Toxicol.*, 2008, **21**, 1107–1119.
30. A. T. Banks, H. J. Zimmerman, K. G. Ishak and J. G. Harter, *Hepatology*, 1995, **22**, 820–827.
31. E. G. Breen, J. McNicholl, D. Cosgrove, J. McCabe and F. M. Stevens, *Gut*, 1986, **27**, 1390–1393.
32. P. Purcell, D. Henry and G. Melville, *Gut*, 1991, **32**, 1381–1385.
33. R. Bort, K. Mace, A. Boobis, M. J. Gómez-Lechón, A. Pfeifer and J. Castell, *Biochem. Pharmacol.*, 1999, **58**, 787–796.
34. S. Shen, M. R. Marchick, M. R. Davis, G. A. Doss and L. R. Pohl, *Chem. Res. Toxicol.*, 1999, **12**, 214–222.
35. T. Y. Aw, *News Physiol. Sci.*, 2003, **18**, 201–204.
36. M. E. Rodríguez-García, A. G. Quiroga, J. Castro, A. Ortiz, P. Aller and F. Mata, *Toxicol. Sci.*, 2009, **111**, 413–423.
37. J. Dong, S. Ramachandiran, K. Tikoo, Z. Jia, S. S. Lau and T. J. Monks, *Am. J. Physiol. Renal Physiol.*, 2004, **287**, F1049–F1058.
38. N. Yamamoto, H. Sawada, Y. Izumi, T. Kume, H. Katsuki, S. Shimohama and A. Akaike, *J. Biol. Chem.*, 2007, **282**, 4364–4372.
39. H. Zhang, C. D. Davis, M. W. Sinz and A. D. Rodrigues, *Expert Opin. Drug Metab. Toxicol.*, 2007, **3**, 667–687.
40. N. Masubuchi, C. Makino and N. Murayama, *Chem. Res. Toxicol.*, 2007, **20**, 455–464.
41. Y. Masubuchi, C. Suda and T. Horie, *J. Hepatol.*, 2005, **42**, 110–116.
42. M. E. Marshall, J. L. Mohler, K. Edmonds, B. Williams, K. Butler, M. Ryles, L. Weiss, D. Urban, A. Bueschen and M. Markiewicz, *J. Cancer Res. Clin. Oncol.*, 1994, **120**, S39–S42.
43. J. D. Vassallo, S. M. Hicks, G. P. Daston and L. D. Lehman-McKeeman, *Toxicol. Sci.*, 2004, **80**, 249–257.
44. S. L. Born, D. Caudill, B. J. Smith and L. D. Lehman-McKeeman, *Toxicol. Sci.*, 2000, **58**, 23–31.
45. A. E. Vickers, *Chem.–Biol. Interact.*, 2009, **179**, 9–16.
46. S. J. Gee, C. E. Green and C. A. Tyson, *Drug Metab. Dispos.*, 1984, **12**, 174–178.
47. P. Dogterom and J. Rothuizen, *Drug Metab. Dispos.*, 1993, **21**, 705–709.
48. A. Y. Lu, R. W. Wang and J. H. Lin, *Drug Metab. Dispos.*, 2003, **31**, 345–350.
49. L. Wang, D. Zhang, N. Raghavan, M. Yao, L. Ma, C. E. Frost, B. D. Maxwell, S. Y. Chen, K. He, T. C. Goosen, W. G. Humphreys and S. J. Grossman, *Drug Metab. Dispos.*, 2010, **38**, 448–458.
50. A. P. Li, *Methods Mol. Biol.*, 2010, **640**, 281–294.
51. R. J. Weaver, M. Dickins and M. D. Burke, *Biochem. Pharmacol.*, 1995, **49**, 997–1004.
52. S. A. Benetton, C. Fang, Y. O. Yang, R. Alox, M. Year, C. C. Lin and L. T. Yeh, *Drug Metab. Pharmacokinet.*, 2007, **22**, 78–87.
53. A. D. Rodrigues, *Biochem. Pharmacol.*, 1999, **57**, 465–480.
54. S. S. Singh, *Curr. Drug Metab.*, 2006, **7**, 165–182.

55. H. Zhang, C. D. Davis, M. W. Sinz and A. D. Rodrigues, *Expert Opin. Drug Metab. Toxicol.*, 2007, **3**, 667–687.
56. B. C. Jones, R. Hyland, M. Ackland, C. A. Tyman and D. A. Smith, *Drug Metab. Dispos.*, 1998, **26**, 875–882.
57. Y. Shibata, H. Takahashi, M. Chiba and Y. Ishii, *Drug Metab. Pharmacokinet.*, 2008, **23**, 328–339.
58. K. E. Riley, B. T. Op't Holt and K. M. Merz, *J. Chem. Theory Comput.*, 2007, **3**, 407–433.
59. Z. W. Zhou and S. F. Zhou, *Expert Opin. Drug Metab. Toxicol.*, 2009, **5**, 579–605.
60. M. L. Turpeinen and L. E. Korhonen, *Eur. J. Pharm. Sci.*, 2006, **29**, 130–138.
61. N. J. Hewitt, E. L. Lecluyse and S. S. Ferguson, *Xenobiotica*, 2007, **37**, 1196–1224.
62. A. Madan, R. A. Graham, K. M. Carroll, D. R. Mudra, L. A. Burton, L. A. Krueger, A. D. Downey, M. Czerwinski, J. Forster, M. D. Ribadeneira, L. S. Gan, E. L. LeCluyse, K. Zech, P. Robertson Jr, P. Koch, L. Antonian, G. Wagner, L. Yu and A. Parkinson, *Drug Metab. Dispos.*, 2003, **31**, 421–431.
63. E. L. LeCluyse, K. L. Audus and J. H. Hochman, *Am. J. Physiol.*, 1994, **266**, C1764–C1774.
64. S. M. Huang, J. M. Strong, L. Zhang, K. S. Reynolds, S. Nallani, R. Temple, S. Abraham, S. A. Habet, R. K. Baweja, G. J. Burckart, S. Chung, P. Colangelo, D. Frucht, M. D. Green, P. Hepp, E. Karnaukhova, H. S. Ko, J. I. Lee, P. J. Marroum, J. M. Norden, W. Qiu, A. Rahman, S. Sobel, T. Stifano, K. Thummel, X. X. Wei, S. Yasuda, J. H. Zheng, H. Zhao and L. J. Lesko, *J. Clin. Pharmacol.*, 2008, **48**, 662–670.
65. A. P. Li, P. Maurel, M. J. Gomez-Lechon, L. C. Cheng and M. Jurima-Romet, *Chem.–Biol. Interact.*, 1997, **107**, 5–16.
66. N. J. Hewitt, M. J. Lechón, J. B. Houston, D. Hallifax, H. S. Brown, P. Maurel, J. G. Kenna, L. Gustavsson, C. Lohmann, C. Skonberg, A. Guillouzo, G. Tuschl, A. P. Li, E. LeCluyse, G. M. Groothuis and J. G. Hengstler, *Drug Metab. Rev.*, 2007, **39**, 159–234.
67. R. E. Pearce, W. Lu, Y. Wang, J. P. Uetrecht, M. A. Correia and J. S. Leeder, *Drug Metab. Dispos.*, 2008, **36**, 1637–1649.
68. R. E. Pearce, J. P. Uetrecht and J. S. Leeder, *Drug Metab. Dispos.*, 2005, **33**, 1819–1826.
69. B. K. Park, N. R. Kitteringham, J. L. Maggs, M. Pirmohamed and D. P. Williams, *Annu. Rev. Pharmacol. Toxicol.*, 2005, **45**, 177–202.
70. G. A. Doss and T. A. Baillie, *Drug Metab. Rev.*, 2006, **38**, 641–649.
71. A. Natsch and R. Emter, *Toxicol. Sci.*, 2008, **102**, 110–119.
72. J. M. McKim Jr, *Comb. Chem. High Throughput Screening*, 2010, **13**, 188–206.
73. H. Takakusa, H. Masumoto, A. Mitsuru, O. Okazaki and K. Sudo, *Drug Metab. Dispos.*, 2008, **36**, 816–823.
74. M. Wagner, E. Halilbasic, H. U. Marschall, G. Zollner, P. Fickert, C. Langner, K. Zatloukal, H. Denk and M. Trauner, *Hepatology*, 2005, **42**, 420–430.

75. J. Miao, Z. Xiao, D. Kanamaluru, G. Min, P. M. Yau, T. D. Veenstra, E. Ellis, S. Strom, K. Suino-Powell, H. E. Xu and J. K. Kemper, *Genes Dev.*, 2009, **23**, 986–996.
76. B. Goodwin, S. A. Jones, R. R. Price, M. A. Watson, D. D. McKee, L. B. Moore, C. Galardi, J. G. Wilson, M. C. Lewis, M. E. Roth, P. R. Maloney, T. M. Willson and S. A. Kliewer, *Mol. Cell.*, 2000, **6**, 517–526.
77. L. A. Denson, E. Sturm, W. Echevarria, T. L. Zimmerman, M. Makishima, D. J. Mangelsdorf and S. J. Karpen, *Gastroenterology*, 2001, **121**, 140–147.
78. H. R. Kast, B. Goodwin, P. T. Tarr, S. A. Jones, A. M. Anisfeld, C. M. Stoltz, P. Tontonoz, S. Kliewer, T. M. Willson and P. A. Edwards, *J. Biol. Chem.*, 2002, **277**, 2908–2915.
79. S. Teng, V. Jekerle and M. Piquette-Miller, *Drug Metab. Dispos.*, 2003, **31**, 1296–1299.
80. A. Geick, M. Eichelbaum and O. Burk, *J. Biol. Chem.*, 2001, **276**, 14581–14587.
81. J. L. Staudinger, B. Goodwin, S. A. Jones, D. Hawkins-Brown, K. I. MacKenzie, A. LaTour, Y. Liu, C. D. Klaassen, K. K. Brown, J. Reinhard, T. M. Willson, B. H. Koller and S. A. Kliewer, *Proc. Natl. Acad. Sci. U. S. A.*, 2001, **98**, 3369–3374.
82. J. L. Staudinger, X. Ding and K. Lichti, *Expert Opin. Drug Metab. Toxicol.*, 2006, **2**, 847–857.
83. W. Xie, A. Radominska-Pandya, Y. Shi, C. M. Simon, M. C. Nelson, E. S. Ong, D. J. Waxman and R. M. Evans, *Proc. Natl. Acad. Sci. U. S. A.*, 2001, **98**, 3375–3380.
84. J. F. Glickman, X. Wu, R. Mercuri, C. Illy, B. R. Bowen, Y. He and M. Sills, *J. Biomol. Screen.*, 2002, **7**, 3–10.
85. S. Westin, R. A. Heyman and R. Martin, *Mini Rev. Med. Chem.*, 2005, **5**, 719–727.
86. H. Yabuuchi, K. Tanaka, M. Maeda, M. Takemura, M. Oka, R. Ohashi and I. Tamai, *Biopharm. Drug Dispos.*, 2008, **29**, 441–448.
87. P. J. O'Brien, W. Irwin, D. Diaz, E. Howard-Cofield, C. M. Krejsa, M. R. Slaughter, B. Gao, N. Kaludercic, A. Angeline, P. Bernardi, P. Brain and C. Hougham, *Arch. Toxicol.*, 2006, **80**, 580–604.
88. L. D. Marroquin, J. Hynes, J. A. Dykens, J. D. Jamieson and Y. Will, *Toxicol. Sci.*, 2007, **97**, 539–547.
89. G. L. Cockerell, J. M. McKim and S. L. Vonderfecht, *Toxicol. Pathol.*, 2002, **30**, 4–7.
90. C. Montagut, A. Rovira, B. Mellado, P. Gascon, J. S. Ross and J. Albanell, *Drugs Today*, 2005, **41**, 299–315.
91. C. Lu, R. Gallegos, P. Li, C. Q. Xia, S. Pusalkar, V. Uttamsingh, D. Nix, G. T. Miwa and L. S. Gan, *Drug Metab. Dispos.*, 2006, **34**, 702–708.
92. A. Hemeryck, R. Geerts, J. Monbaliu, S. Hassler, T. Verhaeghe, L. Diels, W. Verluyten, L. van Beijsterveldt, R. N. Mamidi, C. Janssen and R. De Coster, *Cancer Chemother. Pharmacol.*, 2007, **60**, 777–787.
93. T. Asakura and K. Ohkawa, *Curr. Cancer Drug Targets*, 2004, **4**, 577–590.

94. G. Kroemer, B. Dallaporta and M. Resche-Rigon, *Annu. Rev. Physiol.*, 1998, **60**, 619–642.
95. G. Kroemer, N. Zamzami and S. A. Susin, *Immunol. Today*, 1997, **18**, 44–51.
96. P. Kovacic, R. S. Pozos, R. Somanathan, N. Shangari and P. J. O'Brien, *Curr. Med. Chem.*, 2005, **12**, 2601–2623.
97. K. Chan, D. Truong, N. Shangari and P. J. O'Brien, *Expert Opin. Drug Metab. Toxicol.*, 2005, **1**, 655–669.
98. J. P. Mehta, J. L. Campian, J. Guardiola, J. A. Cabrera, E. K. Weir and J. W. Eaton, *Chest*, 2008, **133**, 1410–1414.
99. S. S. Korshunov, O. V. Korkina, E. K. Ruuge, V. P. Skulachev and A. A. Starkov, *FEBS Lett.*, 1998, **435**, 215–218.
100. B. Qu, Q. T. Li, K. P. Wong, T. M. Tan and B. Halliwell, *Free Radic. Biol. Med.*, 2001, **31**, 659–669.
101. R. K. Emaus, R. Grunwald and J. J. Lemasters, *Biochim. Biophys. Acta*, 1986, **850**, 436–448.
102. J. Sakanoue, K. Ichikawa, Y. Nomura and M. Tamura, *J. Biochem.*, 1997, **121**, 29–37.
103. O. Jilkina, H. J. Kong, L. Hwi, B. Kuzio, B. Xiang, D. Manley, M. Jackson and V. V. Kupriyanov, *J. Biomed. Opt.*, 2006, **11**, 014009.
104. C. M. Palmeira, A. J. Moreno, V. M. Madeira and K. B. Wallace, *J. Pharmacol. Toxicol. Methods*, 1996, **35**, 35–43.
105. J. C. Fernández-Checa, M. Ookhtens and N. Kaplowitz, *J. Biol. Chem.*, 1993, **268**, 10836–10841.
106. H. Jaeschke and J. R. Mitchell, *Methods Enzymol.*, 1990, **186**, 752–759.
107. A. I. Cederbaum, *J. Gastroenterol. Hepatol.*, 2006, **21**, S22–S25.
108. R. Sekura and A. Meister, *Proc. Natl. Acad. Sci. U. S. A.*, 1974, **71**, 2969–2972.
109. O. W. Griffith and A. Meister, *Proc. Natl. Acad. Sci. U. S. A.*, 1977, **74**, 3330–3334.
110. N. Kaplowitz, J. Kuhlenkamp, L. Goldstein and J. Reeve, *J. Pharmacol. Exp. Ther.*, 1980, **212**, 240–245.
111. H. J. Majima, T. D. Oberley, K. Furukawa, M. P. Mattson, H. C. Yen, L. I. Szweda and D. K. St Clair, *J. Biol. Chem.*, 1998, **273**, 8217–8224.
112. M. L. Bajt, T. R. Knight, J. J. Lemasters and H. Jaeschke, *Toxicol. Sci.*, 2004, **80**, 343–349.
113. C. Martín, R. Martínez, R. Navarro, J. I. Ruiz-Sanz, M. Lacort and M. B. Ruiz-Larrea, *Biochem. Pharmacol.*, 2001, **62**, 705–712.
114. J. Das, J. Ghosh, P. Manna and P. C. Sil, *Pathophysiology*, 2008, **15**, 181–190.
115. P. J. de Bleser, P. Jannes, S. C. van Buul-Offers, C. M. Hoogerbrugge, C. F. van Schravendijk, T. Niki, V. Rogiers, J. L. van den Brande, E. Wisse and A. Geerts, *Hepatology*, 1995, **21**, 1429–1437.
116. K. H. Hoebe, R. F. Witkamp, J. Fink-Gremmels, A. S. Van Miert and M. Monshouwer, *Am. J. Physiol. Gastrointestinal Liver Physiol.*, 2001, **280**, G720–G728.

117. K. H. Hoebe, M. Monshouwer, R. F. Witkamp, J. Fink-Gremmels and A. S. van Miert, *Vet. Q.*, 2000, **22**, 21–25.
118. J. G. Scharf, T. Braulke, H. Hartmann and G. Ramadori, *J. Cell. Physiol.*, 2001, **186**, 425–436.
119. A. L. Arnaud, L. Fontana, A. J. Angulo, A. Gill and J. M. López-Pedrosa, *Dig. Dis. Sci.*, 2003, **48**, 1406–1413.
120. A. T. Drahushuk, B. P. McGarrigle, H. L. Tai, S. Kitareewan, J. A. Goldstein and J. R. Olson, *Toxicol. Appl. Pharmacol.*, 1996, **140**, 393–403.
121. A. T. Drahushuk, B. P. McGarrigle, K. E. Larsen, J. J. Stegeman and J. R. Olson, *Carcinogenesis*, 1998, **19**, 1361–1368.
122. A. T. Drahushuk, B. P. McGarrigle, B. P. Slezak, J. J. Stegeman and J. R. Olson, *Toxicol. Appl. Pharmacol.*, 1999, **155**, 127–138.
123. J. M. Catania, A. M. Pershing and A. J. Gandolfi, *Toxicol. in Vitro*, 2007, **21**, 956–961.
124. I. A. de Graaf, P. Olinga, M. H. de Jager, M. T. Merema, R. de Kanter, E. G. van de Kerkhof and G. Groothuis, *Nat. Protoc.*, 2010, **5**, 1540–1551.
125. A. Lupp, R. Glöckner, M. Danz and D. Müller, *Toxicol. in Vitro*, 2002, **16**, 749–758.
126. R. Gebhardt, J. G. Hengstler, D. Müller, R. Glöckner, P. Buenning, B. Laube, E. Schmelzer, M. Ullrich, D. Utesch, N. Hewitt, M. Ringel, B. R. Hilz, A. Bader, A. Langsch, T. Koose, H. J. Burger, J. Maas and F. Oesch, *Drug Metab. Rev.*, 2003, **35**, 145–213.
127. J. T. Heinonen, J. S. Sidhu, M. T. Reilly, F. M. Farin, C. J. Omiecinski, D. L. Eaton and T. J. Kavanagh, *Environ. Health Perspect.*, 1996, **104**, 536–543.
128. R. C. Onderwater, J. N. Commandeur and N. P. Vermeulen, *Toxicology*, 2004, **197**, 81–91.
129. M. Van de Bovenkamp, G. M. Groothuis, D. K. Meijer and P. Olinga, *Toxicol. in Vitro*, 2007, **21**, 545–557.
130. I. A. M. de Graff, P. Olinga, M. H. de Jager, M. T. Merema, R. de Kanter, E. G. van de Kerkhof and G. M. M. Groothuis, *Nature Protocols*, 2010, **5**(9), 1540–1551.
131. S. Wilkening, F. Stahl and A. Bader, *Drug Metab. Disp.*, 2003, **31**(8), 1035–1042.

CHAPTER 10

# *Human-based* In Vitro *Experimental Systems for the Assessment of Human-Specific Adverse Drug Effects: Scientific Concepts, Current Applications and Promising Approaches*

ALBERT P. LI

In vitro ADMET Laboratories LLC and Advanced Pharmaceutical Sciences Inc., 9221 Rumsey Road, Suite 8, Columbia, MD 21045, USA

## 10.1 Introduction

Drug development is a costly and time-consuming process. DiMasi *et al.*[1] have estimated that for R&D initiated in 2001 with approval 12 years later (based on the average time required for approval), the out-of-pocket cost for a single approved drug is estimated to be $970 million, equivalent to a capitalized cost of $1.9 billion.

A major challenge in drug development is the low clinical-phase success rate. The most recent published estimation of the clinical approval success rate for investigational drugs is 16%.[2] Lack of efficacy and the occurrence of unacceptable adverse effects are the two principle reasons of failure. Furthermore, marketed drugs continue to be withdrawn or have their use limited due to

RSC Drug Discovery Series No. 12
New Horizons in Predictive Toxicology: Current Status and Application
Edited by Alan G. E. Wilson

Published by the Royal Society of Chemistry, www.rsc.org

adverse effects. Although the number of drugs required to be withdrawn is relatively small comparing to all marketed drugs, the economical impact on the company of the withdrawn drug can be astronomical.[3]

Efficacy and safety are therefore two co-dependent requirements for successful drug development—clinical failure will result if the drug candidate possesses only one of these two properties. Drug discovery should not only emphasize pharmacological effects, but should also take into account drug safety to allow the selection of drug candidates with the highest probability of success.

## 10.2 Human-Specific Drug Toxicity as a Major Reason for the Failure of Prediction of Human Drug Toxicity with Pre-clinical Non-Human Animal Models

The fact that drug candidates fail in clinical trials due to unacceptable safety illustrates that the old paradigm of drug safety testing, namely, the use of laboratory animals to predict human safety, is not adequate. Safety testing in non-human laboratory animals can be used to remove chemical entities which are toxic to both laboratory animals and humans, but would not be useful in the detection of toxicities that are human-specific.

There are two major reasons for human/animal differences in drug toxicity.

### 10.2.1 Species–Species Differences in Drug Metabolism

Species differences in drug-metabolizing enzymes is a major factor for species differences in drug metabolism, and therefore a determinant for species differences in drug toxicity that involves drug metabolism. For instance, of the key P450 isoforms for drug metabolism: 1A, 2A, 2B, 2C, 2D, 2E and 3A, human and the four commonly used laboratory animals: mouse, rat, dog and monkey are different with the exception of CYP1A and CYP2E.[4,5] This difference is known to lead to species differences in drug metabolism, and may contribute to species differences in drug toxicity.

Species differences in metabolite formation are believed to be one of the major contributors to species differences in xenobiotic toxicity for the following reasons:

1) A toxic metabolite that is formed in humans but not in non-human animals would lead to underestimation of the toxicity of the parent xenobiotic.
2) A toxic metabolite that is formed in non-human animals but not in humans would lead to the overestimation of the toxicity of the parent xenobiotic.

An example of rat/human differences in drug metabolism can be illustrated by a study in our laboratory using rat and human liver microsomes. In this study,[6] we evaluated the formation of human metabolites using rat and human liver microsomes from substrates of the major human P450 isoforms. Aroclor 1254-induced and un-induced rat liver microsomes were compared with human liver microsomes in phenytoin *O*-deethylation, coumarin 7-hydroxylation, tolbutamide 4-hydroxylation, *S*-mephenytoin 4′-hydroxylation, chloroxazone 6-hydroxylation and testosterone 6-β-hydroxylation. We found that both induced and un-induced rat liver microsomes were active in all the pathways studied with the exception of coumarin 7-hydroxylation. Coumarin 7-hydroxylation was observed with human liver microsomes but not the rat liver microsomes.

That drug candidates can form human-specific metabolites is now a well-established phenomenon. Due to this concept of possible species differences in drug toxicity due to drug metabolism, the FDA recently recommended independent *in vivo* safety studies for major human metabolites. The testing of unique human metabolites is required if the metabolite in question represents $>10\%$ of the total systemic exposure.[7]

## 10.2.2 Species Differences in Toxicological Mechanisms

Besides differences in metabolism, species differences in xenobiotic toxicity can also be due to differences in pathways perturbed by toxicants, leading to the ultimate toxicology effects. The following are well-defined examples of this phenomenon.

1) Peroxisome proliferation receptor ligands: Antilipidemic agents such as the fibrates are agonists of PPAR-α, leading to the up-regulation of lipid metabolism pathways. These agents have been found be non-genotoxic hepatocarcinogens in rodents but generally not believed to be carcinogenic in primates, including humans.[8]
2) Ah-receptor ligands: the aryl hydrocarbon receptor (AhR) is a ligand-activated transcription factor that mediates many of the biological and toxic effects of halogenated aromatic hydrocarbons (HAHs), polycyclic aromatic hydrocarbons (PAHs), and other structurally diverse ligands. Species differences in toxicity of these ligands, for instance, 2,3,7,8-tetrachlorodibenzo-p-dioxin (TCDD) and poly-brominated biphenol (PBB), are well established.[9]
3) PXR-ligands: pregnane-X receptor (PXR) is an orphan nuclear receptor that regulates the expression of genes encoding drug-metabolizing enzymes and transporters. Activation of PXR leads to up-regulation of drug-metabolizing enzymes including cytochrome P450 isoforms and the transporter Pgp. Although the consequences are mainly in drug–drug interactions, there is an apparent correlation between enzyme induction potential and hepatotoxicity for drugs that are known to cause

idiosyncratic toxicity. Human/rodent differences in PXR activation are well established.[10] For instance, rifampin has a higher affinity for human PXR than for rodent PXR, while pregnenolone 16-α-carbonitrile (PCN), has a higher affinity for rodent PXR than human PXR, with CYP3A induction potential reflecting these differences.

4) Anticancer agents: species–species differences in target cell sensitivity have been illustrated with direct-acting cytotoxicants evaluated *in vitro* using metabolically incompetent cells such as bone-marrow cells. An example of this is the species differences of the toxicity of various anticancer agents on myeloid progenitor cells. Erickson-Miller *et al.*[11] evaluated the toxicity of ercamptothecin (CAM), topotecan (TPT) and 9-aminocamptothecin (AC) to human, canine, and murine myeloid progenitors (CFU-GM) *in vitro* and found that the murine $IC_{90}$ values were 2.6-, 2.3-, 10-, 21-, 5.9-, and 11-fold higher than human values for CAM lactone (NSC-94600) and sodium salt (NSC-100880), TPT (NSC-609699), and racemic (NSC-629971), semisynthetic and synthetic preparations (NSC-603071) of 9AC, respectively. In contrast, canine $IC_{90}$ values were the same as, or lower than, the human $IC_{90}$ values for all six compounds. The results illustrate that species–species differences can also exist at the target cells in the absence of hepatic metabolism.

## 10.3 Overcoming Species–Species Differences

Experimental systems that can provide information towards human-specific toxicity therefore should be valuable in the prediction of human drug toxicity *in vivo*. As *in vivo* experimentation with humans during pre-clinical phases is neither practical nor ethical, surrogates for humans *in vivo* need to be applied. For the past decade, human-based *in vitro* experimental systems have been developed and applied routinely for the evaluation of drug metabolism and drug–drug interactions.[12,13] The ready acceptance of the *in vitro* systems can be attributed to the well-defined disciplines of drug metabolism. As the liver is the major organ for xenobiotic metabolism, *in vitro* hepatic systems such as liver microsomes and hepatocytes are found to readily reproduce *in vivo* hepatic metabolism. The FDA[14] has endorsed the use of *in vitro* human-based experimental systems in the definition of human metabolic fate and drug–drug interaction potential of drugs. Furthermore, the FDA has recommended that *in vitro* results with human-based systems such as liver microsomes and hepatocytes can be used to define human drug–drug interaction potential, without further clinical trials (clinical trials are recommended only if the results suggest significant drug–drug interaction potential). It is interesting to note that the application of *in vitro* drug metabolism technologies using human-based experimental systems has been attributed to the removal of pharmacokinetics as a major reason for clinical trial failure.

### 10.3.1 *In Vitro–In Vivo* Strategy (IVIVS) for the Prediction of Human Drug Toxicity

The success in the application of *in vitro* drug metabolism systems, in combination with data from relevant *in vivo* animal models, in the prediction of human metabolism suggest that the same approach will also be successful for safety evaluation.[15,16] Based on the premise that the inability to accurately predict human drug toxicity is due to species–species differences, *i.e.*, there are human-specific drug properties that cannot be revealed by non-human animal studies, a safety evaluation strategy is proposed here for the pre-clinical evaluation of human drug toxicity:

1) Application of **human**-based *in vitro* systems to provide human-specific toxicity data;
2) Select a relevant animal species to develop ***in vivo*** parameters;
3) Predict **human *in vivo*** drug toxicity *via* a combination of human-specific information obtained *in vitro*, and *in vivo* parameters obtained from non-human animals *in vivo*.

This IVIVS will require the development of *in vitro* experimental systems with human-specific properties to cover the key toxic drug effects in humans, and a vigorous set of parameters defining the relevant non-human animal species.

### 10.3.2 Selection of Human *In Vitro* Experimental Systems

For the *in vitro–in vivo* paradigm to serve the intended purpose of accurate prediction of human drug toxicity, one has to careful in the choice experimental systems. The following are guidelines for the choice of *in vitro* systems:

1) Human-specific properties: as the purpose is to derive human-specific information, the system used should have the desired human properties. Examples of human-specific properties include human drug-metabolism enzymes, transporters, and cellular targets relevant to drug toxicity.
2) Physiologically relevant experimental conditions: *in vitro* systems, when used under experimental conditions that would not be achieved *in vivo*, may yield information that is difficult to extrapolate to the *in vivo* situation. Examples of irrelevant experimental conditions include the use of too high a drug concentration, interaction of the test substance with media ingredients that are not present in human body fluids, and the use of cells with properties irrelevant to the target cells *in vivo*.
3) Appropriate endpoints: the endpoints used in conjunction with a chosen experimental system must be scientifically proven to be representative of the *in vivo* toxic events.

### 10.3.3 The MTE Requirement for the Selection of Human *In Vitro* Systems

It is proposed here that experimental systems used for the assessment of human drug effects should have the following properties (the MTE requirement):

1) Human drug-metabolizing enzyme pathways (M);
2) Human target cells with cellular and biochemical pathways, the perturbation of which would lead to toxicity observed *in vivo* (T);
3) Appropriate endpoints which would reflect toxicity found *in vivo* (E).

## 10.4 Human Hepatocytes as an *In Vitro* Experimental System for the Evaluation of Human-Specific Drug Properties

Hepatocytes are the parenchymal cells of the liver which are responsible for hepatic biotransformation of xenobiotics. Isolated hepatocytes represent the most physiologically relevant experimental system for drug metabolism studies as they contain all the major hepatic drug-metabolizing enzyme pathways which are not undisrupted such as cell-free fractions. Further, the drug-metabolizing enzymes and cofactors in the hepatocytes are present at physiological concentrations. Freshly isolated hepatocytes and cryopreserved hepatocytes are generally believed to represent the most complete *in vitro* system for the evaluation of hepatic drug metabolism.[17–19] This cell system satisfies the MTE requirement described above:

1) Human xenobiotic metabolism: fresh isolates or cryopreserved fresh isolates of human hepatocytes are known to contain most, if not all, of the *in vivo* hepatic xenobiotic metabolism capacity.
2) Human target cells: the hepatocytes are the cells in the human liver that are damaged by hepatotoxicants, leading ultimately to liver failure.
3) Endpoints: myriad of toxicological endpoints allowing measurements of necrosis, apoptosis, nuclear receptor interactions, P450 functions, transporter functions *etc.* have been developed in hepatocytes for the evaluation of adverse drug properties.

It is to be emphasized that the use of cell lines without human metabolism and not representative of *in vivo* target cells will not have any advantage over the use of laboratory animals in the evaluation of human drug toxicity. For instance, a commonly used cell line, the HepG2 cells, does not have these properties, and therefore would not represent a relevant *in vitro* model for the investigation of hepatotoxicity:

1) Human xenobiotic metabolism: HepG2 cells only retain a minimal capacity (estimated to be less than 1%) of the normal hepatic xenobiotic metabolism.

2) Human target cells: HepG2 cells are derived from a human adenocarcinoma of the liver, not the parenchymal cells which are the *in vivo* target of hepatotoxicants.

An *in vitro* experimental system such as human hepatocytes that satisfies the MTE requirement is scientifically likely to provide information that is useful for the prediction of adverse drug effects in humans *in vivo*. The following are successful applications of human hepatocytes in the evaluation of drug properties.

### 10.4.1 Human Hepatocyte Cryopreservation as an Enabling Technology

In the past, the use of human hepatocytes has been severely limited by their availability, as studies would be performed only if human livers were available for hepatocyte isolation. Furthermore, hepatocyte isolation from human livers is not a technology available to most drug-metabolism laboratories. This limitation has been overcome in the past decade due to the advancements in the procurement of human livers for research, and the commercial availability of isolated human hepatocytes. The application of human hepatocytes in drug-metabolism studies is also greatly aided by the successful cryopreservation of human hepatocytes to retain drug-metabolism activities.[18–20] Recently, the usefulness of cryopreserved human hepatocytes is further extended through the development of technologies to cryopreserve human hepatocytes to retain their ability to be cultured as attached cultures (plateable cryopreserved hepatocytes) which can be used for longer term studies such as enzyme induction studies.[18]

Cryopreserved human hepatocytes have several advantages over the use of freshly isolated cells:

1) Experimentation can be readily scheduled;
2) There are little or no deleterious effects of cryopreservation on key hepatocyte properties;
3) **Repeat of experimentation** can be performed at different times or by different laboratories with cells from the same donor;
4) The hepatocytes can be pre-characterized for properties relevant to a specific study before they are used for experimentation;
5) Hepatocytes from multiple donors can be used in the same study.

## 10.5 Cryopreserved Human Hepatocyte Assays for the Evaluation of Drug–Drug Interactions

Undesired drug–drug interactions can lead to serious toxicity or loss of drug efficacy. This adverse drug effect is one of the major reasons for black box warnings and withdrawal of marketed drugs. Due to species differences in drug metabolism, *in vitro* human-based systems such as human liver fractions and human hepatocytes are preferred over *in vivo* animal models for the assessment of drug–drug interactions.

### 10.5.1 Mechanisms of Metabolic Drug–Drug Interactions

Metabolic drug–drug interaction results from the alteration of the metabolic clearance of one drug by a co-administered drug. There are two major pathways of metabolic drug–drug interactions:

*Inhibitory drug–drug interaction:* when one drug inhibits the drug-metabolism enzyme responsible for the metabolism of a co-administered drug, the result is a decreased metabolic clearance of the affected drug, resulting in a higher than desired systemic burden. For drugs with a narrow therapeutic index, this may lead to serious toxicological concerns. Most fatal drug–drug interactions are due to inhibitory drug–drug interactions.

*Inductive drug–drug interactions:* drug–drug interactions can also be a result of the acceleration of the metabolism of a drug by a co-administered drug. Acceleration of metabolism is usually due to the induction of the gene expression, leading to higher rates of protein synthesis and therefore higher cellular content of the induced drug-metabolizing enzyme and a higher rate of metabolism of the substrates of the induced enzyme. Inductive drug–drug interactions can lead to a higher metabolic clearance of the affected drug, leading to a decrease in plasma concentration and loss of efficacy. Inductive drug–drug interactions can also lead to a higher systemic burden of metabolites, which, if toxic, may lead to safety concerns.

### 10.5.2 Mechanism-Based Approach for the Evaluation of Drug–Drug Interaction Potential

Due to the realization that it is physically impossible to evaluate empirically the possible interaction between one drug and all marketed drugs, and that most drug-metabolizing enzyme pathways are well defined, a mechanism-based approach is used for the evaluation of drug–drug interaction potential of a new drug or drug candidate,[12,21,22] This mechanism-based approach is endorsed and required by the FDA (www.fda.gov/cber/gdlns/interactstud.htm) for new drug applications. The approach consists of the following major studies:

#### *10.5.2.1 Metabolic Phenotyping*

Metabolic phenotyping is defined as the identification of the major pathways involved in the metabolism of the drug in question. The reasoning is that if the pathways are known, then one can estimate potential interaction of the drug in questions with known inhibitors or inducers of the pathway.

#### *10.5.2.2 Evaluation of Inhibitory Potential for Drug-Metabolizing Enzymes*

The ability of the drug in question to inhibit the activities of known pathways for drug metabolism is evaluated. If a drug is an inhibitor of a drug-metabolizing enzyme pathway, it will have the potential to cause inhibitory drug interactions with co-administered drugs that are substrates of the inhibited pathway.

#### *10.5.2.3 Evaluation of Induction Potential for Drug-Metabolizing Enzymes*

The ability of the drug in question to induce drug-metabolizing enzyme activities is evaluated. If the drug in question is an inducer of a specific pathway, it will have the potential to cause inductive drug interactions with co-administered drugs that are substrates of the induced pathway.

The *in vitro* approaches for the evaluation of drug–drug interactions are now standardized. We have previously reviewed approaches to evaluate drug–drug interactions using human-based *in vitro* systems, including the use of human hepatocytes, human liver microsomes, and recombinant P450.[21,23] We describe here the most recent approaches developed in our laboratory for the evaluation of drug–drug interactions.

## 10.6 Higher Throughput Human Hepatocyte-Based Drug–Drug Interaction Studies

Cytochrome P450s represent an important family of enzymes responsible for xenobiotic metabolism. Of the multiple isoforms, cytochrome P450 isoform 3A4 (CYP3A4) is the most abundant of the isoforms in the human liver. CYP3A4 has been found to be responsible for the metabolism of a large variety of exogenous and endogenous substrates.[5,24] In drug development, there is a need to evaluate the inhibitory and inductive potential of drug candidates towards CYP3A4 to estimate their drug–drug interaction potential with the myriad of drugs that are substrates of this important P450 isoform.[25–27] In our laboratory, we have developed cost- and time-effective higher throughput screening assays for the evaluation of drug–drug interaction potentials of drug candidates involving CYP3A4. The assays are as follows:

1) 384-well CYP3A4 inhibition assay;
2) 96-well time-dependent CYP3A4 inhibition assay;
3) 96-well CYP3A4 induction assay.

The throughput of the assays is increased *via* use of the following technologies:

1) Cryopreserved human hepatocytes cultured in microwell cell culture plates: The properties and advantages of cryopreserved human

hepatocytes have been discussed earlier. The use of microwell (96- and 384-well plates) allows the ease of sample organization, decreased cost of cells and reagents, and allows the use of automation.

2) Luciferin-isopropyl acetal (LIPA) as CYP3A4 substrate: LIPA is metabolized to luciferin specifically by CYP3A4. The use of this substrate allows CYP3A4 activity to be quantified using a plate-reader, thereby eliminating the need for the time-consuming and costly LC-MS assays that are used with conventional substrates.

### 10.6.1 384-Well CYP3A Inhibition Assay with Intact Human Hepatocytes

Evaluation of P450 inhibition is traditionally performed with liver microsomes and recombinant CYP enzymes.[28,29] Intact hepatocytes represent an additional experimental system that may provide useful information to improve the accuracy of the prediction of *in vivo* effects. A chemical, for instance, may be metabolized by non-CYP pathways to a metabolite that is a potent P450 inhibitor and therefore would be inhibitory in hepatocytes but not in microsomes or recombinant CYP enzymes. Gemfibrozil, for instance, requires glucuronidation for its CYP3A4 inhibitory effects and is found to be a potent CYP3A4 inhibitor in hepatocytes but not in liver microsomes nor recombinant CYP3A4.[30] Hepatocytes can also be used for the modeling of differential inhibitor distribution between plasma and intracellular compartments. Lu *et al.* reported the use of hepatocytes suspended in 100% human plasma to accurately predict CYP3A4 inhibitory effects of several CYP3A inhibitors *in vivo*.[31] The presence of active transporters in human hepatocytes, including cryopreserved hepatocytes, also suggest that an inhibitor may be actively accumulated inside the cells, leading to substantially higher concentration and a correspondingly higher inhibitory effect which would not be observed using cell-free systems.[32,33]

We have previously introduced the use of human hepatocytes in P450 inhibition studies.[22,34,35] In the HTS human hepatocyte CYP3A4 inhibition assay described here, 384-well plates were used to reduce the quantity of hepatocytes, reagents, as well as the chemical to be evaluated. The use of LIPA as CYP3A4 substrate substantially enhances the efficiency of the assay, as its metabolism can be quantified based on luminescence using a plate-reader,[35] thereby eliminating the need for HPLC and mass spectrometry, which are routinely required with conventional substrates such as testosterone and midazolam. The use of robotics allows rapid and accurate delivery of relatively small volumes of reagents into the 384-well plates. The accuracy of the assay is demonstrated by the relatively low coefficient of variation (standard deviations $<10\%$ of mean values) of the results.

A homogenous (addition assay) has been developed in our laboratory using cryopreserved human hepatocytes cultured in 384-well plates. An automated workstation is used for the performance of the assay. The workstation is programmed to perform serial dilutions of the model inhibitors and for the initiation of the assay. White opaque 384-well plates are used. The workstation is programmed to add into each of the wells of the 384-well plates 10 μL of hepatocytes (containing 10 000 cells) and 10 μL of Hepatocyte Metabolism Medium containing either solvent (0.1% v/v of acetonitrile) or P450 inhibitors at the designated concentrations (at 3 × of the designated concentrations). The assay is initiated by the addition of 10 μL of 3 μM LIPA (final concentration 1 μM). The plates are returned to a cell culture incubator maintained at 37 °C, in a highly humidified atmosphere of 95% air and 5% carbon dioxide. After an incubation period of 120 min, the plates are returned to the workstation for the addition of 10 μL of Luciferin Detection Reagent. Luminescence is quantified using a multi-channel plate-reader.

Results with 10 CYP3A4 inhibitors and non-inhibitors with this 384-well assay are presented here (Figure 10.1). Extensive (>80% inhibition), statistically significant, and dose-dependent inhibition is observed for the known CYP3A4 inhibitors 1-aminobenzotriazole, erythromycin, ketoconazole and verapamil.Substantially less (<50%) inhibition was observed for the non-CYP3A4 inhibitors diethyldithiocarbamate, quercetin, quinidine, sulfaphenazole, ticlopidine and tranylcypromine. The standard deviation values are consistently <10% of that of the mean values. The results demonstrate the ability of this HTS assay to generate highly accurate and specific results and therefore can be applied routinely as a screening assay for CYP3A4 inhibitory potential of compounds.

## 10.6.2 96-Well Time-Dependent Inhibition Assay for CYP3A4 in Human Hepatocytes

In terms of P450 inhibition, time-dependent inhibition (TDI) or mechanism-based P450 inhibition is of particular concern. In TDI, the inactivated P450 needs to be replaced by newly synthesized proteins to return to its normal activity. After cessation of administration with the TDI inhibitor, the patient would continue to have decreased drug metabolizing capacity before the inactivated enzymes are fully replaced.[27,36]

While TDI is generally studied using liver microsomes or recombinant CYP,[37,38] there are substantial efforts in the evaluation of this important mechanism of drug–drug interaction in human hepatocytes.[39,40] Human hepatocytes, because of the intact plasma membrane, complete and uninterrupted drug metabolism enzymes and cofactors, represent a desirable *in vitro* experimental system for the evaluation of human drug properties.

Traditionally, TDI studies with hepatocytes utilize suspension cultures.[40] The use of hepatocytes in suspension culture is a common practice with cryopreserved cells as most preparations of cryopreserved hepatocytes would have compromised ability to be cultured as monolayer cultures. Due to our success in cryopreservation of human hepatocytes to retain their ability to be cultured, a convenient and quantitative approach for the evaluation of TDI using

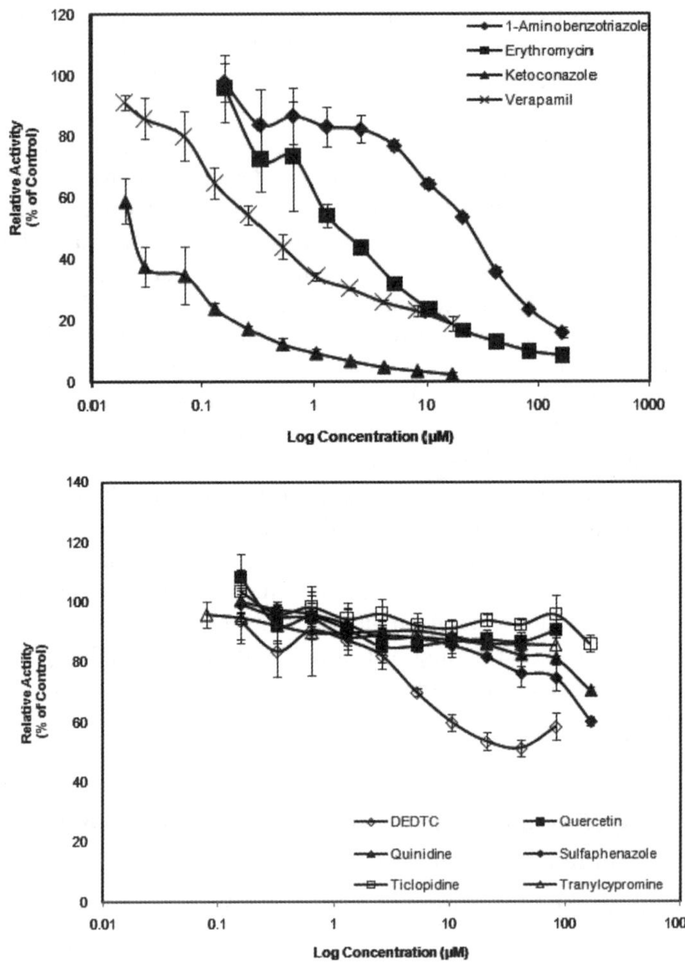


**Figure 10.1** Results of higher throughput 384-well plate human hepatocyte CYP3A4 inhibition assay. Top: known CYP3A4 inhibitors 1-aminobenzotriazole; erythromycin; ketoconazole; verapamil. Bottom: known non-CYP3A4 inhibitors diethyldithiocarbamate (DEDTC; CYP2E1 inhibitor); quercetin (CYP2C8 inhibitor); quinidine (CYP2D6 inhibitor); sulfaphenazole (CYP2C9 inhibitor); and tranylcypromine (CYP2A6 inhibitor).

monolayer cultures of plateable cryopreserved human hepatocytes has been developed in our laboratory.

In this assay, the cryopreserved human hepatocytes are thawed from cryopreservation using Cryopreserved Hepatocytes Recovery Medium and plated at 50 000 cells per well in 96-well collagen coated plates in Cryopreserved Hepatocytes Plating Medium at a volume of 100 μL per well. The cells are cultured for 24 h in a cell culture incubator maintained at 37 °C with a highly humidified atmosphere of 5% carbon dioxide and 95% air. The cells on the day after plating (24 h cultures) are used for the evaluation of TDI. On the day of treatment, the plating medium is removed and the cells are washed three times with Hepatocyte Metabolism Medium (HMM), followed by the addition of 50 μL of HMM per well. At designated times, treatment media consisting of HMM containing 2 × concentrated solutions of the inhibitors or medium control is added. At designated periods after treatment, media are removed by quickly inverting the 96-well plates on absorbent paper. The cells are washed five times with 100 μL of HMM to remove the inhibitors. The cells are incubated at 37 °C with 100 μL per well of HMM for a 60 min "washout" period to allow removal of intracellular inhibitors by diffusion, to minimize competitive inhibition with CYP3A4 substrate. After the washout period, medium is replaced with that containing 3 μM of the CYP3A4-specific substrate LIPA. After an incubation period of 30 min, 50 μL of the incubated substrate solution from each well is removed and placed into a white 96-well plate. After all the solutions are collected from the various time points, 50 μL of Luciferin Detection Reagent is added to each well containing incubated substrate solution followed by quantification of luminescence using a Wallac Victor-3 plate-reader. Luminescence signals were converted to pmoles of luciferin based on a standard curve generated from luciferin. Viability of the hepatocytes after treatment is determined after CYP3A4 activity quantification using cellular ATP as an endpoint using a commercially available ATP kit consisting of lysis buffer and ATP detection reagent.

Results are expressed as % remaining activity, which is calculated as a ratio of the activity in the presence of inhibitors to that of the solvent control using the following equation:

$$\text{Remaining activity (\%)} = [\text{normalized activity (treatment)/normalized activity (solvent control)}] \times 100;$$

where 'activity' represents luciferin generated in each well quantified by luminescence normalized by relative activity based on ATP content using the following equations:

$$\text{Normalized activity} = \text{CYP3A4 activity/relative viability}$$
$$\text{Relative viability (\%)} = \text{ATP content (treatment)/ATP content (solvent control)}$$

Enzyme kinetic parameters for TDI are derived as follows: The observed rate of enzyme inactivation ($k_{obs}$) is determined as the initial slope of the linear regression line of a semi-logarithmic plot of the natural logarithm of remaining activity *versus* pre-incubation time. $k_{inact}$ and $K_i$ values are determined based on the double-reciprocal Lineweaver–Burk plot ($1/k_{obs}$ *versus* 1/[I], whereas [I] represents inhibitor concentration), where $k_{inact}$ is estimated as the reciprocal of the $y$-intercept and $K_i$ as the negative reciprocal of the $x$-intercept.

Results with the model time-dependent inhibitors of CYP3A, 1-aminobenzotriazole, are presented here (Figure 10.2). Time and concentration-dependent loss of CYP3A4 activity was observed. The plots of the natural logarithm of remaining activity *versus* inhibitor yielded linear plots for both inhibitors. The double-reciprocal Lineweaver–Burk plot is used for the calculation time-dependent inhibition kinetics constants. The calculated $K_i$ and $k_{inact}$ values are 64.5 μM and 0.60 $min^{-1}$.

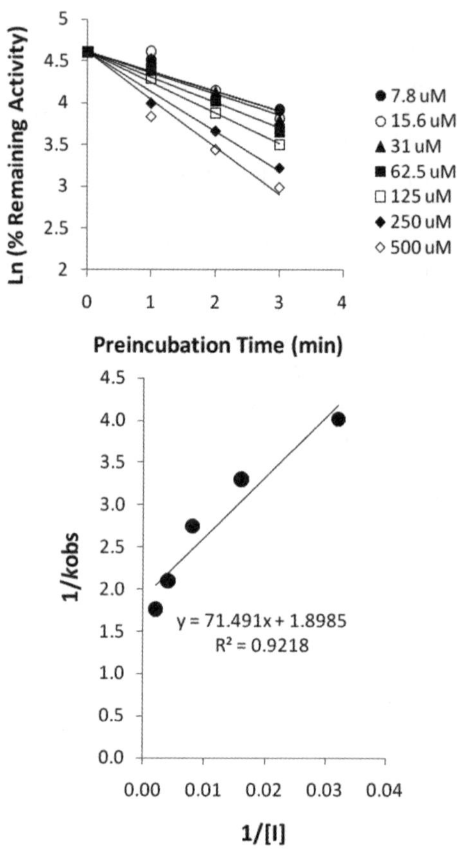


**Figure 10.2** Higher throughput 96-well plate human hepatocyte time-dependent CYP3A4 inhibition assay. The application of this assay to evaluate a known time-dependent inhibitor, 1-aminobenzotriazole, is shown here. A plot of the natural logarithm of the % remaining activity (activity as a percent of solvent control) *versus* time (top) illustrates the time-dependent inhibitory effects. The Lineweaver–Burk double-reciprocal plot of the rates of decrease ($1/k_{obs}$) *versus* inhibitor concentration (1/[I]) (bottom) allows the calculation of $k_{inact}$ (as 1/*y*-intercept) and $K_i$ (as -1/*x*-intercept), two key parameters for time-dependent inhibition.

### 10.6.3 96-Well CYP3A4 Induction Assay with Human Hepatocytes

Enzyme induction is a major mechanism for drug–drug interactions. Induction of a drug- metabolizing enzyme by one drug would lead to the enhanced metabolism of co-administered drugs that are substrates of the induced enzyme.

Experimental evaluation of enzyme induction involves the treatment of human hepatocytes for several days with the test article followed by evaluation of enzyme activities using P450 isoform-specific substrates.[22] As freshly isolated hepatocytes possess endogenous activities which may be the result of inducers present in the donor's systemic circulation, the isolated hepatocytes are cultured for two to three days to allow the P450 enzyme activities to return to a basal level. Testing for induction potential is that initiated by treatment of the cultured hepatocytes for two to three days to allow full expression of the induced enzyme. Induction is generally evaluated by measuring enzyme activity as activity represents the most relevant endpoint for drug–drug interaction. Both freshly isolated and plateable cryopreserved human hepatocytes can be used for the induction study.

At the time of writing, all known inducers of P450 isoforms *in vivo* are inducers *in vitro*.[18]

The typical experimental procedures for an enzyme induction study are as follows:

1) Day 0: plate human hepatocytes (freshly isolated or plateable cryopreserved human hepatocytes), overlay with Matrigel® (0.3 mg $mL^{-1}$) at approximately 4 h after plating.
2) Day 1: refresh medium.
3) Day 2: refresh medium.
4) Day 3: change medium to that containing test article, solvent control, or positive control, *i.e.*
   i) minimum of three test article concentrations, with the high concentration at least one order of magnitude greater than expected plasma concentration;
   ii) if plasma concentration not known, evaluate concentrations ranging over at least two orders of magnitude (*e.g.*, 1, 10, 100 μM).
5) Day 4: refresh treatment medium.
6) Day 5: refresh treatment medium.
7) Day 6: measure activity (*in situ* incubation with isoform-specific substrates).

Traditionally, P450 induction studies are performed in 24-well plates, with approximately 0.35 million cells plated into each well to achieve a confluent monolayer culture. Cell density is critical: 85% or higher confluence is needed for maximal responsiveness to CYP3A inducers.

In our laboratory, we have developed a higher throughput P450 induction assay using 96-well plates. The procedures are as follows:

1) Day 0: plate human hepatocytes (freshly isolated or plateable cryopreserved human hepatocytes) with 50 μL of cell suspension per well, at a cell density of 1 million cells per mL thereby delivering 50 000 cells per well.
2) Day 1: change medium to cold (4 to 10 °C) medium containing 0.25 mg $mL^{-1}$ of Matrigel®.
3) Day 2: change medium to treatment medium containing test articles at the desired concentrations.
4) Days 3–5: continue treatment—medium change is not necessary unless the test article is known to be unstable under the culturing conditions.
5) Day 6: measure activity (*in situ* incubation with isoform-specific substrates)

We routinely evaluate the induction of CYP1A2 and CYP3A4, using substrates that are metabolized to metabolites that can be quantified using a plate-reader to increase the throughput of the assay. CYP1A2 is evaluated by the metabolism of 7-ethoxyresorufin to resorufin which can be quantified based on fluorescence. CYP3A4 is evaluated by the metabolism of luciferin-IPA to luciferin which can be quantified based on luminescence. The known CYP inducers are now known to induce either CYP1A and/or CYP3A, with inducers of other inducible isoforms such as CYP2A6, CYP2C9, CYP2C19 found also to be CYP3A inducers. For general enzyme induction evaluation for drug–drug interaction evaluation, it may be adequate to simply screen for CYP1A and CYP3A induction. If CYP3A induction is observed, then investigations into CYP2A6, CYP2C9 and CYP2C19 induction are warranted.

The two most common confounding factors for P450 induction studies are as follows:

1) Inducers that are also inhibitors: the co-occurrence of P450 inhibition and induction (*i.e.*, the compound is both an inhibitor and inducer) can confound induction results. Ritonavir is an example of a CYP3A4 inducer[41] which is also a potent CYP3A4 inhibitor.[42] The inhibitory effects can overcome any induction effects using activity as an endpoint. For the evaluation of enzyme induction potential of inhibitors, Western blotting for the amount of enzyme proteins would be most appropriate. Studies with mRNA expression would provide data to distinguish between induction of gene expression or protein stabilization as mechanisms. As in the case of ritonavir, induction effects persist after the clearance of the drug from the systemic circulation, leading to enhanced clearance of drugs that are substrates of the induced pathways. It is important to define the induction potential of a drug even if it is found to be an enzyme inhibitor.

2) Cytotoxic compounds: induction effects can be masked by the decrease of cell viability, as most induction assay quantify substrate metabolism *in situ* (in the same cell culture plate that the cells are cultured) and assume that there is no change in cell number. Cytotoxicity evaluation therefore should always be performed concurrently with induction studies. In the presence of cytotoxicity, activity should be corrected by the viability for comparison with negative control activity to assess induction potential.

A compound is concluded to be an inducer if reproducible, statistically significant, and dose-dependent induction effects are observed. The FDA recommends the use of the criterion of "40% of higher of the activity of positive controls" as a positive response (www.fda.gov/cber/gdlns/interactstud.htm).

Results of this higher throughput CYP3A induction assay with model CYP3A4 inducers are shown in Figure 10.3.

## 10.7 *In Vitro* Evaluation of Drug Toxicity

The current success in the application of human-based *in vitro* experimental models in the evaluation of drug metabolism and drug–drug interactions paves the way for a similar approach to evaluate drug toxicity, especially human-specific toxic events that cannot be observed in laboratory animals. *In vitro* toxicity assays can be applied during various phases of drug development:

1) **Early screening of intrinsic toxicity**: Cell-based systems are used for rapid screening of drug candidates, especially structural analogs, to allow the selection of less toxic structures for further development. The screening assay can allow logical evaluation of structures responsible for toxicity (toxicophore) which, hopefully, can be separated from structures for pharmacological activity (pharmacophore). Toxicity screening with *in vitro* systems requires only limited amount of test articles, and is rapid and quantitative. Toxicity screening is most effective when one has an indication for *in vivo* toxicity (*e.g.*, hepatotoxicity or nephrotoxicity) for a lead molecule, therefore allowing the selection of the most appropriate *in vitro* system for screening (*e.g.*, hepatocytes for hepatotoxicity and renal proximal tubule cells for nephrotoxicity).
2) **Mechanistic evaluations**: Mechanistic understanding is critical to drug development. It allows a better understanding of human health risks, defines potential risk factors, and evaluates the relationship between efficacy and adverse effects. Mechanistic studies may be performed after adverse effects are observed in non-human animals to aid the prediction of human toxicity as well as the development of approaches for a more acceptable replacement. The defined experimental conditions and the availability of reagents and approaches for multiple endpoints of *in vitro*

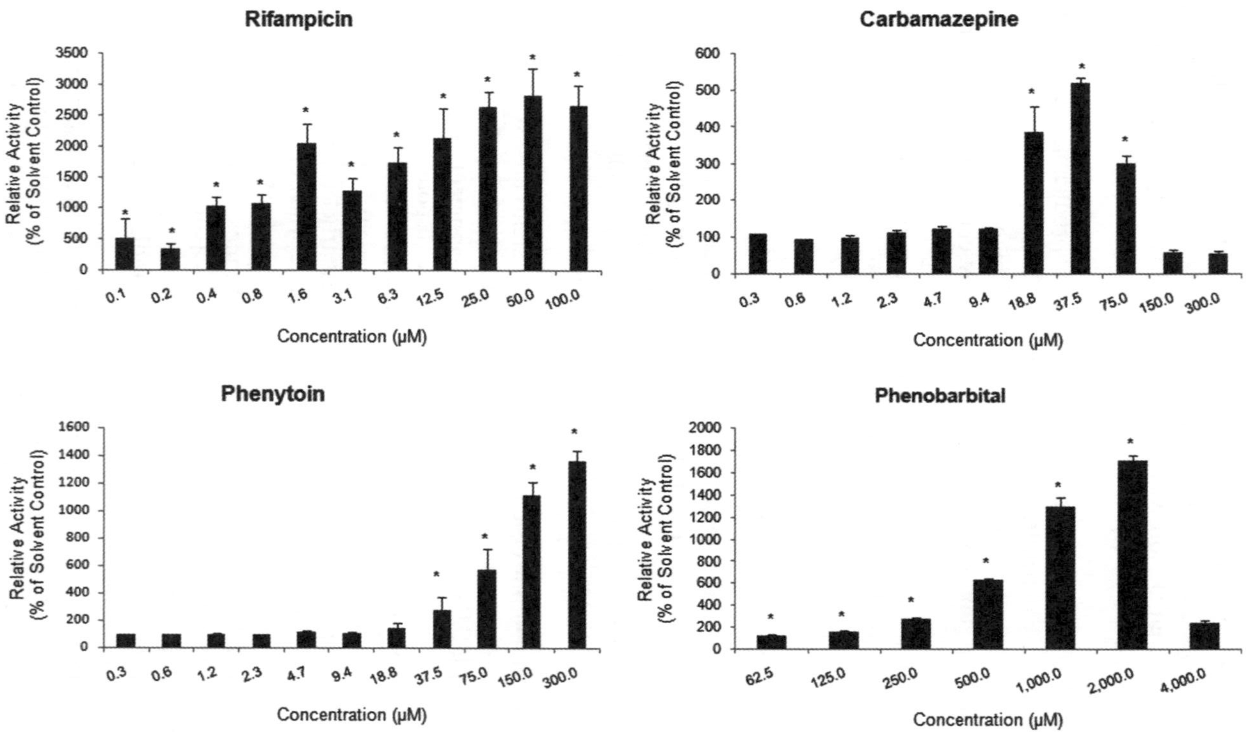


**Figure 10.3** Higher throughput 96-well human hepatocyte CYP3A4 induction assay. Results with the known CYP3A4-inducing drugs: rifampicin, carbamazepine, phenytoin, and phenobarbital are shown. Asterisks represent statistically significant ($p<0.05$) induction over the activity of solvent control (shown as 100% relative activity).

experimental systems allow one to define the key pathways involved in a toxicology phenomenon.

The preferred human *in vitro* systems for the evaluation of drug toxicity are primary cells derived from human organs, used within a period that the cells would retain differentiated functions, thereby serving as surrogates of the similar cells *in vivo*.

Primary cell culture systems, including stem-cell-derived differentiated cells representative of the key cell types in each organ, are currently available and the respective organ-specific toxicity is as follows:

i) Hepatocytes (hepatotoxicity)
ii) Renal proximal tubule epithelial cells (nephrotoxicity)
iii) Vascular endothelial cells (vascular toxicity)
iv) Neuronal cells, glial cells and astrocytes (neurotoxicity)
v) Cardiomyocytes (cardiotoxicity)
vi) Bone-marrow cells (bone-marrow toxicity).

## 10.8 Overcoming the Major Deficiencies of *In Vitro* Systems

An argument routinely raised against the application of *in vitro* systems in safety evaluation is that toxicity is a complex phenomenon and therefore cannot be adequately modeled by simple *in vitro* systems such as cell culture assays.

The major deficiencies of *in vitro* experimental systems can be defined as follows:

1) **Lack of systemic effects**: *in vitro* experimental systems in general consist of single cell types. Toxic effects are evaluated in the absence of influences from systemic effects that may be critical to drug toxicity. An example is the participation of the immune system in organ toxicity. One hypothesis for idiosyncratic hepatotoxicity, for instance, is the hapten-hypothesis which postulates that liver failure arises from the cytotoxicity of antibodies towards antigens developed between the idiosyncratic drug (or its metabolites) on the plasma membrane of the hepatocytes.
2) **Absence of chronic dosing**: It is generally believed that drug toxicity due to acute cytotoxic events can be studied effectively with *in vitro* systems. However, toxic effects due to chronic, low-dose treatments may require multiple events that may or may not be obtained with *in vitro* studies, with cells treated for a relatively short time period (*e.g.*, 24 h). Long-term treatments (*e.g.*, months to years) of cells in culture is theoretically possible but in practice near impossible. Furthermore, it is extremely difficult to maintain primary cells, the preferred cell system, in a differentiated state for a long time period.

For *in vitro* systems to be useful, one needs to develop experimental approaches to overcome these deficiencies.

### 10.8.1 Target Cell Initiation Theory for Drug-Induced Organ Failure (TACIT)

It is well established that the final manifestation of organ failure may require systemic, multiple-organ interactions. For instance, damage to a cell population in an organ may lead to the recruitment of inflammatory cells which in turn may secrete cytotoxic cytokines, leading to further damage to the organ. The involvement of inflammation in liver toxicity has been suggested by one line of evidence that hepatotoxicity is enhanced in animals treated with pro-inflammatory agents.

However, it can be visualized that organ toxicity may be due to a cascade of events, starting with a toxicant causing perturbations in a specific cell populations, initiating the cascade. The Target Cell Initiation Theory of Organ Toxicity (TACIT) is proposed here (Figure 10.4):

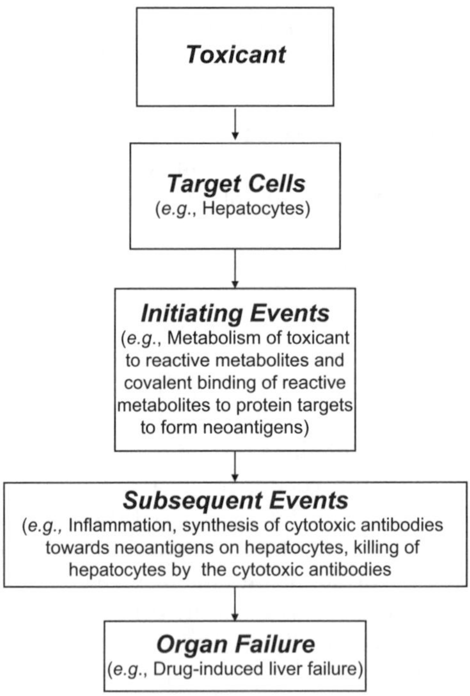


**Figure 10.4** The Target Cell Initiation of Organ Toxicity (TACIT) Hypothesis, which argues that there are key initiating events that are triggered by the toxicants in a target cell, followed by a sequence of events that would lead to the final toxic effects. Based on TACIT, one can predict complicated organ toxicity using an *in vitro* system by measuring the occurrence of the initiating events in appropriate target cells.

Drug-induced organ failure is caused by drug-induced changes in a target cell population which have the potential to initiate a cascade of events, and may or may not involve different cell types within the organ, or mechanisms involving non-target organs, leading ultimately to extensive damage to the organ in question.

A corollary to the TACIT is that although organ failure may involve multiple cell types and multiple organs, one can identify toxicants that can cause organ failure if the following critical factors are identified:

1) The initiating target cells for the toxicant in questions;
2) The critical initiation events which would cause the organ-failure cascade.

### 10.8.2 Practical Application of TACIT

TACIT states that one can use the target cells in isolation in combination with critical endpoints reflecting initiating events to detect agents that can cause organ failure, regardless of the subsequent pathways which may involve non-target cells and organs.

An example of an application of the hypothesis is the evaluation of hepatotoxic potential using primary hepatocytes:

1) **Target cell selection**: For most toxic drugs, liver parenchymal cells are the cells that are initially damaged. The parenchymal cells represent the major cell type of the liver, with all the drug-metabolizing enzymes of the liver. The cells can be damaged by the drugs directly (*e.g.*, high, bolus concentration after oral administration) or the metabolites (*e.g.*, cytotoxic or highly reactive metabolites). Primary hepatocytes, as fresh or cryopreserved isolates, represent the most appropriate cell system for the evaluation of hepatotoxicity.
2) **Endpoint selection**: Hepatotoxicity is known to be initiated by both cytotoxic and non-cytotoxic events (Table 10.1). Endpoints based on these known events can be selected to be used with hepatocytes for the evaluation of hepatotoxicity.

**Table 10.1** Mechanisms of action of various types of hepatotoxicants. These mechanisms can be used to designed screening assays for the early evaluation of hepatotoxicity.

| *Hepatotoxic mechanism* | *Toxicants* |
|---|---|
| Direct cytotoxicity | Cadmium chloride; *cis*-platinum |
| Toxic/reactive metabolite formation | Acetaminophen; cocaine; cyclophosphamide; ethanol |
| Toxic antibodies towards neoantigens | Amineptine, erythromycin derivatives, halothane, imipramine, isaxonine, alpha-methyldopa, tienilic acid |
| Cholestasis | Rifampin, glibenclamide, cyclosporin A |
| Steatosis | Carbamazepine; cycloheximide; tetracycline |
| Phospholipidosis | Amiodarone; diethylaminoethoxyhexestrol; perhexiline |

i) *Direct cytotoxicity:* liver toxicity is known to be preceded with cytotoxicity to the hepatocytes. Cytotoxicity can be using endpoints such as leakage of cytoplasmic enzymes, cellular ATP content, and mitochondrial metabolic activities as described earlier.

ii) *Indirect cytotoxic effects:* toxicity of a substance to the liver may result from effects that may not lead to cytotoxicity directly, but will precipitate subsequent events which will lead to severe hepatotoxicity. These pre-lethal effects include the following:

a) Formation of reactive metabolites: Reactive metabolites formed in the hepatocytes react with cellular macromolecules which may lead to direct toxicity due to inactivation of key biochemical pathways. The reactive metabolites may also react with cellular proteins to form neoantigens, leading to cytotoxic inflammatory events. Reactive metabolites can be identified as glutathione (GSH) conjugates (e.g., using LC/MS).[43,44] An indirect indication of reactive metabolite formation is the depletion of cellular GSH in the absence of cytotoxicity.

b) Steatosis: microvesicular steatosis, abnormal accumulation of intracellular lipid, is known to occur with exposure to hepatotoxic drugs. Accumulation of lipid vesicles and subsequent rupture of the lipid-laden hepatocytes is believed to be a key step towards severe liver damage. Steatosis can be measured in cultured hepatocytes *via* the quantification of intracellular triglyceride accumulation and light microscopic examination of cells with lipid-specific stains such as Nile red.[45–47]

c) Cholestasis: bile acid retention in hepatocytes as a result of compromised efflux is known to be related to liver damage. The basolateral and apical transporters for bile acids are thought to be targets of drugs that induce cholestasis. Inhibition of bile acid transporters therefore is a relevant endpoint for the screening of drugs with cholestatic potential.[48]

d) Phospholipidosis: impaired phospholipid metabolism is known to be related to inflammatory events and histopathological changes. Some hepatotoxic drugs are known to cause phospholipidosis in hepatocytes which can be detected morphologically using electron microscopy as cytoplasmic lamella bodies. Screening for lipidosis can be performed also using a dye for intracellular lipids such as Nile red.[49] Unlike steatosis, the relationship between phospholipidosis and hepatotoxicity is not yet established. However, this endpoint is a frequently used histopathological endpoint used to suggest hepatotoxic potential.[50]

### 10.8.3 High-Content Endpoint Assays

High-content assays such as toxicogenomics for gene expression, proteomics for protein expression, metabonomics for natural metabolite synthesis, and cellomics for cell morphology changes, are relative novel technologies with potential application in the definition of drug toxicity. It is anticipated that these high-content assays, which allow one to evaluate the effect of a test substance on myriad events (*e.g.*, expression of 20 000 human genes), one may achieve the following:

1) Discover response patterns (response profiles) that can be used to define toxicity.
2) Discover new biomarkers for specific types of toxicity.
3) Discover early indicators of chronic toxicity.

High-content assays may represent a powerful tool for the TACIT approach. They allow the evaluation of initiating events that may be linked to toxicity that are difficult to evaluate such as idiosyncratic drug toxicity. These events may be uncovered, for instance, by the treatment of a target cell (*e.g.*, hepatocytes) with drugs that are known to cause idiosyncratic drug toxicity (*e.g.*, troglitazone), using their non-toxic or less toxic structural analogs (*e.g.*, rosiglitazone and pioglitazone as non-toxic analogs of troglitazone) to aid in identifying the key initiating events. It needs to be cautioned, however, that data interpretation for high-content assays needs to include not only statistics, but also mechanistic reasoning. Perhaps the value of high-content assays is in hypothesis development. Vigorous experiments performed to further substantiate the hypothesis may allow the elucidation of toxic mechanisms, leading to better risk assessment. Events that have proven to be mechanistically linked to the ultimate toxicity may be used as early biomarkers for clinical toxicity, and also can be used to design cost-efficient screening assays for the development of non-toxic analogs to replace a toxic drug candidate.[51–54]

### 10.8.4 *In Vitro* Experimental Model for Multiple Organ Interactions: Integrated Discrete Multiple Organ Co-Culture (IdMOC)

One major drawback of *in vitro* system is that each cell type is studied in isolation. In the human body, multiple organ interactions may be critical to drug toxicity. An example of multiple-organ interactions is a drug which is firstly metabolized by one organ (*e.g.*, the liver) to form metabolites which then may enter the general systemic circulation to cause toxicity in a distant organ (*e.g.*, the heart).

The multiple-organ interaction is not covered by the TACIT approach using a single cell type, as the initiating events may include effects of a toxicant on a non-target cell. To overcome this deficiency, we have developed the IdMOC (Independent Discrete Multiple Organ Co-Culture) system.[55–57] The IdMOC allows the co-culturing of cells from different organs as physically separated cultures that are interconnected by an overlying medium, akin to the blood circulation connecting the multiple organs in the human body (Figure 10.5).

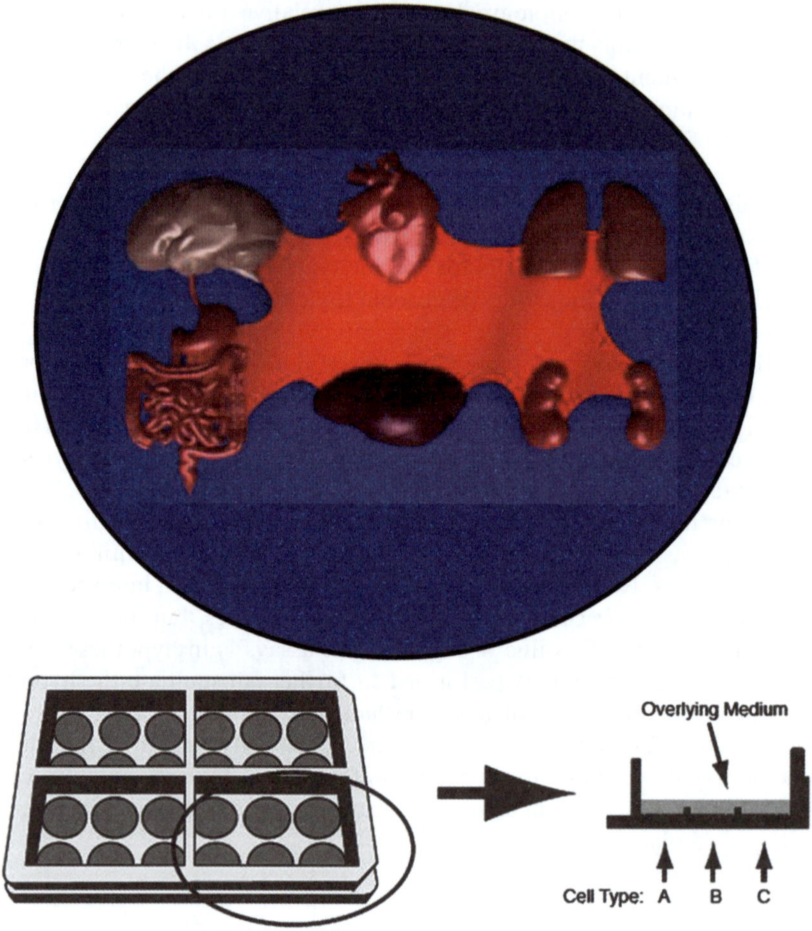


**Figure 10.5** The Integrated Discrete Multiple Organ Co-culture (IdMOC) experiment system is based on the concept that in the human body consists of multiple organs interacting *via* the systemic circulation (top figure). A toxicant may be metabolized by one or more of the organs, and the resulting metabolites may interact with one or more organs *via* the systemic circulation. This concept is reduced to practice as an IdMOC plate (bottom left), with multiple wells within a chamber. Cells from individual organs are cultured physically separated in the wells, with the cells of the multiple organs interconnected *via* an overlying medium (bottom right).

The IdMOC models the multiple-organ interaction in the whole organism *in vivo*, allowing the evaluation of organ-specific effects a drug and its metabolites. The IdMOC represents an improved *in vitro* experimental system for routine screening of ADMET drug properties.

The IdMOC involves the "wells-in-a-well" concept. The typical IdMOC plate consists of a chamber within which are several wells (Figure 10.5). Cells of different origins (*e.g.*, from different organs) are initially cultured, each in its specific medium, in the wells. When the cells are established, the wells are flooded with an overlying medium, thereby connecting all the wells. The multiple cell types now can interact *via* the overlying medium, akin to the multiple organs in a human body interacting *via* the systemic circulation.

The IdMOC system can be used for the following:

1) Differential cytotoxicity: evaluation of the toxicity of a substance on different cell types (*e.g.*, cells from different organs) under virtually identical experimental conditions with multiple cell-type interactions. Aflatoxin B1, a know hepatotoxicant in humans *in vivo*, is shown to have selectively higher cytotoxicity in hepatocytes in the IdMOC co-culture of hepatocytes, renal proximal tubule cells, and small airway epithelial cells.
2) Differential distribution: evaluation of the differential accumulation/distribution of a substance among multiple cell types. This application is especially useful for the development of cytotoxic anticancer agent with selective affinity towards cancer cells.
3) Multiple-organ metabolism: evaluate the ultimate metabolic fate of a substance upon metabolism by cells representing multiple organs with metabolic functions (*e.g.*, liver, kidney, lung). This application allows the development of metabolite profiling of drugs which are subjected to both hepatic and extrahepatic metabolism.

The evaluation of organ-specific toxicity is illustrated by the treatment of IdMOC with a known hepatotoxicant, aflatoxin B1, in IdMOC with three human primary cell types: hepatocytes, renal proximal tubule epithelial cells,

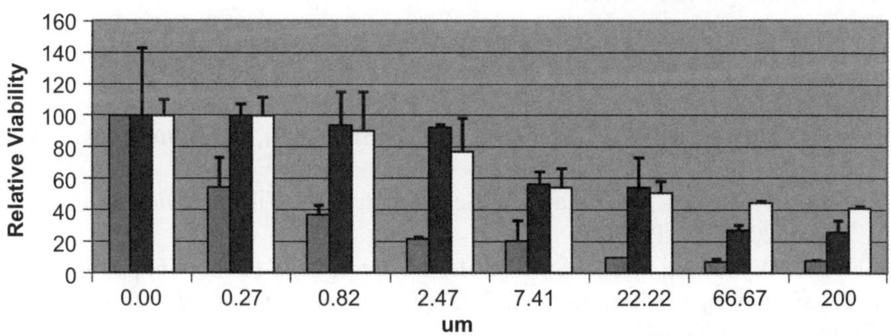


**Figure 10.6** Evaluation of organ-specific toxicity using IdMOC. Aflatoxin B1 is a known hepatotoxicant and hepatocarcinogen. IdMOC with co-cultures of human hepatocytes (left bar), human renal proximal tubule epithelial cells (middle bar), and human pulmonary epithelial cells (right bar) were treated with aflatoxin B1 at the various concentrations shown for 48 h. Viability of the cells after treatment was determined based on cellular ATP content. Aflatoxin B1 was found to be significantly more cytotoxic towards human hepatocytes than the other two cell types. The results illustrate the usefulness of this novel technology for the identification of organ-specific toxicants.

and pulmonary (small airway) epithelial cells. Aflatoxin B1 was found to be significantly more cytotoxic towards human hepatocytes, presumably due to the higher P450 activities of the cells *versus* the other two cell types (Figure 10.6), as it is known that aflatoxin requires P450 metabolism to toxic metabolites to exert its toxicity.

## 10.9 Conclusions

Accurate prediction of human drug toxicity represents a major challenge for drug development. The high rate of clinical failure of drug candidates that have been carefully selected from preclinical studies illustrates clearly that the routine, "classical" approach of pre-clinical safety evaluation is inadequate. It has been argued here that species–species differences in drug toxicity is a major reason—human-specific toxicity, by definition, cannot be predicted with non-human laboratory animals. It is proposed here that human *in vivo* drug toxicity can be predicted using a combination of human-based *in vitro* experimental systems and appropriate *in vivo* laboratory animals—the *in vitro–in vivo* strategy (IVIVS). The success of IVIVS will depend on the selection of appropriate *in vitro* models. Human-specific drug metabolism, appropriate target cell populations, and relevant endpoints are three key parameters for the selection of an appropriate *in vitro* model. Human hepatocytes represent an appropriate experimental model to evaluate liver-specific events such as hepatic metabolism, drug–drug interactions, and hepatotoxicity. IdMOC allows the co-culturing of multiple cell types modeling *in vivo* multiple organ interactions and thereby represent a more complete *in vitro* experimental system for the prediction of *in vivo* toxic effects.

## References


1. J. A. DiMasi, R. W. Hansen and H. G. Grabowski, *J. Health Econ.*, 2003, **22**, 151–185.
2. J. A. DiMasi, L. Feldman, A. Seckler and A. Wilson, *Clin. Pharmacol. Ther.*, 2010, **87**, 272–277.
3. D. K. Wysowski and L. Swartz, *Arch. Intern. Med.*, 2005, **165**, 1363–1369.
4. D. F. Lewis, C. Ioannides and D. V. Parke, *Environ. Health Perspect.*, 1998, **106**, 633–641.
5. F. P. Guengerich, *Drug Metab. Rev.*, 2004, **36**, 159–197.
6. J. Easterbrook, C. Lu, Y. Sakai and A. P. Li, *Drug Metab. Dispos.*, 2001, **29**, 141–144.
7. T. A. Baillie, M. N. Cayen, H. Fouda, R. J. Gerson, J. D. Green, S. J. Grossman, L. J. Klunk, B. LeBlanc, D. G. Perkins and L. A. Shipley, *Toxicol. Appl. Pharmacol.*, 2002, **182**, 188–196.
8. R. C. Cattley, J. DeLuca, C. Elcombe, P. Fenner-Crisp, B. G. Lake, D. S. Marsman, T. A. Pastoor, J. A. Popp, D. E. Robinson, B. Schwetz, J. Tugwood and W. Wahli, *Regul. Toxicol. Pharmacol.*, 1998, **27**, 47–60.

9. J. B. Hengstler, B. Van der Burg, P. Steinberg and F. Oesch, *Drug Metab. Rev.*, 1999, **31**, 917–970.
10. E. L. LeCluyse, *Chem.–Biol. Interact.*, 2001, **134**, 283–289.
11. C. L. Erickson-Miller, R. D. May, J. Tomaszewski, B. Osborn, M. J. Murphy, J. G. Page and R. E. Parchment, *Cancer Chemother. Pharmacol.*, 1997, **39**, 467–472.
12. A. P. Li, *Adv. Pharmacol.*, 1997, **43**, 103–130.
13. B. Davit, K. Reynolds, R. Yuan, F. Ajayi, D. Conner, E. Fadiran, B. Gillespie, C. Sahajwalla, S. M. Huang and L. J. Lesko, *J. Clin. Pharmacol.*, 1999, **39**, 899–910.
14. L. Zhang, Y. Zhang, P. Zhao and S.-M. Huang, *AAPS J.* 2009, **11**, 300–306.
15. J. T. MacGregor and J. M. Collins, *Toxicol. Sci.*, 2001, **59**, 17–36.
16. A. P. Li, *Curr. Drug Saf.*, 2007, **2**, 193–199.
17. N. J. Hewitt, M. J G. Lechón, J. B. Houston, D. Hallifax, H. S. Brown, P. Maurel, J. G. Kenna, L. Gustavsson, C. Lohmann, C. Skonberg, A. Guillouzo, G. Tuschl, A. P. Li, E. LeCluyse, G. M. M. Groothuis and J. G. Hengstler, *Drug Metab. Rev.*, 2007, **39**, 159–234.
18. A. P. Li, *Chem.–Biol. Interact.*, 2007, **168**, 16–29.
19. A. P. Li, *ALTEX*, 2008, **25**, 33–42.
20. L. J. Loretz, A. P. Li, M. W. Flye and A. G. E. Wilson, *Xenobiotica*, 1989, **19**, 489–498.
21. A. P. Li, *IDrugs,* 1998, **1**, 311–314.
22. A. P. Li, *Methods Mol. Biol.*, 2010, **640**, 281–294.
23. A. P. Li and M. Jurima-Romet, *Adv. Pharmacol.*, 1997, **43**, 1–6.
24. A. P. Li, D. L. Kaminski and A. Rasmussen, *Toxicology*, 1995, **104**, 1–8.
25. D. A. Flockhart and J. R. Oesterheld, *Child. Adolesc. Psychiatr. Clin. North Am.,* 2000, **9**, 43–76.
26. K. Fujita, *Drug Metab. Drug Interact.*, 2004, **20**, 195–217.
27. S. F. Zhou, C. C. Xue, *Ther. Drug Monit.*, 2007, **29**, 687–710.
28. C. L. Crespi and B. W. Penman, *Adv. Pharmacol.*, 1997, **43**, 171–188.
29. N. Chauret, N. Tremblay, R. L. Lackman, J.-Y. Gauthier, J. M. Silva, J. Marois, J. A. Yergey and D. A. Nicoll-Griffith, *Anal. Biochem.*, 1999, **276**, 215–226.
30. B. W. Ogilvie, D. Zhang, Wenying Li, A. D. Rodrigues, A. E. Gipson, J. Holsapple, P. Toren and A. Parkinson, *Drug Metab. Dispos.*, 2006, **34**, 191–197.
31. C. Lu, P. Hatsis, C. Berg, F. W. Lee and S. K. Balani, *Drug Metab. Dispos.*, 2008, **36**, 1255–1260.
32. Y. Shitara, A. P. Li, Y. Kato, C. Lu, K. Ito, T. Itoh and Y. Sugiyama, *Drug Metab. Pharmacokinet.*, 2003, **18**, 33–41.
33. K. Maeda and M. Kambara, *Mol. Pharm.*, 2006, **3**, 70–77.
34. A. P. Li, C. Lu, J. A. Brent, C. Pham, A. Fackett, C. E. Ruegg, P. M. Silber, *Chem.–Biol. Interact.*, 1999, **121**, 17–35.
35. A. P. Li, *Drug Metab. Dispos.*, 2009, **37**,1598–1603.
36. Z. W. Zhou and S. F. Zhou, *Expert Opin. Drug Metab. Toxicol.*, 2009, **5**, 579–605.

37. X. Wang, Y. Wang, Y. Chunsheng, L. Wang and S. Han, *Arch. Environ. Contam. Toxicol.*, 2002, **42**, 29–35.
38. K. Mori, H. Hashimoto, H. Takatsu, M. Tsuda-Tsukimoto and T. Kume, *Xenobiotica*, 2009, **39**, 415–422.
39. D. F. McGinnity, A. J. Berry, J. R. Kenny, K. Grime and R. J. Riley, *Drug Metab. Dispos.*, 2006, **34**, 1291–1300.
40. J. Mao, M. A. Mohutsky, John P. Harrelson, S. A. Wrighton and S. D. Hall, *Drug Metab. Dispos.*, 2011, **39**, 591–602.
41. N. Hariparsad, S. C. Nallani, R. S. Sane, D. J. Buckley, A. R. Buckley and P. B. Desai, *J. Clin. Pharmacol.*, 2004, **44**, 1273–1281.
42. J. H. Lillibridge, B. H. Liang, B. M. Kerr, S. Webber, B. Quart, B. V. Shetty and C. A. Lee, *Drug Metab. Dispos.*, 1998, **26**, 609–616.
43. J. Gan, T. W. Harper, M.-M. Hsueh, Q. Qu and W. G. Humphreys, *Chem. Res. Toxicol.* 2005, **18**, 896–903.
44. A. Leblanc, T. C. Shiao, *Rapid Commun. Mass Spectrom.*, 2010, **24**, 1241–1250.
45. D. E. Amacher and B. A. Martin, *Fundam. Appl. Toxicol.*, 1997, **40**, 256–263.
46. M. Neumeier, J. Weigert, A. Schäffler, T. S. Weiss, C. Schmidl, R. Büttner, C. Bollheimer, C. Aslanidis, J. Schölmerich and C. Buechler, *Biochem. Biophys. Res. Commun.*, 2006, **350**, 731–735.
47. D. E. Amacher, *Toxicology,* 2011, **279**, 10–18.
48. J. H. Ansede, W. R. Smith, C. H. Perry, R. L. St. Claire III and K. R. Brouwer, *Drug Metab. Dispos.*, 2010, **38**, 276–280.
49. T. Kasahara, K. Tomita, H. Murano, T. Harada, K. Tsubakimoto, T. Ogihara, S. Ohnishi and C. Kakinuma, *Toxicol. Sci.,* 2006, **90**, 133–141.
50. M. J. Reasor, K. L. Hastings and R. G. Ulrich, *Expert Opin. Drug Saf.*, 2006, **5**, 567–583.
51. L. D. Kier, R. Neft, L. Tang, R. Suizu, T. Cook, K. Onsurez, K. Tiegler, Y. Sakai, M. Ortiz, T. Nolan, U. Sankar and A. P. Li, *Mutat. Res.*, 2004, **549**, 101–113.
52. T. Uehara, A. Ono, T. Maruyama, I. Kato, H. Yamada, Y. Ohno and T. Urushidani, *Mol. Nutr. Food Res.*, 2010, **54**, 218–227.
53. C. A. Afshari, H. K. Hamadeh and P. R. Bushel, *Toxicol. Sci.*, 2010, **120**, S225–S237.
54. A. S. Kienhuis, J. G. Bessems, J. L.A. Pennings, M. Driessen, M. Luijten, J. H. M. van Delft, A. A. C. M. Peijnenburg and L. T. M. van der Ven, *Toxicol. Appl. Pharmacol.*, 2011, **250**, 96–107.
55. A. P. Li, C. Bode and Y. Sakai, *Chem.–Biol. Interact.* 2004, **150**, 129–136.
56. A. P. Li, *ALTEX*, 2008, **25**, 43–49.
57. A. P. Li, *Altern. Lab. Anim.* 2009, **37**, 377–385.

CHAPTER 11

# *Pathways of Organ Injury to Define Human Response in Organotypic Cultures*

ALISON E. M. VICKERS

Allergan Inc., Investigative Sciences, 2525 Dupont Drive, Irvine, CA 92612, USA

## 11.1 Introduction

### 11.1.1 Insight on Mechanism Will Lead to Better Candidate Selection

While listening to a drug advertisement, one hears many potential side-effects listed, some of which are quite terrifying, especially if you become part of the percentage of individuals that manifests the side-effect. Regulatory authorities, including the FDA and EMEA, are increasingly scrutinizing safety data of pharmaceuticals, which has led to an increased number of black box warnings, an extension of post-marketing safety oversight, and the withdrawal of drugs from the market.[1–3] To minimize safety concerns on drug candidates progressing from discovery through non-clinical and clinical development, a continuum of knowledge gained about the mechanisms of the side-effects, human response and risk, will aid in better decisions about the best drug candidate to market. Currently, molecular approaches applied to human tissue models to characterize key pathways that are causal to organ dysfunction and injury, prior to changes in morphology and frank clinical symptoms are improving the

RSC Drug Discovery Series No. 12
New Horizons in Predictive Toxicology: Current Status and Application
Edited by Alan G. E. Wilson

Published by the Royal Society of Chemistry, www.rsc.org

extrapolation of safety data for humans and broadening the scope of translational toxicology in drug safety evaluation.

Publications from recent initiatives in the area of toxicogenomics and in the area of understanding human response for improving toxicity testing have stimulated further discussions within the scientific community. For toxicogenomics, a survey written and distributed by the Health and Environmental Institute (HESI) Committee on the application of genomics to mechanism-based risk assessment, was sent to users and decision makers in the field of toxicogenomics of the pharmaceutical industry, academia and government regulatory agencies. Identification of the major areas where toxicogenomics is having an impact included: 1) understanding biological mechanisms, 2) identification of biomarker candidates, and 3) identifying species differences. The major hurdle for further implementation of toxicogenomics is the limited biological understanding of toxicogenomic data, which is inherent to its impact and consequently relates to the other hurdles identified, including the concern of data interpretation by regulatory agencies and the conservative nature of organizations.[4] Hence, the challenge to accepting toxicogenomic data is in understanding the link of pathways and mechanisms within the biological context; and ultimately, the potential risk of drugs relates to the uncertainty of its biological significance.[5]

On the topic of improving toxicity testing based on a new approach grounded in human biology, the National Research Council published the report *A Vision of Toxicity Testing in the 21st Century*[6,7] and Toxicological Sciences has followed with a Forum Series.[8–12] Even though these papers focus on environmental chemicals, the concepts can be readily applied to risk assessment of pharmaceuticals. This shift towards gaining insight into human mechanism of action and response focuses on identifying the critical perturbations that lead to organ injury based on human biology with the purpose of defining dose–response relationships, such that if maintained above a particular concentration and duration, the outcome would be expected to lead to adverse drug effects. The extrapolation of the human *in vitro* results to predict *in vivo* outcomes will rely on understanding the mode of action, pharmacokinetic models to extrapolate *in vitro* concentrations to relevant human blood and tissue concentrations, as well as systems capable of mapping cell and tissue pathways leading to organ injury. It will also become important to understand the spectrum of adverse effects from multiple cell or organ processes. Although *in vitro* models cannot fully address the whole-body outcome, many key characteristics of organs are retained within the *in vitro* models, including drug metabolism, transport, and combinations of cell types and interactions. Multiple organ interactions are beginning to be addressed with organ co-cultures and interconnected microfluidic compartmental systems for the purpose of combining the organ of initial exposure to the compound with the organ that manifests toxicity.[13–16] The evaluation of human toxicity will incorporate knowledge of human compound metabolism, human target organ pathways, and the consequence of multiple organ interactions. The ability to systematically evaluate toxicity prior to testing *in vivo*, will lead to a refinement of the endpoints determined in both animal and clinical studies, as well as impact the selection of more specific and sensitive safety biomarkers. In spite of significant progress made with *in vitro* models that predict *in vivo* outcomes, these *in vitro* approaches still need to overcome the barriers within organizations to new ways of identifying risk targets, plus be properly resourced and integrated into the evaluation of drug safety assessment.[17–26]

In the pharmaceutical industry, drug candidate attrition due to safety in terms of pharmacokinetics and metabolism has in part been addressed by evaluating compound disposition earlier in the lead selection phase to achieve a desirable exposure and treatment duration. For example, implementation of human *in vitro* models has improved the prediction about metabolic pathways, drug induction or inhibition, and drug–drug interactions which then serve to guide the necessary clinical drug–drug interaction studies.[27–29] Toxicity-related failures, however, remain a challenge since the target organ is often not identified in the discovery efficacy models. Early assessments of drug-induced injury often focus on *in vitro* cell viability. The harmful compounds are readily rejected, however such models do not discriminate amongst compounds with some effects on cell viability, and it is not known at this point how well the concentration-dependent effects translate to *in vivo* exposure. Identification of organ-specific toxicities usually occurs in short-term (1–2 week) repeat-dose toxicity rodent studies. Dose-limiting toxicities, however, are more often identified in the one-month rodent toxicology studies. Even though the drug candidate enters into the development stage, it is important to begin understanding the mechanism of toxicity to provide feedback to research for selection of a back-up compound. Structural modifications to the molecule could minimize the safety liability, resulting in a wider safety margin between efficacy and potential side-effects.

Non-clinical animal and human tissue models that truly provide insight into the mechanism of organ injury and human relevance will contribute to bridging the gap in the extrapolation of animal data to predicting human safety. The existing approaches to safety testing in non-clinical drug development are not powerful enough to reliably identify potential toxic liabilities for humans. Current animal models are about 50–70% predictive of human response, which includes hematological, gastrointestinal, cardiovascular, and urinary tract toxicities (~70%), and hepatic, skin and neurological toxicities (~50%), making these approaches limited in their ability to fully characterize human risk.[1,30,31] Additionally, the primary reasons for drug withdrawals in the United States, European, or Asian markets from 1998–2008 were liver (29%), cardiac/cardiovascular (33%), psychiatric/addiction (8%), gastrointestinal (2%), muscle (2%) and other (22%) which includes renal and drug–drug interactions, which further emphasizes the need to maximize the safety profile of the drug.[23] To improve the current situation, a hybrid approach is emerging in many pharmaceutical companies, combining the use of conventional methods of assessing toxic potential, along with identifying molecular signals linked to organ dysfunction and injury plus employing human tissue models in a targeted, focused manner to define whether the mechanism of organ injury is similar across species, as well as define which species is more sensitive. Identification of specific and sensitive biomarkers will likely come from the mechanistic data for use in bridging the non-clinical and clinical safety evaluation of the therapy. The pharmaceutical industry also has a unique opportunity in that human data collected on compound classes in clinical studies could provide feedback to the non-clinical investigators, to aid in advancing the development and validation of human *in vitro* models or human blood sample analyses, to enhance our understanding of the inter-individual differences which determine susceptibility to adverse drug reactions.[5,18,23,32–35]

Drug-induced organ injury is complex, involving numerous mediators, organelles and cell types. The histological evaluation of tissue from *in vivo* studies identifies the cell types involved, regions and cell-matrix changes. It is also realized that organ toxicities, such as hepatotoxicity may be a culmination of specific molecular events including mitochondrial toxicity, cholestasis, reactive metabolite formation, binding to macromolecules, and the disruption of cell pathways. A means to investigate mechanisms is to utilize organotypic models with genomic, proteomic and metabolomic technologies to provide a means to link tissue specific cellular pathways with drug-specific organ injury and repair processes, as well as provide concentrations at which the perturbation of tissue function occurs. Drug candidate profiling using complex human organotypic models is a means to gain knowledge of human response and susceptibility.[36–39] Additionally, knowledge on compound pharmacology, and side-effect profiles of drugs, often reveal common targets to anticipate for comparative pharmacology and side-effect profiling to help establish a link between non-clinical and clinical drug-induced effects. The safety assessment field is working toward integrating knowledge on chemical structures, target affinities, biological pathways of efficacy and safety, along with individual genomic data, for a systems approach to drug therapy and patient stratification.[40]

### 11.1.2 Translational Mechanistic Models

To accurately characterize drug-induced mechanisms of organ injury and to predict species sensitivity, then the model needs to comprise organ complexity, function and morphology. Organotypic cultures, such as tissue explants and organ slices, are proving that three-dimensional multicellular complexity in concert with organ architecture mimics organ dynamics like *in vivo*. Furthermore, it is essential that such models utilize human tissue to predict human response for comparison with animal tissue response.[31,37,38,41,42] The unit of function is the tissue, and it is increasingly recognized that cells combined with matrices or co-cultured as three-dimensional cultures mimic biologically functional cells from tissues far better than cell monolayers or cell lines. Cells communicate *via* chemical signals, and *via* cell–extracellular matrix interactions to maintain cell differentiation, and to regulate organ function to changes in the microenvironment, both quiescence and responsiveness.[43–49] For instance, macrophages, such as kupffer cells, when activated can trigger either an inflammatory response by the release of pro-inflammatory mediators and subsequent activation of death and survival pathways, or trigger a suppression of inflammation and the release of anti-inflammatory cytokines and inhibition of wound repair.[50,51] In the presence of injury, the tissue response may include aspects of both repair and regeneration with the outcome determined by the extent of injury.[52]

To establish and verify organotypic cultures for characterizing pathways of drug-induced specific organ injury, compounds known to induce liver or kidney injury were initially selected, since information about the mechanism of drug-induced injury was available in the literature or from in-house studies. The approach was to establish liver and kidney rat slice cultures to reproduce the morphology in culture as that described from the *in vivo* studies. The advantage of *in vitro* models is that time-courses at several concentrations can be investigated, to define concentrations at which no effect is detected *versus* concentrations that affect cell pathways and compromise cell function prior to changes in morphology. The mechanistic profile obtained captures the sequence of events culminating in toxicity, such as mitochondrial injury and cholestasis. Generally, it is possible to correlate the *in vitro* concentration of drug-induced effects with *in vivo* drug exposure levels or tissue concentrations to demonstrate that the *in vitro* model is responding in a similar manner to *in vivo*. Once the organotypic culture is established, typically with rat tissue, and the concentration effects defined, it is then possible to compare the response in human, dog or monkey tissue. Questions addressed include whether the pathways of organ injury are similar or different, and determine the concentrations where significant alterations in tissue function are affected to characterize species specificity and sensitivity (Figure 11.1).

## 11.2 Demonstration of *In Vitro–In Vivo* Correlations

### 11.2.1 Liver

Mechanistic studies which employ *in vivo* and *in vitro* models can provide insight into the mechanism of the organ injury as well as discriminate compounds to aid in candidate selection for development. An example is provided here in which four fatty acid oxidation inhibitors were evaluated for effects on liver mitochondrial function and the consequences on overall liver function, as well as the relevance for human by comparing data from a rat *in vivo* study, rat and human liver slices.Impairment of liver mitochondrial β-oxidation of fatty acid metabolism is an important mechanism of drug-induced liver injury, which can lead to microvesicular steatosis, inflammation, and necrosis in rats and man.[53,54] Short-term rat *in vivo* studies (1–4 days) revealed that the inhibitors (etomoxir, CPI975, FOX988, and SDZ51-641) affected serum transaminase values, and caused hepatocellular vacuolation, representing ultrastructural mitochondrial changes. Urine analysis revealed a dicarboxylic aciduria, as

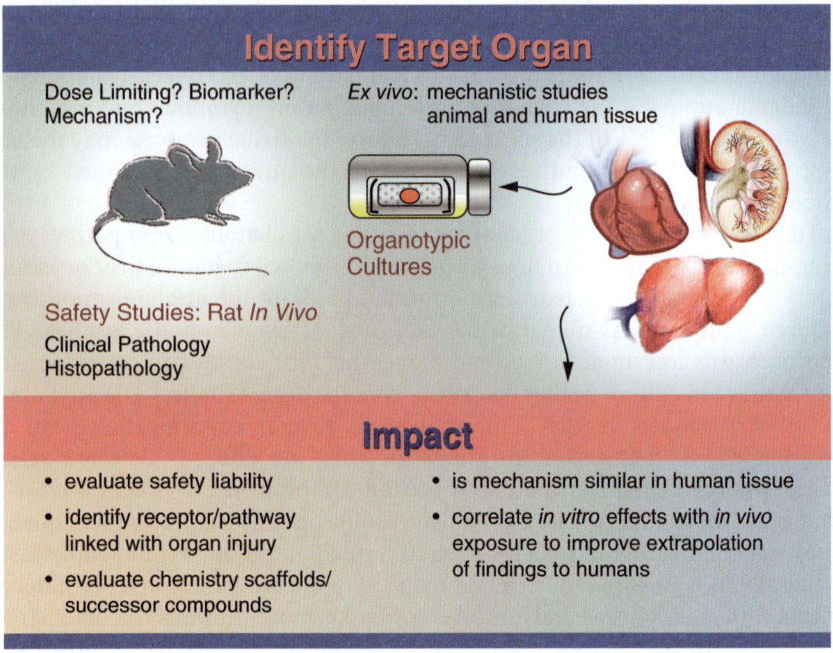


**Figure 11.1** Following identification of the target organs from *in vivo* animal studies, *in vitro* organotypic models are used to evaluate human responses in comparison to animal of drug-induced organ injury. These studies aid in drug candidate selection and risk evaluation of side-effects.

determined by nuclear magnetic resonance (NMR) spectroscopy, indicating incomplete liver fatty acid metabolism, that was either transient or more persistent depending on the compound. Gene expression profiling of livers from the *in vivo* studies demonstrated an up-regulation of genes linked with mitochondrial function, and pathways of fatty acid metabolism, general and oxidative stress.[55] Many of the gene expression changes demonstrating a perturbation of liver function preceded changes in mitochondrial morphology. One compound, CPI, caused less of an effect as marked by fewer gene expression changes in the absence of clinical chemistry, histopathology or urine NMR changes (Table 11.1). Urine analysis in clinical studies to detect dicarboxylic acids as in this example, could serve as a biomarker prior to hepatotoxicity, in that an altered excretion pattern would parallel the altered lipid metabolism at the cellular level.

*In vitro* studies with rat and human tissue allowed for a species comparison to demonstrate that the pathways leading to a change of liver function and hepatotoxicity were similar in rat and in human. The compounds were differentiated on the number of gene expression changes. The *in vitro–in vivo* correlation revealed that many of the gene expression changes in the rat liver slices paralleled the changes detected in the livers obtained from the

**Table 11.1** Summary of rat *in vivo* functional changes *via* clinical pathology and urine metabonomic profile, and pathway and organelle analysis of organ injury by liver gene expression and histopathology, to discriminate mitochondrial effects of four fatty acid oxidation inhibitors.

| *Fatty acid oxidation inhibitors* | *Clinical pathology* | | *Urine metabonomics* | *Liver gene expression changes* | *Histopathology* |
|---|---|---|---|---|---|
| | *Liver dysfunction* | | | | |
| | *SD* | *MD* | *Dicarboxylic aciduria (h)* | *SD[a] and MD[b]* | *Mitochondrial injury* |
| Etomoxir | ↑ AST<br>↑ ALT | NC | 0–48 | Mitochondrial fatty acid metabolism<br>ω-oxidation | Myelin figures (1/5, MD) |
| CPI975 | NC | NC | NC | ω-Oxidation general stress | NC |
| FOX988 | ↓ ALT<br>↑ ALP<br>↑ TBIL | ↓ TP<br>↓ ALB<br>↓ GLU | 0–96 | Mitochondrial ribotoxic cell matrix | Megamitochondria (4/5, MD);<br>enlarged mitochondria (2/5, SD) |
| SDZ51-641 | | ↑ ALT | 0–48 | Mitochondrial fatty acid metabolism<br>general stress<br>ribotoxic cell matrix | Megamitochondria (4/5, MD);<br>single cell necrosis (1/5, SD) |

[a]SD, single dose;
[b]MD, multiple dose;
ALB, albumin; ALP, alkaline phosphatase; ALT, alanine aminotransferase; AST, aspartate aminotransferase; GLU, glucose; NC, no change to baseline; TBIL, total bilirubin; TP, total protein.

*in vivo* study. An up-regulation of general and oxidative stress gene expression, including mitochondrial genes, preceded the functional decline of ATP and GSH levels in the liver slices. Additional gene expression changes detected with the *in vitro* studies included changes in genes linked with a ribotoxic response, apoptosis, proliferation, cell matrix, and inflammation. Associated functional changes included an increase in caspases-3 and -9 activity, markers of apoptosis. The increase in the pro-inflammatory response marker, IL-8, produced by the endothelial cells, demonstrates the value of using an organotypic culture to obtain the full network of events induced by such compounds, which may also have been a useful biomarker.[55,56] A clinical consequence of severe loss of energy by the mitochondria and organelle injury, leads to a decrease in the metabolism of pyruvate from glucose by mitochondrial enzymes, and an increase in the conversion of pyruvate to lactic acid in the cytoplasm, which may progress clinically to lactic acidosis, and if not treated to liver failure (Figure 11.2).

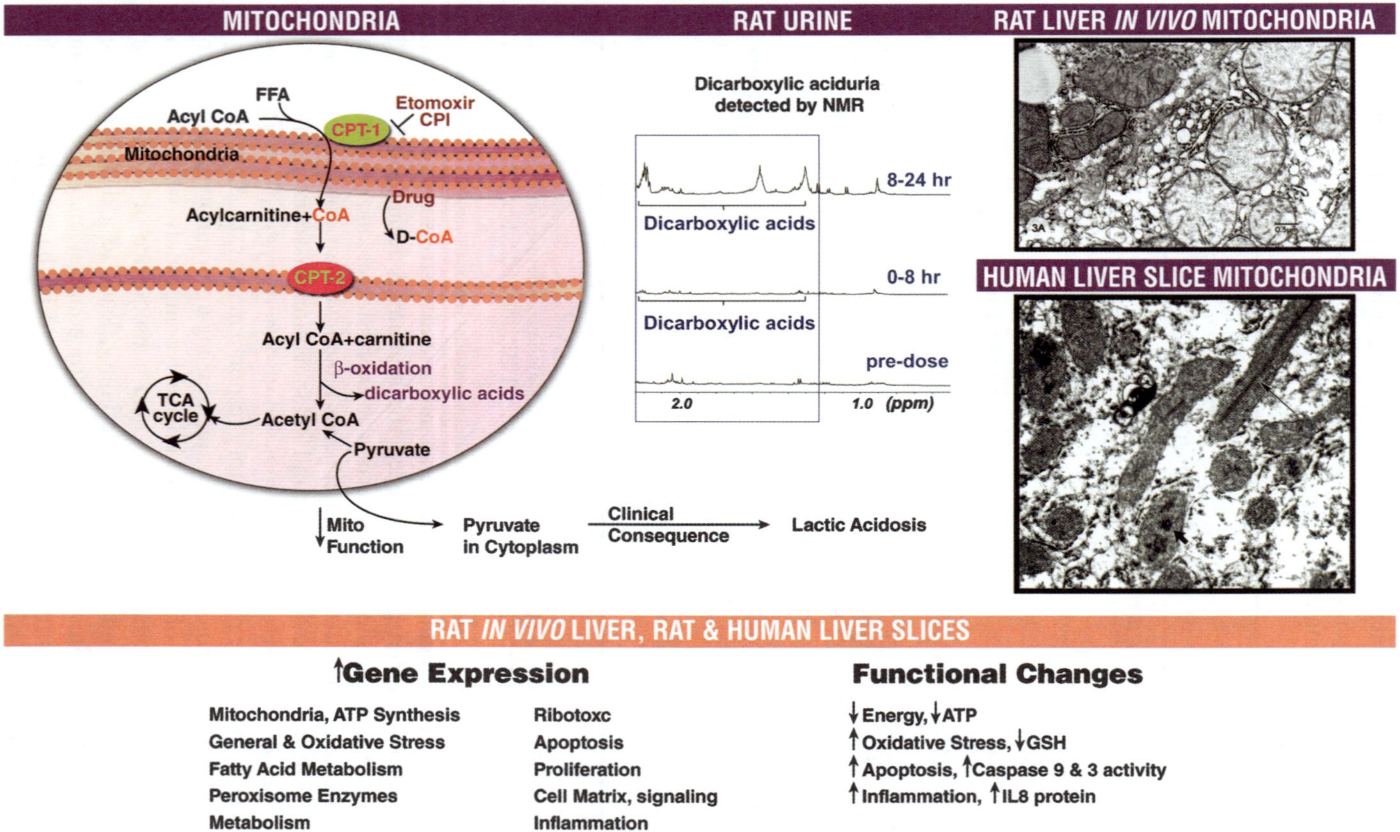


**Figure 11.2** Inhibition of mitochondrial β-oxidation by etomoxir and CPI leads to incomplete fatty acid metabolism and detection of dicarboxylic acids in urine. The up-regulation of liver genes indicative of mitochondria, fatty acid metabolism, stress, apoptosis, and inflammation preceded and coincided with functional changes in mitochondrial energy levels (ATP), stress (GSH levels), apoptosis (caspase activity) and inflammation (IL-8 levels), and changes in mitochondrial morphology in rat and human liver slices.

Other types of liver injury have been reproduced in organ slices. For example, alcoholic liver injury, designated by known hallmarks from animal and human studies, has been reproduced in rat liver slices. Ethanol is metabolized to acetaldehyde, leading to oxidative stress, acute inflammation, reduced albumin secretion, and the development of a fatty liver.[57] The interaction of ethanol on cocaine hepatotoxicity, and known potentiation, has been demonstrated by combination treatments of cocaine (0.5 mM) plus ethanol (0.3%). Significant decreases in human liver slice viability occurred as compared to either treatment alone.[58] The sensitivity of young children towards valproic acid associated hepatotoxicity has been studied in liver slices from weanling and adult rats, and from a limited number of human livers. Liver slices from the donors less than 20 years of age exhibited more toxicity toward valproic acid than liver slices from older donors.[59] Exposure of thioacetamide to rat liver slices resulted in specific centrilobular localization of apoptosis, confirmed by caspase-3 cleavage products and DNA fragmentation in centrilobular hepatocytes, matching the findings of *in vivo* studies.[60] The potential interaction of an antiemesis agent with the chemotherapeutic agent *cis*-platin was demonstrated by the lack of effect on the pharmacological action of *cis*-platin-induced apoptosis in liver slices.[61] Demonstration that measles virus strains from vaccines can penetrated into the deep cell layers of tumor areas within human liver slices establishes the potential of this model for evaluating oncolytic agents on patient tissue prior to virotherapy.[62]

Toxicogenomic profiling of hepatotoxic compounds with different mechanisms, including inflammation induced by lipopolysaccharide, necrosis by paracetamol, fibrosis and necrosis with carbon tetrachloride, and apoptosis with gliotoxin, in rat liver slices correlated with liver profiles from *in vivo* studies of a commercial gene expression database. Specific genes, representative of the different mechanisms however, are not provided.[63] The concordance of organ slice gene expression changes to *in vivo* tissue gene expression changes is expected to be high, since organ slices encompass the various cell types of *in vivo* tissue. Comparative studies will continue to improve as tissue handling and culturing continue to improve, including preparation of slices in a preservation buffer rather than Krebs–Henseleit buffer, and incubation in a dynamic culture exposing the slices to air and medium to maintain differentiation. The number of pathways perturbed depends on the dose of the compound, so comparing drug exposure to outcome will be an important aspect to incorporate into models for predictive purposes.

### 11.2.2 Kidney

An *in vitro–in vivo* comparison of kidney molecular pathways and functional changes associated with toxicity has been demonstrated with *cis*-platin. The mechanism of *cis*-platin nephrotoxicity is complex and progressive, involving several pathways of altered function involving growth arrest, apoptosis, repair, inflammation and necrosis. A comparison of rat kidney slices to rat kidney obtained from an *in vivo* study aided in establishing the human model and verified the advantage of the *in vitro* model for extrapolating animal findings and identifying *cis*-platin effects in human tissue. In the kidney slices, regional differences of *cis*-platin nephrotoxicity could be demonstrated as described with *in vivo* studies.[64,65] A progressive involvement of the tubular epithelium was reproduced morphologically in both human and rat kidney slices, while the glomerulus appeared resistant even at high concentrations.

The gene expression changes induced by *cis*-platin reflected multiple cellular pathways and functions. Both concentration- and time-dependent gene expression changes preceded and coincided with the morphological change. The panel of gene expression changes detected in both the rat *in vivo* kidney and *in vitro* kidney slices were indicative of transcription, DNA damage, cell cycle, proliferation and apoptosis, which is in agreement with the known mechanism of *cis*-platin causing DNA damage, growth arrest and apoptosis.[66–71] Gene expression changes indicative of protein damage, the disruption of transport and calcium homeostasis, cellular metabolism and oxidative stress are pathways linked with *cis*-platin binding to various cellular proteins and macromolecules.[72,73] Apoptosis and mitochondrial involvement was evident by the up-regulation of p53 gene expression which coincided and preceded an increase of p53 protein expression, an increased activity of caspase-9 and -3, decreases of slice ATP and GSH levels, and a characteristic DNA laddering pattern. The comparison of effects in rat and human kidney slices demonstrated differences in the sensitivity toward the injury with the rat being more sensitive than human[74] (Figure 11.3). The integration of gene expression pathway profiling linking with functional assays and morphology strengthens the *in vitro* models for predicting cellular pathways of organ injury. Recently, studies in Nrf2-null mice demonstrate that *cis*-platin toxicity is exacerbated and linked with the lack of induction of cytoprotective genes (heme oxygenase-1, NADPH:quinone oxidoreductase 1, and glutamate cysteine ligase), drug transporters (Mrp2 and Mrp4) and suppression of inflammation which are key events in wild-type mice associated with proximal tubule cell recovery.[75]

In other kidney-slice studies, the nephrotoxicity of clinically relevant concentrations of chloroacetaldehyde, a major metabolite of the chemotherapeutic prodrug ifosfamide, was demonstrated in rat renal cortical slices. Both total GSH and ATP levels were decreased, which affected oxidative phosphorylation at complex I of the mitochondrial respiratory chain. The decrease of glucose synthesis and lactate utilization, revealed that the inhibition of the glycolytic pathway might play a role in the therapeutic efficacy of ifosfamide against tumor cells.[76]

The mechanism of chlorotrifluoroethylene (CTFE) nephrotoxicity involves the sequential liver metabolism of CTFE to the glutathione conjugate (CTFG) followed by further metabolism in rat kidney cortical slices to reactive thiols, which subsequently bind to the cellular macromolecules and ultimately resulting in necrosis.[77] An additional study, showing the further processing of glutathione-conjugated metabolites produced in the liver to mercapturic acid metabolites in the kidney, demonstrates that the hepatorenal cooperation of multistep metabolic processing can be modeled *in vitro*.[78]

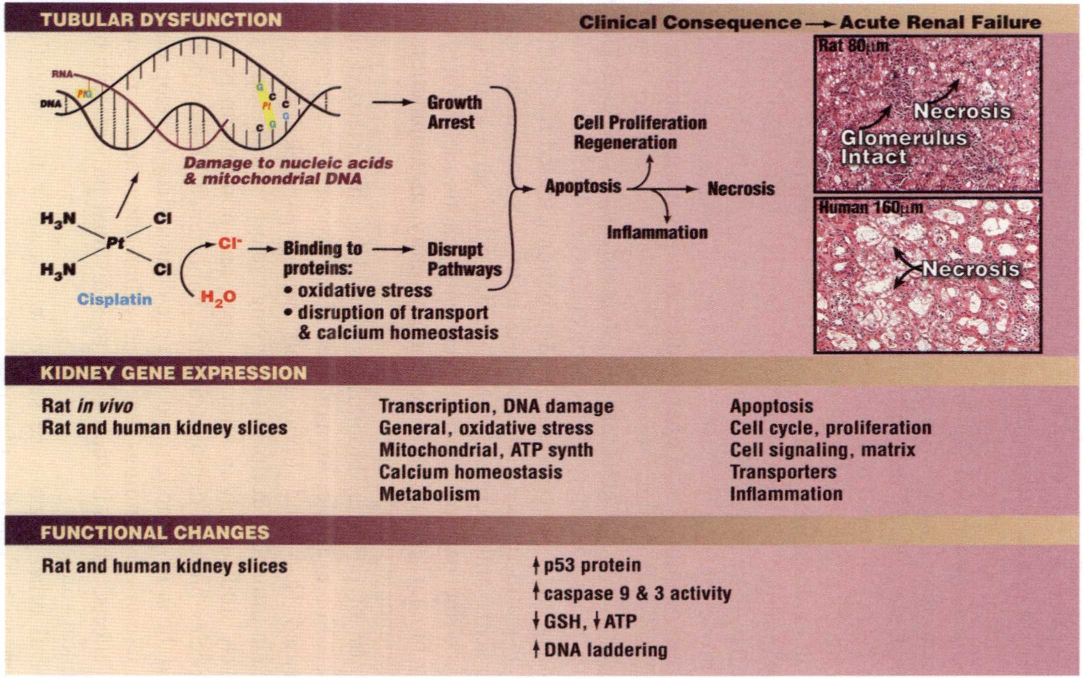


**Figure 11.3** Acute nephrosis of tubular epithelium induced by cisplatin was reproduced in rat and human kidney slices while the glomerulus remained unaffected. In agreement with the mechanism of cisplatin was the up-regulation of genes indicative of DNA damage, growth arrest, and apoptosis; while genes indicative of protein damage, disruption of transport and calcium homeostasis, cellular metabolism and oxidative stress are pathways linked with cisplatin binding to various cellular proteins and macromolecules. Functional changes in ATP and GSH levels, caspase activation, p53 levels and DNA laddering confirmed cellular stress and the activation of apoptotic pathways.

## 11.3 Bridging Biomarkers in Mechanistic Studies

A promising goal for *in vitro* models is the ability to identify tissue or cellular markers which can be used *in vivo* to monitor the onset or progression of a drug-induced side-effect or toxicity. Biomarkers exhibiting regional differences within the liver and kidney include β-glutathione-*S*-transferases (αGST) and β-glutathione-*S*-transferases (πGST). These relatively new biomarkers of liver and kidney cellular status and integrity, have shown clinical utility in the field of organ transplantation,[79] and liver and kidney slices.[80] The HESI nephrotoxicity biomarker consortia demonstrated that in rats treated with *cis*-platin, urinary β-GST and clusterin were detected within 48 h of proximal tubular injury, and were more sensitive than bleed urea nitrogen (BUN) and serum creatinine; while, changes in β-GST or renal papillary antigen 1 (RPA-1) were considered to represent secondary minor effects of proximal tubular injury. The combination of clusterin, kidney injury marker 1 (KIM-1), cystatin C, $\beta_2$-microglobulin, recently qualified by the Critical-Path Institute PSTC and approved for detection of early acute drug-induced renal toxicity in rats by the FDA and EMEA , will improve the non-invasive monitoring of renal damage and discriminate the region of injury.[81,82] Other studies in rats with gentamicin have demonstrated KIM-1 and clusterin to be useful kidney biomarkers prior to functional changes.[83,84] In progress are the steps to qualify several kidney injury biomarkers in clinical safety studies for evaluating human risk toward drug-induced kidney injury *via* consortia.[85] Metabonomic-based rat studies of gentamicin and *cis*-platin suggest that increases in urinary polyamines, phosphate and amino acids, and decreases in nucleosides, could serve as indicators of kidney injury. Urine patterns of particular endogenous metabolites may prove to be early biomarkers indicative of kidney injury, in conjunction with the ability to discriminate injury types.[86]

The identification of potential biomarkers should be characterized in the species of interest. For example, human liver slices exposed to cyclosporine derivatives increased IL-6, and Lp(a) levels, which paralleled the serum increases reported in transplant recipients receiving cyclosporine therapy. Lp(a) levels are effectively studied only in humans, apes, and non-human primates. Differences in species biology demonstrate the importance of incorporating human tissue into the *in vitro* models and into pre-clinical drug development.[80] Furthermore, human *in vitro* findings reveal individual differences in responses to drug-induced effects, which is analogous to individual patients exhibiting side-effects in clinical studies.

There are several other organ-slice studies which show the potential of linking mechanisms with biomarker identification. Increased cytokine secretion (IL-1, IL-6 and TNFα) induced by endotoxin was revealed in human liver slices. This study demonstrated that the importance of non-parenchymal cell involvement in endotoxemia. Depletion of the liver-slice kupffer cells by a liposome-mediated macrophage suicide technique resulted in a loss of IL-1α and TNFα secretion, indicating kupffer cell origin of the cytokines.[87] Investigations with a known hepatobiliary toxicant, geldanamycin, led to decreased rat liver slice transaminase and alkaline phosphatase levels concomitant with an increase of slice bilirubin levels. The tissue biomarker changes were indicative of hepatocellular and biliary injury, which is consistent with the target cell effects from *in vivo* studies.[88–90] The metabolic function of human renal cortical slices has been determined by NMR. The utilization of [$^{13}$C]-labeled glutamines to form ammonia, alanine and lactate increased dose-dependently in the presence of valproate, an established stimulator of renal glutamine metabolism. This ammoniagenic effect of the slices to valproate was retained over the 48 h incubation period.[91]

A challenge of working with human tissue is the variability of response following compound exposure. The human *in vitro* studies become analogous to mini-clinical studies, whereby organ slices derived from some individuals may exhibit an exaggerated response while slices from other individuals may exhibit no response. Understanding the differences and variability of human drug response can in part be studied in organ slices. In the future, a genetic profile of the tissues may in part aid in clarifying the differences seen and to define inter-individual differences. Future studies will also likely include diseased human tissue. It is also feasible to pre-stress the organ slices, by reducing the anti-oxidant status or causing an inflammatory response, prior to drug exposure, in order to mimic individuals with compromised organ function and to study the possible outcomes.

## 11.4 Extension of Organ Slice Cultures: Evidence of Repair Pathways

The multi-cellular three-dimensional complexity of organ slices has distinct requirements for maintaining slice survival in culture. Advances continue to be made in defining optimal incubation conditions and in obtaining higher quality human tissue. Improvements to extend organ slice culture for days enhances the ability to perform mechanistic studies with lower drug concentrations, employ a daily dosing regime, and to investigate both injury and repair. Furthermore, assessment of tissue repair following compound exposure will provide additional functional information regarding doses whereby the drug-induced effect could be reversible *versus* doses in which repair no longer occurs and the toxicity is irreversible. For example, the liver has an extraordinary capacity to regenerate and recover from mechanical or chemical injury. Tissue response to injury may include aspects of repair, including the activation of fibrotic pathways, and regeneration with the outcome determined by the extent of injury and the cross-talk and orchestration between the different cell types and the extracellular matrix.[92–96] Tissue repair increases with dose until a threshold dose is reached and beyond which repair is delayed or impaired. Discerning between an adaptive *versus* a non-reversible response to a drug insult will be valuable for drug selection in the drug-development process.[52] Recent improvements in organ acquisition, organ slice preparation and culturing methods demonstrate that organ slice viability, integrity and morphology is extended for several days in culture which allows for the investigation of injury and repair processes.[97]

Repair processes are evident in organ slices by an increased expression of extracellular matrix genes, the activation of stellate cells, the proliferation of myofibroblast-like cells, and an increased deposition of collagen. The increased gene expression of collagens, particularly I, IV, V, laminins, ninjurin and growth factors is evidence for the activation of regeneration pathways. Liver injury, such as wound healing from the preparation of organ slices, can lead to the activation of hepatic stellate cells and fibrosis pathways. Stellate cell activation is verified by the up-regulation of marker genes, β-smooth muscle actin and collagen 1A1, and the positive staining for β-smooth muscle actin protein.[97,98]

Toxicity-induced repair and hepatic stellate cell activation have been demonstrated by a time- and concentration-dependent increase in mRNA expression of stellate cell markers following $CCl_4$ exposure to rat liver slices.[95] It has also been demonstrated that high doses of ethanol (25 mM) in rat liver slices, induce oxidative stress and sustained IL-6 expression which precedes and coincides with myofibroblast activation.[99] In rat lung slices, fibrinogenesis, evident by extracellular matrix accumulation, myofibroblast transdifferentiation and activation of microvascular endothelial cells, is induced following treatment with $CdCl_2$ plus TGF-$\beta_1$.[100]

The feasibility of using either cold or cryopreserved organ slices has developed substantially. Further refinement is needed to ensure that the function of cold or cryopreserved tissue is truly equivalent to freshly prepared tissue, in order for the methodologies to become common practice. Cryopreservation by freezing with varying amounts of DMSO reveals that organ slice morphology does not change; however the response to apoptotic stimuli is dampened.[101] Cryopreservation of tissue slices by vitrification, a process which prevents the formation of both intra- and extracellular ice crystals while an amorphous glass is formed, has also shown success.[102–104] However, the major hurdle facing cryopreservation by freezing or by vitrification is the toxicity induced by the cryoprotectant and finding a means to neutralize the effects.[105] Organ quality is extremely important and more easily solvable. Organ slices best suited for either cold preservation or cryopreservation are slices obtained from highly viable organs. Additionally, organ slices prepared from transplant quality tissue show significantly greater metabolic function and viability than slices prepared from partial-hepatectomized livers.[106,107]

## 11.5 Liver Screen: Integration of Metabolism and Functional Endpoints

Liver slices are a useful initial screen of organ injury, since compound metabolism is an integral function of the liver, and metabolite formation is often associated with organ toxicity. Tissue regional differences in the expression and inducibility of CYPs, Phase II enzymes and transporters known to exist *in vivo*, and operating *via* the CAR, PXR and AhR pathways are reproducible in human liver slices.[108,109] Penetration of model compounds, exhibiting varied lipophilicity, size, and uptake mechanisms, has been demonstrated with rat and human liver slices. Passive diffusion of a lipophilic compound, rhodamine B, or [$^3$H]-$H_2O$ occurs throughout liver slices (250 μm thickness) within 5 min. Endocytosis, an energy-dependent process, was demonstrated by the uptake of the hydrophilic compound lucigenin into the inner cell layers within 15 min. Specific carrier-mediated uptake with digoxin was shown to be stereoselectively inhibited by quinine, while sinusoidal staining of the inner cell layers of liver slices has been demonstrated for large molecules, like FITC-aconylated human serum albumin.[110] Transport processes have been demonstrated by the differential transport and metabolism of structurally related compounds,[111] as well as the excretion of bile acid derivatives from liver slices into the incubation medium.[112]

An example for using liver slices to investigate drug-induced hepatotoxicity has been shown with diclofenac, a nonsteroidal anti-inflammatory drug. Diclofenac is associated with the formation of reactive metabolites, protein binding, oxidative stress, and mitochondrial injury.[113] Protein adducts have been identified in rat and human primary hepatocytes, and toxicity is evident at lower concentrations than in cell lines because of the increased metabolic capacity of the primary cultures.[114–117]

Liver slice studies revealed a concentration- and time-dependent increase in specific protein binding which preceded changes in function. By 72 h lower concentrations of diclofenac induced toxicity, demonstrating that continued metabolism and the accumulation of specific protein binding was associated with altered liver slice function. The decline of liver slice ATP levels at concentrations not affecting GSH levels implicates mitochondrial dysfunction as a primary factor of hepatotoxicity, of which oxidative stress may be a contributing cause. The species differences in the extent of diclofenac metabolism (rat > monkey > human) correlated with the extent of toxicity.[118]

Binding patterns are beginning to be associated with biological and toxic outcomes. Through the advancement of analyzing protein damage induced by compounds it is recognized that different reactive electrophiles can exhibit a high selectivity for alkylation of different proteins, and for specific nucleophilic sites within these proteins.[27,119] Idiosyncratic drug reactions will also benefit from a greater understanding of the interaction between reactive drug metabolites with proteins, resulting in a varied human response. A major impediment to predicting idiosyncratic drug reactions is the development of valid models and the limited mechanistic understanding.[120,121] Recent studies reveal that acetaminophen triggers the release of inflammatory mediators from kupffer cells which in turn induces a stress response, while neutrophil sequestration is not involved in the initiation of the injury.[122] Hence, a more complex *in vitro* model like liver slices may be more predictive in correlating tissue binding with altered cell function.

## 11.6 Stressed Liver Model

Drug exposure may initiate an oxidative stress response in cells and tissues, leading to an imbalance between oxidant and antioxidant reactions, and resulting in altered cell signaling pathways and function. The major antioxidant and redox regulator in cells is reduced glutathione (GSH). Cellular ATP levels can also be reduced as a consequence of the depletion of the mitochondrial GSH pool. During the metabolism of a drug, a reduction of GSH levels can occur *via* direct conjugation of GSH with a compound/metabolite or by oxidation of GSH from the formation of pro-oxidant radicals.[123–126] In the case of acetaminophen (APAP), the metabolite *N*-acetyl-*p*-benzoquinone imine (NAPQI) is detoxified *via* conjugation with GSH; however high doses of APAP can cause hepatotoxicity and are linked with NAPQI formation. Urine metabolite profiles obtained shortly after APAP administration can distinguish individuals that will develop mild liver injury, prior to an elevation in alanine aminotransferase (ALT) levels, from non-responders.[35] Peripheral blood gene expression profiles revealed a down-regulation of oxidative phosphorylation, which is linked with altered mitochondrial function, in APAP-treated (4 g) subjects but not placebo. Metabonomic data revealed increases of serum lactate levels. The timing of the changes correlated with the percentage of APAP converted to NAPQI.[127]

The mitochondria are important targets for APAP-induced hepatotoxicity. Mitochondria GSH levels become greatly reduced prior to depletion of the cytoplasm pool.[128,129] Additionally, many of the proteins which modulate cell survival and death are redox regulated, such that as tissue levels of GSH are affected, so is the redox status of the tissue. For example, caspases are induced by reactive oxygen species, however high levels of $H_2O_2$ or severe GSH or ATP depletion, can overwhelm the caspases, resulting in mitochondrial dysfunction and a switching of signaling from apoptotic pathways in favor of necrosis.[130–135]

Establishing a stressed liver model in which tissue GSH levels are compromised, allows for the investigation of drugs that induce oxidative stress and whether a poor liver GSH status would lower the concentration of the drug to induce liver injury. Liver-slice GSH levels can be decreased by: 1) BSO (L-buthionine-*S*-sulfoximine) a selective inhibitor of β-glutamylcysteine synthetase, the first and rate-limiting enzyme in GSH synthesis,[136] and by 2) APAP, a drug whereby metabolism involves conjugation with GSH, and reduction of liver GSH levels. An example of a compound that induces oxidative stress *via* the co-oxidation of GSH is methimazole (MMI), the antithyroid agent. Structurally, MMI contains a thione moiety, which is associated with hepatotoxic, hematologic and dermatologic adverse effects.[137–142] It is proposed that metabolism of the MMI thione moiety leads to reactive intermediates, sulfenic acid and sulfinic acid, which co-oxidize GSH to GSSG in the process, resulting in reduced GSH tissue levels, binding to proteins and the subsequent toxic effects.[124,130,141,143,144]

Both BSO and APAP decrease human-liver-slice GSH levels, while in control slices GSH and ATP continue to be synthesized and well maintained. BSO induces a concentration-dependent reduction of GSH levels in human liver slices. For APAP, a concentration associated with hepatotoxicity in humans and subtoxic for cultured hepatocytes is 1 mM.[126,145] Human variability between donor tissue and a progression of injury with time was evident by the variable decreases of GSH and ATP in 1 mM APAP exposed human liver slices (Table 11.2). Co-incubation of MMI with BSO or APAP led to further decreases of GSH and ATP levels in some human livers, at time points and concentrations not detected with MMI alone (Figure 11.4). The combination of MMI with BSO altered the gene expression of oxidative stress related genes and an up-regulation of heat-shock genes. The combination of MMI with APAP increased the expression of genes involved with oxidative stress and anti-oxidant defense, likely to protect the cells from mitochondrial injury.

**Table 11.2** Acetaminophen, at a hepatoxic concentration (1 mM), decreased human liver slice GSH and ATP levels of some donor livers exposed for 24–72 h.

| | *GSH % decrease to control (nmol mg$^{-1}$ wet weight)* | | | *ATP % decrease to control (nmol mg$^{-1}$ wet weight)* | | |
|---|---|---|---|---|---|---|
| Human donor livers | *24 h* | *48 h* | *72 h* | *24 h* | *48 h* | *72 h* |
| HL-1 AST 67; ALT 60; ALP 27 | nd | 19 | 8 | 2 | 20[a] | 37[a] |
| HL-2 AST 30; ALT 36; ALP 39 | 7[a] | 62[a] | 65[a] | 58[a] | 64[a] | 77[a] |
| HL-3 AST 46; ALT 66; ALP 73 | 23 | 38 | 40 | 44[a] | 85[a] | 52[a] |
| HL-4 AST 74; ALT 42; ALP 31 | 21[a] | nd | 77[a] | 24 | 37[a] | 91[a] |

nd = no decrease compared to control; AST = aspartate aminotransferase; ALT = alanine aminotransferase; ALP = alkaline phosphatase.
[a]Significantly different to control.

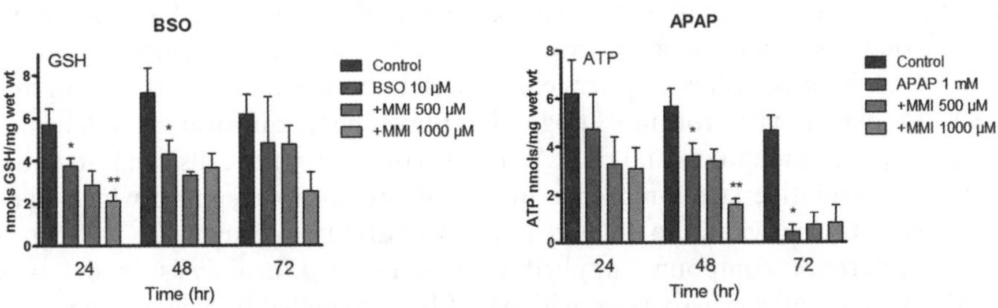


**Figure 11.4** Exposure of human liver slices to the GSH modulating agents, L-buthionine-*S*-sulfoximine (BSO) and inhibitor of GSH synthesis or acetaminophen (APAP) in which a metabolite is conjugated with GSH, causes decreases in slice GSH and ATP levels to generate a stressed liver model. In control slices both ATP and GSH levels are well maintained *via* synthesis. Co-incubation of BSO or APAP with an agent that causes oxidative stress, methimazole (MMI), can lead to a further reduction of GSH or ATP levels.

Generation of a stressed model *via* modulation of the GSH levels with both BSO or APAP reflected the consequences of a poor liver GSH status, as well as human variability in response amongst the human donor livers.[146] Within the field of cellular stress, the monitoring of pathway-based assays which participate in cell activation or death commitments, can serve as indicators in disruption of the tissue homeostatic response and toxicant mechanism of action profiles to screen potentially toxic compounds.[135]

## 11.7 Hemolysis: Co-Culture of Liver and Blood

Hematologic disorders are a major safety concern within drug development, and are a reason for the withdrawal of drugs from the market.[147] In general, compounds that induce changes in hematology parameters, do so in a time–, dose- and route-dependent manner, suggesting that following oral drug exposure metabolites of the compound, generated by the liver, contribute to the hemolytic syndromes.[144,148] Metabolism-induced oxidative stress within the blood cells is often cited as a major mechanism of hemolytic-induced injury, resulting in red blood cell hemolysis, in conjunction with platelet and leukocyte numbers being repressed.[149–152] It is imperative to compare animal and human tissue response of drug-induced hemolytic effects, since species differences exist in the proportion of blood cell types, and in the proportion of compound metabolites generated.[153]

Recently, an *in vitro* model has been developed to provide a means for investigating the mechanism of drug-induced hemotoxicity in animal and human tissue.[154] The model incorporates whole blood co-cultured with a liver slice for several days, allowing for time-dependent responses, such as the generation of sufficient amounts of metabolites which contribute to the outcome. The value of using whole blood and a liver slice is that various cell types, including blood neutrophils and the resident liver macrophages kupffer cells, may participate in the metabolism of a compound.[155] Peroxidase-catalyzed drug oxidation is linked with blood, liver, and bone marrow toxicities due to the prevalence of myeloperoxidase in neutrophils, kupffer cells, as well as bone marrow cells.[124] Kupffer cells also play a major role in hemoglobin uptake, heme turnover, as well as the stress response in humans and rats. Activation of the kupffer cells can lead to an increased oxidative stress response or an inflammatory response which may predispose the individual to an increased susceptibility to drugs.[124,156,157]

The reference compound applied to this *in vitro* hemolysis model was MMI. Adverse effects associated with MMI have included transient leucopenia in about 12% of adults, agranulocytosis (0.1–0.5%), thrombocytopenia and aplastic anemia.[158,159] Hepatotoxicity and dermatological adverse effects are reported for MMI and other thionamides like propylthiouracil.[137–140,142] It is hypothesized that the effects on blood cells and bone marrow cells, may in part be the result of oxidative stress induced *via* the metabolism of MMI. Structure–toxicity relationships of MMI have revealed that analogues without the free sulfhydryl group, or methylation of the thiol group reduces MMI hepatotoxicity in rats.[143] In addition to cytochrome P450s and flavin-containing monooxygenase (FMO), the peroxidase-catalyzed oxidation of MMI by myeloperoxidase (MPO) has been demonstrated. The resultant MMI-thiyl radicals co-oxidize GSH to form reactive oxygen species by redox cycling.[130,160] It has also been reported that human leukocytes accumulate MMI and propylthiouracil.[161]

An oxidative stress response in the blood cells preceded frank hemolysis. A concentration-dependent decline of GSH in blood cells occurred in the rat, dog and human tissue; while, a decline of blood cell ATP occurred in human tissue, and to a lesser extent in the rat with no change in the dog. Hemolysis was time-dependent and progressive in both the rat and human. Hemolysis was evident at 48 h at equivalent MMI concentrations, then by 72 h the extent of hemolysis increased and human tissue exhibited hemolysis at a lower concentration compared to the rat. No hemolysis occurred with the dog tissue. The extent of oxidative stress, the proportion of blood cell types and the proportion of metabolites formed are likely key components leading to red blood cell injury and eventual hemolysis, and are key to species susceptibility (Figure 11.5).

| | %Neutrophils | %Lymphocytes |
|---|---|---|
| Human | 59 | 34 |
| Rat | 15 | 81 |

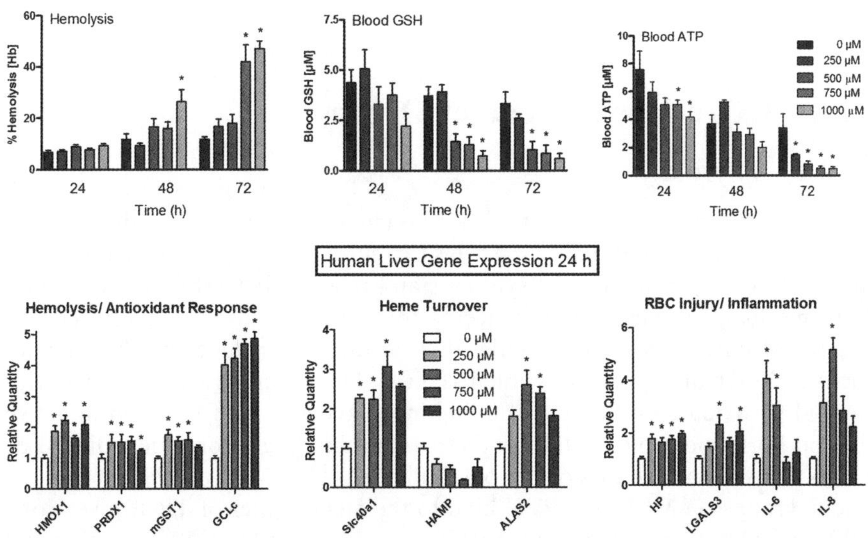


**Figure 11.5** Exposure of human blood–liver slice co-cultures to methimazole (MMI) resulted in time- and concentration-dependent decreases of blood cell GSH and ATP levels prior to frank hemolysis. An up-regulation of liver biomarker genes for heme degradation (*Hmox1, Prdx1*), GSH synthesis and utilization (*mGST1, Gclc*), iron transport (*Slc40a*), uptake of damaged red blood cells or hemoglobin (*Lgals3, Hp*), and activation of an inflammatory response (*IL-6, IL-8*) revealed the dynamic events leading to hemolysis.

MMI is metabolized by FMO and P450s in hepatocytes, and by MPO in kupffer cells and neutrophils. The formation of reactive intermediates co-oxidizes GSH, and the decline of GSH stimulates and up-regulation of GSH synthesis genes (glutathione-*S*-transferase mGST1a and glutamate-cysteine ligase GCLc). A decline of GSH in red blood cells (RBCs) is more evident than in liver cells, since the liver has a greater capacity to synthesize and to store GSH. The reactive metabolites could also bind to hemoglobin (Hb) and lead to RBC shape change. Damaged RBCs bind to lectin on kupffer cells and are phagocytized; while hemoglobin from ruptured RBCs are complexed with haptaglobin and taken up by the kupffer cells. Both pathways lead into heme degradation within the kupffer cells by heme oxygenase 1 (Hmox1) and peroxiredoxin 1 (Prdx1). An up-regulation of Hmox1 and Prdx1 gene expression in liver slices, is a mechanism to protect the cells from heme-mediated oxidative damage. The resultant free iron is then transported from the kupffer cells into the hepatocytes *via* the transporter ferroportin (Slc40a1) which is regulated by hepcidin. Heme synthesis occurs in hepatocytes by the rate-limiting enzyme aminolevulinic acid synthase (Alas2), involved in the maintenance of iron homeostasis. Free Hb and met Hb activates an inflammatory response—release of IL-8 from endothelial cells. Up-regulation of these marker genes prior to and in the presence of hemolysis verified the dynamics of oxidative stress, pre-hemolytic and hemolytic pathways, present in the various cell types of the liver slices (Figure 11.6).

## 11.8 Extra-Hepatic Target Organs

### 11.8.1 Thyroid

The thyroid, one of the largest endocrine glands, can become a drug target, thereby altering thyroid function. Drugs can either accumulate in the thyroid to disrupt function or inhibit the synthesis and release of the thyroid hormones. Both mechanisms raise safety concerns for potential adverse thyroid effects. Classes of chemicals that effect the thyroid directly include the thionamides such as MMI and propylthiouracil (PTU). These compounds interact with thyroid peroxidase (TPO), the rate-limiting enzyme in the formation of active thyroid hormone, which catalyzes the covalent binding of organic iodide (I or $I^+$) to the tyrosine residues of thyroglobulin (Tg).[162,163] It is postulated that the thione groups on MMI and PTU bind to the metal center of TPO, since iron–sulfur coordination is common in metalloenzymes, to inhibit TPO function and decrease thyroid hormone synthesis.[124,130,160] There is also evidence to suggest that these drugs may act to divert oxidized iodides away from Tg through the formation of stable donor–acceptor electron complexes with diiodine, essentially depleting iodine for the iodination of Tg.[164,165]

To evaluate the direct effect of drugs on thyroid function, organotypic thyroid models are utilized. The model employs the *in vitro* incubation of whole rat thyroid lobes or human thyroid slices with test compounds. Both

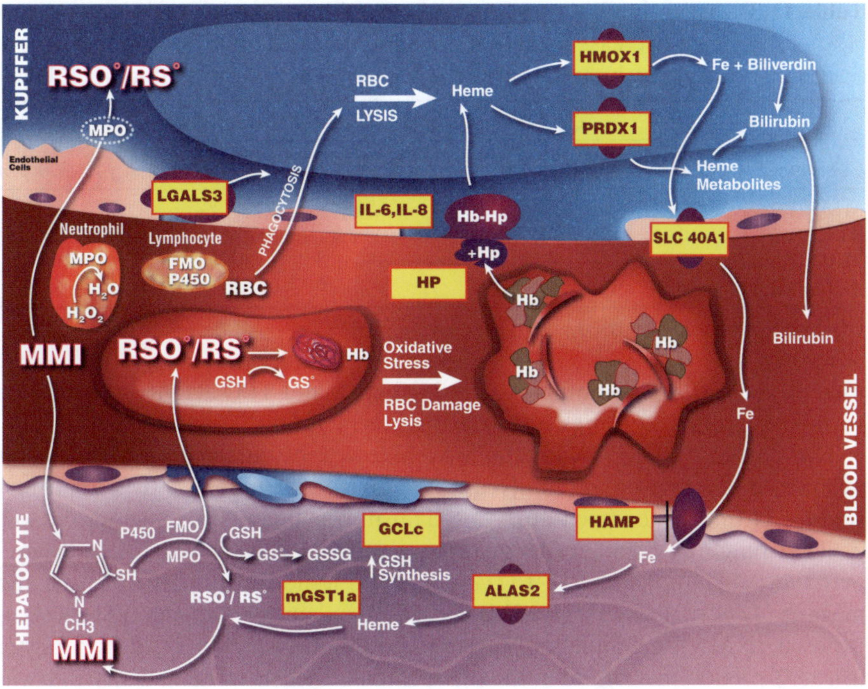


**Figure 11.6** Schematic of MMI metabolism by FMO, MPO, or P450 to reactive intermediates in liver or blood cells which results in a co-oxidation of GSH, particularly in blood cells, followed by the uptake of damaged red blood cells or hemolglobin by kupffer cells, the degradation of heme, and recycling of iron. The dynamics of oxidative stress, heme homeostasis and hemolytic pathways were monitored by gene expression and functional measurements in blood–liver slice co-cultures.

concentration- and time-dependent changes in TPO activity can be measured, as well as the expression changes in thyroid genes involved in thyroid hormone synthesis and release.[166] The models also facilitate a comparison of species sensitivity, rat *versus* human, in terms of the drug concentrations that alter thyroid function to aid in the extrapolation of its safety in humans.

Both MMI and PTU caused a concentration-dependent inhibition of TPO activity in the organotypic cultures. A similar mechanism was evident in both rat and human thyroid tissue. MMI is considered a specific and more potent inhibitor of TPO and thyroid function than PTU.[162] This was reflected in the organotypic cultures in that the extent of TPO enzymatic inhibition by PTU was less than MMI (Table 11.3). Further verification that the organotypic thyroid model is predictive of *in vivo* outcome was demonstrated with an *in vivo* and *in vitro* comparison of TPO activity following MMI exposure. Rats, administered single oral doses of MMI (0–1000 mg $kg^{-1}$), demonstrated significant TPO inhibition in thyroids collected 48 h post dose. Thyroid tissue levels of MMI from the *in vivo* study were within the range of concentrations

**Table 11.3** Mean inhibition of thyroid peroxidase activity, expressed as percent decrease compared to control values, following 24 h exposure of rat or human thyroid *in vitro* to MMI or propylthiouracil PTU.

| | *Concentration of MMI or PTU* | | | |
|---|---|---|---|---|
| *Compound, species* | *0.1 μM* | *1 μM* | *10 μM* | *100 μM* |
| MMI, rat | 26% | 26% | 70% | 100% |
| PTU, rat | 0% | 0% | 45% | nd |
| MMI, human | 19% | 33% | 47% | 100% |
| PTU, human | 8% | 3% | 62% | 86% |

nd = not determined.

used in the *in vitro* organotypic thyroid cultures, and TPO activity was affected with comparable exposures to MMI (Figure 11.7).

The decrease in TPO function was followed by an increase in the gene expression of key proteins involved in the thyroid hormone synthesis pathway (Figure 11.8). This compensatory mechanism was likely to counteract the loss of TPO function. Changes in rat thyroid gene expression profiles of thyroid peroxidase (*Tpo*), deiodinase-1 (*Dio1*), sodium iodide symporter (*Slc5a5*), and megalin (*Lrp2*) occurred with MMI and PTU. In contrast, human thyroid slices exposed to MMI exhibited an up-regulation of the sodium iodide symporter (*Slc5a5*) predominately. The findings demonstrated that human thyroid was less responsive to short-term inhibition of TPO activity than rat thyroid. Human thyroid is also known to have greater iodine and T4 storage capacity than rat, as well as longer half-lives for enzymes like TPO.[167]

The *in vitro–in vivo* correlation with rat tissue demonstrated that the drug-induced changes in the organotypic thyroid cultures closely mimic *in vivo* effects. Effects on thyroid peroxidase activity were comparable and identified concentrations that would alter thyroid function. The perturbation of thyroid hormone synthesis and release is demonstrated *via* gene expression changes in these pathways. Hence, the organotypic model provided value through gaining insight into the mechanism of compound-induced effects on thyroid function, as well as a comparison of species sensitivity. The ultimate goal is that the data generated from such models will serve as a good predictor of drug-induced thyroid effects that will translate to *in vivo* studies.

### 11.8.2 Lung

Lung slice organotypic models are demonstrating that the effects of chemicals, allergens, drugs, gases, nanoparticles on lung function; inflammation and injury can be investigated.[168] Exposure of alveolar ducts, which contain many cell types required for immune responses, such as macrophages, dendritic cells, endothelial and epithelial cells, contribute to the ability to measure the induced release of inflammatory cytokines in response to injury in lung slices.[169–171] To understand the innate immune response, human lung slices were exposed to lipopolysaccharides (LPS) the established immune modulator. LPS triggered a

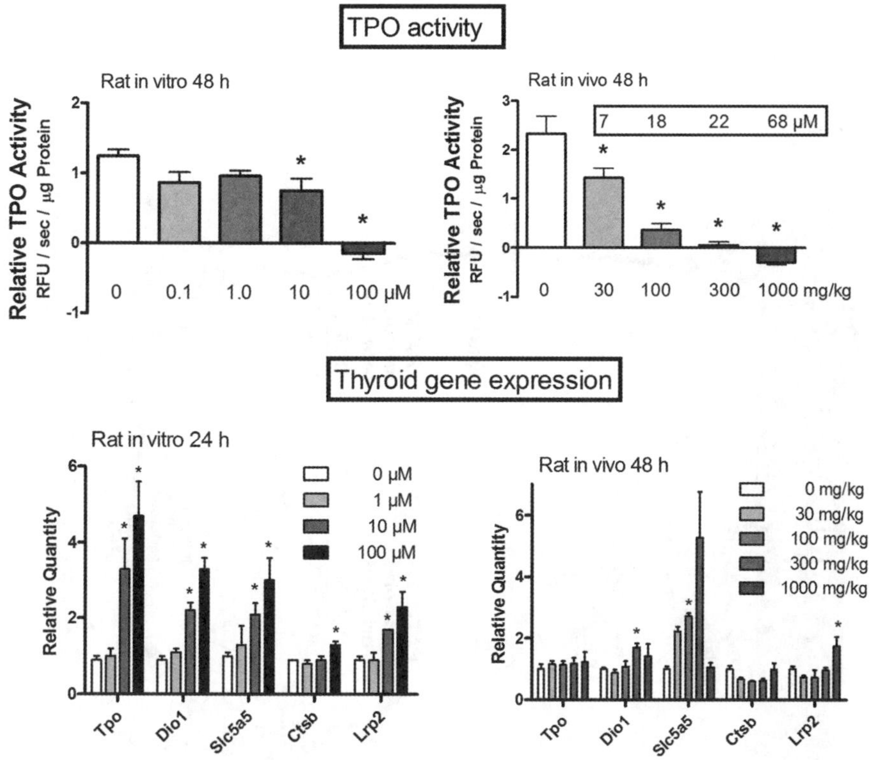


**Figure 11.7** Concentration-dependent decline of TPO activity following exposure to MMI in rat whole thyroid cultures, or in thyroid tissue obtained from a rat *in vivo* study whereby MMI concentrations were comparable to the *in vitro* culture concentrations. An up-regulation of thyroid thyroid hormone synthesis gene (*Tpo*), the iodine transporter (*Slc5a5*) and the pathways of hormone release (*Dio1, Ctsb, Lrp2*) reveal a perturbation of these pathways due to TPO inhibition.

dose-dependent release of pro-inflammatory cytokines, which correlated with several of the cytokine levels measured in human bronchoalveolar lavage (BAL) fluid from subjects exposed to endotoxins. Addition of the immunosuppressive drug dexamethasone significantly decreased the LPS-induced cytokine burst in the human lung slices, demonstrating that therapeutic intervention could be studied.[172]

Early allergic responses in human airways have been demonstrated by the functional changes in airway tonic responses. Both ciliary beat frequency and airway contraction were affected by the induction of an allergic response in human lung slices.[173] Furthermore, the simultaneous responses of airways and vessels to agents have been investigated in rat lung slices. The pulmonary arteries run alongside the airways, branching and changing in diameter, such that endothelial-dependent vessel responses can be studied in parallel to airway responses in lung slices. Addition of acetylcholine to lung slices to

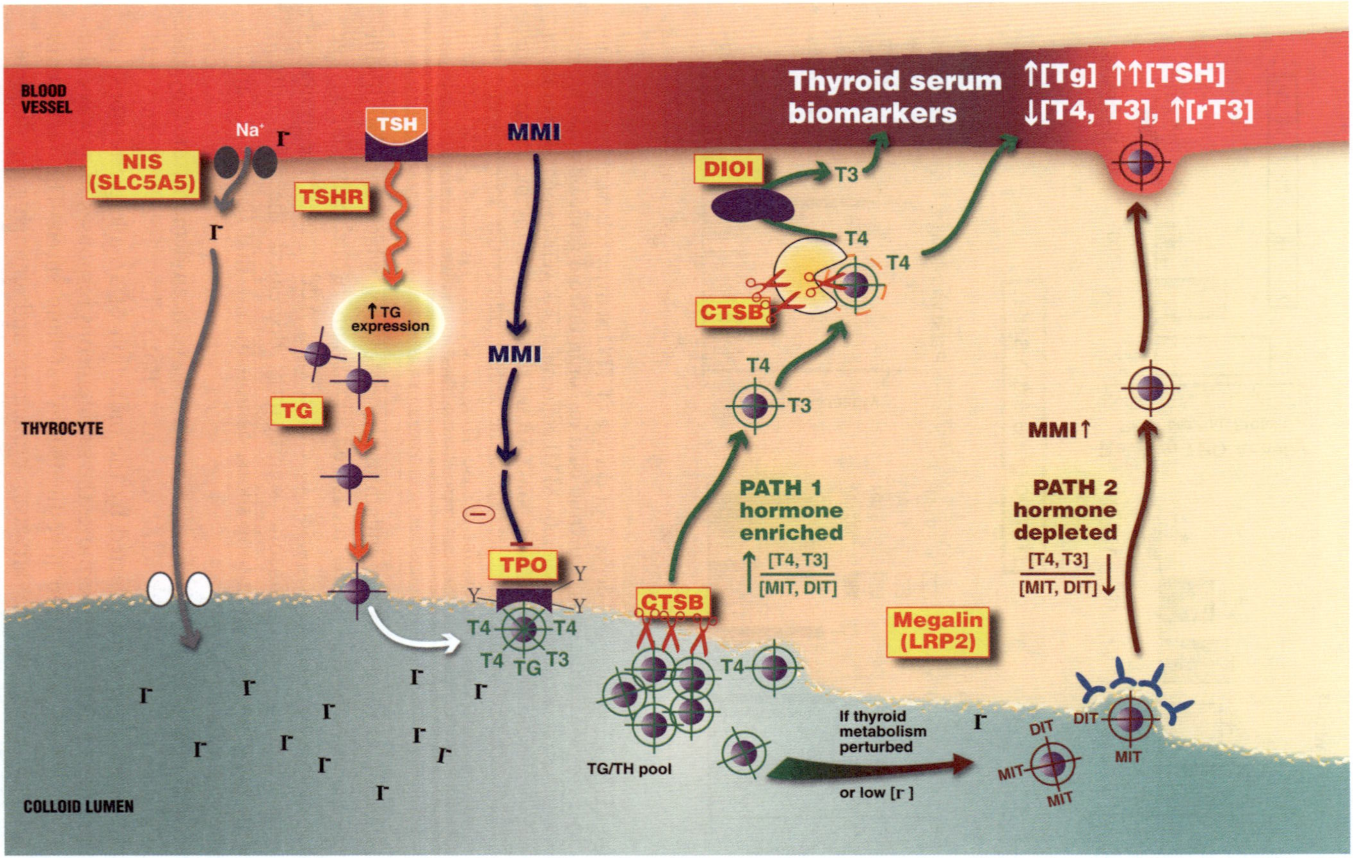


**Figure 11.8** Schematic of thyroid hormone synthesis and release pathways. MMI inhibits TPO activity and traps iodide which triggers an up-regulation of the sodium iodide symporter (*Slc5a5*), TPO, and the pathways of hormone elimination (*Ctsb, Dio1, Lrp2*).

pre-constricted pulmonary artery and airway cells of the lung slice by a thromboxane mimetic agent, caused a relaxation of the artery as measured by wire myographs and image analysis. The dilator effects induced by acetylcholine on the thromboxane mimetic agent was inhibited by L-NAME, a selective inhibitor of NOSIII in the endothelium.[174] Airway contraction and bronchial hyper-reactivity induced by acetylcholine is reversed by cigarette smoke or chronic exposure to nicotine in mouse lung slices.[175] Modeling the inhalation of complex atmospheres such as diesel exhaust, nitrogen dioxide and ozone have been performed with rat or murine lung slices. The lung slices are maintained as biphasic air–liquid organotypic cultures, exposed to continuous flows, and the toxicity response profile and pro-inflammatory responses were determined.[176,177]

## 11.9 Outlook

Drug induced side-effects, which affect organ function or cause organ injury, continue to be a significant clinical issue, leading to increased post-marketing monitoring, black box warnings and the withdrawal of drugs from the market. A gap within the non-clinical and clinical development of drugs is the limited knowledge on human response and mechanism of organ injury for improving risk assessment, as well as the detection and monitoring of organ injury with sensitive and discriminating biomarkers. Within the pharmaceutical industry a hybrid approach is emerging, combining the use of conventional animal models for assessing toxicity, along with identifying molecular signals within the tissues of the *in vivo* studies and with employing human tissue models in a targeted, focused manner to define whether the mechanism of organ injury is similar or different across species, and to define the dose–response relationships and species sensitivity.

Greater use of test methods which provide human mode of action information and exposure data will improve the evaluation of drug candidates. Human organotypic models are advancing our ability to assess the relevance of potential side-effects, by providing mechanistic insight about the key pathways and by identifying concentrations at which dysfunction or injury could become a safety issue. A major goal is to correlate dose–response effects from the human models to facilitate the understanding of risks posed to humans at relevant exposure levels clinically.

Evaluation of target organ risks earlier in drug development, to compare compound structures with a toxic mechanism of action in animal and human organotypic models, will also contribute to drug candidate selection. Feedback can be provided to the research programs as to whether the drug induced toxic effect is linked with a chemical moiety of the molecule, or whether the effect represents an exaggerated pharmacology or an off-target effect. Such investigations should not hinder clinical proof of concept studies to determine drug efficacy, however the human organotypic models will aid in selecting the best drug candidate to market.

Human organotypic models provide an opportunity for a greater understanding of human response, and represent performing clinical studies in a dish. The diversity of donor tissue health status reflects lifestyle, underlying diseases, drug biotransformation capability, and genetic disposition. Responders *versus* non-responders to a drug are detected in these *in vitro* models. Gaining knowledge about human response and the range of responses (normal, stressed, diseased) will aid in defining human variability and susceptibility of drug-induced organ injury in comparison with animal models. Establishing organotypic stressed models, such as a reduced glutathione status to mimic the range of variation in the patient population, can be achieved with the partial depletion of cellular protective pathways, cell types, or by triggering inflammation prior to drug exposure. Cryopreservation of organ slices will increase our ability to assess human variation and response, as well as investigate organ–organ interactions.

## 11.10 Conclusions

In summary, molecular approaches and dose–response relationships applied to human tissue models to characterize key pathways that are causal to organ dysfunction and injury, prior to changes in morphology and frank clinical symptoms are improving the extrapolation of safety data for humans and broadening the scope of translational toxicology in drug safety evaluation.

## References

1. I. Kola and J. Landis, *Nat. Rev. Drug Discovery*, 2004, **3**, 711.
2. T. Agres, Finding Blockbusters a Struggle, *Drug Discovery Dev.*, 2005, March.
3. D. A. Smith and E. F. Schmid, *Curr. Opin. Drug Discovery Dev.*, 2006, **9**, 38.
4. S. Pettit, S. A. des Etages, L. Mylecraine, R. Snyder, J. Fostel, R. T. Dunn, K. Haymes, M. Duval, J. Stevens, C. Afshari and A. Vickers, *Environ. Health Perspect.*, 2010, **118**, 992.
5. A. H. Harrill and I. Rusyn, *Expert Opin. Drug Metab. Toxicol.*, 2008, **4**, 1379.
6. Committee on Toxicity Testing and Assessment of Environmental Agents, National Research Council, *Toxicity Testing in the 21st Century: a Vision and a Strategy,* The National Academies Press, Washington, DC, 2007.
7. D. Krewski, D. Acosta Jr, M. Andersen, H. Anderson, J. C. Bailar III, K. Boekelheide, R. Brent, G. Charnley, V. G. Cheung, S. Green Jr, K. T. Kelsey, N. I. Kerkvliet, A. A. Li, L. McCray, O. Meyer, R. D. Patterson, W. Pennie, R. A. Scala, G. M. Solomon, M. Stephens, J. Yager and L. Zeise, *J. Toxicol. Environ. Health, Part B*, 2010, **13**, 51.

8. M. P. Holsapple, C. A. Afshari and L. D. Lehman-McKeeman, *Toxicol. Sci.*, 2009, **107**, 307.
9. M. E. Andersen and D. Krewski, *Toxicol. Sci.*, 2009, **107**, 324.
10. D. Krewski, M. E. Andersen, E. Mantus and L. Zeise, *Risk Anal.*, 2009, **29**, 474.
11. M. E. Andersen, M. Al-Zoughool, M. Croteau, M. Westphal and D. Krewski, *J. Toxicol. Environ. Health, Part B*, 2010, **13**, 163.
12. M. E. Andersen and D. Krewski, *Toxicol Sci.*, 2010, **117**, 17.
13. K. Viravaidya, A. Sin and M. L. Shuler, *Biotechnol. Prog.*, 2004, **20**, 316.
14. S. Kidambi, R. S. Yarmush, E. Novik, P. Chao, M. L. Yarmush and Y. Nahmias, *Proc. Natl. Acad. Sci. U.S.A.*, 2009, **106**, 15714.
15. E. Novik, T. J. Maguire, P. Chao, K. C. Cheng and M. L. Yarmush, *Biochem. Pharmacol.*, 2010, **79**, 1036.
16. P. M. van Midwoud and G. M. M. Groothuis, M. T. Merema and E. Verpoorte, *Biotechnol. Bioeng.*, 2010, **105**, 184.
17. J. Seed, E. W. Carney, R. A. Corley, K. M. Crofton, J. M. DeSesso, P. M. Foster, R. Kavlock, G. Kimmel, J. Klaunig, M. E. Meek, R. J. Preston, W. Slikker Jr, S. Tabacova, G. M. Williams, J. Wiltse, R. T. Zoeller, P. Fenner-Crisp and D. E. Patton, *Crit. Rev. Toxicol.*, 2005, **35**, 664.
18. S. W. Edwards and R. J. Preston, *Toxicol. Sci.*, 2008, **106**, 312.
19. T. Hartung and G. Daston, *Toxicol. Sci.*, 2009, **111**, 233.
20. T. Hartung, *Toxicol. Sci.*, 2009, **109**, 18.
21. E. A. Hubal, *Toxicol. Sci.*, 2009, **111**, 226.
22. B. Meek and J. Doull, *Toxicol. Sci.*, 2009, **108**, 19.
23. J. S. MacDonald and R. T. Robertson, *Toxicol. Sci.*, 2009, **110**, 40.
24. D. A. Price, J. Blagg, L. Jones, N. Greene and T. Wager, *Expert Opin. Drug Metab. Toxicol.*, 2009, **5**, 921.
25. K. Boekelheide and S. N. Campion, *Toxicol. Sci.*, 2010, **114**, 20.
26. T. Moeller, From in *in vitro* to *in vivo, Drug Discovery Dev.*, 2010, June.
27. T. A. Baillie, *Chem. Res. Toxicol.*, 2008, **21**, 129.
28. S. W. Grimm, H. J. Einolf, S. D. Hall, K. He, H. K. Lim, K. H. Ling, C. Lu, A. A. Nomeir, E. Seibert, K. W. Skordos, G. R. Tonn, H. R. Van, R. W. Wang, Y. N. Wong, T. J. Yang and R. S. Obach, *Drug Metab. Dispos.*, 2009, **37**, 1355.
29. N. Greene, L. Fisk, R. T. Naven, R. R. Note, M. L. Patel and D. J. Pelletier, *Chem. Res. Toxicol.*, 2010, **23**, 1215.
30. H. Olson, G. Betton, D. Robinson, K. Thomas, A. Monro, G. Kolaja, P. Lilly, J. Sanders, G. Sipes, W. Bracken, M. Dorato, D. K. Van, P. Smith, B. Berger and A. Heller, *Regul. Toxicol. Pharmacol.*, 2000, **32**, 56.
31. D. L. Taylor, Human *vs.* rodent, *Drug Discovery Dev.*, 2009, March.
32. J. A. Kramer, J. E. Sagartz and D. L. Morris, *Nat. Rev. Drug Discovery*, 2007, **6**, 636.
33. J. M. McKim Jr., *Comb. Chem. High Throughput Screening*, 2010, **13**, 188.

34. B. A. Wetmore, D. J. Brees, R. Singh, P. B. Watkins, M. E. Andersen, J. Loy and R. S. Thomas, *Hepatology.*, 2010, **51**, 2127.
35. J. H. Winnike, Z. Li, F. A. Wright, J. M. Macdonald, T. M. O'Connell and P. B. Watkins, *Clin. Pharmacol. Ther.*, 2010, **88**, 45.
36. P. H. Bach, A. E. M. Vickers, R. Fisher, A. Baumann, D. C. E Brittebo, H. J. Koster, B. G. Lake, F. Salmon, T. W. Sawyer and G. Skibinski, *ATLA, Altern. Lab. Anim.*, 1996, **24**, 893.
37. A. E. Vickers and R. L. Fisher, *Expert Opin. Drug Metab. Toxicol.*, 2005, **1**, 687.
38. A. E. Vickers and R. L. Fisher, *Chem.–Biol. Interact.*, 2004, **150**, 87.
39. M. Schmolz, *Expert Opin. Drug Discovery*, 2007, **2**, 935.
40. R. Garcia-Serna and J. Mestres, *Expert Opin. Drug Metab. Toxicol.*, 2010, **6**, 1253.
41. C. Hillier and D. Bunton, *Drug Discovery Today.*, 2007, **12**, 382.
42. P. Barry, *Sci. News*, 2008, **173**, 218.
43. G. K. Michalopoulos, W. C. Bowen, K. Mule and D. B. Stolz, *Am. J. Pathol.*, 2001, **159**, 1877.
44. K. L. Schmeichel and M. J. Bissell, *J. Cell Sci.*, 2003, **116**, 2377.
45. G. Y. Lee, P. A. Kenny, E. H. Lee and M. J. Bissell, *Nat. Methods*, 2007, **4**, 359.
46. A. Guillouzo and C. Guguen-Guillouzo, *Expert Opin. Drug Metab. Toxicol.*, 2008, **4**, 1279.
47. S. F. Badylak, D. O. Freytes and T. W. Gilbert, *Acta Biomater.*, 2009, **5**, 1.
48. A. Dash, W. Inman, K. Hoffmaster, S. Sevidal, J. Kelly, R. S. Obach, L. G. Griffith and S. R. Tannenbaum, *Expert Opin. Drug Metab. Toxicol.*, 2009, **5**, 1159.
49. B. A. Justice, N. A. Badr and R. A. Felder, *Drug Discovery Today*, 2009, **14**, 102.
50. R. A. Roberts, P. E. Ganey, C. Ju, L. M. Kamendulis, I. Rusyn and J. E. Klaunig, *Toxicol. Sci.*, 2007, **96**, 2.
51. D. L. Laskin, *Chem. Res. Toxicol.*, 2009, **22**, 1376.
52. H. M. Mehendale, *Toxicol. Pathol.*, 2005, **33**, 41.
53. W. C. Stanley, G. D. Lopaschuk, J. L. Hall and J. G. McCormack, *Cardiovasc. Res.*, 1997, **33**, 243.
54. D. Pessayre, A. Mansouri, D. Haouzi and B. Fromenty, *Cell Biol. Toxicol.*, 1999, **15**, 367.
55. A. E. Vickers, *Toxicol. Pathol.*, 2009, **37**, 78.
56. A. E. Vickers, P. Bentley and R. L. Fisher, *Toxicol. in Vitro*, 2006, **20**, 1173.
57. L. W. Klassen, G. M. Thiele, M. J. Duryee, C. S. Schaffert, A. L. DeVeney, C. D. Hunter, P. Olinga and D. J. Tuma, *Biochem. Pharmacol.*, 2008, **76**, 426.
58. S. Connors, D. Rankin, C. Krumdieck and K. Brendel, *Proc. West Pharmacol. Soc.*, 1989, **32**, 205.
59. R. L. Fisher, J. T. Sanuik, H. Nau, A. J. Gandolfi and K. Brendel, *Toxicol. in Vitro,* 1994, **8**, 371.

60. V. Moronvalle-Halley, B. Sacre-Salem, V. Sallez, G. Labbe and J. C. Gautier, *Toxicology*, 2005, **207**, 203.
61. K. Rose, K. Dooling, A. Pollack and A. Vickers, *Toxicologist*, 1998, **48**, 1278.
62. M. Zimmermann, S. Armeanu, I. Smirnow, S. Kupka, S. Wagner, M. Wehrmann, M. Rots, G. Groothuis, T. Weiss, A. Koenigsrainer, M. Gregor, M. Bitzer and U. Lauer, *Int. J. Oncol.*, 2009, **34**, 1247.
63. M. G. Elferink, P. Olinga, A. L. Draaisma, M. T. Merema, S. Bauerschmidt, J. Polman, W. G. Schoonen and G. M. Groothuis, *Toxicol. Appl. Pharmacol.*, 2008, **229**, 300.
64. D. D. Choie, D. S. Longnecker and A. A. del Campo, *Lab. Invest.*, 1981, **44**, 397.
65. H. Tanaka, E. Ishikawa, S. Teshima and E. Shimizu, *Toxicol. Pathol.*, 1986, **14**, 247.
66. V. M. Gonzalez, M. A. Fuertes, C. Alonso and J. M. Perez, *Mol. Pharmacol.*, 2001, **59**, 657.
67. Q. Huang, R. T. Dunn, S. Jayadev, O. DiSorbo, F. D. Pack, S. B. Farr, R. E. Stoll and K. T. Blanchard, *Toxicol. Sci.*, 2001, **63**, 196.
68. H. Niedner, R. Christen, X. Lin, A. Kondo and S. B. Howell, *Mol. Pharmacol.*, 2001, **60**, 1153.
69. R. P. Amin, A. E. Vickers, F. Sistare, K. L. Thompson, R. J. Roman, M. Lawton, J. Kramer, H. K. Hamadeh, J. Collins, S. Grissom, L. Bennett, C. J. Tucker, S. Wild, C. Kind, V. Oreffo, J. W. Davis, S. Curtiss, J. M. Naciff, M. Cunningham, R. Tennant, J. Stevens, B. Car, T. A. Bertram and C. A. Afshari, *Environ. Health Perspect.*, 2004, **112**, 465.
70. J. A. Kramer, S. D. Pettit, R. P. Amin, T. A. Bertram, B. Car, M. Cunningham, S. W. Curtiss, J. W. Davis, C. Kind, M. Lawton, J. M. Naciff, V. Oreffo, R. J. Roman, F. D. Sistare, J. Stevens, K. Thompson, A. E. Vickers, S. Wild and C. A. Afshari, *Environ. Health Perspect.*, 2004, **112**, 460.
71. K. L. Thompson, C. A. Afshari, R. P. Amin, T. A. Bertram, B. Car, M. Cunningham, C. Kind, J. A. Kramer, M. Lawton, M. Mirsky, J. M. Naciff, V. Oreffo, P. S. Pine and F. D. Sistare, *Environ. Health Perspect.*, 2004, **112**, 488.
72. K. Zhang, M. Chew, E. B. Yang, K. P. Wong and P. Mack, *Mol. Pharmacol.*, 2001, **59**, 837.
73. T. Endo, O. Kimura and M. Sakata, *Toxicology*, 2002, **146**, 187.
74. A. E. Vickers, K. Rose, R. Fisher, M. Saulnier, P. Sahota and P. Bentley, *Toxicol. Pathol.*, 2004, **32**, 577.
75. L. M. Aleksunes, M. J. Goedken, C. E. Rockwell, J. Thomale, J. E. Manautou and C. D. Klaassen, *J. Pharmacol. Exp. Ther.*, 2010, **335**, 2.
76. B. Knouzy, L. Dubourg, G. Baverel and C. Michoudet, *Toxicol. in Vitro*, 2010, **24**, 99.
77. S. Hasal, R. Fisher, A. Gandolfi and K. Brendel, *Toxicologist*, 1998, **42**, 420.
78. O. Kretz, C. Guenat, P. Beilstein and G. Gross, *J. Pharmacol. Toxicol. Methods*, 2002, **48**, 119.

79. A. K. Trull, S. P. Facey, G. W. Rees, D. G. Wight, G. Noble-Jamieson, C. Joughin, P. J. Friend and G. J. Alexander, *Transplantation*, 1994, **58**, 1345.
80. A. Vickers, M. Alegret, R. Jimenez, V. Pflimlin, R. Fisher, C. Spaans and K. Brendel, *In Vitro Mol. Toxicol.*, 1998, **11**, 119.
81. J. C. Gautier, B. Riefke, J. Walter, P. Kurth, L. Mylecraine, V. Guilpin, N. Barlow, T. Gury, D. Hoffman, D. Ennulat, K. Schuster, E. Harpur and S. Pettit, *Toxicol. Pathol.*, 2010.
82. E. A. Lock, *Toxicol. Sci.*, 2010, **116**, 1.
83. M. Sieber, D. Hoffmann, M. Adler, V. S. Vaidya, M. Clement, J. V. Bonventre, N. Zidek, E. Rached, A. Amberg, J. J. Callanan, W. Dekant and A. Mally, *Toxicol. Sci.*, 2009, **109**, 336.
84. D. Hoffmann, M. Adler, V. S. Vaidya, E. Rached, L. Mulrane, W. M. Gallagher, J. J. Callanan, J. C. Gautier, K. Matheis, F. Staedtler, F. Dieterle, A. Brandenburg, A. Sposny, P. Hewitt, H. Ellinger-Ziegelbauer, J. V. Bonventre, W. Dekant and A. Mally, *Toxicol. Sci.*, 2010, **116**, 8.
85. E. Marrer and F. Dieterle, *Toxicol. Appl. Pharmacol.*, 2010, **243**, 167.
86. K. J. Boudonck, M. W. Mitchell, L. Nemet, L. Keresztes, A. Nyska, D. Shinar and M. Rosenstock, *Toxicol. Pathol.*, 2009, **37**, 280.
87. M. I. Luster, D. R. Germolec, T. Yoshida, F. Kayama and M. Thompson, *Hepatology*, 1994, **19**, 480.
88. H. P. Behrsing, A. E. Vickers and C. A. Tyson, *Biochem. Biophys. Res. Commun.*, 2003, **312**, 209.
89. H. P. Behrsing, K. Amin, C. Ip, L. Jimenez and C. A. Tyson, *Toxicol. in Vitro*, 2005, **19**, 1079.
90. K. Amin, C. Ip, L. Jimenez, C. Tyson and H. Behrsing, *Toxicol. Sci.*, 2005, **87**, 442.
91. A. Vittorelli, C. Gauthier, C. Michoudet and G. Baverel, *Toxicol. In Vitro*, 2004, **18**, 285.
92. R. Bataller and D. A. Brenner, *Semin. Liver Dis.*, 2001, **21**, 437.
93. R. Safadi and S. L. Friedman, *MedGenMed*, 2002, **4**, 27.
94. G. K. Michalopoulos and M. C. DeFrances, *Science*, 1997, **276**, 60.
95. M. van de Bovenkamp, G. M. Groothuis, A. L. Draaisma, M. T. Merema, J. I. Bezuijen, M. J. van Gils, D. K. Meijer, S. L. Friedman and P. Olinga, *Toxicol. Sci.*, 2005, **85**, 632.
96. M. van de Bovenkamp, G. M. Groothuis, D. K. Meijer and P. Olinga, *Toxicol. in Vitro*, 2007, **21**, 545.
97. A. E. Vickers, M. Saulnier, E. Cruz, M. T. Merema, K. Rose, P. Bentley and P. Olinga, *Toxicol. Sci.*, 2004, **82**, 534.
98. M. van de Bovenkamp, G. M. Groothuis, D. K. Meijer and P. Olinga, *Toxicol. in Vitro*, 2008, **22**, 771.
99. C. S. Schaffert, M. J. Duryee, R. G. Bennett, A. L. DeVeney, D. J. Tuma, P. Olinga, K. C. Easterling, G. M. Thiele and L. W. Klassen, *Am. J. Physiol Gastrointest. Liver Physiol.*, 2010, **299**, G661.
100. M. Kasper, D. Seidel, L. Knels, N. Morishima, A. Neisser, S. Bramke and R. Koslowski, *Histochem. Cell Biol.*, 2004, **121**, 131.

101. H.-U. Kasper, E. Konze, N. K. Canová, H. P. Dienes and V. Dries, *Exp. Toxicol. Pathol.*, 2010, **20**, DOI: 10.1016/j.etp.2010.04.010.
102. S. M. Wishnies, A. R. Parrish, I. G. Sipes, A. J. Gandolfi, C. W. Putnam, C. L. Krumdieck and K. Brendel, *Cryobiology*, 1991, **28**, 216.
103. R. L. Fisher, S. J. Hasal, J. T. Sanuik, K. S. Scott, A. J. Gandolfi and K. Brendel, *Cryobiology*, 1993, **30**, 250.
104. I. A. de Graaf and H. J. Koster, *Toxicol. in Vitro*, 2003, **17**, 1.
105. G. M. Fahy, B. Wowk, R. Pagotan, A. Chang, J. Phan, B. Thomson and L. Phan, *Organogenesis*, 2009, **5**, 167.
106. P. Olinga, M. Merema, I. H. Hof, K. P. de Jong, M. J. Slooff, D. K. Meijer and G. M. Groothuis, *Drug Metab. Dispos.*, 1998, **26**, 5.
107. R. L. Fisher, A. J. Gandolfi and K. Brendel, *Cell Biol. Toxicol.*, 2001, **17**, 179.
108. H. Martin, J.-P. Sarsat, I. de Waziers, C. Housset, P. Balladur, P. Beaune, V. Albaladejo and C. Lerche-Langrand, *Pharm. Res.*, 2003, **20**, 557.
109. P. Olinga, M. G. Elferink, A. L. Draaisma, M. T. Merema, J. V. Castell, G. Perez and G. M. Groothuis, *Eur. J. Pharm. Sci.*, 2008, **33**, 380.
110. P. Olinga, I. H. Hof, M. T. Merema, M. Smit, M. H. de Jager, P. J. Swart, M. J. Slooff, D. K. Meijer and G. M. Groothuis, *J. Pharmacol. Toxicol. Methods*, 2001, **45**, 55.
111. G. H. Wolfgang, A. J. Gandolfi, J. L. Stevens and K. Brendel, *Toxicol. Appl. Pharmacol.*, 1989, **101**, 205.
112. M. B. Thompson, D. G. Davis and R. W. Morris, *J. Lipid Res.*, 1993, **34**, 553.
113. U. A. Boelsterli and P. L. Lim, *Toxicol. Appl. Pharmacol.*, 2007, **220**, 92.
114. S. J. Hargus, H. R. Amouzedeh, N. R. Pumford, T. G. Myers, S. C. McCoy and L. R. Pohl, *Chem. Res. Toxicol.*, 1994, **7**, 575.
115. A. Kretz-Rommel and U. A. Boelsterli, *Mol. Pharmacol.*, 1994, **45**, 237.
116. M. L. Gil, M. C. Ramirez, M. C. Terencio and J. V. Castell, *Biochim. Biophys. Acta.*, 1995, **1272**, 140.
117. R. Bort, X. Ponsoda, R. Jover, M. J. Gomez-Lechon and J. V. Castell, *J. Pharmacol. Exp. Ther.*, 1999, **288**, 65.
118. A. E. Vickers, *Chem.–Biol. Interact.*, 2009, **179**, 9.
119. D. C. Liebler, *Chem. Res. Toxicol.*, 2008, **21**, 117.
120. J. Uetrecht, *Chem. Res. Toxicol.*, 2008, **21**, 84.
121. G. Liss, S. Rattan and J. H. Lewis, *Expert Opin. Drug Metab. Toxicol.*, 2010, **6**, 1047.
122. C. Saito, H. M. Yan, A. Artigues, M. T. Villar, A. Farhood and H. Jaeschke, *Toxicol. Appl. Pharmacol.*, 2010, **242**, 182.
123. B. K. Park, N. R. Kitteringham, J. L. Maggs, M. Pirmohamed and D. P. Williams, *Annu. Rev. Pharmacol. Toxicol.*, 2005, **45**, 177.
124. S. Tafazoli and P. J. O'Brien, *Drug Discovery Today*, 2005, **10**, 617.
125. W. Tang, Expert Opin. Drug Metab. Toxicol., 2007, **3**, 407.
126. P. B. Watkins, N. Kaplowitz, J. T. Slattery, C. R. Colonese, S. V. Colucci, P. W. Stewart and S. C. Harris, *JAMA, J. Am. Med. Assoc.*, 2006, **296**, 87.
127. R. D. Fannin, M. Russo, T. M. O'Connell, K. Gerrish, J. H. Winnike, J. Macdonald, J. Newton, S. Malik, S. O. Sieber, J. Parker, R. Shah, T. Zhou, P. B. Watkins and R. S. Paules, *Hepatology*, 2010, **51**, 227.

128. G. Vendemiale, I. Grattagliano, E. Altomare, N. Turturro and F. Guerrieri, *Biochem. Pharmacol.*, 1996, **52**, 1147.
129. K. D. Welch, B. Wen, D. R. Goodlett, E. C. Yi, H. Lee, T. P. Reilly, S. D. Nelson and L. R. Pohl, *Chem. Res. Toxicol.*, 2005, **18**, 924.
130. P. J. O'Brien, *Chem.–Biol. Interact.*, 2000, **129**, 113.
131. T. O'Brien, G. Babcock, J. Cornelius, M. Dingeldein, G. Talaska, D. Warshawsky and K. Mitchell, *Toxicol. Appl. Pharmacol.*, 2000, **164**, 280.
132. D. E. Amacher, *Curr. Drug Metab.*, 2006, **7**, 219.
133. D. Han, N. Hanawa, B. Saberi and N. Kaplowitz, *Am. J. Physiol. Gastrointest. Liver Physiol.*, 2006, **291**, G1.
134. R. A. Roberts, D. L. Laskin, C. V. Smith, F. M. Robertson, E. M. Allen, J. A. Doorn and W. Slikker, *Toxicol. Sci.*, 2009, **112**, 4.
135. S. O. Simmons, C. Y. Fan and R. Ramabhadran, *Toxicol. Sci.*, 2009, **111**, 202.
136. D. Wu and A. Cederbaum, *Mol. Pharmacol.*, 2004, **66**, 749.
137. D. S. Cooper, *N. Engl. J. Med.*, 1984, **311**, 1353.
138. A. Bartalen, F. Bogazzi and M. Enio, *Drug Exp.*, 1996, **15**, 53.
139. K. A. Woeber, *Endocr. Pract.*, 2002, **8**, 222.
140. S. H. Pearce, *Clin. Endocrinol.*, 2004, **61**, 589.
141. A. S. Kalgutkar, I. Gardner, R. S. Obach, C. L. Shaffer, E. Callegari, K. R. Henne, A. E. Mutlib, D. K. Dalvie, J. S. Lee, Y. Nakai, J. P. O'Donnell, J. Boer and S. P. Harriman, *Curr. Drug Metab.*, 2005, **6**, 161.
142. M. Benyounes, C. Sempoux, C. Daumerie, J. Rahier and A. P. Geubel, *World J. Gastroenterol.*, 2006, **12**, 6232.
143. T. Mizutani, M. Murakami, M. Shirai, M. Tanaka and K. Nakanishi, *J. Appl. Toxicol.*, 1999, **19**, 193.
144. J. C. Erve, *Expert. Opin. Drug Metab. Toxicol.*, 2006, **2**, 923.
145. G. Esteban-Pretel and M. Pilar Lopez-Garcia, *Free Radic. Biol. Med.*, 2006, **41**, 610.
146. A. E. M. Vickers, R. L. Fisher and J. R. Sinclair, *Curr. Drug Discovery Technol.*, 2010, **7**, 154.
147. M. Fung, A. Thornton, K. Mybeck, J. Hsiao-Hui, K. Hornbuckle and E. Muniz, *Drug. Info. J.*, 2001, **35**, 293.
148. T. P. Bradshaw, D. C. McMillan, R. K. Crouch and D. J. Jollow, *Free Radical Biol. Med.*, 1995, **18**, 279.
149. S. J. Grossman, J. Simson and D. J. Jollow, *Toxicol. Appl. Pharmacol.*, 1992, **117**, 208.
150. T. P. Reilly, P. M. Woster and C. K. Svensson, *J. Pharmacol. Exp. Ther.*, 1999, **288**, 951.
151. D. J. Jollow and D. C. McMillan, *Adv. Exp. Med. Biol.*, 2001, **500**, 595.
152. D. C. McMillan, C. L. Powell, Z. S. Bowman, J. D. Morrow and D. J. Jollow, *Toxicol. Sci.*, 2005, **88**, 274.
153. S. Geaghan, in *Hematology Basic Principles and Practice*, ed. R. Hoffman, E. Benz, S. Shattil, B. Furie, H. Cohen, L. Silberstein and P. MGlave, Churchill Livingstone, New York, 3rd edn, 1999, pp. 2520–2521.

154. A. E. Vickers, J. R. Sinclair, R. L. Fisher, S. R. Morris and W. Way, *Toxicol. Appl. Pharmacol.*, 2010, **244**, 354.
155. H. D. Fahimi, *J. Cell Biol.*, 1970, **47**, 247.
156. F. L. Willekens, J. M. Werre, J. K. Kruijt, B. Roerdinkholder-Stoelwinder, Y. A. Groenen-Dopp, A. G. van den Bos, G. J. Bosman and T. J. van Berkel, *Blood*, 2005, **105**, 2141.
157. M. Rokushima, K. Omi, A. Araki, Y. Kyokawa, N. Furukawa, F. Itoh, K. Imura, K. Takeuchi, M. Okada, I. Kato and J. Ishizaki, *Toxicol. Sci.*, 2007, **95**, 474.
158. H. Nakamura, J. Noh, K. Itoh, S. Fukata, A. Miyauchi and N. Hamada, *J. Clin. Endocrinol. Metab.*, 2007, **92**, 2157.
159. D. M. Mintzer, S. N. Billet and L. Chmielewski, *Adv. Hematol.*, 2009, 495863.
160. L. G. McGirr, S. D. Jatoe and P. J. O'Brien, *Chem–Biol. Interact.*, 1990, **73**, 279.
161. D. C. Lam and R. H. Lindsay, *Biochem. Pharmacol.*, 1979, **28**, 2289.
162. A. Nagasaka and H. Hidaka, *J. Clin. Endocrinol. Metab.*, 1976, **43**, 152.
163. C. C. Capen, *Toxicol. Pathol.*, 1997, **25**, 39.
164. C. Raby, J. F. Lagorce, A. C. Jambut-Absil, J. Buxeraud and G. Catanzano, *Endocrinology*, 1990, **126**, 1683.
165. F. Isaia, M. C. Aragoni, M. Arca, F. Demartin, F. A. Devillanova, G. Floris, A. Garau, M. B. Hursthouse, V. Lippolis, R. Medda, F. Oppo, M. Pira and G. Verani, *J. Med. Chem.*, 2008, **51**, 4050.
166. J. Sinclair, S. Morris, J. Heale, W. Way, R. Fisher and A. Vickers, *The Toxicologist*, 2008, **102**, 92.
167. A. C. Bianco, D. Salvatore, B. Gereben, M. J. Berry and P. R. Larsen, *Endocr. Rev.*, 2002, **23**, 38.
168. T. A. Liberati, M. R. Randle and L. A. Toth, *Expert Rev. Mol. Diagn.*, 2010, **10**, 501.
169. M. Henjakovic, C. Martin, H. G. Hoymann, K. Sewald, A. R. Ressmeyer, C. Dassow, G. Pohlmann, N. Krug, S. Uhlig and A. Braun, *Toxicol. Sci.*, 2008, **106**, 444.
170. M. Henjakovic, K. Sewald, S. Switalla, D. Kaiser, M. Muller, T. Z. Veres, C. Martin, S. Uhlig, N. Krug and A. Braun, *Toxicol. Appl. Pharmacol.*, 2008, **231**, 68.
171. M. Nassimi, C. Schleh, H. D. Lauenstein, R. Hussein, K. Lubbers, G. Pohlmann, S. Switalla, K. Sewald, M. Muller, N. Krug, C. C. Muller-Goymann and A. Braun, *Inhal. Toxicol.*, 2009, **21**, 104.
172. S. Switalla, L. Lauenstein, F. Prenzler, S. Knothe, C. Forster, H. G. Fieguth, O. Pfennig, F. Schaumann, C. Martin, C. A. Guzman, T. Ebensen, M. Muller, J. M. Hohlfeld, N. Krug, A. Braun and K. Sewald, *Toxicol. Appl. Pharmacol.*, 2010, **246**, 107.
173. A. Wohlsen, C. Martin, E. Vollmer, D. Branscheid, H. Magnussen, W. M. Becker, U. Lepp and S. Uhlig, *Eur. Respir. J.*, 2003, **21**, 1024.

174. L. Moreno, F. Perez-Vizcaino, L. Harrington, R. Faro, G. Sturton, P. J. Barnes and J. A. Mitchell, *Respir. Res.*, 2006, **7**, 111.
175. E. Streck, R. A. Jorres, R. M. Huber and A. Bergner, *J. Invest. Allergol. Clin Immunol.*, 2010, **20**, 324.
176. A. Bion, M. Fal, F. Gouriou, P. E. Le, F. Dionnet and J. P. Morin, *Cell Biol. Toxicol.*, 2002, **18**, 301.
177. S. Switalla, J. Knebel, D. Ritter, N. Krug, A. Braun and K. Sewald, *Toxicol. Lett.*, 2010, **196**, 117.

CHAPTER 12

# *Predicting Drug-Induced Mitochondrial Dysfunction*

SASHI NADANACIVA AND YVONNE WILL*

Pfizer Global R&D, Compound Safety Prediction, Eastern Point Road, Groton CT, 06340, USA

## 12.1 Introduction

"Prediction is very difficult, especially about the future" quipped the Danish physicist, Niels Bohr. However, this has not deterred those of us working in the toxicology field within the pharmaceutical industry from championing methods for predicting safety outcomes in patients. The reasons for this are many. Firstly, the pharmaceutical industry faces enormous economic pressure to decrease costs, billions of dollars often being incurred as a result of late-stage compound attrition due to toxicity. Secondly, adverse drug reactions are estimated to be the fourth–sixth leading cause of death in the USA, causing approximately 100 000 deaths each year in hospitalized patients.[1] Thirdly, adverse drug reactions are estimated to cause hospitalization or serious injury in more than two million people in the USA each year, leading to increasing health care costs.[1]

Drug-induced mitochondrial impairment as a contributor to toxicity has now become "the new kid on the block". Until a few years ago, the terms "mitochondrial toxicity", "mitochondrial impairment", and "mitochondrial dysfunction" were considered germane to those in the pharmaceutical industry only in connection with anti-retrovirals, drugs given in the treatment of HIV (human immunodeficiency virus) infection. However, the withdrawal of

RSC Drug Discovery Series No. 12
New Horizons in Predictive Toxicology: Current Status and Application
Edited by Alan G. E. Wilson

Published by the Royal Society of Chemistry, www.rsc.org

cerivastatin and troglitazone and a black box warning for tolcapone have highlighted the necessity for testing many different drug classes for potential mitochondrial impairment.[2] Moreover, recent technological advances in high-throughput screening for mitochondrial impairment have fueled efforts to incorporate mitochondrial toxicity testing early in the drug-discovery process.[2–5] This chapter provides a brief overview of mitochondrial function, discusses some of the mechanisms that cause drugs to impair these organelles, and describes *in vitro* methods that are currently being used to identify drug-induced mitochondrial dysfunction (DIMD). We also describe animal models and techniques that can potentially be used to study DIMD *in vivo* and discuss the hurdles that lie ahead in this field of toxicity.

## 12.2 Overview of Mitochondrial Physiology

Mitochondria are the primary source of energy production in the cell, providing approximately 95% of adenosine triphosphate (ATP) during aerobic respiration. Moreover, they are also involved in many other roles such as fatty acid oxidation, heme synthesis, steroid synthesis, calcium signaling, and apoptosis.[6] These functions are carried out by an armory of proteins, of which there are estimated to be at least a thousand.[7,8]

Mitochondria are found in most eukaryotic cells, the number in each cell varying from one to several thousand depending on the cell type and tissue type. Morphologically and functionally complex, mitochondria are dynamic in nature, undergoing fusion and fission events.[9] This fluidity is essential for the cell's physiology since mitochondria move to regions of the cell which require either high amounts of ATP or regulation by calcium signaling.[10] Highly compartmentalized organelles, mitochondria have two membranes, the outer one being rich in cholesterol and the inner one being rich in cardiolipin.[11] The outer membrane has several pores composed of a voltage-dependent anion channel which transiently opens, enabling ions and molecules of less than 1.5 kDa to cross this barrier. In contrast, the inner membrane is impermeable to ions and polar molecules and has many transporters allowing the export/import of molecules such as ATP, ADP (adenosine diphosphate), malate and aspartate. The inner membrane is invaginated, forming structures called cristae and contains five protein complexes, Complexes I, II, III, IV and V. These enzymes are involved in a process known as oxidative phosphorylation, where electron transfer is tightly coupled to ATP synthesis.[11] The space between the inner membrane and outer membrane is referred to as the inter-membrane space and contains proteins such as creatine kinase and adenylate kinase. Within the space enclosed by the inner membrane, a region known as the mitochondrial matrix, lie proteins involved in fatty acid oxidation, heme synthesis, steroid synthesis, and the citric acid cycle. Some mitochondrial proteins such as cytochrome *c* and the apoptosis-inducing factor have dual locations, moving from the inter-membrane space to the cytoplasm during apoptosis. In addition to the hundreds of proteins permanently located within mitochondria, there is increasing evidence that many proteins such as the nuclear transcription factors, p53 and NF-κB, and the pro-apoptotic cytosolic protein, bax, temporarily translocate to mitochondria to carry out their signaling roles.[12,13]

With the exception of the nucleus, mitochondria are the only organelles in animal cells to possess their own genome. Mitochondrial DNA (mtDNA) is maternally inherited and is present as several copies within the mitochondrial matrix, the number varying according to the type of the cell. Moreover, mtDNA shows some similarity to bacterial genomes in being circular and lacking histones.[14] Each copy of mtDNA encodes 13 proteins, as well as 22 types of tRNAs and two rRNAs. The 13 proteins are subunits of Complex I, Complex III, Complex IV and Complex V, and are essential for oxidative phosphorylation. MtDNA often contains many mutations, known as polymorphisms, which gives rise to a situation known as heteroplasmy where both mutated mtDNA and wild-type mtDNA co-exist within the same cell. Some of these mutations can cause serious disorders such as MELAS (mitochondrial encephalomyopathy with lactic acidosis and stroke-like episodes), MERRF (myoclonic epilepsy with ragged red fibers), LHON (Leber hereditary optic neuropathy), and NARP (neuropathy, ataxia, and retinitis pigmentosa).[15] Many of these disorders are multi-systemic due to the ubiquitous presence of mitochondria. Not all mitochondrial diseases are due to mutations in mtDNA however; some occur as a result of mutations in nuclear DNA and are inherited in a Mendelian fashion. A common characteristic of mitochondrial disorders is an inadequate supply of ATP for the energy demands of the cell. This can lead to lactic acidosis, muscle weakness, developmental disorders of the brain, optic neuropathy, neuropathic pain, hearing loss, and cardiomyopathy. Moreover, mitochondrial dysfunction has been implicated in Parkinson's disease, Alzheimer's disease, Huntington's disease, bipolar disorder, schizophrenia, and type II diabetes, and is also thought to play a key role in the aging process.[16]

In addition to having their own DNA, mitochondria also have their own ribosomes which share structural similarities to bacterial ribosomes.[17] This has given rise to the theory that, more than a billion years ago, mitochondria were free-living aerobic bacteria that were engulfed by eukaryotic cells. The bacterial origin of mitochondria has implications in the drug-discovery process since drugs designed to impair protein synthesis in bacterial ribosomes may have the potential to cause an adverse effect in the host's mitochondrial ribosomes as well.

### 12.2.1 ATP Production in Mitochondria

ATP production in mitochondria occurs *via* a complex series of reactions which initially commences with the oxidation of carbohydrates, fats and proteins. Carbohydrates are oxidized in the cytoplasm to eventually form pyruvate which is actively transported to mitochondria where it is oxidatively decarboxylated to acetyl coenzyme A and carbon dioxide. During oxidation of fats, triglycerides are broken down to fatty acids and glycerol in the cytoplasm with the subsequent transportation of fatty acids to the mitochondrial matrix where they are oxidized to acetyl coenzyme A. The mitochondrion is also the site at which the terminal steps of amino acid degradation occur, resulting in the production of acetyl coenzyme A. Acetyl coenzyme A is, thus, a converging point for many of the catabolic pathways, and enters the citric acid cycle where energy-rich electrons abstracted from the oxidation of food are used to reduce NAD (nicotinamide adenine dinucleotide) and FAD (flavin adenine dinucleotide).

The energy-rich reducing equivalent, NADH, transfers electrons to the inner mitochondrial membrane protein, Complex I (also known as NADH ubiquinone oxidoreductase) which donates electrons to a mobile electron carrier, ubiquinone.[11] Meanwhile, the reduced form of FAD, a prosthetic group within Complex II (succinate dehydrogenase) also donates electrons to ubiquinone. Ubiquinone, in its reduced form (ubiquinol), donates electrons to Complex III (ubiquinol cytochrome *c* oxidoreductase) which donates electrons to a water-soluble electron carrier, cytochrome *c*. Reduced cytochrome *c* transfers electrons to the membrane-embedded Complex IV (cytochrome *c* oxidase) which, finally, donates electrons to oxygen with the production of water. The transfer of electrons down an energy gradient is concomitant with the process of proton pumping from the matrix to the inter-membrane space by Complex I, III and IV. This results in an electrochemical gradient, also known as the proton-motive force, comprised of a pH gradient and a membrane potential. The energy contained in the electrochemical gradient is used by Complex V (the ATP synthase) to make ATP from ADP and inorganic phosphate. ATP synthesis is tightly coupled to electron transport, the entire process being known as 'oxidative phosphorylation'. Since the proton-motive force is essential for driving ATP synthesis, an inner membrane that is impermeable to protons is crucial for ATP production in mitochondria.

### 12.2.2 Mitochondria and Reactive Oxygen Species

The process of electron transfer along Complex I, II, III and IV inevitably leads to a low leakage of electrons that are directly donated to oxygen. This results in the formation of a highly reactive oxygen species, such as superoxide, which can react with, and damage, phospholipids, proteins and DNA within the cell.[18] Under normal physiological conditions, cells are able to counteract the harmful effects of reactive oxygen species (ROS) by several antioxidant defense systems. For instance, superoxide dismutase located within mitochondria breaks down superoxide to hydrogen peroxide which, in turn, is converted to water by glutathione peroxidase. Other players in the antioxidant defense system include cytosolic superoxide dismutase and catalase. However, when overproduction of ROS exceeds the capacity of the defense mechanisms, oxidative stress ensues, particularly during aging, inflammation and in the presence of certain drugs. Since the main sources of reactive oxygen species, Complex I, Complex III, and monoamine oxidase, are mitochondrial components, other mitochondrial proteins and mtDNA which are in close proximity to these ROS sources are in danger of being impaired by oxidative stress.[19] Moreover, impairment of Complex I and Complex III by oxidative stress can result in a further increase in ROS and, hence, a vicious cycle ensues.

## 12.2.3 The Heterogeneous Nature of Mitochondria

Mitochondria exemplify the saying "Variety is the spice of life". Different tissues have different energy demands and this is reflected in the diversity of structure and composition found in mitochondria. In an elegant study done on mitochondria isolated from rat heart, muscle, liver, kidney and brain, Benard *et al.* showed that mitochondrial content varies with each tissue, with the heart containing the most mitochondria, the rank order being heart > muscle > brain > kidney > liver.[20] The study also showed that there were structural differences in mitochondria from the five tissues; for instance, heart mitochondria contained more cristae and also had the highest density of the mitochondrial matrix in comparison with mitochondria from the other four tissues, with the hierarchy being heart > muscle > brain > kidney > liver. Furthermore, mitochondria from heart and muscle were enriched in the protein complexes involved in oxidative phosphorylation in comparison with brain, kidney or liver. Enzyme-activity measurements done on mitochondria isolated from the five organs showed that heart mitochondria had higher apparent $V_{max}$ (the maximum velocity of an enzyme) values for Complex IV than mitochondria from the other tissues, with liver and kidney showing the lowest apparent $V_{max}$ values for this enzyme. Since $V_{max}$ values are dependent on both the amount of enzyme and the catalytic constant (the catalytic constant is the number of reactions catalyzed per unit of time by each active site), Benard *et al.* determined the catalytic constant for Complex IV and found that it was highest in brain mitochondria, with the rank order being brain > liver > heart > muscle > kidney. Similarly, for Complex III, brain mitochondria had the highest catalytic constant in comparison with mitochondria from the other four tissues. Thus, the study showed that, while the heart contains the highest amount of protein complexes involved in oxidative phosphorylation (OXPHOS) in comparison with other tissues, the brain contains the most active OXPHOS complexes.

Proteomic analysis of mitochondria during the past few years has gained increasing popularity, revealing novel aspects of these organelles. A quantitative proteomic comparison of mitochondria from rat heart, skeletal muscle and liver by Forner *et al.* showed that the protein complexes involved in oxidative phosphorylation are more abundant in heart than in skeletal muscle and liver, regulatory enzymes such as pyruvate dehydrogenase phosphatase were most abundant in skeletal muscle, and enzymes involved in the urea cycle were abundant in the liver.[21] These differences in mitochondria from different organs may be relevant during mitochondrial toxicity testing.

One of the intriguing aspects of mitochondria with regard to heterogeneity is that Complexes I, II, III, IV and V are present far in excess of what is actually required for oxidative phosphorylation. Each of these protein complexes has to be inhibited by a certain percentage before respiration and ATP synthesis are compromised, and this threshold varies with each complex and varies with each tissue. Davey *et al.* have shown that, in rat synaptic mitochondria, Complex I, III, and IV have to be inhibited by 25, 80 and 70%, respectively before respiration and ATP synthesis are impaired, *i.e.*, Complex I has a lower threshold than Complex III and IV.[22] In contrast, Complex I in non-synaptic mitochondria has a much higher threshold of 72% than its synaptic counterpart.[23] These differences in threshold effects highlight some of the complexities that arise when translating *in vitro* results to *in vivo* outcomes.

## 12.3 Many Mechanisms Can Lead to DIMD

Given the structural and functional intricacies of mitochondria, it comes as no surprise that many mechanisms can lead to DIMD.[2–5] Some drugs can inhibit the activity of the protein complexes involved in oxidative phosphorylation, thereby having the ultimate effect of impairing mitochondrial ATP production. Drugs can also uncouple electron transport from ATP synthesis by shuttling protons across the inner mitochondrial membrane, or by forming channels through the lipid bilayer or by simply disrupting the bilayer. Mitochondrial dysfunction can also occur as a result of inhibition of transporters such as the adenine nucleotide translocator and carnitine palmitoyltransferases I and II. Drugs can also inhibit enzymes involved in fatty acid oxidation or the citric acid cycle, leading to depletion of substrates. Oxidative stress caused by redox cycling or depletion of antioxidants such as glutathione can also lead to mitochondrial dysfunction. In addition, drugs can induce irreversible opening of the mitochondrial permeability transition pore, resulting in loss of mitochondrial components such as ATP, $NAD^+$, and glutathione. The result is intrusion of water into the mitochondria, leading to osmotic swelling which can subsequently result in cell death. Some drugs can impair mtDNA replication while others impair mtDNA-encoded protein synthesis, both mechanisms eventually leading to a reduction in mtDNA-encoded protein levels and hence to a decrease in ATP levels.

## 12.4 *In Vitro* Methods to Detect DIMD

No single assay identifies *all* mechanisms of DIMD, thus necessitating a panel of assays for identifying DIMD. We describe here some of the current *in vitro* methods (summarized in Table 12.1) that are being utilized to identify DIMD, although the list is not meant to be exhaustive.

### 12.4.1 Measurement of ATP Levels in Cells Grown in Glucose- and Galactose-Containing Media

Cell viability assays, where ATP levels are measured, are routinely used to identify compound-induced toxicity. Often, this is done with immortalized cell lines due to the ease with which these cells can be handled. Paradoxically, most immortalized cell lines, although possessing the capacity to be aerobic, have a preference for making ATP *via* glycolysis when grown in glucose-rich media. This phenomenon, known as the Crabtree effect, makes identification of

**Table 12.1** *In vitro* methods to detect drug-induced mitochondrial dysfunction.

| *In vitro methods* | *Throughput* |
|---|---|
| Cellular ATP content measurement of immortalized cell lines grown in media containing (a) galactose and (b) glucose | +++ 96- or 384-well plate-based format |
| Mitochondrial membrane potential measurement of cells using fluorescent dyes (*e.g.*, MitoTracker Red, JC-1) | +++ 96- or 384-well plate-based format |
| Oxygen consumption measurement of isolated mitochondria using water-soluble fluorescent probes[a] | +++ 96- or 384-well plate-based format |
| Oxygen consumption and extracellular acidification measurements of cells using water-soluble fluorescent probes[a] | +++ 96- or 384-well plate-based format |
| Oxygen consumption and extracellular acidification measurements of cells using solid state fluorescent probes[b] | ++ 96-well plate-based format |
| Activity measurement of protein complexes involved in oxidative phosphorylation either by immunocapture from cells/tissues[c] or by classical biochemical methods | ++ 96-well plate-based format |
| MtDNA-encoded protein level measurement in cells using high-content imaging | ++ 96-well plate-based format |

+++ high throughput; ++ medium throughput
[a]Luxcel Biosciences Ltd. www.luxcel.com
[b]Seahorse Bioscience, www.seahorsebio.com
[c]MitoSciences Inc., www.mitosciences.com

mitochondrial toxicants difficult. In order to overcome this, cells can be grown in media containing galactose instead of glucose.[24] Since the net yield of ATP from galactose to pyruvate *via* glycolysis is zero, galactose-grown cells are forced to rely on mitochondria for their ATP production and are, hence, more susceptible than glucose-grown cells to compounds which are un-couplers or inhibitors of oxidative phosphorylation. We routinely use galactose-grown and glucose-grown HepG2 cells in our laboratory to distinguish compounds (*e.g.*, nefazodone) which cause toxicity primarily through mitochondrial targets from those (*e.g.*, tamoxifen) that cause toxicity through multiple targets.[24,25]

## 12.4.2 Mitochondrial Membrane Potential Measurements

One of the most common methods to detect mitochondrial dysfunction has been to monitor the mitochondrial membrane potential of cells. A variety of fluorescent dyes such as tetramethylrhodamine methyl ester, JC-1, rhodamine 123, and MitoTracker Red have been used in traditional fluorescence microscopy, automated high-content imaging, or high-throughput screening assays utilizing fluorescence plate readers.[26] These dyes are cations that distribute to the mitochondrial matrix as a function of the Nernst equation. The drawback of mitochondrial membrane potential measurements in investigating drug-induced mitochondrial impairment is that a decrease in the membrane potential is not necessarily due to a direct impairment on mitochondria: cells undergoing apoptosis or necrosis will show a decrease in mitochondrial membrane potential even in the absence of direct mitochondrial impairment.

### 12.4.3 Oxygen Consumption Measurements of Mitochondria

Traditionally, oxygen uptake of isolated mitochondria was determined with the Clark electrode, but throughput was limited to approximately 10–20 compounds per day at a single dose. In recent years, a conjugated Pt–porphyrin probe with long-decay phosphorescence that is quenched by molecular oxygen has been used extensively in a plate-based format to assess oxygen consumption of isolated mitochondria.[27,28] This soluble oxygen sensor allows measurements both in 96-well format and 384-well format, enabling high-throughput screening of compounds. We have used the oxygen sensor to test the effect of several hundreds of compounds, including thiazolidinediones, statins, and biguanides on mitochondria isolated from rat liver.

### 12.4.4 Oxygen Consumption and Extracellular Acidification Measurements of Cells

While oxygen sensors are sufficient for investigating acute effects of compounds on oxidative phosphorylation in isolated mitochondria, a decrease in oxygen consumption in cells cannot be interpreted as mitochondrial toxicity *per se* since a dying cell, regardless of the mechanism of toxicity, will also display a decrease in oxygen consumption. Hence, soluble pH sensors have been developed for measuring the extracellular acidification rate, and hence, glycolytic rate, of cells.[29] This measurement provides the necessary information to delineate between compounds that directly impair mitochondrial function from those that cause general cytotoxicity since there is, generally, a compensatory increase in the glycolytic rate of cells when compounds impair oxidative phosphorylation whereas this effect is not seen with compounds that merely cause cytotoxicity. Another recent technology for measuring oxygen consumption and extracellular acidification of cells is a fully integrated instrument which utilizes a disposable sensor cartridge containing either 24 pairs or 96 pairs of fluorescent biosensors for oxygen and pH.[30,31]

### 12.4.5 Assays for Measuring the Activity of Enzymes Involved in Oxidative Phosphorylation

If inhibition of oxygen consumption is observed with either isolated mitochondria or cells, the specific target of inhibition of oxidative phosphorylation can be identified either by classical biochemical methods[32] or by immunocapturing the individual protein complexes (Complexes I, II, III, IV, V) from the cells/tissue of interest in 96-well plates and determining each enzyme's activity in the presence of the test compounds.[33] We have used the latter technique to identify the off-target of several drugs including the biguanides, thiazolidinediones, and statins.[34,35]

### 12.4.6 Measurement of mtDNA-Encoded Protein Levels in Cells

Compounds which impair mtDNA replication (*e.g.*, nucleoside reverse transcriptase inhibitors) or mtDNA-encoded protein synthesis (*e.g.*, some antibiotics) are seldom identified in 24–72 h cell viability assays since both mtDNA and the 13 proteins they encode have low turnover rates. Furthermore, the protein complexes involved in oxidative phosphorylation have to fall below a critical threshold in order for mitochondrial ATP synthesis to be impaired, the threshold varying for each cell type. Since the 13 mtDNA-encoded proteins are subunits of the protein complexes involved in oxidative phosphorylation, they too have to fall below a critical threshold before ATP synthesis is impaired. Until recently, identification of compounds that impair mtDNA replication or mtDNA-encoded protein synthesis has required lengthy treatment of cells with the test compounds followed by techniques such as Western blotting or lateral-flow immunoassays.[36,37] However, these techniques are not ideal for high-throughput screening. We have recently developed a 96-well high-content imaging assay that measures the level of a mtDNA-encoded protein (subunit 1 of Complex IV) synthesized on mitochondrial ribosomes and the level of a nuclear DNA-encoded protein (Complex V-$\alpha$ subunit) synthesized on cytosolic ribosomes to assess the effect of several antibiotics and anti-retrovirals over a six-day treatment in adherent eukaryotic cells.[38]

## 12.5 What Do *In Vitro* Methods Tell Us About Drugs That Impair Mitochondrial Function?

The *in vitro* methods discussed in the previous section and other techniques which are beyond the scope of this chapter have demonstrated that a variety of drugs (Table 12.2) have the potential to impair mitochondrial function depending on their potency and length of exposure. We discuss some of these drugs in greater detail here.

### 12.5.1 Drugs Given in the Treatment of Type II Diabetes

The major oral drugs currently used in the treatment of type 2 diabetes include the biguanide, metformin, and the thiazolidinediones, rosiglitazone and pioglitazone.

*In vitro* assessment of metformin and two other biguanides, phenformin and buformin, showed that HepG2 cells grown in galactose are more susceptible to biguanide toxicity than cells grown in glucose.[34] Moreover, the rank order of cytotoxicity seen with the galactose-grown cells was phenformin > buformin > metformin. In addition, the same rank order of toxicity was observed when oxygen consumption of both isolated mitochondria and HepG2 cells was

**Table 12.2** Drugs which have been implicated in mitochondrial dysfunction.

| *Drug* | *Drug class* | *Therapeutic action* | *Mitochondrial off-target* | *Organ affected* | *Clinical observations* |
|---|---|---|---|---|---|
| Phenformin, buformin, metformin | Biguanide | Anti-diabetic | Complex I | — | Lactic acidosis[89] |
| Troglitazone | Thiazolidinedione | Anti-diabetic | Complexes I, II, III, IV, V; Permeability transition pore | Liver | Steatosis,[90] bile duct hyperplasia,[91] apoptosis,[92] hepatic necrosis,[93] hepatotoxicity[94] |
| Ciglitazone | Thiazolidinedione | Anti-diabetic | Complexes I, II, III, IV, V; permeability transition pore | Eye | — |
| Fenofibrate, ciprofibrate, clofibrate, gemfibrozil | Fibrate | Anti-lipidemic | Complex I | Muscle, liver | Hepatocarcinogenesis,[95] hepatic cell death[96] |
| Simvastatin, lovastatin, cerivastatin | Statin | Cholesterol lowering agent | Permeability transition pore | Muscle, heart | Myopathy[97] |
| Linezolid | Oxazolidinone | Antibiotic | MtDNA-encoded protein synthesis | Blood, eye | Myelosuppression, optic neuropathy, peripheral neuropathy[58] |
| Chloramphenicol | — | Antibiotic | MtDNA-encoded protein synthesis | Blood | Myelosuppression[59] |
| Tetracycline | Tetracyclines | Antibiotic | MtDNA-encoded protein synthesis; fatty acid oxidation | Liver | Hepatotoxicity[98] |
| Gentamicin | Aminoglycoside | Antibiotic | MtDNA-encoded protein synthesis | Kidney, ear | Nephrotoxicity,[62] ototoxicity[61] |
| Trovafloxacin | Fluoroquinolone | Antibiotic | Oxidative stress, mtDNA-encoded protein loss | Liver | Acute hepatitis[99] |

| | | | | | |
|---|---|---|---|---|---|
| Zalcitabine, didanosine, stavudine | Nucleoside reverse transcriptase inhibitors | Anti-retroviral | MtDNA synthesis | Liver, heart, muscle, kidney, pancreas | Steatohepatitis[100] |
| Nimesulide, diclofenac | Non-steroidal anti-inflammatory drugs | Analgesic | Uncouples electron transport from ATP synthesis; permeability transition pore | Liver, gastrointestinal tract | Acute hepatic failure,[101] hepatotoxicity,[73] intestinal inflammation[102] |
| Chlorpromazine | Typical antipsychotic | Antipsychotic | Complexes I and V; uncouples electron transport from ATP synthesis | CNS, heart | QT prolongation[103] |
| Nefazodone | Antidepressant | Antidepressant | Complex I | Liver | Hepatic necrosis, hepatitis[104] |
| Amineptine, tianeptine | Tricyclic antidepressant | Antidepressant | Fatty acid oxidation | Liver | Hepatic steatosis[105] |
| Tolcapone | Catechol-*O*-methyl transferase inhibitor | Parkinson's disease | Uncouple electron transport from ATP synthesis | Liver | Fulminant hepatitis[106] |
| Amiodarone, perhexiline | — | Anti-anginal | Uncouple electron transport from ATP synthesis; oxidative stress | Liver | Hepatotoxicity,[107] hepatitis[108] |
| Valproic acid | — | Anti-epileptic | Fatty acid oxidation | Liver | Hepatic steatosis[109] |
| Tamoxifen | Estrogen receptor antagonist | Anti-cancer | Uncouple electron transport from ATP synthesis; complex IV | Liver | Steatohepatitis,[110] hepatic necrosis[111] |
| Flutamide | Non-steroidal anti-androgen | Anti-cancer | Complex I | Liver | Acute hepatitis, hepatic failure[112] |
| Doxorubicin | Anthracycline | Anti-cancer | Oxidative stress | Heart | Cardiomyopathy[113] |

measured.[34] Overall, these results show that mitochondrial impairment is a key component in the toxicity caused by biguanides.

The *in vitro* results on the biguanides are in direct accord with clinical observations. Metformin is one of the most widely prescribed anti-diabetic drugs in the USA and is, in general, well-tolerated. However, phenformin and buformin, were withdrawn from the market several years ago due to reports of lactic acidosis.[39] The *in vitro* results suggest that biguanide-induced lactic acidosis can be attributed to acceleration of glycolysis in response to mitochondrial impairment. It is conceivable that the desired clinical outcome of decreased blood glucose in the treatment of type II diabetes could be due to increased glucose uptake as a result of increased glycolytic flux in response to DIMD.

The other major drugs given in the treatment of type II diabetes, the thiazolidinediones, improve insulin sensitivity and lower blood glucose levels by activating the γ-isoform of peroxisome proliferator-activated receptors (PPARγ). Several *in vitro* studies have implicated some of the thiazolidinediones in mitochondrial impairment. Studies performed on isolated rat liver mitochondria within our group show that troglitazone, ciglitazone, and darglitazone increase basal respiration and inhibit ADP-driven respiration whereas rosiglitazone and pioglitazone cause little impairment.[35] Further analysis on mitochondrial enzymes showed that troglitazone, ciglitazone, and darglitazone strongly inhibit Complexes II + III, IV, and V, whereas rosiglitazone and pioglitazone cause little impairment. Recently, Kwon *et al.* showed that ciglitazone causes activation of p38 MAPK (mitogen-activated protein kinase) and nuclear translocation of AIF (apoptosis inducing factor) through a ROS- and intracellular $Ca^{2+}$ dependent-pathway.[40] Rachek *et al.* have demonstrated that troglitazone induces mtDNA damage which then leads to cell death in human hepatocytes.[41] Hence, most of the *in vitro* assessments on thiazolidinediones indicate that, depending on potency, troglitazone, ciglitazone, and darglitazone, can perturb mitochondrial function.

The identification of a novel mitochondrial protein, mitoNEET, which has the ability to bind to the thiazolidinediones raises the question of what the actual off-target of these drugs is.[42] Although the physiological role of mitoNEET is not known, it has been reported that it is an iron–sulfur containing outer mitochondrial membrane protein; in addition, studies comparing mitochondria from wild-type mice and mitoNEET null mice suggest that the protein may be involved in controlling the maximal respiratory capacity of these organelles.[43] Geldenhuys *et al.* have shown that rosiglitazone, pioglitazone, and a novel ligand which they refer to as NL-1, containing a thiazolidinedione group, are able to bind mitoNEET; moreover, NL-1 was able to uncouple mitochondrial respiration as well as inhibit ADP-driven respiration.[44] It remains to be seen whether the thiazolidinediones can cause impairment on mitochondria from mitoNEET null mice.

The rank order of potency of the thiazolidinediones on mitochondrial impairment *in vitro* appears to be in accord with the toxicity outcomes seen with these drugs in the clinic. Troglitazone, the first thiazolidinedione launched on the market in the USA, was withdrawn after three years, because of several incidents of hepatotoxicity.[45,46] Development of darglitazone and ciglitazone was discontinued, with the latter showing cataractogenic potential in rats.[47] The development of muraglitazar, the first drug to activate both the α- and γ-isoforms of PPARs, was dropped because of increased cardiotoxicity.[48] Recently, amidst much controversy, there have been reports of cardiac failure associated with rosiglitazone.[49] Whether there is any link between rosiglitazone-associated cardiac failure and mitochondrial impairment is not known.

### 12.5.2 Drugs Given in the Treatment of Dyslipidemia

Since an elevated plasma lipid level is often a problem in Type II diabetes, patients are often prescribed a combination therapy to reduce plasma lipid levels as well as blood glucose levels. The major drugs used in lowering lipid levels are the fibrates, which target the PPAR-α isoform, thereby reducing triglyceride levels, and the statins, which inhibit HMG-CoA (3-hydroxy-3-methylglutaryl-coenzyme A) reductase, thereby lowering circulating cholesterol levels.

*In vitro* assessments of fibrates and statins implicate some of them in mitochondrial impairment. Our group,[35] as well as Brunmair *et al.*,[50] has shown that some of the fibrates such as fenofibrate can affect the activity of the protein complexes involved in oxidative phosphorylation. Kaufmann *et al.* have reported that cerivastatin, fluvastatin, atorvastatin, and simvastatin dissipate membrane potential and repress glutamate-driven respiration in isolated rat skeletal muscle mitochondria, whereas pravastatin does not.[51] Velho *et al.* have shown that lovastatin and simvastatin induce the irreversible opening of the permeability transition pore in isolated rat liver mitochondria whereas pravastatin does not.[52] Simvastatin and lovastatin have been reported to cause more potent mitochondrial impairment than atorvastatin and pravastatin, increasing basal respiration and inhibiting Complexes II, III, IV, and V.[35]

Most fibrates cause some level of myopathy, including pain and creatine phosphokinase release, a consequence of muscle death.[53] This is also the case for most statins where serious side-effects include hepatotoxicity and myotoxicity.[53] Rhabdomyolysis (muscle deterioration) forced the withdrawal of cerivastatin in 2001.[54] Recently, the FDA warned patients and physicians of the risk of rhabdomyolysis associated with high levels (80 mg per day) of simvastatin based on information received from clinical trials, adverse event reports, observational studies and prescription-use data. Moreover, clinical experience with various combinations of statins prescribed with either thiazolidinediones or fibrates suggests drug–drug interactions.[54,56] For example, the majority of the deaths during the cerivastatin trial were in patients also taking gemfibrozil.[54]

### 12.5.3 Antibiotics and Anti-Retrovirals

Because of the bacterial origin of mitochondria, antibiotics which target the bacterial ribosome can potentially impair protein synthesis on mitochondrial ribosomes.

*In vitro* results indicate that linezolid and chloramphenicol, antibiotics that prevent bacterial protein synthesis by binding to the 50S subunit of the bacterial ribosome, impair mtDNA-encoded protein synthesis.[36–38,57] These *in vitro* results are in agreement with clinical observations including myelosuppression, lactic acidosis, optic neuropathy, and peripheral neuropathy that have been observed with both antibiotics.[58,59]

The aminoglycoside antibiotics (*e.g.*, gentamicin, kanamycin) bind to the 30S subunit of the bacterial ribosome and prevent protein synthesis.[60] They are known to cause ototoxicity and nephrotoxicity in some patients.[61,62] For instance, patients with the mutations A1555G or C1494T within the rRNA of the small subunit of mitochondrial ribosomes are susceptible to aminoglycoside-induced hearing loss.[63] Böttger and colleagues have shown, by *in vitro* experiments, that ribosomes containing either of these mutations are susceptible to aminoglyoside-induced inhibition of protein synthesis whereas ribosomes containing the wild-type mitochondrial rRNA sequence are not.[64]

The fluoroquinolone antibiotics impair bacterial type II topoisomerases in their primary mode of action.[60] *In vitro* studies with some of the fluoroquinolones, ciprofloxacin, levofloxacin, ofloxacin, and trovafloxacin, have shown that they can decrease mtDNA-encoded protein levels in eukaryotic cells.[38] Furthermore, Lawrence *et al.* have shown that ciprofloxacin makes site-specific double-stranded DNA breaks and depletes mtDNA in eukaryotic cells.[65] Mammalian mitochondria have a type II topoisomerase, an enzyme that cleaves both strands of DNA duplex.[66] Although the homology between this enzyme and its bacterial counterpart is not known, it is possible that fluoroquinolones impair mtDNA which in turn leads to a decrease in mtDNA-encoded protein levels.

Anti-retrovirals, in particular nucleoside reverse transcriptase inhibitors (NRTIs), are known to cause mitochondrial toxicity.[67] NRTIs are phosphorylated by cellular kinases to a triphosphate form which act as competitive inhibitors of the HIV reverse transcriptase and terminate elongation of the viral DNA chain. DNA polymerase-$\gamma$, the enzyme responsible for replicating mtDNA, is highly sensitive to certain NRTIs[67] and, hence, impairment of mtDNA replication leads to decreased levels of the proteins encoded by mtDNA.[67] Adverse effects of NRTIs include lactic acidosis, lipodystrophy, peripheral neuropathy, optic neuropathy, and cardiomyopathy.[68] *In vitro* results show that some of the NRTIs impair mtDNA synthesis and, thereby, decrease mtDNA-encoded protein levels with a rank order of potency zalcitabine > didanosine > stavudine > lamivudine = abacavir = tenofovir.[69]

## 12.5.4 Non-Steroidal Anti-Inflammatory Drugs

The widespread use of non-steroidal anti-inflammatory drugs (NSAIDs) has lead to reports of upper gastrointestinal injury and, less frequently, to reports of hepatotoxicity.[70] Bromfenac and benoxaprofen were withdrawn from the market due to idiosyncratic hepatotoxicity while nimesulide and diclofenac, although still on the market in some countries, are also associated with idiosyncratic liver injury.[71–73] In addition, diclofenac is also reported to cause gastrointestinal injury. Although the causes of hepatotoxicity and gastrointestinal injury associated with NSAIDs are still not clear, mitochondrial impairment has been implicated as a possible mechanism. The lipophilic and weakly acidic characteristics of NSAIDs make many of these drugs potent uncouplers of oxidative phosphorylation in isolated mitochondria.[74]

## 12.6 Challenges That Lie Ahead in Detecting DIMD

While the wealth of *in vitro* assays has revealed much about drug-induced mitochondrial dysfunction, there are many challenges that lie ahead. We briefly discuss some of these difficulties here.

### 12.6.1 Lack of *In Silico* Methods to Predict DIMD

*In silico* methods to predict DIMD are still in their infancy, one of the reasons being that there are potentially many mechanisms by which a compound could impair mitochondrial function. However, one of the areas where a considerable amount of work has been done pertains to protonophoric uncouplers. These compounds shuttle protons across the inner mitochondrial membrane, thereby dissipating the pH gradient and hence, inhibiting ATP synthesis. They tend to have an acidic dissociable group, an electron withdrawing moiety and a large hydrophobic group.[75] Compounds in this category include DNP (2,4-dinitrophenol), FCCP (carbonyl cyanide *p*-trifluoromethoxyphenylhydrazone), CCCP (carbonylcyanide *m*-chlorophenylhydrazone), phenols, benzimidazoles, *N*-phenylanthranilates, phenylhydrazones, and salicylic acids. As mentioned in an earlier section, many non-steroidal anti-inflammatory drugs such as diflunisal, flufenamic acid, tolfenamic acid and mefenamic acid are weak acids and have strong uncoupling properties in isolated mitochondria. Interestingly, Brand and colleagues[76] have reported that some compounds such as substituted triphenylphosphonium molecules cause uncoupling *via* the adenine nucleotide translocase (ANT), a protein which imports ADP and exports ATP across the inner mitochondrial membrane.[76] Compounds which uncouple *via* ANT are not necessarily weak acids and lose their uncoupling properties when the ANT is inhibited, for example by carboxyatractylate (CAT).[76] The mechanism by which CAT-sensitive uncouplers act through ANT is not known.

Horobin *et al.* have used physicochemical classification and quantitative structure–activity relationship models to analyze more than 100 "mitochondriotropics", compounds which target mitochondria.[77] Their analysis showed that approximately 36% of mitochondriotropics were lipophilic cations, approximately 39% were anions of which most were weak acids whose free acidic species were lipophilic, 14% were hydrophilic cations, and 10% were electrically neutral. These observations indicate that most compounds which target mitochondria do not share a common set of physicochemical properties, highlighting the difficulties we currently face in predicting, by *in silico* methods, whether a compound will enter mitochondria.

### 12.6.2 Paucity of Suitable Animal Models to Detect Mitochondrial Dysfunction

Routine pathology and clinical chemistry done on rodent or non-rodent models have so far failed to identify DIMD. Mitochondrial capacity decreases with age or lack of exercise, suggesting that aged, sedentary rodents may be more appropriate models for studying DIMD than young, active rodents. Recently, Thyfault *et al.* showed that rats which were artificially selected to be low-capacity runners over several generations had reduced mitochondrial content (cytochrome *c* protein levels and citrate synthase activity) and reduced oxidative capacity in their livers and were more prone to hepatic steatosis and liver injury than their counterparts who were high-capacity runners.[78] Clearly, there is a need for physiologically or pathologically realistic animal models in order for drug-induced mitochondrial function to be identified *in vivo*.

Although there are various mouse models (Table 12.3) that exhibit impaired mitochondrial function, few have been used within the pharmaceutical industry for toxicity studies. An exception is the Sod2$^{+/-}$ mouse which is heterozygous for mitochondrial manganese superoxide dismutase. The Sod2$^{+/-}$ mouse appears phenotypically normal but has only 50% of the MnSod2 enzyme and, hence, shows increased oxidative stress. In contrast to wild-type mice which are not susceptible to hepatotoxicity caused by troglitazone, Sod2$^{+/-}$ mice show symptoms of liver injury when dosed with troglitazone.[79] The Sod2$^{+/-}$ mouse model has also been used to investigate the potential toxic effects of nimesulide, flutamide, and trovafloxacin, drugs known to cause idiosyncratic liver injury and impair mitochondrial function.[80–82] Interestingly, the effect of Sod2 knockdown has also been analyzed in *Drosophila*, where mutants with low Sod2 expression show reduced mitochondrial aconitase activity and shorter life spans than the wild-type flies.[83] However, the use of *Drosophila* in toxicity studies has not become prevalent, despite researchers using transgenic fruit flies in the study of diseases such as Alzheimer's and Huntington's disease.

Harrill *et al.* have used a panel of 36 inbred mouse strains to study inter-individual variability to hepatotoxicity caused by acetaminophen.[84] If these mouse strains have inherent differences in mitochondrial function, they could potentially be used to study DIMD.

### 12.6.3 Lack of Validated Biomarkers for Identifying DIMD in Patients

Through its Critical Path Initiative, the FDA, together with other organizations, has set up a Biomarkers Consortium to search and validate new biomarkers. However, to date, there are no *validated* biomarkers of drug-induced mitochondrial dysfunction.

**Table 12.3** Mouse models that show impaired mitochondrial function.

| *Mouse model* | *Mutation* | *Phenotype* |
|---|---|---|
| *Sod2*$^{+/-}$ mouse[114] | Heterozygous for mitochondrial manganese superoxide dismutase | Phenotypically normal; shows increased oxidative stress |
| Mito-mouse[114] | MtDNA deletion that removes six tRNA genes and seven structural genes | Low body weight, lactic acidosis, ischemia, myopathy |
| *ANT1*$^{-/-}$ mouse[114] | Lacks an isoform of the adenosine nucleotide translocator | Increased serum lactate levels, decreased oxygen consumption, cardiomyopathy |
| *Tfam*$^{+/-}$ mouse[114] | Heterozygous for the mitochondrial transcription factor A | Reduced mtDNA copy number, decreased Complex I and IV activities, cardiomyopathy |
| POLG mouse[114] | Contains mutated DNA polymerase γ | Premature aging |
| *Neil1*$^{-/-}$ mouse[115] | Lacks Neil1 DNA glycosylase | Severe obesity, dyslipidemia, fatty liver disease, hyperinsulinemia, increased damage and deletions in mtDNA |
| *Cisd2*$^{-/-}$ mouse[116] | Lacks the Cisd2 protein which is an outer mitochondrial membrane protein | Mitochondrial breakdown and dysfunction, autophagic cell death, nerve and muscle degeneration, premature aging |

A recent study describes the use of lateral-flow dipstick immunoassays to detect mtDNA-encoded proteins in peripheral fat and peripheral blood mononuclear cells (PBMCs) from HIV-positive individuals who were on anti-retroviral therapy.[85] The results showed that individuals on anti-retroviral therapy with adverse symptoms of lipodystrophy have lower mtDNA-encoded protein levels (Complexes I and IV) than individuals who were HIV negative. The authors of the study also showed that there was a significant correlation between the levels of these proteins in PBMCs with that in peripheral fat, suggesting that mtDNA-encoded proteins in blood could be used as a biomarker for monitoring mitochondrial impairment caused by anti-retroviral therapy.

An intriguing report by Zhang *et al.* discusses how certain types of cellular injury such as major trauma results in the release of mtDNA into the peripheral circulation. The authors demonstrate that mtDNA as well as mitochondrial formyl peptides which are released into the circulation as a result of trauma, activate neutrophil-mediated organ injury.[86] Whether mtDNA is released into the circulation after DIMD remains to be seen. The use of transcriptomic analysis of blood in identifying potential "signatures" of drug-induced liver injury was recently demonstrated in a proof-of-concept study where genes involved in oxidative phosphorylation were found to be down-regulated 48 h after a supratherapeutic level of acetaminophen was administered in six healthy adults.[87] Concomitant with the down-regulation of these genes was an increase in serum lactate. Since acetaminophen is known to affect mitochondria by depleting the anti-oxidant, glutathione, *via* a reactive metabolite, these results suggest that gene expression analysis of blood could be a potential method for detecting DIMD *in vivo*.

### 12.6.4 Complexities in Conclusively Attributing Mitochondrial Dysfunction to a Particular Drug in the Real World

Perhaps the most daunting challenge that we face in the field of drug-induced mitochondrial dysfunction is demonstrating that *in vitro* observations actually predict clinical outcomes in humans. Given the lack of validated biomarkers for DIMD, mitochondrial impairment is rarely tested in patients, with the exception of those on highly active anti-retroviral therapy. A classical hallmark of mitochondrial impairment is lactic acidosis, a condition in which the lactate level in blood rises above 5 mmol $L^{-1}$.[88] The resting lactate level in humans lies between 0.5–1.5 mmol $L^{-1}$. If, however, mitochondria are impaired by drugs, cells try to compensate for decreased ATP production by increasing glycolysis in order to make more ATP in the cytoplasm. An increase in glycolysis, however, results in an increase in the byproduct, lactate. High levels of lactate decrease the pH of the blood and this can have fatal consequences. Lactic acidosis can occur as a result of lack of oxygen or poor tissue perfusion, as a result of renal and liver failure, as a result of certain drugs, and as a result of inborn errors of metabolism.

As an exercise in finding out if lactic acidosis diagnosed in patients was associated with drugs that cause mitochondrial impairment *in vitro*, we explored the FDA's Adverse Event Reporting System (AERS) database to identify drugs associated with lactic acidosis. AERS is a computerized information database designed to support the FDA's post-marketing safety surveillance program for all approved drugs and therapeutic biologic products. The adverse event reports in AERS are provided either voluntarily by physicians and the public or *via* a mandatory route by drug manufacturers. The reports that we found were dated between the last quarter of 1997 to the last quarter of 2009. Each of the reports contained an AERS report number, the age and gender of the patient, the adverse events that were observed in the patient, the outcome (for example, hospitalization, life threatening situation and/or death), the primary suspected drug, secondary suspected drugs, co-medications, the date the adverse event occurred or began, the manufacturer's unique report identifier and the name of manufacturer (if the report had been sent by the drug's manufacturer), the date the FDA received the report, and the report type ("expedited" when sent by the manufacturer, "direct" when sent by a physician or consumer). We found that the drugs most frequently associated with lactic acidosis were metformin (1955 reports), anti-retrovirals (1604 reports), anti-diabetic drugs other than metformin (114 reports), linezolid (78 reports), fluoroquinolone antibiotics (31 reports), diclofenac (24 reports), and valproic acid (21 reports).

There are certain caveats when drawing conclusions from the AERS database. Firstly, submission of post-marketing reports by physicians and patients is voluntary in the USA and is unverified. Since the reports are obtained *via* a passive surveillance system, it is very likely that the number of cases of lactic acidosis that we identified is an underestimate of drug-induced lactic acidosis that actually occurs within the USA. Secondly, the AERS database provides no information on the number of patients who are prescribed a drug. Thus, although there were many more reports on lactic acidosis associated with metformin than with linezolid, there is no indication as to what percentage of patients on metformin experience lactic acidosis in comparison with those prescribed linezolid.

While many of the drugs that we found to be associated with lactic acidosis in the AERS reports have, indeed, been shown to cause mitochondrial impairment *in vitro*, the AERS reports highlight difficulties in conclusively attributing mitochondrial dysfunction to a particular drug in the real world. Unlike in the controlled environment of *in vitro* experiments, there is rarely any certainty that the primary suspected drug caused the adverse event in patients. Hence, lactic acidosis could have occurred because of the underlying medical condition or a concurrent disease rather than because of the drug. Moreover, in many of the adverse event reports, we found that patients were prescribed more than one medication, often six to 10. For example, most of the patients who were prescribed diclofenac were also prescribed metformin, thus making it difficult to identify which of the two drugs, if either, contributed to lactic acidosis. Conversely, the information in the reports provides scope for further research, both in the laboratory and in the clinic. Thus, one could investigate if there is a drug–drug interaction between diclofenac and metformin which exacerbates mitochondrial impairment.

## 12.7 Conclusions

In conclusion, drug-induced mitochondrial dysfunction (DIMD) is rapidly gaining recognition within the pharmaceutical industry as a contributor to compound attrition and post-market withdrawals. The development of high-throughput assays to screen for mitochondrial impairment *in vitro* has been instrumental in uncovering the importance of DIMD. Demonstrating the physiological relevance of these assays, identifying mitochondrial dysfunction in appropriate animal models and predicting safety outcomes in patients are the next challenges on the horizon. Simply put, drug-induced mitochondrial dysfunction is a new frontier we have just begun to explore.

## References

1. J. Lazarou, B. H. Pomeranz and P. N. Corey, *JAMA, J. Am. Med. Assoc.*, 1998, **279**, 1200.
2. J. A. Dykens and Y. Will, *Drug Discovery Today*, 2007, **12**, 777.
3. J. A. Dykens, L. D. Marroquin and Y. Will, *Expert Rev. Mol. Diagn.*, 2007, **7**, 161.

4. K. Chan, D. Truong, N. Shangari and P. J. O'Brien, *Expert Opin. Drug Metab. Toxicol.*, 2005, **1**, 655.
5. K. B. Wallace, *Trends Pharmacol. Sci.*, 2008, **29**, 361.
6. L. Wojtczak and K. Zablocki, in *Drug-Induced Mitochondrial Dysfunction*, ed. J. A. Dykens and Y. Will, John Wiley & Sons, Hoboken, New Jersey, 2008, p. 3.
7. D. J. Pagliarini, S. E. Calvo, B. Chang, S. A. Sheth, S. B. Vafai, S. E. Ong, G. A. Walford, C. Sugiana, A. Boneh, W. K. Chen, D. E. Hill, M. Vidal, J. G. Evans, D. R. Thorburn, S. A. Carr and V. K. Mootha, *Cell*, 2008, **134**, 112.
8. S. W. Taylor, E. Fahy, B. Zhang, G. M. Glenn, D. E. Warnock, S. Wiley, A. N. Murphy, S. P. Gaucher, R. A. Capaldi, B. W. Gibson and S. S. Ghosh, *Nat. Biotechnol.*, 2003, **21**, 281.
9. S. B. Berman, F. J. Pineda and J. M. Hardwick, *Cell Death Differ.*, 2008, **15**, 1147.
10. S. Campello and L. Scorrano, *EMBO Rep.*, 2010, **11**, 678.
11. I. E. Scheffler, *Mitochondria*, John Wiley & Sons, Hoboken, New Jersey, 2008.
12. A. M. Psarra and C. E. Sekeris, *Biochim. Biophys. Acta*, 2008, **1783**, 1.
13. J. Lee, S. Sharma, J. Kim, R. J. Ferrante and H. Ryu, *J. Neurosci. Res.*, 2008, **86**, 961.
14. I. E. Scheffler in *Drug-Induced Mitochondrial Dysfunction*, ed. J. A. Dykens and Y. Will, John Wiley & Sons, Hoboken, New Jersey, 2008, p. 37.
15. H. A. Tuppen, E. L. Blakely, D. M. Turnbull and R. W. Taylor, *Biochim. Biophys. Acta*, 2010, **1797**, 113.
16. D. C. Wallace, *Annu. Rev. Genet.*, 2005, **39**, 359.
17. E. C. Bottger, *Cell. Mol. Life Sci.*, 2007, **64**, 791.
18. J. F. Turrens, *J. Physiol.*, 2003, **552**, 335.
19. V. Adam-Vizi and C. Chinopoulos, *Trends Pharmacol. Sci.*, 2006, **27**, 639.
20. G. Benard, B. Faustin, E. Passerieux, A. Galinier, C. Rocher, N. Bellance, J. P. Delage, L. Casteilla, T. Letellier and R. Rossignol, *Am. J. Physiol. Cell. Physiol.*, 2006, **291**, C1172.
21. F. Forner, L. J. Foster, S. Campanaro, G. Valle and M. Mann, *Mol. Cell Proteomics*, 2006, **5**, 608.
22. G. P. Davey, S. Peuchen and J. B. Clark, *J. Biol. Chem.*, 1998, **273**, 12753.
23. G. P. Davey and J. B. Clark, *J. Neurochem.*, 1996, **66**, 1617.
24. L. D. Marroquin, J. Hynes, J. A. Dykens, J. D. Jamieson and Y. Will, *Toxicol. Sci.*, 2007, **97**, 539.
25. J. A. Dykens, J. D. Jamieson, L. D. Marroquin, S. Nadanaciva, J. J. Xu, M. C. Dunn, A. R. Smith and Y. Will, *Toxicol. Sci.*, 2008, **103**, 335.
26. A. Nieminen, V. K. Ramesh and J. J. Lemasters in *Drug-Induced Mitochondrial Dysfunction*, ed. J. A. Dykens and Y. Will, John Wiley & Sons, Hoboken, New Jersey, 2008, p. 413.
27. J. Hynes, L. D. Marroquin, V. I. Ogurtsov, K. N. Christiansen, G. J. Stevens, D. B. Papkovsky and Y. Will, *Toxicol. Sci.*, 2006, **92**, 186.
28. Y. Will, J. Hynes, V. I. Ogurtsov and D. B. Papkovsky, *Nat. Protoc.*, 2006, **1**, 2563.

29. J. Hynes, T. C. O'Riordan, A. V. Zhdanov, G. Uray, Y. Will and D. B. Papkovsky, *Anal. Biochem.*, 2009, **390**, 21.
30. D. A. Ferrick, A. Neilson and C. Beeson, *Drug Discovery Today*, 2008, **13**, 268.
31. M. Wu, A. Neilson, A. L. Swift, R. Moran, J. Tamagnine, D. Parslow, S. Armistead, K. Lemire, J. Orrell, J. Teich, S. Chomicz and D. A. Ferrick, *Am. J. Physiol. Cell Physiol.*, 2007, **292**, C125.
32. M. A. Birch-Machin in *Drug-Induced Mitochondrial Dysfunction*, ed. J. A. Dykens and Y. Will, John Wiley & Sons, Hoboken, New Jersey, 2008, p. 383.
33. S. Nadanaciva, A. Bernal, R. Aggeler, R. Capaldi and Y. Will, *Toxicol. in Vitro*, 2007, **21**, 902.
34. J. A. Dykens, J. Jamieson, L. Marroquin, S. Nadanaciva, P. A. Billis and Y. Will, *Toxicol. Appl. Pharmacol.*, 2008, **233**, 203.
35. S. Nadanaciva, J. A. Dykens, A. Bernal, R. A. Capaldi and Y. Will, *Toxicol. Appl. Pharmacol.*, 2007, **223**, 277.
36. E. E. Nagiec, L. Wu, S. M. Swaney, J. G. Chosay, D. E. Ross, J. K. Brieland and K. L. Leach, *Antimicrob. Agents Chemother.*, 2005, **49**, 3896.
37. S. Nadanaciva, J. H. Willis, M. L. Barker, D. Gharaibeh, R. A. Capaldi, M. F. Marusich and Y. Will, *J. Immunol. Methods*, 2009, **343**, 1.
38. S. Nadanaciva, K. Dillman, D. F. Gebhard, A. Shrikhande and Y. Will, *J. Biomol. Screening,* 2010, **15**, 937.
39. R. Mehta, K. Chan, O. Lee, S. Tafazoli and P. J. O'Brien in *Drug-Induced Mitochondrial Dysfunction*, ed. J. A. Dykens and Y. Will, John Wiley & Sons, Hoboken, New Jersey, 2008, p. 71.
40. C. H. Kwon, J. Y. Park, T. H. Kim, J. S. Woo and Y. K. Kim, *Toxicology*, 2009, **257**, 1.
41. L. I. Rachek, L. V. Yuzefovych, S. P. Ledoux, N. L. Julie and G. L. Wilson, *Toxicol. Appl. Pharmacol.*, 2009, **240**, 348.
42. J. R. Colca, W. G. McDonald, D. J. Waldon, J. W. Leone, J. M. Lull, C. A. Bannow, E. T. Lund and W. R. Mathews, *Am. J. Physiol. Endocrinol. Metab.*, 2004, **286**, E252.
43. S. E. Wiley, A. N. Murphy, S. A. Ross, P. van der Geer and J. E. Dixon, *Proc. Natl. Acad. Sci. U. S. A.*, 2007, **104**, 5318.
44. W. J. Geldenhuys, M. O. Funk, K. F. Barnes and R. T. Carroll, *Bioorg. Med. Chem. Lett.*, 2010, **20**, 819.
45. W. L. Isley, *Expert Opin. Drug Saf.*, 2003, **2**, 581.
46. H. E. Lebovitz, *Diabetes. Metab. Res. Rev.*, 2002, **18**, S23.
47. M. D. Aleo, C. M. Doshna and K. A. Navetta, *J. Pharmacol. Exp. Ther.*, 2005, **312**, 1027.
48. S. E. Nissen, K. Wolski and E. J. Topol, *JAMA, J. Am. Med. Assoc.*, 2005, **294**, 2581.
49. S. E. Nissen, *Eur. Heart J.*, 2010, **31**, 773.
50. B. Brunmair, A. Lest, K. Staniek, F. Gras, N. Scharf, M. Roden, H. Nohl, W. Waldhausl and C. Furnsinn, *J. Pharmacol. Exp. Ther.*, 2004, **311**, 109.

51. P. Kaufmann, M. Torok, A. Zahno, K. M. Waldhauser, K. Brecht and S. Krahenbuhl, *Cell. Mol. Life Sci.*, 2006, **63**, 2415.
52. J. A. Velho, H. Okanobo, G. R. Degasperi, M. Y. Matsumoto, L. C. Alberici, R. G. Cosso, H. C. Oliveira and A. E. Vercesi, *Toxicology*, 2006, **219**, 124.
53. T. E. Johnson in *Drug-Induced Mitochondrial Dysfunction*, ed. J. A. Dykens and Y. Will, John Wiley & Sons, Hoboken, New Jersey, 2008, p. 235.
54. M. Evans and A. Rees, *Drug Saf.*, 2002, **25**, 649.
55. D. J. Graham, J. A. Staffa, D. Shatin, S. E. Andrade, S. D. Schech, L. La Grenade, J. H. Gurwitz, K. A. Chan, M. J. Goodman and R. Platt, *JAMA, J. Am. Med. Assoc.*, 2004, **292**, 2585.
56. J. T. Chang, J. A. Staffa, M. Parks and L. Green, *Pharmacoepidemiol. Drug Saf.*, 2004, **13**, 417.
57. E. E. McKee, M. Ferguson, A. T. Bentley and T. A. Marks, *Antimicrob. Agents Chemother.*, 2006, **50**, 2042.
58. D. J. Kuter and G. S. Tillotson, *Pharmacotherapy*, 2001, **21**, 1010.
59. H. M. Feder, *South. Med. J.*, 1986, **79**, 1129.
60. C. T. Walsh, *Antibiotics: actions, origins, resistance*, ASM Press, Washington, DC, 2003.
61. L. P. Rybak and V. Ramkumar, *Kidney Int.*, 2007, **72**, 931.
62. W. M. Sweileh, *Fundam. Clin. Pharmacol.*, 2009, **23**, 515.
63. D. Pacheu-Grau, A. Gomez-Duran, M. J. Lopez-Perez, J. Montoya and E. Ruiz-Pesini, *Drug Discovery Today*, 2010, **15**, 33.
64. S. N. Hobbie, S. Akshay, S. K. Kalapala, C. M. Bruell, D. Shcherbakov and E. C. Bottger, *Proc. Natl. Acad. Sci. U. S. A.*, 2008, **105**, 20888.
65. J. W. Lawrence, D. C. Claire, V. Weissig and T. C. Rowe, *Mol. Pharmacol.*, 1996, **50**, 1178.
66. H. Zhang, L. H. Meng and Y. Pommier, *Biochimie*, 2007, **89**, 474.
67. W. Lewis, B. J. Day and W. C. Copeland, *Nat. Rev. Drug Discovery*, 2003, **2**, 812.
68. A. Carr, *Nat. Rev. Drug Discovery*, 2003, **2**, 624.
69. G. Birkus, M. J. Hitchcock and T. Cihlar, *Antimicrob. Agents Chemother.*, 2002, **46**, 716.
70. G. P. Aithal and C. P. Day, *Clin. Liver Dis.*, 2007, **11**, 563.
71. E. B. Hunter, P. E. Johnston, G. Tanner, C. W. Pinson and J. A. Awad, *Am. J. Gastroenterol.*, 1999, **94**, 2299.
72. A. Duthie, A. Nicholls, M. Freeth, P. Moorhead and D. Triger, *Br. Med. J.*, 1982, **285**, 62.
73. A. T. Banks, H. J. Zimmerman, K. G. Ishak and J. G. Harter, *Hepatology*, 1995, **22**, 820.
74. R. Moreno-Sanchez, C. Bravo, C. Vasquez, G. Ayala, L. H. Silveira and M. Martinez-Lavin, *Biochem. Pharmacol.*, 1999, **57**, 743.
75. H. Terada, *Environ. Health Perspect.*, 1990, **87**, 213.
76. P. H. Lou, B. S. Hansen, P. H. Olsen, S. Tullin, M. P. Murphy and M. D. Brand, *Biochem. J.*, 2007, **407**, 129.

77. R. W. Horobin, S. Trapp and V. Weissig, *J. Control. Release*, 2007, **121**, 125.
78. J. P. Thyfault, R. S. Rector, G. M. Uptergrove, S. J. Borengasser, E. M. Morris, Y. Wei, M. J. Laye, C. F. Burant, N. R. Qi, S. E. Ridenhour, L. G. Koch, S. L. Britton and J. A. Ibdah, *J. Physiol.*, 2009, **587**, 1805.
79. M. M. Ong, C. Latchoumycandane and U. A. Boelsterli, *Toxicol. Sci.*, 2007, **97**, 205.
80. M. M. Ong, A. S. Wang, K. Y. Leow, Y. M. Khoo and U. A. Boelsterli, *Free Radical Biol. Med.*, 2006, **40**, 420.
81. R. Kashimshetty, V. G. Desai, V. M. Kale, T. Lee, C. L. Moland, W. S. Branham, L. S. New, E. C. Chan, H. Younis and U. A. Boelsterli, *Toxicol. Appl. Pharmacol.*, 2009, **238**, 150.
82. C. J. Hsiao, H. Younis and U. A. Boelsterli, *Chem.–Biol. Interact.*, 2010, **188**, 204.
83. A. Paul, A. Belton, S. Nag, I. Martin, M. S. Grotewiel and A. Duttaroy, *Mech. Ageing Dev.*, 2007, **128**, 706.
84. A. H. Harrill, P. B. Watkins, S. Su, P. K. Ross, D. E. Harbourt, I. M. Stylianou, G. A. Boorman, M. W. Russo, R. S. Sackler, S. C. Harris, P. C. Smith, R. Tennant, M. Bogue, K. Paigen, C. Harris, T. Contractor, T. Wiltshire, I. Rusyn and D. W. Threadgill, *Genome Res.*, 2009, **19**, 1507.
85. C. M. Shikuma, M. Gerschenson, D. Chow, D. E. Libutti, J. H. Willis, J. Murray, R. A. Capaldi and M. Marusich, *AIDS Res. Hum. Retroviruses*, 2008, **24**, 1255.
86. Q. Zhang, M. Raoof, Y. Chen, Y. Sumi, T. Sursal, W. Junger, K. Brohi, K. Itagaki and C. J. Hauser, *Nature*, 2010, **464**, 104.
87. R. D. Fannin, M. Russo, T. M. O'Connell, K. Gerrish, J. H. Winnike, J. Macdonald, J. Newton, S. Malik, S. O. Sieber, J. Parker, R. Shah, T. Zhou, P. B. Watkins and R. S. Paules, *Hepatology*, 2010, **51**, 227.
88. R. D. Cohen and H. F. Woods, *Clinical and Biochemical Aspects of Lactic Acidosis*, Blackwell, Oxford, 1976.
89. A. Protti, R. Russo, P. Tagliabue, S. Vecchio, M. Singer, A. Rudiger, G. Foti, A. Rossi, G. Mistraletti and L. Gattinoni, *Crit. Care*, 2010, **14**, R22.
90. S. E. Schadinger, N. L. Bucher, B. M. Schreiber and S. R. Farmer, *Am. J. Physiol. Endocrinol. Metab.*, 2005, **288**, E1195.
91. C. Rothwell, E. J. McGuire, D. M. Altrogge, H. Masuda and F. A. de la Iglesia, *J. Toxicol. Sci.*, 2002, **27**, 35.
92. Y. Yamamoto, M. Nakajima, H. Yamazaki and T. Yokoi, *Life Sci.*, 2001, **70**, 471.
93. H. Li, D. S. Heller, C. B. Leevy, K. G. Zierer and K. M. Klein, *J. Diabetes Complications*, 2000, **14**, 175.
94. S. K. Herrine and C. Choudhary, *Ann. Intern. Med.*, 1999, **130**, 163.
95. J. Nishimura, Y. Dewa, T. Okamura, M. Muguruma, M. Jin, Y. Saegusa, T. Umemura and K. Mitsumori, *Arch. Toxicol.*, 2008, **82**, 641.
96. B. J. Keller, H. Yamanaka, D. C. Liang and R. G. Thurman, *Toxicol. Appl. Pharmacol.*, 1990, **104**, 259.

97. J. Hanai, P. Cao, P. Tanksale, S. Imamura, E. Koshimizu, J. Zhao, S. Kishi, M. Yamashita, P. S. Phillips, V. P. Sukhatme and S. H. Lecker, *J. Clin. Invest.*, 2007, **117**, 3940.
98. P. C. Heaton, S. R. Fenwick and D. E. Brewer, *J. Clin. Phar. Ther.*, 2007, **32**, 483.
99. M. I. Lucena, R. J. Andrade, L. Rodrigo, J. Salmeron, A. Alvarez, M. J. Lopez-Garrido, R. Camargo and R. Alcantara, *Clin. Infect. Dis.*, 2000, **30**, 400.
100. P. Chariot, I. Drogou, I. de Lacroix-Szmania, M. C. Eliezer-Vanerot, B. Chazaud, A. Lombes, A. Schaeffer and E. S. Zafrani, *J. Hepatol.*, 1999, **30**, 156.
101. H. H. Tan, W. M. Ong, S. H. Lai and W. C. Chow, *Singapore Med. J.*, 2007, **48**, 582.
102. L. Maiden, B. Thjodleifsson, A. Theodors, J. Gonzalez and I. Bjarnason, *Gastroenterology*, 2005, **128**, 1172.
103. E. M. Strachan, C. A. Kelly and D. N. Bateman, *Eur. J. Clin. Pharmacol.*, 2004, **60**, 541.
104. D. E. Stewart, *Can. J. Psychiatry*, 2002, **47**, 375.
105. S. Ricca Rosellini, F. Grilli, M. Gaudio, A. Saragoni and F. Miglio, *Ital. J. Gastroenterol.*, 1990, **22**, 40.
106. N. Borges, *Expert Opin. Drug Saf.*, 2005, **4**, 69.
107. M. Babatin, S. S. Lee and P. T. Pollak, *Curr. Vasc. Pharmacol.*, 2008, **6**, 228.
108. D. Lewis, H. C. Wainwright, M. C. Kew, S. Zwi and C. Isaacson, *Gut*, 1979, **20**, 186.
109. K. Sato, Y. Ueda, K. Ueno, K. Okamoto, H. Iizuka and S. Katsuda, *Virchows Arch.*, 2005, **447**, 996.
110. K. A. Osman, M. M. Osman and M. H. Ahmed, *Expert Opin. Drug Saf.*, 2007, **6**, 1.
111. E. C. Storen, J. E. Hay, J. Kaur, K. Zahasky and L. Hartmann, *Cancer J.*, 2000, **6**, 58.
112. M. Garcia Cortes, R. J. Andrade, M. I. Lucena, H. Sanchez Martinez, M. C. Fernandez, T. Ferrer, R. Martin-Vivaldi, G. Pelaez, F. Suarez, M. Romero-Gomez, J. L. Montero, E. Fraga, R. Camargo, R. Alcantara, M. A. Pizarro, E. Garcia-Ruiz and M. Rosemary-Gomez, *Rev. Esp. Enferm. Dig.*, 2001, **93**, 423.
113. D. L. Keefe, *Semin. Oncol.*, 2001, **28**, 2.
114. A. Torraco, F. Diaz, U. D. Vempati and C. T. Moraes, *Biochim. Biophys. Acta*, 2009, **1793**, 171.
115. V. Vartanian, B. Lowell, I. G. Minko, T. G. Wood, J. D. Ceci, S. George, S. W. Ballinger, C. L. Corless, A. K. McCullough and R. S. Lloyd, *Proc. Natl. Acad. Sci. U. S. A.*, 2006, **103**, 1864.
116. Y. F. Chen, C. H. Kao, Y. T. Chen, C. H. Wang, C. Y. Wu, C. Y. Tsai, F. C. Liu, C. W. Yang, Y. H. Wei, M. T. Hsu, S. F. Tsai and T. F. Tsai, *Genes Dev.*, 2009, **23**, 1183.

CHAPTER 13

# *Non-Clinical Models for the Evaluation of Mechanisms of Toxicity*

JEFFREY A. KRAMER

Alcon Research Ltd., Department of Preclinical Safety, 6201 South Freeway, Fort Worth, TX 76134, USA

## 13.1 Introduction

Advancing a new molecular entity (NME), biological agent, or medical device into human clinical trials requires non-clinical safety evaluation in regulated studies using one or more non-clinical animal model species. For a small molecule, such studies minimally include mammalian toxicity, safety pharmacology, and genetic toxicity studies. Depending on the intended indication, duration of treatment, and patient population, additional non-clinical studies may include reproductive toxicology, immunotoxicology, and additional safety pharmacology studies over and above those required for all small molecule NMEs. For non-oral dose routes and for evaluations of pharmacology/efficacy, animal models other than the standard species may be most appropriate. In the early stages of drug discovery, some non-mammalian species are increasingly used for early whole organism screens. Finally, understanding and managing toxicity findings may often be accomplished most readily in still other animal models. Although these model species are typically used infrequently to support regulatory submissions, they may provide invaluable mechanistic information for the management of toxicology issues.

RSC Drug Discovery Series No. 12
New Horizons in Predictive Toxicology: Current Status and Application
Edited by Alan G. E. Wilson

Published by the Royal Society of Chemistry, www.rsc.org

The purpose of performing early preclinical safety assessments is not to show that a compound is "safe," but rather to identify the dose-limiting toxicity. Failure to identify dose-limiting toxicity in a pivotal GLP toxicology study can mean having to re-run the study at higher doses. Furthermore, the early identification of dose-limiting toxicities allows for characterization during the early stages of lead optimization, when the synthetic chemistry effort is active and a Structure–Toxicity Relationship (STR) can be developed. The key information in choosing to advance a compound into development is not the presence or absence of toxicity, but the nature of the toxicity (*i.e.*, reversibility and "monitorability"), and the margin relative to an efficacious dose or exposure at which the toxicity is observed (*i.e.*, the preclinical safety margin). Understanding the dose-limiting toxicity in non-clinical animal models allows clinicians to develop a clinical plan that allows for more rapid dose escalation to efficacious levels, while armed with evidence that, based on the non-clinical studies, the most likely dose-limiting adverse events in the clinic, when observed, will be monitorable and reversible. Since all compounds are toxic at some dose or exposure level, a key question is whether the dose-limiting toxicity is potentially limiting for further development. "Development-limiting" toxicity can be difficult to define, and depends on factors such as the safety margin (therapeutic index in the clinic); the nature of the toxicity (*i.e.*, reversibility, availability of monitorable biomarkers); the route of administration, duration of treatment and intended therapeutic indication being sought (*i.e.*, risk to benefit); and potential for occurrence in the human population at large.

Just as adverse drug reactions (ADR) in the clinic have been divided into broad categories,[1] toxicities identified in non-clinical animal models during the evaluation of NMEs can typically be divided into three broad types of dose limiting toxicity, each of which can best be managed and/or minimized by different means.[2] The three types of dose-limiting toxicity are: 1) adverse primary pharmacology, 2) secondary pharmacology, and 3) chemically mediated toxicity. Similar to type-A clinical ADRs in Park *et al.*, adverse primary pharmacology or "target-mediated toxicity" represents toxicity that results from modulation of the drug target. Since adverse primary pharmacology, like the efficacy being sought, is mediated by the primary drug target, this type of toxicity can be nearly impossible to avoid. Some adverse primary pharmacology may reflect exaggerated pharmacology, such as that seen with many antithrombotics, which at supra-efficacious exposures can cause hemorrhage.[3] In such cases, exaggerated pharmacology may be dealt with in the clinic through careful attention to dosage. With some types of adverse primary pharmacology, controlling the patient population may allow for the control of adverse primary pharmacology. For example, non-steroidal anti-inflammatory drugs (NSAIDs) that target cyclooxygenase I may cause severe gastrointestinal toxicity. Avoiding NSAID-sensitive populations or treating with cyclooxygenase II selective agents can be an effective way to manage this type of adverse primary pharmacology.[4] Due to their typically high specificity to their primary target, biologics often elicit only primary pharmacology mediated toxicity *in vivo*; but the humanized clinical test articles may also induce immunologic effects in non-clinical animal models, requiring the development of alternative approaches to the development of such agents. Regardless, adverse primary pharmacology is often impossible to avoid completely short of selecting a completely new drug target.

Secondary pharmacology is the result of a compound interacting with a secondary target, usually one that is structurally, functionally, or evolutionarily related to the primary therapeutic target. As with adverse primary pharmacologically mediated toxicity, secondary pharmacology can be predicted from the established pharmacology of the secondary target, provided the identity of that target is known. Dealing with adverse secondary pharmacology is often as easy as including an assay for the relevant secondary target in the testing funnel. However, it can be difficult to distinguish secondary pharmacology from other types of toxicity, and it is often difficult to identify the actual target responsible for the adverse effects observed *in vivo*, and the structure–activity relationships for the primary and secondary targets can be very similar, making it difficult to "design away from" the offending secondary pharmacology. For example, it took nearly 50 years to demonstrate that the gynaecomastia associated with spironolactone, a mineralocorticoid-receptor agonist, was associated with a second structurally related nuclear receptor; and then design a new MR agonist that spared the secondary target.[5,6]

Chemically mediated toxicity is independent of the pharmacologic targets with which a compound interacts, and is similar to the type-C ADRs described by Park *et al.*[1] These toxicities often exhibit discreet STRs, and can typically be screened out of a lead chemical series when identified early in the drug discovery process. In fact, *in vitro* assays exist for several specific types of toxicity, including steatosis,[7] phospholipidosis,[8,9] apoptosis,[10–13] reactive oxygen species,[14] cellular stress (please see Chapter 6), and mitochondrial toxicities[15] (please see Chapter 12). Although it may be impractical to screen every promising lead compound through all of these *in vitro* assays prospectively, upon identification in early *in vivo* toxicity studies, these relatively high-throughput cell-based assays can prove invaluable in understanding STR and screening out the liability in future leads. Regardless, in all of these types of toxicity management, non-clinical animal models play a significant role.

## 13.2 Standard Non-Clinical Toxicology Models

### 13.2.1 Mammalian Toxicity

Advancing a "typical" orally administered NME into first-in-human clinical trials minimally requires mammalian toxicity, safety pharmacology, and genetic toxicity studies. Mammalian toxicology studies must be performed in two species, one rodent and one non-rodent, by the same dosing route and at least equal duration to that intended for use in human trials.[16,17] Historically, the species of choice for these studies have included the rat almost exclusively as the rodent species, and the beagle dog or *cynomolgus* monkey as the non-rodent species. For these "hallmark" non-clinical model species there exists a significant body of knowledge of spontaneous lesions, many years of accumulated data on baseline clinical chemistry and hematology ranges, standardization and broad agreement regarding parameters for dose administration and blood collection (Table 13.1), and a prodigious database of compounds that have been assayed in single and repeat dose toxicology studies. This is particularly true for the mammalian toxicity assays in the rodent, where the volume of background data on the rat makes the use of the mouse or any other rodent for routine IND-enabling GLP toxicology studies unattractive in all but the most compelling cases. However, there are several reasons why the mouse might be considered a suitable model for the early *in vivo* toxicology signal generation studies. One obvious advantage of the mouse over the rat is the significantly lower compound requirement to conduct *in vivo* toxicology testing. This is of particular value in the early stages of drug discovery, when a project team may have multiple lead candidates and compound supply is limiting. One recent evaluation of an individual laboratory's experience and an exhaustive evaluation of the literature have suggested that the mouse is a suitable alternative to the rat for mammalian (rodent) toxicology studies.[18]

When selecting the non-rodent ("second") species for mammalian toxicity assessment, several factors must be considered. Perhaps the single most critical consideration in selecting an appropriate non-rodent animal model when

**Table 13.1** Recommendations for substance administration and blood removal.[a]

| *Dose volumes (mL kg$^{-1}$)* | | | | | *Blood volume and recommended sites* | |
|---|---|---|---|---|---|---|
| *Species* | *Oral* | *Subcutaneous* | *Intraperitoneal* | *Intravenous (bolus)* | *Volume (mL) kg$^{-1}$* | *Recommended site(s) for blood collection by species* |
| Mouse | 10 (50)[b] | 10 (40) | 20 (80) | 5 | 72 | Saphenous, tail |
| Rat | 10 (40) | 5 (10) | 10 (20) | 5 | 64 | Saphenous, tail |
| Hamster | 10 (20) | 10 (20) | 20 | 5 | [d] | [d] |
| Guinea pig | 10 (20) | [c] | 10 | 5 | [d] | [d] |
| Rabbit | 10 (15) | 1 (2) | 5 (20) | 2 | 56 | Marginal ear, central ear artery, jugular |
| Dog | 5 (15) | 1 (2) | 1 (20) | 2.5 | 85 | Cephalic, jugular, saphenous |
| Monkey | 5 (15) | 2 (5) | (10)[c] | 2 | 65 | Cephalic, saphenous, femoral |
| Minipig | 10 (15) | 1 (2) | 1 (20) | 2.5 | 65 | Cranial vena cava |

[a]Data collected from refs. 89 and 90.
[b]The first number is a maximum volume (per kg of body weight) considered good practice and recommended for repeated dose administration. The number in parentheses is a maximum volume for a single dose administration.
[c]No data is available for subcutaneous dosing in the guinea pig, or for repeated intraperitoneal dosing in the non-human primate.
[d]Blood volume data and recommended collection site information was not found for hamster and guinea pig.

advancing a NME is the ADME (absorption, distribution, metabolism, elimination) profile. Knowledge of the metabolic profile in humans and the non-clinical species from *in vitro* studies with liver preparations (S9 fractions, microsomes, and/or primary hepatocytes) are particularly useful. Non-rodent species selection may also be based in part on *in vivo* pharmacokinetic studies to determine bioavailability and metabolic profile. Additionally, pharmacology and pilot toxicity studies in rodent and non-rodent animal models may provide valuable information for selecting the most appropriate second species for mammalian safety assessment. Although generally less expensive and more readily available, it has been recommended that the dog should be selected as the non-rodent species for pharmacodynamic, pharmacokinetic, metabolic and other scientific reasons, and not solely for practical considerations.[19] Similarly, a simple assumption that the non-human primate, being evolutionary closer to human than is the dog, is more predictive for human safety, may be an overly simplistic view in the absence of pharmacodynamic, pharmacokinetic, and metabolic data.

The primary outcome of standard mammalian toxicology studies is the identification and characterization of dose-limiting toxicity. Information on the dose-limiting toxicity (or toxicities) in the most sensitive species is used to determine several key parameters that are in turn used for later safety assessments and for clinical trial design. Among these parameters are the no-observed-effect level (NOEL), the no-observed-adverse-effect level (NOAEL), the lowest-observed-adverse-effect level (LOAEL), the maximum-tolerated dose (MTD), and the safety margin.[20,21] The NOEL is routinely defined as the highest dose (or exposure) at which no statistically or biologically significant effects are observed in the treated population compared to the appropriate control population. Since not all observed effects are clearly compound mediated and/or adverse, the NOAEL has been used to identify the dose (or exposure) at which no statistically or toxicologically significant adverse effects are observed in the treated population compared to the appropriate control population. The LOAEL is the lowest tested dose (or exposure) at which statistically or toxicologically adverse findings are observed. The MTD is historically defined as the dose that causes a 10% weight loss in a repeated dose sub-chronic toxicology study, however parameters other than weight loss may be used to determine the MTD. Although there is debate regarding the utility of the MTD, this concept is still among those used in setting doses for carcinogenicity studies and other IND- and NDA-enabling non-clinical studies. In order to determine a safety margin, some indication of toxicity (typically the NOAEL) is compared to the predicted human efficacious exposure or the exposure at a fully efficacious dose in a widely accepted non-clinical model of disease.[20,21] These parameters are used for several key decisions within pharmaceutical companies, but more importantly, the NOAEL in the most sensitive species (unless mechanistic toxicology studies convincingly suggest that a particular non-clinical dose-limiting toxicity is not relevant for humans), along with pharmacokinetic (PK) and pharmacodynamic (PD) data and modeling are used to estimate the human equivalent dose (HED) and select a maximum recommended starting dose (MRSD) for first-in-human clinical trials.[22] Since the MRSD can determine the number of dose escalation groups needed to achieve sufficient exposure for the demonstration of a desired effect (and for the identification of the dose-limiting adverse effect), the determination of a MRSD can have significant implications for the cost and duration of the first phase of clinical development.

### 13.2.2 Genetic Toxicity and Carcinogenicity

Among the non-clinical safety studies that must be performed on NMEs prior to advancement into clinical trials are a standard battery of genetic toxicity evaluations.[23] Additional carcinogenicity assays may be required for some NMEs prior to registration.[24] The standard battery of genetic toxicology assays required to support an investigational new drug (IND) application comprises a bacterial gene mutation assay, an *in vitro* cytogenetic test for chromosomal damage or mouse lymphoma tk gene mutation assay, and an *in vivo* test for genotoxicity. An alternative option has been proposed that is comprised of the bacterial gene mutation test along with an *in vivo* assessment of genotoxicity with two tissues, and a second *in vivo* assay.[25] In both standard battery options, the *in vivo* genotoxicity assays can often be integrated into repeat-dose mammalian toxicity studies, provided that the dose levels are sufficient to meet the criteria delineated in the regulatory guidance. As such, selection of the most appropriate non-clinical animal model for IND-enabling mammalian toxicity studies may also include the possibility of adding genetic toxicity assessments. For an additional and more detailed review of *in vivo* approaches to genetic toxicity, please see Chapter 15 of this book. Carcinogenicity assessments prior to registration are typically performed only in rodents, and these have increasingly utilized genetic mouse models (please see section 13.4, below).

### 13.2.3 Safety Pharmacology

The core battery of safety pharmacology studies typically required prior to advancement of a NME into human trials includes an assessment of effects on cardiovascular, central nervous, and respiratory systems in accordance with regulatory guidelines ICH S7A and S7B.[26] An assessment of cardiovascular effects must include an evaluation of cardiac output, ventricular contractility, vascular resistance, and effects on cardiovascular responses to endogenous or exogenous substances. The QT interval of the ECG is widely accepted as an endpoint to gauge effects of a test substance on ventricular repolarization. The telemeterized dog model has gained broad acceptance in the pharmaceutical industry. In one reported comparison of conscious *vs.* anesthetized dogs, both models detected QT interval prolongation with similar sensitivity.[27] These investigators favored the conscious dog model, due in part to the opportunity for extended continuous ECG recording, and to a lower sensitivity in the anesthetized dogs with at least one positive control agent. However, several factors should be considered when deciding on the non-clinical animal model used to conduct these studies. These include factors such as heart rate (particularly in conscious *vs.* anesthetized animals) that may confound interpretation of QT interval data, and potential inter-species and gender differences in cardiac electrophysiology, hemodynamics, and/or metabolism.

Central nervous system effects are typically evaluated in the rat or mouse. These include the functional observation battery (FOB) in rats[28] or the modified Irwin assay, performed in the mouse.[29] The CNS effects that ought to be evaluated include motor activity, behavioral changes, coordination, sensory/motor reflex responses and body temperature. The evaluation of respiratory function ought to include an assessment of airway resistance, compliance, pulmonary arterial pressure, blood gas, and blood pH, and are most commonly performed in the rat. However, respiratory function can also be assessed in the species used for the pivotal non-rodent mammalian toxicology studies. Additional studies may be required when there is a cause for concern to evaluate potential effects on organ systems not addressed by the core battery or by the standard repeat-dose mammalian toxicity studies. These may include specific assessments of renal function, which can typically be accomplished by examination of the appropriate analytes in urine and blood collected as part of the pivotal mammalian toxicology studies,[30] or gastrointestinal function (*e.g.*, charcoal meal test in the rat,[31] among others).

As with genetic toxicity endpoints (see above), there have recently been efforts aimed at integrating safety pharmacology endpoints into mammalian toxicology studies.[32] For example, endpoints related to behavior (*i.e.*, FOB) and cardiovascular toxicity may be integrated into the standard mammalian toxicology studies. Such studies can also allow interpretation of safety pharmacology endpoints along with clinical chemistry, hematology, and histopathology data. However, the limitations of conducting safety pharmacology measurements in IND-enabling mammalian toxicology studies must be acknowledged. Although technical progress in non-invasive methodologies has been made, there is as yet no replacement for telemetry. The potential complications in data analysis presented by surgically implanting telemetry units into animals intended for pivotal mammalian toxicology studies make this option undesirable. However, simple veterinary health observations of heart rate, respiration, behavior, and GI effects including food consumption and bowel movements in the mammalian toxicity studies can direct and inform dose selection for safety pharmacology studies. For this reason, safety pharmacology studies should ideally complement toxicity studies where possible with respect to species and dose regimen.

### 13.2.4 Reproductive Toxicology

An assessment of the potential of a NME to cause reproductive and/or developmental toxicity must include an evaluation of the test agent's effects on six stages of fertility, reproduction and development. As defined in ICH S5A,[33] these stages are pre-mating to conception (adult male and female reproductive functions, development and maturation of gametes, mating behavior, fertilization); conception to implantation (adult female reproductive functions, pre-implantation development, implantation); organogenesis (defined as implantation to closure of the hard palate); perinatal development (closure of the hard palate to the end of pregnancy); birth to weaning (adult female reproductive functions, neonate adaption to extra uterine life, pre-weaning development and growth); and weaning to sexual maturity (post weaning development and growth, adaption to independent life, attainment of full sexual function). An assessment of the effects of a NME on these processes is most often accomplished by three categories of *in vivo* study, the so-called segment I, segment II, and segment III assays. The selection of appropriate non-clinical *in vivo* models for reproductive toxicology evaluations relies on the same considerations as for other non-clinical safety studies (*e.g.*, bioavailability, pharmacokinetics, pharmacologic response); but also depends upon a knowledge of the reproductive biology of the species to be utilized.

The segment I fertility study includes administration of test article to both genders for a period of time sufficient to span the period of gametogenesis, and continues with treatment of the female until implantation.[34] The rodent is a particularly convenient model for an assessment of drug mediated effects of fertility due to the relatively brief gestation time (~3 weeks) and rapid spermatogenesis (~3 weeks). Additionally, spermatogenesis in the rodent tends to occur in waves, such that an entire follicle in the testis contains a single population of gametes at the same developmental stage, making visualization of stage specific effects simpler. Segment II developmental toxicity studies are typically performed in two species, a rodent, and a non-rodent (often the rabbit). Test article administration can be performed from implantation through the end of the major period of organogenesis. In the mouse or rat this period is from gestational day (g.d.) 5 until g.d. 17. In the rabbit, the period spans g.d. 6 to g.d. 19. Segment III studies are usually performed in a single rodent species. Except for considerations of test article needs (often not an issue at the late stage in pharmaceutical development at which segment III studies are performed), the rat typically provides significant advantages over the mouse, including the fact that in most cases the earlier pivotal rodent mammalian toxicology studies were most likely performed in the rat.

None of the non-clinical species commonly used for reproductive toxicology assessment are a perfect model for human reproduction and development, and all species have advantages and disadvantages. The ICH S5A guidance lists a number of disadvantages for common non-clinical models that may impact their utility for understanding mechanisms of reproductive toxicology. Some of these disadvantages have been summarized in Table 13.2. As noted in Table 13.2, the non-human primate, though often unsuitable for detecting a reproductive toxicology liability due to low animal numbers, may be the best model when characterizing a known or suspected reproductive toxicant. For additional information detailing *in vivo* models for the assessment of reproductive and developmental toxicology, please see Chapter 18 of this book.

**Table 13.2** Disadvantages of common non-clinical animal models for reproductive toxicology.

| *Species* | *Issue/disadvantage* |
|---|---|
| Rat | Sensitivity to sex hormones, unsuitable for dopamine agonists (prolactin dependence during early pregnancy), highly susceptibility to NSAIDs late in pregnancy. |
| Mouse | Rapid metabolic rate, sensitivity to stress, small fetus. |
| Rabbit | Often little kinetic and toxicity data, susceptible to some antibiotics and to disturbance of the alimentary tract, clinical signs can be difficult to interpret. |
| Guinea pig | Often little kinetic and toxicity data, susceptibility to some antibiotics and to disturbance of the alimentary tract, long fetal period, limited historical background data. |
| Pig/minipig | Malformation clusters with variable background rate, large amounts of compound required, limited historical background data. |
| Ferret | Typically a seasonal breeder, limited historical background data. |
| Hamster | Intravenous dose route very difficult, can hide doses in the cheek pouches, sensitive to intestinal disturbance, overly sensitive teratogenic response to many chemicals, small fetus. |
| Dog | Seasonal breeders, inbreeding factors, limited historical background data. |
| NHP | Non-human primates can differ kinetically from humans as much as other species, limited historical background data, numbers often too low for risk detection. May be most suitable when the objective is to characterize a relatively certain reproductive toxicant. |

## 13.2.5 Immunotoxicology

For the purposes of seeking regulatory approval, immunotoxicity can be defined as either unintended immunosuppression or enhancement, and agents can be divided into those that are intended to modulate immune function, and those that are not.[35] Regardless, all NMEs should be evaluated for the potential to produce immunotoxicity. The earliest signal(s) of immunotoxic potential may be obtained from the standard mammalian toxicity studies. These include: hematological changes in particular white blood cell populations (such as leukocytopenia/leukocytosis, granulocytopenia/granulocytosis, or lymphopenia/lymphocytosis); alterations in immune system organ weights and/or histology (*e.g.*, thymus, spleen, lymph nodes, bone marrow); and/or changes in serum globulins that occur without other plausible explanations. Any statistically significant and dose-dependent change in the above parameters in IND-enabling studies in any species may signal an effect on immune function.

If a weight-of-evidence evaluation suggests immunotoxic potential, additional immunotoxicity studies may be required. The primary non-clinical immune function study specifically detailed in the regulatory guidance[35] is the T-cell dependent antibody response (TDAR). The generally accepted TDAR study design is in the rodent, although adaptations have been described using non-rodent species.[36] Where possible, the species and strain used (along with dose, duration, and route of administration) should be consistent with the mammalian toxicity study in which the immunotoxic potential was first identified. Additional non-clinical studies that may be required include immunophenotyping, natural killer cell activity assays, host resistance studies, macrophage/neutrophil function assays, and cell-mediated immunity assays such as the delayed-type hypersensitivity assay. For additional details on *in vivo* models for the assessment of immunotoxicology, please see Chapter 17 of this book.

## 13.3 Non-Standard and Mechanistic Non-Clinical Toxicology Models

With few exceptions, the non-clinical species and assays described in the previous section are intended for the identification of toxicity, rather than for the evaluation and management of known toxic liabilities. These assays often provide little information on the nature (*i.e.*, mechanism) of the toxicity observed. Upon identification in the "standard" IND enabling studies, toxicology issues are managed by evaluating the risk to human subjects. In order to determine if the findings are development limiting, the answers to a number of questions about the toxicity are critical. These "issue management" questions revolve around safety margin (*i.e.*, the window between a fully efficacious dose or exposure and the highest safe dose/exposure of NOAEL), reversibility, monitorability, and mechanism. The answers to these questions are key in determining the relevance of the finding to humans. The first two questions are typically addressed in the standard *in vivo* toxicology studies, and established clinical pathology (*i.e.*, hematology, clinical chemistry, urinalysis, coagulation) endpoints. Ongoing efforts at the identification of novel toxicity biomarkers (please see Chapter 19 of this book) can address the third question. However, an understanding of the mechanism by which toxicity is mediated can be key to positioning the finding with respect to human relevance. When designing studies to understand the nature of a particular dose-limiting toxicity, and when toxicity is related directly to the primary pharmacology, and when evaluating NMEs for non-oral dose routes, species other than the "standard" species detailed above are often used.

The *in vivo* pharmacology of a NME or drug target is often studied in an *in vivo* model other than one of the standard non-clinical toxicology species. In many cases this is because the model used has a particular similarity to human biology in a key biological system being studied. In such cases, the species in which pharmacology is evaluated may be most suitable for delineating the mechanism of toxicity. If the observed toxicity is related to the pharmacology of the target and NME, then minimal severity (or absence) of the toxicity in standard non-clinical species may not signal the lack of risk for human subjects, since the non-standard animal model was presumably selected based upon similarity to humans for some key system or function. When using non-standard animal models for toxicity assessments, it is critical to understand the issues and limitations of those models. Perhaps most common among these is the lack of ADME/PK data. As described earlier, an evaluation of the metabolic fate of a NME in the common non-clinical species is key to species selection and study design. The differences in xenobiotic metabolism in the more common non-clinical species are fairly well characterized. This is less true for the less common species. Thus, the significance of the paucity of ADME/PK data is even more compelling in light of the often incomplete understanding of the metabolic capacity of these atypical animal models. For example, McConkey *et al.*[37] hypothesize that a deficiency in *N*-acetyltransferase activity in cats may contribute to species-dependent metabolism-mediated toxicity of acetaminophen in this species. In spite of this and other limitations, Sekis *et al.*[38] used the cat to perform the Comet assay to address a positive result observed in one of the standard battery of genetic toxicity assays.

Another significant issue with the use of non-standard animal models is the lack of historical comparator data, along with limited historical ranges for common clinical pathology parameters, and a general lack of reagents (*e.g.*, species-specific antibodies, DNA sequence information, validated kits, reagents, and methods). Finally, it can be difficult to find contract research organizations familiar with these less-common species or thought leaders on the use of these species that also have significant industry and drug safety experience. In spite of these limitations, there exists a number of *in vivo* models for evaluating specific safety issues in non-standard species. One such example is the ferret emesis model. In situations where safety pharmacology studies of GI function are called for, the ferret emesis model has gained broad acceptance.[39,40]

### 13.3.1 *In Vivo* Models for Toxicity Screening

Along with their use for mechanistic studies and non-oral dose routes, a number of non-standard non-clinical models have been developed for *in vivo* screening. As well as its utility in the emesis model (above), the ferret has also been used as a model for electrophysiology and cardiac safety.[41,42] When compared to the dog, one significant advantage of the ferret is its small size, making it ideal for comparing several NMEs after a safety pharmacology issue was previously identified with an early lead in the more standard safety pharmacology battery. The use of non-standard species for retrospective evaluations to "screen out" known safety liabilities can result in savings of time, money and resources. Similarly, there have been efforts to introduce *in vivo* safety studies earlier in project testing funnels, to identify dose-limiting toxicity, understand STR, and prioritize the most promising leads while the synthetic chemistry effort is fully engaged. One approach to move *in vivo* screening earlier in the testing funnel is the use of early whole-organism screens. For this application, small organisms such as the zebrafish have gained popularity.[43] For additional information on models for whole organism toxicity screening, please see Chapter 14 of this book.

### 13.3.2 Models for Non-Oral Dose Routes

Although a significant proportion of NMEs evaluated in regulated non-clinical toxicology studies are intended for oral administration in the clinic, other routes of administration are not uncommon. Many of these non-orally-delivered agents are evaluated non-clinically in animal models that were selected based on biological and structural/morphological similarities to humans in key parameters. For example, differences in ocular structure between humans and rodents make the rat or mouse less than ideal for the prediction of human ocular toxicity risk. Specifically, vitreous volume is approximately 0.02 ml in rats, 1.5 ml in rabbits, 3.0 ml in *cynomolgus* monkeys, and 4.0 ml in humans.[44] Overall eye size in the rodent is much smaller than in the other common non-clinical species, whereas it is quite similar between rabbit, nonhuman primate, and human. The rabbit anterior chamber and lens are larger than in the monkey, whereas the vitreous is larger in the monkey than in the rabbit.[44] These features, along with the lower cost and ready availability of the rabbit relative to the non-human primate, make the rabbit the most common non-clinical model for safety assessment *via* ocular routes. This is true both for topical ocular administration,[45] as well as intracameral and intravitreal routes.[46–48] Since test article amount is not typically a factor in ocular studies, the size of the non-clinical animal models is less of an issue, and species can be selected based on ocular morphology rather than test article requirements. For this reason, large species such as the minipig are more commonly used in ocular toxicity assessments[49] than for systemic toxicity. For otic administrations, the chinchilla has been used for non-clinical assessments both of topical otic and middle ear injection studies.[50,51] The suitability of chinchillas is largely due to the otic morphology of this species. In particular, the large bullas and (comparatively) readily accessible middle ear space, along with well characterized hearing thresholds and parameters and sensitivity to drug exposure make this an ideal model for ototoxicity assessments.[52]

### 13.3.3 Models for Idiosyncratic Toxicity

As noted previously, adverse drug reactions (ADRs) in the clinic have been divided into broad categories.[1] The categories include type-A "augmented" ADRs that are a direct result of the pharmacology of the drug target, type-B idiosyncratic reactions, type-C "chemically" mediated ADRs that are a function of the chemical properties of the drug, and type-D "delayed" ADRs (such as carcinogenicity). The type-B idiosyncratic ADRs are typically not predictable from the pharmacology of the drug target, show differences in individual susceptibility, and lack clear dose dependence. Although idiosyncratic ADRs cannot at this time be reliably predicted non-clinically, there have been hypotheses put forward that implicate a role for reactive metabolites and for inflammation and oxidative stress.[53–55] Any model that claims to predict the potential for idiosyncratic toxicity may face significant challenges to gaining broad support in the scientific community, since the resulting assays would be virtually impossible to validate empirically. As a result, such models could only serve to generate largely un-testable concerns around what may be otherwise promising drug candidates. When applied, such assays should be positioned early in the testing funnel to reduce risk amongst a series of leads, rather than used as an attempt to identify an actual safety liability. Additional details concerning the state of the art in predicting idiosyncratic toxicity potential can be found in Chapter 25 of this book.

## 13.4 Genetic Models

Throughout the pharmaceutical industry, researchers routinely seek early confirmation of pharmacologic effect both pre-clinically and in the clinic in an effort to address one of the primary sources of attrition (*i.e.*, lack of efficacy in clinical trials). In the pre-clinical setting, this has increasingly included genetic as well as pharmacologic proof-of-concept (POC). That is, as well as seeking pharmacologic POC *via* systemic exposure of an early lead in a non-clinical model of disease; researchers increasingly use RNA interference, short-interfering RNA, transgenic, and gene knockout technologies. These technologies can be used to achieve genetic POC for a particular drug target by interfering with the function of that target in the absence of any test article in a non-clinical disease model.[56–58] This same approach holds great promise for pre-clinical safety assessment, where differentiating adverse primary pharmacology from secondary pharmacology (so-called "off-target" effects) can be a key to dealing with a toxicologic finding. When advancing NMEs directed against drug targets from very large gene families, such as the kinases, it can be very difficult to identify an active compound that does not also interact with one or more structurally related secondary targets.[59] In such cases a toxicity mediated by secondary pharmacology can seem like adverse primary pharmacology, since the STR for both targets may be highly conserved. The ability to recreate a dose-limiting toxicity in the absence of exposure to the NME in a non-clinical model in which the primary target has been knocked out can provide definitive mechanistic evidence that the toxicity is related to a secondary molecular target. Given the frequency with which any small molecule may interact with "other" molecular targets *in vivo*, such studies will become increasingly valuable as researchers strive to differentiate new pharmaceutical agents based on their safety profiles. Even before screening compound libraries for compounds capable of modulating the activity of a particular drug target, exhaustive characterization of gene knockout models can provide hints regarding the toxicity liabilities likely to be confronted in drug-discovery efforts. Such analyses ought to be included in any process by which new drug targets are evaluated.[60]

### 13.4.1 Carcinogenicity Models

Along with their potential value in understanding the toxicologic liabilities of particular drug targets, genetic models have also been developed and applied to address specific issues in drug development. In particular, genetic models have achieved relevance as alternatives to the two-year rodent carcinogenicity assay, which is typically required prior to registration of any NME intended for chronic or intermittent use over six months of duration.[61] These studies are typically the most expensive non-clinical studies performed. They require a significant amount of active pharmaceutical ingredient, large numbers of animals, and significant amounts of *in vivo* technical and animal husbandry staff support. As such, carcinogenicity studies are often development rate-limiting and are typically not completed until late in the development process. Conducting these studies so late in the development of a NME can increase both the risk and complexity of the development process. A number of these genetic models for carcinogenicity assessment have been characterized in collaborations spanning industry, academia, and regulatory agencies. These include the rasH2 transgenic model, the $p53^{+/-}$ heterozygous mouse, the TgAC transgenic mouse, the $xpa^{-/-}$ knockout mouse, and $xpa/p53^{+/-}$ mouse model.[62] In general, these assessments demonstrated clear benefits to the use of some of these genetic models of carcinogenicity,[63,64] though the models were not without issues and false positive and false negative results.[65,66] Although not fully agreed upon within the scientific community and between different regulatory agencies, there is a consensus building that the $p53^{+/-}$ heterozygous mouse model may be particularly suited to identify hormonally mediated carcinogenic mechanisms, immunosuppressive carcinogens, and genotoxic carcinogens, whereas the TgAC transgenic mouse may predict for topically applied carcinogens.[67] These and other assessments have suggested that the rasH2 transgenic model may be useful in the detection of both nongenotoxic and genotoxic rodent tumorigens, with improved concordance with human response.[67] An additional review of the genetic mouse models for carcinogenicity can be found in Chapters 15 on *in vivo* approaches to genotoxicity assessment.

### 13.4.2 Genetic Models for Mechanistic Toxicity

In addition to genetic models developed specifically to address issues in drug development, genetic models have been used to address specific mechanisms of toxicity for a number of well known toxicants. The increasing availability, variety, and complexity of genetic models make it more possible to evaluate new potential targets for pharmaceutical intervention for safety as well as efficacy. Complex genetic models such as humanized "knock-in" models make it possible to evaluate mechanisms of non-clinical toxicity of NMEs, and to evaluate potential safety liabilities of the drug targets themselves, well in advance of a synthetic effort to identify small molecules that mediate their activity.[68] A thorough characterization of genetic models can identify broad liabilities associated with therapeutic approaches, and even point to ways to address/minimize limitations in predictivity for human risk.

The chemical class known as peroxisome proliferators (PP) includes a number of chemically distinct environmental toxicants, industrial chemicals, and commercially available pharmaceutical agents that express specific pleiotropic effects, including hepatomegaly, increased fatty acid β-oxidation, and an increase in the number and volume of peroxisomes in responsive tissues.[69–71]

These effects are mediated *via* the peroxisome proliferator activated receptor (PPAR)-α, a member of the nuclear hormone receptor family. Upon binding a PP in the cytosol, PPAR-α forms a heterodimer with RXR, another member of the nuclear hormone receptor family, and translocates to the nucleus, where it recognizes and binds to a specific sequence element (the peroxisome proliferator response element or PPRE) in the promoter of PP responsive genes. Upon binding the PPAR-α:RXR heterodimer recruits the transcriptional machinery and brings about the expression of PP responsive genes. A characterization of the PPAR-α knockout mouse line demonstrated that disruption of the gene resulted in a complete abolishment of the pleiotropic effects of the peroxisome proliferators clofibrate and WY-14 643 in adult mice.[70] Additionally, Abbott *et al.*[72] demonstrated that the developmental toxicity of the potent PP perfluorooctanoic acid, including delayed eye opening and post-natal weight gain and lethality, was dependent upon expression of PPAR-α in the mouse. Interestingly, studies in PPAR-α humanized mice support other research suggesting that many of the PP-mediated adverse effects observed in the rodent liver do not translate to human risk.[73–75] Specifically in both PPAR-α null and PPAR-α humanized mice, hepatocyte necrosis observed in response to exposure to PP in wild-type mice was markedly diminished.[76] The ability to use genetic models to identify species-specific drug-induced toxicities represents a potential giant leap forward in the predictivity of non-clinical studies for human risk and safety.

In other experiments, genetic models have demonstrated utility in understanding adaptive responses to how organisms deal with compound mediated toxicity. For example, in a mouse model of Parkinson's disease, estradiol provides protection against the neurotoxic effects of 1-methyl-4-phenyl-1,2,3,6-tetrahydropyridine (MPTP). In estrogen receptor (ER) knockout mice, estradiol treatment did not exhibit significant neuroprotective effects suggesting a greater susceptibility to MPTP toxicity.[77] The protective effects of estradiol corresponded to prevention of MPTP mediated decreases in striatal dopamine and dopamine metabolite concentrations in wild type, but not ER knockout mice, suggesting the possibility of an estradiol : ER mediated effect on transporter and/or metabolic enzyme levels. Several other studies using genetic mouse models in which a specific transporter or cytochrome P450 gene has been knocked out have also demonstrated the utility of this approach for understanding the role of metabolism and distribution in compound mediated toxicity. For example, studies of the toxicant docetaxel in cytochrome P450 (CYP)3A knockout mice demonstrated higher drug exposure levels and increased sensitivity to docetaxel toxicity compared to wild-type mice, suggesting a role for CYP3A in detoxification of this chemotherapeutic agent.[78] In additional characterizations of the CYP3A knockout mice, the utility of genetic models for delineating complex detoxification pathways was demonstrated.[79] Specifically, the metabolism of midazolam, a widely used probe for CYP3A activity was evaluated using CYP3A knockout and wild-type mice. Surprisingly, comparable amounts of midazolam and its major metabolites were observed in the plasma of both CYP3A knockout and wild-type mice.

Additional studies provided evidence that CYP2C enzymes, which were found to be up-regulated in the CYP3A knockout mice, were responsible for the midazolam metabolism observed.[79] Although until recently only mouse genetically engineered models have been readily available, there are now several reports detailing the generation of gene knockout rats.[80–82]

## 13.5 *In Vivo* Technologies

Alongside the non-clinical animal models for mechanistic toxicology are a number of new and developing technologies that bear mention as particularly useful tools for the evaluation of the mechanism(s) of toxicity and the management of dose-limiting toxicities in the drug discovery and development paradigm. The generation of genetic animal models (see previous section) is itself a comparatively young *in vivo* technology with profound impact on mechanistic toxicology. However, there are other technologies, some older, some quite new, that when applied appropriately, hold the potential to aid in our understanding of toxicity mechanisms, and assist with the management of dose-limiting adverse effects.

Although genetic models and their application to mechanistic toxicity have been dealt with earlier in the present chapter, it is worth noting that high-throughput "genome-wide" phenotyping approaches have been described.[83] Although such platforms have been largely developed for the identification of novel disease genes with the primary purpose of target discovery,[84] the potential value for mechanistic toxicity assessment is significant. As noted above, this sort of approach offers the possibility to identify and characterize adverse primary pharmacology before a chemical library is screened or a single new compound is synthesized. Furthermore, several promising targets for a particular disease area can be compared not just with respect to pharmacologic effect (efficacy) and "druggability," but also for safety liabilities, resulting in the selection of superior drug targets. High-throughput knockout phenotyping offers the potential for developing new genetic disease models, and the possibility of studying toxicity in genetic disease models relevant for human health. The approach offers potential models to test not just primary but also secondary pharmacology hypotheses. High-throughput phenotyping of knockout (KO) lines provides a substrate for complex breeding to generate multigenic KO lines, and for generation of humanized lines to assess human risk of toxicities observed pre-clinically. The observation of similar knockout phenotypes may lead to the identification of novel pathway linkages and/or common biological activities of poorly studied genes and gene products.

Similarly, biomarkers have garnered much attention recently. The identification of new biomarkers holds great promise for identifying toxicity earlier in the drug-discovery process. Although "type D" delayed clinical ADRs by definition cannot be identified in short-duration studies, there have been efforts to validate existing biomarkers or identify novel ones for the preclinical prediction of some delayed toxicities.[85,86] This could allow for the opportunity to predict chronic toxicities earlier, possibly facilitating the ability to screen out the liability with short *in vivo* studies rather than identifying the toxicity only after lengthy and expensive repeated dose toxicity studies. If the biomarkers work acutely, or can even be used in primary cell lines where there is no validated *in vitro* screen for the adverse effect, the toxicity (once identified in early *in vivo* signal generation studies), could be rapidly screened out of a lead series while the synthetic chemistry effort is still actively engaged. But perhaps the greatest promise for biomarker research is the identification of "bridging" biomarkers; biomarkers that faithfully predict toxicity (or target interaction or outcome) in both non-clinical models and in human subjects. The ability in the clinic to track changes in a biomarker that has been shown to predict toxicity non-clinically allows for the clinician to withdraw treatment before an adverse event becomes severe and/or irreversible. As noted earlier, the purpose of non-clinical toxicology studies is not to show that the compound is safe, but to identify the dose-limiting toxicity in the most sensitive non-clinical species, and characterize that toxicity with respect to margin of safety, "monitorability," reversibility, and mechanism. Novel biomarkers that improve our ability to predict toxicity pre-clinically and monitor it clinically, hold great value, and are discussed at length in this book (please see Chapter 19).

Another area in which new or existing technologies are adding value to non-clinical safety assessment is the addition of new analyses into toxicology studies. For example, the inclusion of veterinary physical examinations in non-clinical studies provides several potential benefits. Physical exam endpoints such as general health assessments and veterinary evaluations of organ systems are increasingly performed on general toxicology studies. These may include assessments of general health and appearance, eyes and mucous membranes, as well as in-life evaluation of integumentary, musculo-skeletal, circulatory, respiratory, digestive, genito-urinary, otic, neural, and lymphatic systems. Additionally, telemetry and pulse oximetry to evaluate blood pressure, pulse rate, blood oxygen, and other cardiac endpoints in general toxicology studies are increasingly included. Such analyses will not replace the need for additional safety pharmacology studies (when prescribed by the regulatory guidelines), but they may hint at issues that will arise in such studies. Since short-term *in vivo* signal generation studies and standard mammalian toxicity studies are typically completed prior to IND-enabling safety pharmacology studies (which are typically completed immediately prior to preparation of IND documents), earlier identification of potential safety pharmacology "signals" could trigger the more predictive safety pharmacology studies earlier in a drugs' development, before significant resources have been expended. Additionally, ophthalmic examinations have been used with some success as a non-invasive method to assess general health and well-being.[87]

Finally, along with the inclusion telemetry and pulse oximetry (above), several other technologies have demonstrated great value in expanding the utility gleaned from and mechanistic opportunities provided by *in vivo* toxicology studies. Since the advent of mass spectrometry, nearly constant improvement in sensitivity has allowed for increased ease in the determination of exposure and estimation of pharmacokinetic parameters. Although the high doses routinely used in systemic toxicology studies do not require great sensitivity to measure exposure, systemic exposure must also be assessed following dose administration by other routes, such as topical ocular, dermal, otic, nasal, *etc*. Such dosing routes may often result in very low levels of systemic exposure, however systemic toxicity studies are required (along with studies via the route sought for clinical use). In such cases, relating the dose-limiting systemic toxicity to the likely systemic exposure caused by the intended clinical route requires the determination of $C_{max}$ and an estimation of the area under the dose–response curve (AUC) following dosing *via* the intended route. Another particularly useful technological development is the ability to continuously monitor and automatically sample the blood. The Culex system allows for continuous monitoring of selected parameters (notably pulse rate and blood pressure), while also allowing for automated blood sampling. Blood volume constraints, animal care and use guidelines regarding the number of blood collections allowed per animal in a 24 hour period, and the repeated use of anesthesia (required for many of the most common routes of blood collection), make it difficult to collect rich pharmacokinetic datasets. In addition, the time required to collect each time point can make it difficult to collect sufficient data immediately following dose administration to characterize the uptake of rapidly distributed and/or very short half-life compounds, and difficult to accurately calculate $C_{max}$ following intravenous administration. Automated blood sampling holds great potential for collection of several time points in rapid succession immediately after dose administration, and/or the collection of multiple time points during the terminal phase, allowing for more accurate determination of key pharmacokinetic parameters. Automated blood sampling has demonstrated value in *in vivo* studies,[88] and holds great potential for creating PK/PD and TK/TD models linking pharmacokinetic and toxicokinetic data with pharmacodynamic and toxicodynamic effects.

## 13.6 Conclusions

Advancing a new molecular entity into human clinical trials requires safety assessment in non-clinical animal models. With compound attrition increasing at all stages of drug development, and differentiation against marketed agents increasingly important, the mechanistic understanding of toxicity has become critical to successfully advancing NMEs into the clinic and onto the market. The safety evaluation of new molecular entities and devices requires studies in several non-clinical animal models for the identification and characterization of dose-limiting toxicity. Upon identification, positioning toxicity with respect to human relevance is a key component of the risk assessment required to advance drugs into the clinic. In this endeavor, an evaluation of the mechanism of the dose-limiting toxicity is critical. Such non-clinical studies may require the use of "common" animal models such as the rat, mouse, dog, and monkey, as well as less common and "niche" models such as the ferret, pig, guinea pig, hamster, chinchilla, and zebrafish. A full understanding of the strengths and weaknesses of each species will allow for the selections of the most appropriate model to evaluate and understand pharmacology and toxicology *in vivo*. Additional mechanistic studies are increasingly possible using genetic models and novel *in vivo* technologies, and the potential afforded by these models for reducing attrition due to toxicology is significant.

# References


1. B. K. Park, M. Pirmohamed and N. R. Kitteringham, *Chem. Res. Toxicol.*, 1989, **11**, 969–988.
2. J. A. Kramer, J. E. Sagartz and D. L. Morris, *Nat. Rev. Drug Discovery*, 2007, **68**, 636–649.
3. A. A. Adgey, *Haemostasis*, 1996, **26**, 237–246.
4. F. E. Silverstein, G. Faich, J. L. Goldstein, L. S. Simon, T. Pincus, A. Whelton, R. Makuch, G. Eisen, N. M. Agrawal, W. F. Stenson, A. M. Burr, W. W. Zhao, J. D. Kent, J. B. Lefkowith, K. M. Verburg and G. S. Geis, *JAMA, J. Am. Med. Assoc.*, 2000, **284**, 1247–1255.
5. J. Menard, *Mol. Cell Endocrinol.*, 2004, **217**, 45–52.
6. D. A. Sica, *Heart Fail. Rev.*, 2005, **10**, 23–29.
7. M. K. McMillian, E. R. Grant, Z. Zhong, J. B. Parker, L. Li, R. A. Zivin, M. E. Burczynski and M. D. Johnson, *In Vitro Mol. Toxicol.*, 2001, **14**, 177–190.
8. R. J. Gum, D. Hickman, J. A. Fagerland, M. A. Heindel, G. D. Gagne, J. M. Schmidt, M. R. Michaelides, S. K. Davidsen and R. G. Ulrich, *Biochem. Pharmacol.*, 2001, **62**, 1661–1673.
9. J. K. Morelli, M. Buehrle, F. Pognan, L. R. Barone, W. Fieles and P. J. Ciaccio, *Cell Biol. Toxicol.*, 2006, **22**, 15–27.
10. C. Portera-Cailliau, C. H. Sung, J. Nathans and R. Adler, *Proc. Natl. Acad. Sci. U. S. A.*, 1994, **91**, 974–978.
11. D. W. Fairbairn, P. L. Olive and K. L. O'Neill, *Mutat. Res.*, 1995, **339**, 37–59.
12. I. Vermes, C. Haanen, H. Steffens-Nakken and C. Reutelingsperger, *J. Immunol. Methods*, 1995, **184**, 39–51.
13. V. Gurtu, S. R. Kain and G. Zhang, *Anal. Biochem.*, 1997, **251**, 98–102.
14. P. A. Hyslop and L. A. Sklar, *Anal. Biochem.*, 1984, **141**, 280–286.
15. R. A. Capaldi, J. Murray, L. Byrne, M. S. Janes and M. F. Marusich, *Mitochondrion*, 2004, **4**, 417–426.
16. *M3: Non-clinical safety studies for the conduct of human clinical trials for pharmaceuticals*, International Conference on Harmonisation, 1997, Geneva, Switzerland.
17. *M3 (R2): Non-clinical safety studies for the conduct of human clinical trials and marketing authorization for pharmaceuticals*, International Conference on Harmonisation, 2010, Geneva, Switzerland.
18. J. A. Kramer, E. O'Neill, M. E. Phillips, D. Bruce, T. Smith, M. M. Albright, S. Bellum, S. Gopinathan, W. E. Heydorn, X. Liu, A.

Nouraldeen, B. J. Payne, R. Read, P. Vogel, X.-Q. Yu and A. G. E. Wilson, *Toxicol. Pathol.*, 2010, **38**, 452–471.
19. C. Parkinson and P. Grasso, *Hum. Exp. Toxicol.*, 1993, **12**, 99–109.
20. R. W. Lewis, R. Billington, E. Debryune, A. Gamer, B. Lang and F. Carpanini, *Toxicol. Pathol.*, **30**, 66–74.
21. M. A. Dorato and J. A. Engelhardt, *Regul. Toxicol. Pharmacol.*, 2005, **42**, 265–274.
22. *Guidance for Industry: Estimating the Maximum Safe Starting Dose in Initial Clinical Trials for Therapeutics in Adult Healthy Volunteers*, FDA, Silver Spring, MD, 2005.
23. *S2B: Genotoxicity: a standard battery for genotoxicity testing of pharmaceuticals*, International Conference on Harmonisation, Geneva, Switzerland, 1997.
24. (*a*) *S1C(R2): Dose selection for carcinogenicity studies of pharmaceuticals*, International Conference on Harmonisation, Geneva, Switzerland, 2008; (*b*) *S1A: The need for long-term rodent carcinogenicity studies of pharmaceuticals*, International Conference on Harmonisation, Geneva, Switzerland, 1996; (*c*) *S1B: Testing for carcinogenicity of pharmaceuticals*, International Conference on Harmonisation, Geneva, Switzerland, 1998.
25. *S2(R1): Genotoxicity testing and data interpretation for pharmaceuticals intended for human use*, International Conference on Harmonisation, Geneva, Switzerland, 2008.
26. (*a*) *S7A: Safety pharmacology studies for human pharmaceuticals*, International Conference on Harmonisation, Geneva, Switzerland, 2001; (*b*) *S7B: Non-clinical evaluation of QT interval prolongation*, International Conference on Harmonisation, Geneva, Switzerland, 2005.
27. A. Ollerstam, S. A. Visser, G. Duker, T. Forsberg, A. H. Persson, L. B. Nilsson, J. A. Björkman, J. Gabrielsson and A. Al-Saffar, *J. Pharmacol. Toxicol. Methods*, 2007, **56**, 131–144.
28. J. L. Mattsson, P. J. Spencer and R. R. Albee, *J. Am. Coll. Toxicol.*, 1996, **15**, 239–254.
29. S. Irwin, *Psychopharmacologia*, 1968, **13**, 222–257.
30. S. G. Emeigh Hart, *J. Pharmacol. Toxicol. Methods.*, 2005, **52**, 30–45.
31. S. W. Mittelstadt, C. L. Hemenway and R. D. Spruell, *J. Pharmacol. Toxicol. Methods*, 2005, **52**, 154–158.
32. J. Luft and G. Bode, *Fundam. Clin. Pharmacol.*, 2002, **16**, 91–103.
33. *S5A: Guideline for industry: detection of toxicity to reproduction for medicinal products*, International Conference on Harmonisation, Geneva, Switzerland, 1994.
34. *S5B: Guideline for industry: detection of toxicity to reproduction for medicinal products: addendum on toxicity to male fertility*, International Conference on Harmonisation, Geneva, Switzerland, 1996.
35. *S8: Guidance for industry: immunotoxicity studies for human pharmaceuticals*, International Conference on Harmonisation, Geneva, Switzerland, 2006.
36. H. G. Haggerty, *J. Immunotoxicol.*, 2007, **4**, 165–169.

37. S. E. McConkey, D. M. Grant and A. E. Cribb, *J. Vet. Pharmacol. Ther.*, 2009, **32**, 585–595.
38. I. Sekis, K. Ramstead, M. Rishniw, W. S. Schwark, S. P. McDonough, R. E. Goldstein, M. Papich and K. W. Simpson, *J. Feline Med. Surg.*, 2009, **11**, 60–68.
39. A. P. Florczyk, J. E. Schurig and W. T. Bradner, *Cancer Treat. Rep.*, 1982, **66**, 187–189.
40. B. Costall, A. M. Domeney, R. J. Naylor and F. D. Tattersall, *Neuropharmacology*, 1987, **26**, 1321–1326.
41. R. E. Klabunde and L. J. Mulligan, *Lab. Anim. Sci.*, 1998, **48**, 529–532.
42. R. C. Truex, R. Belej, L. M. Ginsberg and R. L. Hartman, *Anat. Rec.*, 1974, **179**, 411–422.
43. R. L. Tanguay and M. J. Reimers, *Methods Mol. Biol.*, 2008, **447**, 63–74.
44. B. G. Short, *Toxicol. Pathol.*, 2008, **36**, 49–62.
45. O. V. Angelov, A. G. Wiese, D. D. Tang-Liu, A. A. Acheampong, I. M. Ismail and B.S. Brar, *Eur. J. Ophthalmol.*, 1996, **6**, 21–25.
46. P. J. Ness, N. Mamalis, L. Werner, S. Maddula, D. K. Davis, E. D. Donnenfeld and R. J. Olson, *Am. J. Ophthalmol.*, 2010, **150**, 498–504.
47. J. Heaton, P. Kastner and R. Hackett, *Surv. Ophthalmol.*, 2007, **52**, S35–S40.
48. D. H. McGee, O. Dembinska and M. M. Gruebbel, *Int. J. Toxicol.*, 2005, **24**, 419–425.
49. J. W. Proksch, J. Y. Driot, P. Vandeberg and K. W. Ward, *J. Ocul. Pharmacol. Ther.*, 2008, **24**, 320–332.
50. S. J. Daniel and R. Munguia, *Otolaryngol. Head Neck Surg.*, 2008, **139**, 840–845.
51. D. M. Kaplan, A. L. James, M. A. Thorp, R. J. Mount and R. V. Harrison, *J. Otolaryngol.*, 2004, **33**, 160–164.
52. P. S. Roland, *Otolaryngol. Head Neck Surg.*, **110**, 598–602.
53. R. A. Roth, J. P. Luyendyk, J. F. Maddox and P. E. Ganey, *J. Pharmacol. Exp. Ther.*, 2003, **307**, 1–8.
54. S. Tafazoli, D. D. Spehar and P. J. O'Brien, *Drug Metab. Rev.*, 2005, **37**, 311–325.
55. J. F. Waring, M. J. Liguori, J. P. Luyendyk, J. F. Maddox, P. E. Ganey, R. F. Stachlewitz, C. North, E. A. Blomme and R. A. Roth, *J. Pharmacol. Exp. Ther.*, 2006, **316**, 1080–1087.
56. B. P. Zambrowicz, C. A. Turner and A. T. Sands, *Curr. Opin. Pharmacol.*, 2003, **3**, 563–570.
57. D. G. Rudmann and S. K. Durham, *Toxicol. Pathol.*, 1999, **27**, 111–114.
58. M. Martin, J. F. Reidhaar-Olson and C. M. Rondinone, *Pharmacogenomics*, 2007, **8**, 455–464.
59. D. L. Morris, S. P. O'Neil, R. V. Devraj, J. P. Portanova, R. W. Gilles, C. J. Gross, S. W. Curtiss, W. J. Komocsar, D. S. Garner, F. A. Happa, L. J. Kraus, K. J. Nikula, J. B. Monahan, S. R. Selness, G. R. Galluppi, K. M. Shevlin, J. A. Kramer, J. K. Walker, D. M. Messing, D. R. Anderson, R. J. Mourey, L. O. Whiteley, J. S. Daniels, J. Z. Yang, P. C. Rowlands, C. L. Alden, J. W. Davis II and J. E. Sagartz, *Toxicol. Pathol.*, 2010, **38**, 606–618.

60. A. L. Berg and Y. M. Bohlooly, *Exp. Toxicol. Pathol.*, 2006, **57**, 383–384.
61. *S1A: Guideline for industry: the need for long-term rodent carcinogenicity studies of pharmaceuticals*, International Conference on Harmonisation, Geneva, Switzerland, 1996.
62. S. M. Cohen, D. Robinson and J. MacDonald, *Toxicol. Sci.*, 2001, **64**, 14–19.
63. T. Usui, M. Mutai, S. Hisada, M. Takoaka, K. A. Soper, B. McCullough and C. Alden, *Toxicol. Pathol.*, 2001, **29**, 90–108.
64. R. D. Storer, F. D. Sistare, M. V. Reddy and J. J. DeGeorge, *Toxicol. Pathol.*, 2010, **38**, 51–61.
65. C. F. van Kreijl, P. A. McAnulty, R. B. Beems, A. Vynckier, H. van Steeg, R. Fransson-Steen, C. L. Alden, R. Forster, J. W. van der Laan and J. Vandenberghe, *Toxicol. Pathol.*, 2001, **29**, 117–127.
66. G. G. Long, D. Morton, T. Peters, B. Short and M. Skydsgaard, *Toxicol. Pathol.*, 2010, **38**, 43–50.
67. C. Alden, P. Smith and D. Morton, *Toxicol. Pathol.*, 2002, **30**, 135–138.
68. S. J. Engle, *Int. Drug Discovery*, 2009, **5**, 17–22.
69. M. A. Belury, S. Y. Moya-Camarena, H. Sun, E. Snyder, J. W. Davis, M. L. Cunningham and J. P. Van den Heuvel, *Toxicol. Appl. Pharmacol.*, 1998, **151**, 254–261.
70. S. S. Lee, T. Pineau, J. Drago, E. J. Lee, J. W. Owens, D. L. Kroetz, P. M. Fernandez-Salguero, H. Westphal and F. J. Gonzalez, *Mol. Cell Biol.*, 1995, **15**, 3012–3022.
71. D. E. Moody, J. K. Reddy, B. G. Lake, J. A. Popp and D. H. Reese, *Fundam. Appl. Toxicol.*, 1991, **16**, 233–248.
72. B. D. Abbott, C. J. Wolf, J. E. Schmid, K. P. Das, R. D. Zehr, L. Helfant, S. Nakayama, A. B. Lindstrom, M. J. Strynar and C. Lau, *Toxicol. Sci.*, 2007, **98**, 571–581.
73. J. Ashby, A. Brady, C. R. Elcombe, B. M. Elliott, J. Ishmael, J. Odum, J. D. Tugwood, S. Kettle and I. F. Purchase, *Hum. Exp. Toxicol.*, 1994, **13**, S1–S117.
74. R. C. Cattley, J. DeLuca, C. Elcombe, P. Fenner-Crisp, B. G. Lake, D. S. Marsman, T. A. Pastoor, J. A. Popp, D. E. Robinson, B. Schwetz, J. Tugwood and W. Wahli, *Regul. Toxicol. Pharmacol.*, 1998, **27**, 47–60.
75. J. D. Tugwood, T. C. Aldridge, K. G. Lambe, N. Macdonald and N. J. Woodyatt, *Ann. NY Acad. Sci.*, 1996, **804**, 252–265.
76. J. E. Foreman, S. C. Chang, D. J. Ehresman, J. L. Butenhoff, C. R. Anderson, P. S. Palkar, B. H. Kang, F. J. Gonzalez and J. M. Peters, *Toxicol. Sci.*, 2009, **110**, 204–211.
77. M. Morissette, S. Jourdain, S. Al Sweidi, F. S. Menniti, A. D. Ramirez and T. Di Paolo, *Neuropharmacology*, 2007, **52**, 1509–1520.
78. A. E. van Herwaarden, E. Wagenaar, C. M. van der Kruijssen, R. A. van Waterschoot, J. W. Smit, J. Y. Song, M. A. van der Valk, O. van Tellingen, J. W. van der Hoorn, H. Rosing, J. H. Beijnen and A. H. Schinkel, *J. Clin. Invest.*, 2007, **117**, 3583–3592.
79. R. A. van Waterschoot, A. E. van Herwaarden, J. S. Lagas, R. W. Sparidans, E. Wagenaar, C. M. van der Kruijssen, J. A. Goldstein, D. C.

Zeldin, J. H. Beijnen and A. H. Schinkel, *Mol. Pharmacol.*, 2008, **73**, 1029–1036.

80. A. M. Geurts, G. J. Cost, Y. Freyvert, B. Zeitler, J. C. Miller, V. M. Choi, S. S. Jenkins, A. Wood, X. Cui, X. Meng, A. Vincent, S. Lam, M. Michalkiewicz, R. Schilling, J. Foeckler, S. Kalloway, H. Weiler, S. Ménoret, I. Anegon, G. D. Davis, L. Zhang, E. J. Rebar, P. D. Gregory, F. D. Urnov, H. J. Jacob and R. Buelow, *Science*, 2009, **325**, 433–435.
81. Z. Izsvák, J. Fröhlich, I. Grabundzija, J. R. Shirley, H. M. Powell, K. M. Chapman, Z. Ivics and F. K. Hamra, *Nat. Methods*, 2010, **7**, 443–445.
82. C. Tong, P. Li, N. L. Wu, Y. Yan and Q. L. Ying, *Nature*, 2010, **467**, 211–213.
83. C. J. Friddle, A. Abuin, R. Ramirez-Solis, L. J. Richter, E. C. Buxton, J. Edwards, R. A. Finch, A. Gupta, G. Hansen, K. H. Holt, Y. Hu, W. Huang, C. Jaing, B. W. Key Jr, P. Kipp, B. Kohlhauff, Z. Q. Ma, D. Markesich, M. Newhouse, T. Perry, K. A. Platt, D. G. Potter, N. Qian, J. Shaw, J. Schrick, Z. Z. Shi, M. J. Sparks, D. Tran, E. R. Wann, W. Walke, J. D. Wallace, N. Xu, Q. Zhu, C. Person, A. T. Sands and B. P. Zambrowicz, *Cold Spring Harbor Symp. Quant. Biol.*, 2003, **68**, 311–315.
84. B. P. Zambrowicz and A. T. Sands, *Nat. Rev. Drug Discovery*, 2003, **2**, 38–51.
85. C. R. Elcombe, J. Odum, J. R. Foster, S. Stone, S. Hasmall, A. R. Soames, I. Kimber and J. Ashby, *Environ. Health Perspect.*, 2002, **110**, 363–375.
86. J. A. Kramer, S. W. Curtiss, K. L. Kolaja, C. L. Alden, E. A. Blomme, W. C. Curtiss, J. C. Davila, C. J. Jackson and R. T. Bunch, *Chem. Res. Toxicol.*, 2004, **17**, 2004, 463–470.
87. B. Kuiper, M. H. Boevé, T. Jansen, M. E. Roelofs-van Emden, J. W. Thuring and M. V. Wijnands, *Lab. Anim.*, 1997, **31**, 177–183.
88. H. Long, Y. Zhu, M. Cregor, F. Tian, L. Coury, C. B. Kissinger and P. T. Kissinger, *J. Chromatogr., B: Biomed. Sci. Appl.*, 2001, **763**, 47–51.
89. K. H. Diehl, R. Hull, D. Morton, R. Pfister, Y. Rabemampianina, D. Smith, J. M. Vidal and C. van de Vorstenbosch, *J. Appl. Toxicol.*, 2001, **21**, 15–23.
90. *The Care and Feeding of an IACUC: The Organization and Management of an Institutional Animal Care and Use Committee*, ed. M. L. Podolsky and V. S. Lukas, CRC Press, Boca Raton, 1999, pp. 187–188.

CHAPTER 14

# *In Vivo Approaches to Predictive Toxicology Using Zebrafish*

MICHAEL T. SIMONICH, JILL A. FRANZOSA AND ROBERT L. TANGUAY*

Oregon State University, Department of Environmental & Molecular Toxicology, the Sinnhuber Aquatic Research Laboratory and the Environmental Health Sciences Center, Corvallis, OR 97333, USA

## 14.1 Introduction: Sustainable Discovery

We are fortunate to live in a time when the pace of chemical discovery, whether combinatorial or natural in origin, is unprecedented. The benefits to humankind from the rate of discovery will be incalculable advances in pharmacologic and materials technology. Faced with a chemical diversity that, in fact, far exceeds any public agency's ability to adequately evaluate the components of for efficacy, utility or hazard, sustainable discovery will increasingly be dependent on massively scaled structure–activity relationships (SARs).[1] One key to sustainable discovery from the astonishing chemical diversity available will be SARs based on vertebrate model responses. Another key, closely linked to the first, will be a shift to greater reliance on predictive toxicology, developed from vertebrate model data. The larger such vertebrate response databases become, the more effectively they will predict the likely biological activity of new chemistries.

RSC Drug Discovery Series No. 12
New Horizons in Predictive Toxicology: Current Status and Application
Edited by Alan G. E. Wilson

Published by the Royal Society of Chemistry, www.rsc.org

## 14.2 The Challenge: Why We Need Better Toxicology

What do we mean by sustainable discovery? The demands for discovery are great. But we can confidently say the discovery and development process for a single drug is unsustainable.[2] Current estimates are a 10–15 year average development timeline at an average cost of \$1.3 billion per compound.[2,3] Involving cutting-edge toxicology early in the discovery process would be a huge leap in efficiency. The FDA reported in 2004 that the rate of new pharmaceutical therapies reaching patients was slowing because the number of new molecular entities submitted to the FDA had declined by half since 1997 (http://www.fda.gov/oc/initiatives/criticalpath/whitepaper/htm).[4,5] The report cited *technological deficits in toxicology* as one of the primary causes of the 'pipeline problem'. The deficits developed, and persist, because toxicology remains largely separate from the discovery process, often not entering the decision making process until Phase III/regulatory review, or after the product has already gone to market.[2,6,7] The use of *in vitro* toxicity assays to prioritize drug leads and eliminate problem moieties from screening libraries has been a step towards reducing attrition of candidate drugs. Still, 20–50% of drug and consumer product discoveries showing promise in early *in vitro* stages often fail in later animal testing (after \$millions have been invested) because the *in vitro* efficacy does not translate to the whole animal, or because of unintended side effects.[8–10] *Prediction of toxicology based on phenotypic and toxicogenomic responses in a vertebrate model would hasten the discovery pipeline by avoiding many leads otherwise destined to fail.* Zebrafish is the emerging choice for such a model.[11] No other vertebrate is better suited to high-throughput chemical screening.[5]

## 14.3 Why Use Zebrafish for Toxicology?

The characteristics of small size, short life cycle, external fertilization, embryo transparency and low husbandry cost established the zebrafish as an important developmental and genetic model over two decades ago. Zebrafish made forward genetic approaches to understanding vertebrate-specific processes a practical possibility. The advantages of the zebrafish for toxicology work have been extensively reviewed.[12–14] A comprehensive suite of tools, developed over the last decade, have further enhanced the utility of the model. The research community has completely sequenced and extensively annotated the zebrafish genome. We can interrogate the expression of the entire genome simultaneously on microarrays to look for molecular signatures of a biological impact. When anomalies occur, we can pinpoint the genomic and molecular mechanism with powerful tools such as antisense morpholino knockdown, chemical genetics, proteomics, and transgenic fish which contain fluorescent protein either in blood vessels or in other specific cellular populations. An entire adult zebrafish section can fit onto a standard histology slide without organ dissection, enabling rapid-throughput adult histopathology. Zebrafish studies provide a quick and inexpensive way to test hypotheses and to generate strategies for complementary integrative research with rodent models, and with human subjects.

## 14.4 Zebrafish Toxicological Endpoints are Complex

The molecular responses of zebrafish to chemicals have a high degree of relevance to human biology. The signal-transduction mechanisms, anatomy, and physiology of zebrafish are homologous to those of humans. Zebrafish possess all the classical sense modalities, including vision, olfaction, taste, touch, balance, and hearing. Thus, toxicity investigations in the zebrafish have included endpoints in reproductive, developmental, neuro, cardio, ocular, otic, gastrointestinal, hepato, endocrine, regenerative and vascular toxicity, and carcinogenicity.[14–27]

As in all vertebrates, zebrafish development is the most sensitive life stage to chemical exposure. Importantly, embryonic zebrafish chemical perturbation is also a reliable predictor of chemical toxicity in the adult stage. The bulk of the model's utility, and hence the bulk of zebrafish toxicology work, is centered on development. Because zebrafish embryos remain transparent throughout much of organogensis, adverse effects of chemical exposure on development of the brain, notochord, heart, jaw, body segmentation, and body size can be continuously assessed in the living animal under low magnification. Advances in high-content imaging are enabling automated collection of these endpoints.[28,29] An important developmental feature is that zebrafish embryos that are malformed, missing organs, or displaying organ dysfunction, usually survive well beyond the point at which those organs normally start to function. This is especially true of the developing zebrafish heart.[30–32] Contrast this feature to rodents where heart and other organ malformations, missing or dysfunctional organs typically cause a generalized *in utero* lethality. In a large-scale (>1000 animal) rodent screen, underlying organ deficits would be missed with anything less than a Herculean effort at detection.

## 14.5 Specific, Rapid Endpoints of Zebrafish Toxicology

### 14.5.1 Cardiotoxicity

Several high-profile instances of cardiotoxicity of non-cardiovascular drugs, and their subsequent removal from the market, are well known.[33] Earlier discovery of cardiac side-effects with better toxicology models could have prevented these examples. The ability to visually assess nuances of cardiotoxicity including aberrant heart rate, arrhythmia, bradycardia, contractility and circulation has attracted much attention to the developing zebrafish heart model. Zebrafish have a two-chambered heart that begins beating around 20 hpf and remains externally visible throughout the first week of development. Much of what is known about cardiotoxicity in zebrafish came from studies of the developmental effects of 2,3,7,8-tetrachlorodibenzo-*p*-dioxin (TCDD).[18,19,34] In embryonic zebrafish, TCDD exposure results in severe heart malformations, reduced peripheral blood flow, pericardial edema, and hemorrhage.[35,36] TCDD also reduces heart size during development in zebrafish and causes compaction of the ventricle, elongation of the heart, and increased incidence of ventricular standstill.[32] Effects on the heart can be seen before any observable effect on blood flow.[32] More recently, transgenic zebrafish lines expressing fluorescent protein restricted to the myocardium have enabled rapid-throughput screening for modulators of QT prolongation, heart rate, cardiac rhythmicity and pharmaceutical-induced membrane voltage dynamics.[37–39]

Despite lacking a pulmonary system, zebrafish cardiac physiology is, in some aspects, more similar to humans than rodents.[33,40–43] Early embryonic cardiomyocytes can be patch clamped, exhibit multiple physiologic currents as early as 3 dpf, recapitulate the majority of cardiac conductances and have a heart rate and action potential duration similar to humans.[44] These parallels have enabled complete modeling of the onset of arrhythmia in the zebrafish embryo. This is possible because all of cardiogenesis is visible under a dissecting scope and calcium and voltage transients can be monitored in heart primordia prior to their migration into the primitive heart tube.[45] Bradycardia in the zebrafish embryo is physiologically similar to prolonged QT interval in humans, a risk factor associated with life-threatening arrhythmia.[43,46,47] Cardiac pharmacology modeling in zebrafish appears to parallel the close electrophysiologic modeling. Several groups have shown that pharmacologic compounds that elicit cardiomyopathy and prolonged QT interval in humans also cause bradycardia, an abnormal atrial/ventricular ratio, decreased contractility and slowed circulation in the developing zebrafish.[48–50] Using bradycardia in zebrafish embryos as an endpoint, another study showed that 22 of 23 drugs known to cause QT prolongation in humans also caused bradycardia in the developing zebrafish heart.[48] Recently, developing zebrafish embryos were used to mimic the heart malformations that occur in humans with fetal alcohol syndrome.[51] Bradycardia and decreased blood flow were observed in zebrafish embryos and larvae exposed to the common cough and cold medication, dextromethorphan.[52] The high correlation observed between human and zebrafish drug toxicities strongly supports the zebrafish as a cardiotoxicology model.[5,43] Electrocardiogram (ECG) analysis indicates that adult zebrafish heart functions are also similar to humans including PR interval, the QRS complex and the QT interval.[53] Zebrafish ECGs can be integrated with other automated assays to rapidly screen drug candidates for cardiotoxicity at about 1% the cost for similar profiling in rodents.[33,53]

## 14.5.2 Hepatotoxicity

Unforeseen liver toxicity is a frequent problem for pharmaceutical development largely because toxicological assessments are dependent on rodent liver assays and hence are expensive, low throughput and necessarily performed late in the development pipeline. Zebrafish complete their primary liver development by 48 hpf with the liver being fully formed and functioning by 72 hpf. Thus, the late embryo–early larval stage is a compact, transparent and inexpensive liver model amenable to some high-throughput chemical profiling assays, especially those based on automated imaging and *in situ* hybridization (ISH), or liver-specific enzymes. Zebrafish respond to xenobiotics similarly to mammals, including Phase I and Phase II enzyme inductions and oxidative stress responses.[54,55] Proteomic analysis of the zebrafish liver has also revealed indicators of xenobiotic response further supporting the model's use in translational/predictive toxicology.[56] Embryonic and adult zebrafish models for acetaminophen liver toxicity were recently used with moderate-throughput assessments of morphometric, liver-specific GFP reporting, ISH and histology to show that prostaglandin E2 acts synergistically with *N*-acetylcysteine to protect the liver.[57] The study reinforced the relevance of the zebrafish liver toxicity model to human and rodent physiology through its consistency with reports that an ortholog of the major APAP-metabolizing enzyme in humans, CYP3A4, is also present in zebrafish, and by showing that a subset of the proteins regulated in this study responded similarly in rodents after acetaminophen injury.[57–59] Conserved indicators of liver toxicity between zebrafish and humans such as GFP reporter enzymes, CYP enzymes, serum alanine transaminase in adults, liver necrosis and histopathology have been reviewed elsewhere.[33]

### 14.5.3 Neurotoxicity

Neurotoxicity is another critical facet of drug and consumer product development that is often inadequately assessed before market or, because of reliance on exceedingly low-throughput behavioral and neurohistopathological assessments in rodent models, is discovered late in the development pipeline. Zebrafish is a practical compromise between system complexity and simplicity with a neurochemistry and brain anatomy fundamentally similar to humans (extensively reviewed by Sager *et al.*[60]). They are sensitive to dopaminergic neurotoxins, a variety of seizure-inducing compounds, acetylcholine agonists and antagonists, NMDA receptor antagonists, human depressants and anti-depressants, and common chemicals such as alcohol and caffeine (reviewed by McGrath[33] and Eimon[61]). The zebrafish has more recently emerged as an excellent model organism for several human diseases of the central nervous system including Alzheimer's, Huntington's, Parkinson's, and several motor neuron diseases, and shown promise for modeling amyotrophic lateral sclerosis, autism spectrum disorders and schizophrenia (reviewed by Kabashi *et al.*[62]). This, combined with a striking level of functional gene orthology to humans, suggests a strong translational relevance of zebrafish neurotoxicity data. A variety of neurotoxicity endpoints, from purely morphological to neurosensory, to locomotion and cognitive changes have been described in zebrafish. For recent reviews see refs. 61, 63 and 64. Here we will briefly profile some of the neurotoxicity endpoints most amenable to assay automation.

#### *14.5.3.1 Neuronal Reporter Fish*

The utility of zebrafish transgenic reporter lines is reviewed in more depth below, but brief mention of commonly used neuronal-specific reporter lines is warranted here. The zebrafish would make an exceptionally convenient neurotoxicity model if for no other reason than the entire nervous system, including the brain, can be stained and imaged on a single slide. But staining methods are time-intensive and transgenics have offered a rapid alternative. Advances in *in vivo* high-content imaging have opened up the rapid-throughput use of neuron-specific, fluorescent protein reporters for direct visual assessment of neuronal development in transparent embryos and larvae.[28,29] Chemical perturbation of neuronal survival, proliferation and pathfinding can now be quantitatively monitored in the whole animal in a 96-well microplate format as one measure of neurotoxicity. For instance, the *gfp:ngn1* (neurogenin 1) line specifically labels the sites of primary neurogenesis in the zebrafish embryo and the *gfp:islet1* line specifically labels sensory and motor neurons in the developing embryo and larvae.[65] An *Engrailed 1* reporter line specifically expresses GFP in inhibitory spinal interneurons and an *alx:gfp* reporter specifically labels excitatory spinal interneurons.[66,67] Recently the live imaging of apoptotic cells in a transgenic zebrafish line was accomplished using secreted annexin V protein fused to yellow fluorescent protein.[68] In the larval stage, neuronal cell apoptosis as a normal part of development was visualized at single-cell resolution in the hind brain, in and around the eye, spinal interneurons and Rohon Beard neurons.[68] This reporter line is highly amenable to automated screening in 96-well format. Combining use of this transgenic line with automated, high-content imaging may provide a powerful model for quickly assessing neurotoxicity as changes in stereotypical apoptotic patterns. We now know that the classes of spinal neurons in swimming larvae represent a functioning network and that larval swimming movements are virtually indistinguishable from adult swimming, and rely on the same motor and interneurons. Thus, chemical perturbation and motor deficits in the more easily assayed larval stage are predictive of motor deficits in the adult stage.

#### *14.5.3.2 Behavior*

The embryonic, larval and adult zebrafish stages all exhibit characteristic behaviors. These range from very simple, early stage movements to cognitive ability in adults. For example, embryos still in the chorion (about 24 hpf) display arrhythmic tail bending. The larval zebrafish (72 hpf to 8 dpf) displays characteristic swimming behavior, optomotor response, photometer and acoustic startle responses, pre-pulse inhibition, epileptic seizure-analogous behavior and rhythmic rest–wake cycles.[69–82] Adult zebrafish swimming and sleep activity shows circadian rhythmicity.[83,84] Adults also display learning and memory, fear and anxiety, and social behavior which have been recently reviewed.[64,85]

The potential applications of rapid-throughput behavior assays are most numerous for the larval stage where behavior complexity and practical throughput strike an optimal balance.[63] The larval stage is easily arrayed in 96 well microplate format, one animal per well, with sufficient space for swimming. The photomotor response to short (several minute) duration light–dark cycles, the visual or acoustic startle response, and pre-pulse inhibition and seizure are all readily automated assays in a microplate format. Typically, all 96 wells can be assayed simultaneously with a CCD camera under visible and infra-red light regimens using computerized motion tracking and quantification software. Several such manual plate load systems are now offered commercially, and robotically accessible systems are expected in forthcoming versions. To date, the few published studies of larval behaviors as phenotype-based chemical profiling have aimed solely at drug discovery.[63,86] But a corollary to this work is that these same phenotypes can be toxicological endpoints. To be a toxicological endpoint, larval behavior only has to be sensitive to neuroactive chemicals. Thus, simple changes in locomotion such as attenuated swimming speed, hyperactive movements indicative of seizure, or aberrant locomotor response to light or startling can indicate potential neurotoxicity.[72,76] Because the molecular targets upon which chemicals typically act to effect neuronal signaling are strongly conserved, simple larval zebrafish chemobehaviors can be used to predict neurotoxic potential of chemicals in higher vertebrates.

### 14.5.4 Developmental Toxicity

The zebrafish has had an enormous impact on developmental biology over the past 20 years. The knowledge gained from that work and the unique advantages of rapid external development, embryo transparency, and amenability to high-throughput assays makes it an attractive model of developmental toxicity. The effect of TCDD on zebrafish development has been extensively studied, as has the developmental toxicology of polycyclic aromatic hydrocarbons, with the result that most of what we know about aryl hydrocarbon receptor (AhR) mediated signaling we have learned from the zebrafish.[19,87] While the more specific toxicology endpoints, reviewed above, are all subsets of developmental toxicology, the more classical endpoints of developmental toxicity and teratogenicity *i.e.*, mortality, malformations, and embryo growth, are amenable to high-throughput assays. This is largely due to the advantages of the model and the advent of automated high-content image analysis. Up until now, a big limitation on the throughput of zebrafish chemical screens has been the inability to automatically process 96-well plates for image analysis. Thus, most published zebrafish chemical screens have relied on visual examination of individual wells by the investigator. This approach is semi-quantitative at best and necessarily restricts recording and archiving of images to just a small sampling of the experimental animals. It also leaves no means by which to conduct retrospective analyses of all endpoints that may have been captured, or to cross-reference endpoint data with past or future screens using the same compound library. This limitation on phenotype-based chemical screens has largely been obviated with the advent of automated high-content image recording and analysis that can be performed at the single-cell level up to the morphology of the entire zebrafish larva in a single confocal optics based system. Several studies have recently appeared making use of automated imaging with the goal of high-throughput chemical screening in transgenic zebrafish reporter lines.[28,29,88,89] The development of automated high-content imaging has placed the zebrafish at the forefront of vertebrate models with which we can rapidly integrate a very large body of developmental knowledge with chemical toxicity. This will be an invaluable tool for predictive toxicology.

### 14.5.5 Ototoxicity

Mechanosensory hair cells of the fish lateral line (LL) are analogous to hair cells of the mammalian inner ear and, like in mammals, are easily damaged by metabolites of chemicals such as *cis*-platin, heavy metals, and aminoglycoside antibiotics.[17,61,90,91] Screening of over 1000 compounds for ototoxicity (hair cell loss) in zebrafish larvae indicated the hair cell response is conserved. Twenty one of the compounds were confirmed to be ototoxic in the zebrafish, nine of which were already known to be ototoxic in humans, while no human ototoxicity data existed for the other 12 compounds.[22] Two of the remaining 12 were toxic to mouse utricle explants. Five compounds in the library appeared to be false negatives, being known human ototoxins that did not disrupt zebrafish hair cells. Possible poor solubility or lack of absorption of these five compounds was not reported.

The zebrafish LL is essential to the fish's ability to orient relative to water current, detect prey and avoid predation, and is thus also an important effector of neurosensory behavior when disrupted.[92,93] The LL has been well studied as a zebrafish model of ototoxicity because it is functional at 3–4 dpf, is easily accessible, easy to stain and image, and extraordinarily sensitive to waterborne chemicals. The LL is composed of rosette-like structures called neuromasts, located on the surface of the fish, which are in turn composed of hair cells and supporting peripheral sensory neurons.[94] Development of the zebrafish LL is well understood as many genes involved in neuromast differentiation have been uncovered using neurosensory mutants and knockdown morphants.[93] Many exposure studies have indicated the applicability of the zebrafish LL for assessing potential mechanosensory deficits or neurotoxicity and these have been recently reviewed.[93] The sensitive hair cells and sensory neurons of the LL are in direct contact with chemicals in the water and necessary for stereotypical swimming behavior. While no transgenic reporter line for neuromast or hair cell disruption has yet been reported, the likely development of such a reporter in the near future will make neuromast toxicity a rapid and powerful endpoint for predictive toxicology.

## 14.6 Toxicogenomics: Filling the Tool Box for Predictive Toxicology

The zebrafish phenotypic endpoints already discussed offer varying degrees of toxicant-specific information and thus, alone, do not fully achieve a predictive toxicology. Nor can a toxicogenomics approach, alone, achieve robust prediction without phenotype data. But in parallel with assessment and databasing of phenomics, toxicogenomics bridges the gap between the whole animal phenotype and subcellular responses *in vivo*. Of course, toxicogenomics can stand alone by uncovering molecular changes elicited from low-dose exposures that have no overt morphological or behavioral effects in the animals.[95,96] But the question of biological significance is raised when expression changes have no discernable effect on the animal. Rather, toxicogenomics is at its most valuable providing a refined and complex view of toxic effects, from which meaningful patterns of response can be discerned and related to animal phenotype. Moreover, analysis of the transcriptome, as well as the proteome and the metabolome, affords the most efficient route to understanding: 1) the mechanism of a chemical's activity in the animal and 2) comparative effects, *i.e.*, it is very easy to compare toxicant-elicited gene expression changes between a zebrafish and a mammal. If those expression changes are accompanied by comprehensive phenotype data, we can predict a likely translation of the toxicant effect to mammals.

### 14.6.1 Zebrafish Supports a Whole-Animal Approach to Toxicogenomics

A ubiquitous consideration in mammalian toxicogenomics is the unknown distribution of toxicant-elicited expression profiles across different tissues, when typically only one tissue is examined, or, the choice of tissue to examine in the first place. These considerations are largely obviated by use of the zebrafish model which has its strength in the whole-animal approach due to its compact size. The strength of the whole-animal approach is even greater with embryos and juveniles. A whole-animal expression approach has the advantage of simultaneous examination of all tissues and transcripts. A corresponding disadvantage is transcript signal dilution from highly tissue-restricted expression, but this has been largely overcome by modern, high-definition microarray approaches and massively parallel RNA sequencing (RNA-seq).[97–99]

### 14.6.2 Toxicogenomics Approaches

The application of RNA-seq to zebrafish transcriptomics is emerging because it does not require pre-defined probes, in theory profiling all transcripts present in a sample. RNA-seq also requires less RNA sample, is generally higher resolution than microarray results with lower background and wider dynamic range.[97,98] While RNA-seq has been used to profile the transcriptome response to several zebrafish pathogens, its use has not yet been reported for profiling expression changes from chemical exposure.[100,101] The advantages of deep sequencing and its widespread use in other species suggests we can anticipate its routine application to zebrafish toxicogenomics. In the microarray arena, most published studies have established transcriptional responses from $\leq$ 300 genes, a small subset relative to the number of probes on most zebrafish arrays. A recent report of high-definition toxicogenomics explored responses to sub-NOEC concentrations of four different ecotoxicants and revealed 3000–5000 responding genes, which is 10–1000 times greater than previously reported, with significance at lower levels of fold change.[99] This level of refinement was achieved by maximizing statistical power using a loop design, increased replication, and optimized analysis of false discovery rates (FDRs), setting a new standard for array-based toxicogenomic approaches to chemicals testing.

### 14.6.3 What Has Toxicogenomics Contributed?

More than 20 studies in zebrafish have been published that present the findings of mechanistic, predictive and comparative -omics approaches in zebrafish. These studies have very recently been comprehensively reviewed with the conclusion that zebrafish transcriptomics, microRNAomics, proteomics and metabolomics are all practical and powerful means to facilitate the translation of zebrafish data across species.[96] Not surprisingly, combining -omics approaches into a systems-level analysis rapidly yields plausible toxicity mechanisms and more informative comparative studies. What might this look like? A recent example in zebrafish combined microarray transcriptome analysis of mercury hepatotoxicity, gene set enrichment analysis and data mining comparison to reported human and mammalian data, phenotype anchoring, and gene expression validation by real-time PCR, in one study.[102] The result from this single study was a plausible *in vivo* mechanism of mercury hepatotoxicity where none existed before.[102] Other toxicogenomics studies in zebrafish have significantly advanced our understanding of the transcriptional changes following AhR activation and, in so doing, have provided much new knowledge about cardiac development and tissue regeneration. Studies aimed at understanding the molecular mechanisms of AhR signaling that lead to cardiovascular dysfunction have identified changes in genes important to xenobiotic metabolism, cell proliferation, heart contractility and heart development.[34,103] Gene-expression studies performed in adult and larval zebrafish regenerating fin tissue (an exception to the whole-animal approach), after AhR activation by TCDD, revealed a cluster of genes important for xenobiotic metabolism, cellular differentiation, signal transduction and extracellular matrix composition.[104,105]

### 14.6.4 Some Considerations

When comparing expression profiles from developmental stage zebrafish to human responses, an obvious consideration is that the developing embryo may confound the toxicological processes that would be observed in an adult with indicators of disruption of developmental processes. Early-stage (4–24 hpf) mRNA expression profiles are generally less robust than alterations in transcript expression patterns observed from animals at later embryonic stages (> 24 hpf), perhaps due to the immature organ physiology during early development.[96] Additionally, recall that a strength of the zebrafish model is that -omics approaches are whole-animal. This will invariably be a comparative consideration between whole-animal zebrafish profiles and higher vertebrates where profiling is generally tissue-specific. But refinements such as high-definition microarray experiments and RNA-seq offer the necessary information-rich profiles and variation control to remove life stage-specific interference. Profile 'hits' uncovered in the zebrafish embryo can then be evaluated by automated ISH to see where the hit is expressed.[106]

## 14.7 Gene Function and Phenotype Screens

Transgenic expression of exogenous genes, transient gene knockdown and the efficient mutation of the genome are invaluable tools that have allowed zebrafish phenotypic screens to ultimately identify the functions of thousands of genes. This has provided completely novel insights into vertebrate development and established a wide array of zebrafish models of human diseases.[107,108]

### 14.7.1 Transgenic Lines

The first stable transgenic zebrafish lines were developed two decades ago.[109] Today hundreds of stable transgenic lines exist and express fluorescent reporter genes in tissue-specific patterns or are under the regulation of exogenous and endogenous, constitutive and inducible promoters. The continuing utility of reporter lines to our understanding of developmental stage- and tissue-specific gene regulation in toxicology and pharmacology is immense. Several reviews comprehensively address their construction, use, and emerging utility for chemical screening and modeling human diseases.[108,110,111] Transgenic zebrafish lines greatly increase the high-throughput predictive power of this model, especially when coupled with high-resolution automated image analysis.[41,108] Several differently colored fluorescent proteins are commonly used so the expression patterns of multiple genes can be imaged in the same animal. Several transgenic lines described are making a significant contribution to toxicology becoming more rapid and predictive.[41] These lines include a *cyp1A1:gfp* line that responds to xenobiotic activation of the AhR, a zebrafish GFP reporter governed by regulatory regions of *neurogenin1* and *sonic hedgehog* that sense low-level dioxin, and the Tg(*eno2:egfp*) line, with widespread neuronal expression, has been used to create several zebrafish models of neurodegenerative disease.[60,112,113] A *Tg(cmlc2:gfp)* reporter restricted to the myocardium at 24 hpf was recently used in an automated high-throughput assay of small molecule cardiotoxicity.[37] Other transgenic zebrafish reporter lines have been developed to query compound effects on developmental signaling by retinoic acid, Delta/Notch, and FGF.[114–116] A host of transgenic zebrafish lines are also available to study angiogenesis through visualization of endothelial cells and their precursors such as *fli:egfp* that expresses EGFP in the vasculature and *flk1:EGFP* that is used to assess angioblast migration and vascular tube formation.[117–119]

### 14.7.2 Transient Knockdown of Gene Expression

Morpholinos are chemically modified antisense oligonucleotides that target and bind to mRNAs. This technology can be custom designed to hybridize to the un-translated region of a mRNA to block translation, or to small nuclear RiboNuceloProtein (snRNP) binding sites and splice junctions to modify pre-mRNA splicing. Morpholinos are typically injected into single-cell stage embryos and cause a substantial transient knockdown of gene expression and function.[5,120] A typical experimental path from post-chemical exposure expression profiling to putative effector/target gene knockdown is: 1) micro-array identification of genes with altered expression profiles, 2) bioinformatic analysis of mammalian orthology and ontology, 3) morpholino design and commercial synthesis (Gene Tools, Philomath, OR, USA), 4) one-cell egg injection and transient knock-down of expression target and phenotype analysis. Most of the hundreds of zebrafish papers that report morpholino knockdown have taken either the above approach or used a targeted knock-down to recapitulate a mutant phenotype uncovered in a forward genetic screen. Another opportunity is to model a disease state in zebrafish by mutation or toxicant exposure and conduct a genome-wide screen to systematically knock down gene targets by morpholino with the goal of uncovering targets that, when suppressed, ameliorate or potentiate the disease. Verification of knockdown by PCR (splice-block type) or Western blot (translation-block and splice block types) indicates morpholino functionality while phenotypic or physiological analysis gauges the impact of suppressing the particular effector/target gene, and the likely signaling pathway affected by the test compound.

### 14.7.3 Zebrafish Mutations

Both forward and reverse genetics approaches have identified thousands of different mutant zebrafish lines, many that recapitulate a human disease or a closely analogous condition, and of potentially great value to drug-discovery interests.[108,121,122] Disease-modeling mutants can be used for predictive purposes in small-molecule screens to detect activities that modulate the phenotype in the embryo/larval zebrafish. Thus, a disease-modulation phenotype, plus extensive evaluation of the compound in zebrafish toxicity assays, is a relatively inexpensive and rapid approach to frontloading efficacy and safety evaluations for compounds with therapeutic promise.[108] Several techniques are commonly used to induce zebrafish mutations. These include: 1) retroviral insertion, an efficient method of genome disruption that 'tags' the site of mutation, obviating the need for positional cloning, 2) TILLING (targeting induced local lesions in genomes) an alkylating-agent mutagenesis followed by high-throughput sequencing to identify mutations in a gene of interest, 3) locus-specific zinc-finger nucleases, engineered to recognize a unique target sequence in any gene of interest, including small RNAs or gene regulatory sequences.[123–129]

## 14.8 The Role of Automation in Predictive Toxicology

The advanced genetics and convenient developmental features of the zebrafish embryo make it the best vertebrate model for high-throughput phenotyping. It is perhaps the only vertebrate model compatible with the predictive toxicology needs of drug discovery to alleviate the pipeline problem. Two key technologies will support the widespread implementation of zebrafish high throughput screens: 1) the application of robotics to embryo handling, and 2) automated, image-based phenotype analysis.

Zebrafish embryo sorting and transfer to 96-well plates is a major bottleneck for chemical screening. A robust and practical method of detecting embryos, picking up and transferring embryos to 96-well plates, and microinjecting reagents at the one-cell stage has yet to be reported. The advantages of automating these tasks in the light of screening say, a 15 000 compound library, with sufficient replication, are obvious. Affordable machine-vision cameras and robotic arms with micron movement accuracy can perform these functions quickly and reliably and are commercially available. The extraordinary movement accuracy and placement precision of modern robotic arms are also a means to automate microinjection at the one-cell stage. Many zebrafish labs routinely perform microinjections of hundreds of eggs per day, typically for antisense gene repression experiments. Microinjections by a machine-vision guided robot would equal or exceed the quality of manual performance, and free several investigator hours per day. Software coding of the hardware functions is a minor hurdle to automated embryo handling, but in our experience this is inexpensively accomplished by non-experts or computer science students. There are no examples to refer to yet except to say that our laboratory and a number of other groups are developing embryo handling automation 'in-house' and as reports are published, more laboratories will implement the technology. We also note that a big impetus for developing *de novo* robotic embryo handling is that most of the downstream robotic shuttling of 96-well plates from robot arms to commercial automation platforms such as liquid handlers, plate washers, plate readers, thermocyclers and incubators has already been developed from intense automation of high-throughput *in vitro* screens.

A major factor limiting the throughput of zebrafish chemical screens is the lack of methodology to automatically scan 96-well plates for phenotype imaging and analysis. Automated, image-based phenotype analysis is emerging as a technology that will dramatically expand the size and information content of zebrafish high-throughput, chemical screens. The basic platform design is variable, low-magnification, confocal image acquisitions of a 96-well plate on a motorized X-Y-Z stage. Flexible and powerful software control allows configuration of the system to acquire bright-field and/or fluorescence images, well-by-well, in rapid succession and to automatically assess morphology parameters and fluorescence localization with a high-resolution, high-sensitivity digital camera. The images can be automatically processed, analyzed and stored. In addition, the platform is robotically accessible, so can function as one station in an automated screening work cell. Most of the zebrafish screens published to date have screened $\geq$ 1000 small-molecule chemicals in libraries by manually performing most aspects of the set-up, phenotype observation and analysis. The advantages of the model alone have permitted the size and number of manual screens reported. But manual phenotype assessment as a component of modern drug discovery and toxicology screens is impractical because it is too labor intensive, slow, does not generate numerical readouts and usually lacks complete archiving of screen images and data. Automated image-based screening addresses these hurdles and preserves the ability to conduct retrospective analyses of screen performance, to examine phenotypic changes that were not the primary focus of the screen, and to cross-reference screening data with past or future screens using the same compound library.[28,29] Automated embryo placement and image analysis will thus eliminate two major impediments to zebrafish whole-animal chemical screening, and, in so doing, vastly expand the accessibility of high-throughput screening and the range of chemical activity that can be explored and databased.

### 14.8.1 Small-Molecule Screens in Zebrafish

A number of zebrafish laboratories have recently reported systematic evaluations of zebrafish toxicity endpoints using many pharmacologically relevant compounds with well-established toxicity profiles in mammals. These studies are thoroughly reviewed and included cardiotoxicity, seizure liability, ototoxicity, developmental toxicity and gut motility assays.[61] The results of these studies indicate that zebrafish chemical screens can attain toxicological predictivity ranging from "sufficient" to "good" based on guidelines established by the European Centre for the Validation of Alternative Methods.[61,130] An article by Redfern *et al.* examined zebrafish assays as early safety pharmacology screens, emphasizing assay validation outcomes and predictive relevance to human toxicity, with an overall positive evaluation of using zebrafish for safety screening.[131]

The first small-molecule screen in zebrafish was published a decade ago, and the nearly 20 screens conducted in zebrafish through 2008, and the libraries used, have been thoroughly reviewed.[132,133] Two recent reviews in particular offer informative perspectives on what has been learned from high-throughput zebrafish screens and the likely future directions of their use in drug discovery.[86,134] We note that nearly all of the zebrafish screens published have been directed at drug discovery, drug toxicity, or small-molecule bioactivity with the resulting identification of important probes of whole-animal processes. They have also yielded a handful of compounds of potentially great therapeutic value.[134] Zebrafish screens have focused primarily on small-molecule suppression of mutations or models of human disease, and on perturbations of defined signaling pathways.[134] Emerging efforts into more complex behavioral and physiologic phenotypes will exploit the power of whole-organism phenotypic screening. This will be fostered, in large part, by automated image analysis.

The advantages of the model and the level of assay automation that can be brought to bear are the tools with which we can access the power of zebrafish pharmacological screens to study more complex physiologic and behavioral phenotypes. Developing behavior as a high-throughput endpoint has already been successfully reported. One behavior-based screen recently used automated motion analysis to define movement during wake and sleep cycles in zebrafish, and screened approximately 4000 unique compounds for modifiers of movement behavior.[79] Another recent screen defined the visual photomotor response to alternating brief periods of light and dark and screened a library of 14 000 compounds for modifiers of the response.[80] Both studies used high-throughput screening platforms and analysis programs that, because of the unique challenges presented by so much data, were developed 'in house' to format analyzed data into barcodes, allowing for hierarchal clustering of the behavior responses into groups of *phenotypically* related molecules. As an example, one phenotypically related cluster of molecules modified the photomotor response to a "slow-to-relax" behavior. The cluster of molecules contained acetylcholinesterase (AChE) inhibitors, along with two structurally unrelated and un-characterized compounds, which, by phenotype alone, were accurately predicted to have AChE-inhibiting activity.[80]

We have discussed above how other physiologic parameters of the zebrafish are amenable to rapid-throughput screening and are becoming accessible for toxicology screening. Transparent and rapid development of the heart, rapid electrocardiogram assessment, and fluorescent reporters allow rapid measurement of heart rate, contractility, rhythm (arrhythmia) and QT interval. Small-scale screens have already used zebrafish embryos to analyze heart rate and ERG function, and to screen drugs that may affect both of these parameters.[48,50] Continued development and application of novel tissue-specific and xenobiotic-responsive reporter lines will be a foundational approach to general screening of new chemistries for cardio, hepato, and neuronal toxicity. Screens that incorporate gene expression profiling with comprehensive phenotype analyses will continue to strengthen the predictivity of zebrafish toxicology data and encourage greater use of the model, especially as a means of frontloading hazard detection and reducing late-stage attrition in drug discovery.

## 14.9 Current Needs and Challenges

### 14.9.1 Metabolic Differences

Metabolism and adsorption, distribution, metabolism and excretion (ADME) modeling is extremely important for both drug development and toxicology. It allows for investigation into the fate of compounds *in vivo* that can be followed up with SAR studies to determine structural changes that improve the potency of a compound without increasing toxicity or adversely impacting ADME. Mammalian models remain the principal standard for metabolic studies in the public and private sector. Though rat and mouse metabolism of some chemicals depart dramatically from humans, rodents offer obvious advantages for ease and accuracy of dosing, monitoring food and water intake, and monitoring excretion. But the high cost of rodent metabolism studies, the much larger compound amounts needed to affect their biology, and continuing regulatory pressure on researchers to reduce the use of mammals in the lab, are shifting attention to the zebrafish for metabolism studies. It is critical to understand the metabolism of a compound to active metabolites, or those that elicit different pharmacological mechanisms, to fully predict the toxicity of a substance.[5,135] Over the last 10 years research has confirmed the presence of a host of important drug-metabolizing enzymes in zebrafish. The following list was reported by Alderton *et al.*: monoamine oxidase, aldehyde and alchohol dehydrogenases, acetyltransferases (*ADH 8A* and *B*), glucuronyltransferases, sulfotransferases (*SULT ST2, 3* and *5*) and glutathione-*S*-tranferases.[54,136–143] Additionally, approximately 90 zebrafish genes have been identified as Phase I, cytochrome P450 family and sub-family members and isoforms.[144] The zebrafish is a promising predictive model of metabolism for drug-safety studies. It is also a metabolic model for environmental toxicants. Examples include *zfCYP1A* and *zfCYP26K* metabolism of benzo(*a*)pyrene and aflatoxin-B1, respectively.[145,146] AhR-mediated CYP1A induction by polychlorinated biphenyls (PCBs) has also been investigated.[147] Zebrafish may also be a good model for studying prevalent diseases such as atherosclerosis, Alzheimer's disease, obesity and type II diabetes, now known to involve deficient lipid metabolism.[148] Lipid deposition, cellular changes and macrophage deposition of lipids were imaged in zebrafish to study atherosclerotic-like lesion development.[148,149] Combining zebrafish behavioral analysis as a phenotype anchor with automated imaging of aberrant lipid accumulation in the CNS will make the zebrafish a powerful model of neurodegenerative diseases.[148] Zebrafish also exhibit hyperglycaemic responses similar to humans after high-glucose exposure, and show decreased blood glucose following administration of glipizide, an anti-diabetic drug.[148,150,151]

#### *14.9.1.1 Chemical Compound Metabolism*

Only a few studies to date have investigated compound metabolism in zebrafish larvae. For example, the metabolism of methimazole, atrazine, ethoxuresorufin, and microcystin-LR have been assessed in zebrafish.[135,152–154] The accumulation and metabolism of several common drugs and CYP gene probe substrates was recently assessed using pharmacologically and toxicologically relevant conditions.[135] When the metabolites of several compounds were quantified, the metabolites accounted for only a small percentage of the amount of parent compound administered, and metabolite quantity was always much lower than that of parent compound. Striking similarities as well as important differences between zebrafish and mammalian metabolic pathways were noted, indicating that for some compounds, metabolites would not significantly contribute to the outcome of safety pharmacology or toxicology studies in zebrafish larvae under typical study paradigms.[135]

#### *14.9.1.2 Sex-Related Differences in Zebrafish Metabolism*

A recent metabolomics study in zebrafish demonstrated sex-related differences in the metabolism of amino acids, unsaturated fatty acids, cholesterol and phospholipids in adult livers. These data highlight another relative unknown in zebrafish metabolism needing further investigation before the widespread use of metabolomics in pharmological and toxicological studies.[96]

#### *14.9.1.3 Metabolism and the Developing Zebrafish*

A recent study profiled the metabolites of dextromethorphan generated over several stages of zebrafish development and suggested that metabolic processes varied with the stage of development.[52] This is a preliminary but valuable insight for future ADME studies aiming to assess metabolic pathways of interest for safety pharmacology.[96,155] More studies that systematically characterize the metabolism of class-representative compounds are needed to optimize use of the developing zebrafish for ADME. Developmental-stage-specific metabolic activity could also present a challenge for large chemical or drug screens in zebrafish which are typically conducted over a fixed exposure time. A way to deal with this caveat would be to simply screen for predicted 'problem' metabolites during the appropriate embryonic state. Another approach is to include induced rat liver microsomes, during the zebrafish embryo exposure, as a mammalian metabolic activation system able to biotransform proteratogenic compounds.[156,157] Mammalian-type metabolites in this approach have been reported to modulate the toxicological responses to a variety of compounds.[156,157]

Zebrafish metabolism may prove to be a predictive model of compound ADME and relative hazard in higher vertebrates, but more characterization of zebrafish metabolic pathways is needed before we have a functional grasp of the metabolic differences and similarities with mammals. When metabolomic data are linked with protein and mRNA expression data from the same or similar studies, we will begin to have a systems biology perspective of zebrafish metabolism from which to gauge the predictive capacity of zebrafish ADME data.[96]

### 14.9.2 Routes of Exposure and Uptake

Differences in routes of exposure and uptake, primarily adsorption and distribution must also be addressed. There is concern whether or not a chemical will target the same site in zebrafish that it does in a mammal. Since zebrafish are relatively dimethyl sulfoxide (DMSO) tolerant, test compounds can be diluted and administered in up to 0.1% DMSO without causing any morphological or genetic alterations in the animal. Therefore, zebrafish can absorb many chemicals soluble in DMSO. During the time frame of most larval zebrafish screening assays (0–5 dpf) oxygen is supplied primarily *via* diffusion across the skin, also a major route of adsorption of chemicals.[158–160]

Approximately 72 hpf is when zebrafish begin to swallow and oral exposure becomes an active route. Gill formation and use occurs after the period of typical larval zebrafish toxicology exposure and is, therefore, not a relevant exposure route. While water-born exposures are the most commonly used administration, compounds can also be administered *via* microinjection. Inexpensive, and commonly used microinjection allows nanoliter volumes of chemicals in solution to be administered to several hundred embryos per hour making it a moderate-throughput exposure method.[159]

Metabolic differences and, to a lesser extent, the nuances of exposure and uptake, present mild challenges to the use of zebrafish for predictive toxicology. The advantages of the zebrafish embryo for transparently monitoring chemical effects on major organ systems, including the brain, liver, nervous and cardiovascular systems, cartilage, notochord, and kidney outweigh the challenges especially in light of the speed with which zebrafish embryo studies can be completed, the cost savings over mammals, and less restrictive regulatory concerns.

## 14.10 Data Management Tools

The identification of predictive endpoints is at the core of modern toxicology. The basic approach to hazard prediction will require statistical inference of toxicity response from either chemical features (*i.e.*, QSAR), embryo/larval response to exposure (phenotype), or gene expression profiling of target tissues. Proteomic and metabolomic profiling from zebrafish will be later additions. The approach has been validated in a few small-scale zebrafish studies, showing a potential for predictive toxicology, but there is still no systematic approach to model the interaction between chemical features, molecular networks and toxicity outcome.[53,72,95,161–163] While much remains to be done, toxicology data frameworks exist into which zebrafish knowledge can be integrated or organizationally modeled after. For example, a large knowledgebase of the toxicological effects of chemicals in higher vertebrates has been organized into a searchable database [Toxicity Reference Database (ToxRefDB)] curated by the US Environmental Protection Agency.[164] The National Institutes of Health's Chemical Genomics Center is focusing on predictive toxicology, conducting high-throughput screening of >1000 compounds to determine which biological processes are targets of environmental chemicals. This effort is part of the ToxCast chemical prioritization program, and the data are being integrated into the ToxCast database.[165,166] ACToR (Aggregated Computational Toxicology Resource) is a database and set of software applications that bring into one central location information on chemical structure, *in vitro* bioassays and *in vivo* toxicology assays derived from more than 150 sources and helps manage large ToxCast data sets.[167] Having a large body of detailed zebrafish phenotype (including behavior), toxicogenomic and tissue spatiotemporal expression data in these databases, along with chemical structure, will provide the much-needed SARs for zebrafish-based hazard prediction. This only reinforces the need for systematic screening of compound libraries by high throughput assays with the most robust and informative endpoints. Zebrafish will become a predictive, computational toxicology model with the availability of large, high-quality data streams from the public and private sector, streams that are necessarily high-information-content, and publicly available. At the level of the investigator, these data streams will require novel biostatistical methods and substantial computational power to analyze. A variety of inexpensive, highly developed, open-source software packages such as MatLab (Mathworks Inc.) and Open Microscopy Environment (OME Inc.) are available and readily configurable for data-formatting analyses and classification. Software to manage the workflow and data acquisition from complex screening protocols is also becoming affordable as open source.[168]

## 14.11 Conclusion: Is Zebrafish Relevant Enough to be Predictive?

The bulk of zebrafish toxicological work suggests that it is a sufficiently relevant model to be predictive. Numerous zebrafish assays and -omics approaches have been developed for evaluating whole-organism responses to many thousands of chemicals and, when specifically examined, the results appear to predict toxic liability in humans. This has been a big step forward for the model and for toxicology. Yet a pressing need remains for large-scale zebrafish studies that systematically evaluate the most promising zebrafish assays against the widest possible range of positive and negative reference compounds, *i.e.*, chemistries with pharmacological relevance and well-known effects in mammals. This will form a much needed foundation of assay validation and distinguish the truly predictive approaches in zebrafish from those that are not.

## References

1. L. G. Valerio Jr., *Toxicol. Appl. Pharmacol.*, 2009, **241**, 356–370.
2. S. M. Paul, D. S. Mytelka, C. T. Dunwiddie, C. C. Persinger, B. H. Munos, S. R. Lindborg and A. L. Schacht, *Nat. Rev. Drug Discovery*, 2010, **9**, 203–214.
3. J. A. DiMasi and H. G. Grabowski, *J. Clin. Oncol.*, 2007, **25**, 209–216.
4. S. Frantz, *Nat. Rev. Drug Discovery*, 2004, **3**, 379.
5. L. I. Zon and R. T. Peterson, *Nat. Rev. Drug Discovery*, 2005, **4**, 35–44.
6. J. A. DiMasi, *Pharmacoeconomics*, 2002, **20**, 1–10.
7. J. Cook, G. Hunter and J. A. Vernon, *Pharmacoeconomics*, 2009, **27**, 355–363.
8. I. Kola and J. Landis, *Nat. Rev. Drug Discovery*, 2004, **3**, 711–715.
9. A. Luhe, L. Suter, S. Ruepp, T. Singer, T. Weiser and S. Albertini, *Mutat. Res.*, 2005, **575**, 102–115.
10. D. R. Boverhof and T. R. Zacharewski, *Toxicol. Sci.*, 2006, **89**, 352–360.

11. T. P. Barros, W. K. Alderton, H. M. Reynolds, A. G. Roach and S. Berghmans, *Br. J. Pharmacol.*, 2008, **154**, 1400–1413.
12. A. L. Rubinstein, *Curr. Opin. Drug Discovery Devel.*, 2003, **6**, 218–223.
13. A. J. Hill, H. Teraoka, W. Heideman and R. E. Peterson, *Toxicol. Sci.*, 2005, **86**, 6–19.
14. A. L. Rubinstein, *Expert Opin. Drug Metab. Toxicol.*, 2006, **2**, 231–240.
15. S. E. Brockerhoff, J. B. Hurley, U. Janssen-Bienhold, S. C. Neuhauss, W. Driever and J. E. Dowling, *Proc. Natl. Acad. Sci. U. S. A.*, 1995, **92**, 10545–10549.
16. S. C. Neuhauss, O. Biehlmaier, M. W. Seeliger, T. Das, K. Kohler, W. A. Harris and H. Baier, *J. Neurosci.*, 1999, **19**, 8603–8615.
17. C. Ton and C. Parng, *Hear. Res.*, 2005, **208**, 79–88.
18. W. Heideman, D. S. Antkiewicz, S. A. Carney and R. E. Peterson, *Cardiovasc. Toxicol.*, 2005, **5**, 203–214.
19. S. A. Carney, A. L. Prasch, W. Heideman and R. E. Peterson, *Birth Defects Res., Part A*, 2006, **76**, 7–18.
20. C. Parng, N. M. Roy, C. Ton, Y. Lin and P. McGrath, *J. Pharmacol. Toxicol. Methods*, 2007, **55**, 103–112.
21. E. A. Andreasen, L. K. Mathew, C. V. Lohr, R. Hasson and R. L. Tanguay, *Toxicol. Sci.*, 2007, **95**, 215–226.
22. L. L. Chiu, L. L. Cunningham, D. W. Raible, E. W. Rubel and H. C. Ou, *J. Assoc. Res. Otolaryngol.*, 2008, **9**, 178–190.
23. F. M. Richards, W. K. Alderton, G. M. Kimber, Z. Liu, I. Strang, W. S. Redfern, J. P. Valentin, M. J. Winter and T. H. Hutchinson, *J. Pharmacol. Toxicol. Methods*, 2008, **58**, 50–58.
24. S. Berghmans, P. Butler, P. Goldsmith, G. Waldron, I. Gardner, Z. Golder, F. M. Richards, G. Kimber, A. Roach, W. Alderton and A. Fleming, *J. Pharmacol. Toxicol. Methods*, 2008, **58**, 59–68.
25. R. Chapin, K. Augustine-Rauch, B. Beyer, G. Daston, R. Finnell, T. Flynn, S. Hunter, P. Mirkes, K. S. O'shea, A. Piersma, D. Sandler, P. Vanparys and G. Van Maele-Fabry, *Birth Defects Res., Part B*, 2008, **83**, 446–456.
26. S. Sun, Y. Gui, Y. Wang, L. Qian, X. Liu, Q. Jiang and H. Song, *Acta Biochim. Biophys. Sin.*, 2009, **41**, 86–96.
27. M. C. Mione and N. S. Trede, *Dis. Model. Mech.*, 2010, **3**, 517–523.
28. A. Vogt, A. Cholewinski, X. Shen, S. G. Nelson, J. S. Lazo, M. Tsang and N. A. Hukriede, *Dev. Dyn.*, 2009, **238**, 656–663.
29. A. Vogt, H. Codore, B. W. Day, N. A. Hukriede and M. Tsang, *J. Vis. Exp.*, 2010.
30. J. N. Chen, P. Haffter, J. Odenthal, E. Vogelsang, M. Brand, F. J. van Eeden, M. Furutani-Seiki, M. Granato, M. Hammerschmidt, C. P. Heisenberg, Y. J. Jiang, D. A. Kane, R. N. Kelsh, M. C. Mullins and C. Nusslein-Volhard, *Development*, 1996, **123**, 293–302.
31. J. P. Incardona, T. K. Collier and N. L. Scholz, *Toxicol. Appl. Pharmacol.*, 2004, **196**, 191–205.
32. D. S. Antkiewicz, C. G. Burns, S. A. Carney, R. E. Peterson and W. Heideman, *Toxicol. Sci.*, 2005, **84**, 368–377.

33. P. McGrath and C. Q. Li, *Drug Discovery Today*, 2008, **13**, 394–401.
34. S. A. Carney, J. Chen, C. G. Burns, K. M. Xiong, R. E. Peterson and W. Heideman, *Mol. Pharmacol.*, 2006, **70**, 549–561.
35. T. R. Henry, J. M. Spitsbergen, M. W. Hornung, C. C. Abnet and R. E. Peterson, *Toxicol. Appl. Pharmacol.*, 1997, **142**, 56–68.
36. H. Teraoka, W. Dong, S. Ogawa, S. Tsukiyama, Y. Okuhara, M. Niiyama, N. Ueno, R. E. Peterson and T. Hiraga, *Toxicol. Sci.*, 2002, **65**, 192–199.
37. C. G. Burns, D. J. Milan, E. J. Grande, W. Rottbauer, C. A. MacRae and M. C. Fishman, *Nat. Chem. Biol.*, 2005, **1**, 263–264.
38. T. C. Tran, B. Sneed, J. Haider, D. Blavo, A. White, T. Aiyejorun, T. C. Baranowski, A. L. Rubinstein, T. N. Doan, R. Dingledine and E. M. Sandberg, *Cancer Res.*, 2007, **67**, 11386–11392.
39. H. Tsutsui, S. Higashijima, A. Miyawaki and Y. Okamura, *J. Physiol.*, 2010, **588**, 2017–2021.
40. D. J. Milan and C. A. Macrae, *Prog. Biophys. Mol. Biol.*, 2008, **98**, 301–308.
41. L. Yang, N. Y. Ho, R. Alshut, J. Legradi, C. Weiss, M. Reischl, R. Mikut, U. Liebel, F. Muller and U. Strahle, *Reprod. Toxicol.*, 2009, **28**, 245–253.
42. D. J. Milan, A. M. Kim, J. R. Winterfield, I. L. Jones, A. Pfeufer, S. Sanna, D. E. Arking, A. H. Amsterdam, K. M. Sabeh, J. D. Mably, D. S. Rosenbaum, R. T. Peterson, A. Chakravarti, S. Kaab, D. M. Roden and C. A. MacRae, *Circulation*, 2009, **120**, 553–559.
43. I. U. Leong, J. R. Skinner, A. N. Shelling and D. R. Love, *Acta Physiol.*, 2010, **199**, 257–276.
44. K. Baker, K. S. Warren, G. Yellen and M. C. Fishman, *Proc. Natl. Acad. Sci. U. S. A.*, 1997, **94**, 4554–4559.
45. R. Creton, J. E. Speksnijder and L. F. Jaffe, *J. Cell Sci.*, 1998, **111**, 1613–1622.
46. M. J. Ackerman, *Mayo Clin. Proc.*, 1998, **73**, 250–269.
47. M. J. Ackerman, *Pediatr. Rev.*, 1998, **19**, 232–238.
48. D. J. Milan, T. A. Peterson, J. N. Ruskin, R. T. Peterson and C. A. MacRae, *Circulation*, 2003, **107**, 1355–1358.
49. U. Langheinrich, *Bioessays*, 2003, **25**, 904–912.
50. U. Langheinrich, G. Vacun and T. Wagner, *Toxicol. Appl. Pharmacol.*, 2003, **193**, 370–382.
51. C. A. Dlugos and R. A. Rabin, *Alcohol Clin. Exp. Res.*, 2010, **34**, 1013–1021.
52. Z. Xu, F. E. Williams and M. C. Liu, *J. Appl. Toxicol.*, 2011, **31**, 157–163.
53. D. J. Milan, I. L. Jones, P. T. Ellinor and C. A. MacRae, *Am. J. Physiol. Heart Circ. Physiol.*, 2006, **291**, H269–H273.
54. C. Wiegand, S. Pflugmacher, M. Giese, H. Frank and C. Steinberg, *Ecotoxicol. Environ. Saf.*, 2000, **45**, 122–131.
55. S. A. Carney, R. E. Peterson and W. Heideman, *Mol. Pharmacol.*, 2004, **66**, 512–521.
56. N. Wang, L. Mackenzie, A. G. De Souza, H. Zhong, G. Goss and L. Li, *J. Proteome Res.*, 2007, **6**, 263–272.

57. T. E. North, I. R. Babu, L. M. Vedder, A. M. Lord, J. S. Wishnok, S. R. Tannenbaum, L. I. Zon and W. Goessling, *Proc. Natl. Acad. Sci. U. S. A.*, 2010, **107**, 17315–17320.
58. T. Bresolin, M. de Freitas Rebelo and A. Celso Dias Bainy, *Comp. Biochem. Physiol., Part C: Toxicol. Pharmacol.,* 2005, **140**, 403–407.
59. H. P. Tseng, T. H. Hseu, D. R. Buhler, W. D. Wang and C. H. Hu, *Toxicol. Appl. Pharmacol.*, 2005, **205**, 247–258.
60. J. J. Sager, Q. Bai and E. A. Burton, *Brain Struct. Funct.*, 2010, **214**, 285–302.
61. P. M. Eimon and A. L. Rubinstein, *Expert Opin. Drug Metab. Toxicol.*, 2009, **5**, 393–401.
62. E. Kabashi, N. Champagne, E. Brustein and P. Drapeau, *Trends Genet.*, 2010, **26**, 373–381.
63. D. Kokel and R. T. Peterson, *Briefings Funct. Genomics Proteomics*, 2008, **7**, 483–490.
64. R. Gerlai, *Molecules*, 2010, **15**, 2609–2622.
65. P. Blader, C. Plessy and U. Strahle, *Mech. Dev.*, 2003, **120**, 211–218.
66. S. Higashijima, M. A. Masino, G. Mandel and J. R. Fetcho, *J. Neurosci.*, 2004, **24**, 5827–5839.
67. Y. Kimura, Y. Okamura and S. Higashijima, *J. Neurosci.*, 2006, **26**, 5684–5697.
68. T. J. van Ham, J. Mapes, D. Kokel and R. T. Peterson, *FASEB J.*, 2010, **24**, 4336–4342.
69. R. C. Eaton, R. A. Bombardieri and D. L. Meyer, *J. Exp. Biol.*, 1977, **66**, 65–81.
70. I. V. Zhdanova, S. Y. Wang, O. U. Leclair and N. P. Danilova, *Brain Res.*, 2001, **903**, 263–268.
71. P. I. Bang, P. C. Yelick, J. J. Malicki and W. F. Sewell, *J. Neurosci. Methods*, 2002, **118**, 177–187.
72. S. C. Baraban, M. R. Taylor, P. A. Castro and H. Baier, *Neuroscience*, 2005, **131**, 759–768.
73. D. G. Zeddies and R. R. Fay, *J. Exp. Biol.*, 2005, **208**, 1363–1372.
74. H. A. Burgess and M. Granato, *J. Neurosci.*, 2007, **27**, 4984–4994.
75. H. A. Burgess and M. Granato, *J. Exp. Biol.*, 2007, **210**, 2526–2539.
76. M. J. Winter, W. S. Redfern, A. J. Hayfield, S. F. Owen, J. P. Valentin and T. H. Hutchinson, *J. Pharmacol. Toxicol. Methods*, 2008, **57**, 176–187.
77. A. Easter, M. E. Bell, J. R. Damewood Jr, W. S. Redfern, J. P. Valentin, M. J. Winter, C. Fonck and R. A. Bialecki, *Drug Discovery Today*, 2009, **14**, 876–884.
78. R. Portugues and F. Engert, *Curr. Opin. Neurobiol.*, 2009, **19**, 644–647.
79. J. Rihel, D. A. Prober, A. Arvanites, K. Lam, S. Zimmerman, S. Jang, S. J. Haggarty, D. Kokel, L. L. Rubin, R. T. Peterson and A. F. Schier, *Science*, **327**, 348–351.
80. D. Kokel, J. Bryan, C. Laggner, R. White, C. Y. Cheung, R. Mateus, D. Healey, S. Kim, A. A. Werdich, S. J. Haggarty, C. A. Macrae, B. Shoichet and R. T. Peterson, *Nat. Chem. Biol.*, **6**, 231–237.
81. K. P. Mueller and S. C. Neuhauss, *Curr. Biol.*, 2010, **20**, R159–R161.

82. G. A. Hortopan, M. T. Dinday and S. C. Baraban, *Dis. Model. Mech.*, 2010, **3**, 144–148.
83. I. V. Zhdanova, *Zebrafish*, 2006, **3**, 215–226.
84. J. E. Zimmerman, N. Naidoo, D. M. Raizen and A. I. Pack, *Trends Neurosci.*, 2008, **31**, 371–376.
85. W. Norton and L. Bally-Cuif, *BMC Neurosci.*, 2010, **11**, 90.
86. K. L. Taylor, N. J. Grant, N. D. Temperley and E. E. Patton, *Cell Commun. Signal.*, 2010, **8**, 11.
87. S. M. Billiard, A. R. Timme-Laragy, D. M. Wassenberg, C. Cockman and R. T. Di Giulio, *Toxicol. Sci.*, 2006, **92**, 526–536.
88. D. Arslanova, T. Yang, X. Xu, S. T. Wong, C. E. Augelli-Szafran and W. Xia, *BMC Biotechnol.*, 2010, **10**, 24.
89. X. Xu, X. Huang, W. Xia and S. Xia, *J. Biomol. Screen.*, 2010, **15**, 1152–1159.
90. S. R. Blechinger, R. C. Kusch, K. Haugo, C. Matz, D. P. Chivers and P. H. Krone, *Toxicol. Appl. Pharmacol.*, 2007, **224**, 72–80.
91. H. C. Ou, D. W. Raible and E. W. Rubel, *Hear. Res.*, 2007, **233**, 46–53.
92. A. Johnson, E. Carew and K. A. Sloman, *Aquat. Toxicol.*, 2007, **84**, 431–438.
93. M. Froehlicher, A. Liedtke, K. J. Groh, S. C. Neuhauss, H. Segner and R. I. Eggen, *Aquat. Toxicol.*, 2009, **95**, 307–319.
94. A. Ghysen, C. Dambly-Chaudiere and D. Raible, *Neural. Dev.*, 2007, **2**, 15.
95. L. Yang, J. R. Kemadjou, C. Zinsmeister, M. Bauer, J. Legradi, F. Muller, M. Pankratz, J. Jakel and U. Strahle, *Genome Biol.*, 2007, **8**, R227.
96. H. Sukardi, C. Y. Ung, Z. Gong and S. H. Lam, *Zebrafish*, 2010, **7**, 41–52.
97. Z. Wang, M. Gerstein and M. Snyder, *Nat. Rev. Genet.*, 2009, **10**, 57–63.
98. B. T. Wilhelm and J. R. Landry, *Methods*, 2009, **48**, 249–257.
99. A. D. Sawle, E. Wit, G. Whale and A. R. Cossins, *Toxicol. Sci.*, 2010, **118**, 128–139.
100. Z. Hegedus, A. Zakrzewska, V. C. Agoston, A. Ordas, P. Racz, M. Mink, H. P. Spaink and A. H. Meijer, *Mol. Immunol.*, 2009, **46**, 2918–2930.
101. A. Ordas, Z. Hegedus, C. V. Henkel, O. W. Stockhammer, D. Butler, H. J. Jansen, P. Racz, M. Mink, H. P. Spaink and A. H. Meijer, *Fish Shellfish Immunol.*, 2010.
102. C. Y. Ung, S. H. Lam, M. M. Hlaing, C. L. Winata, S. Korzh, S. Mathavan and Z. Gong, *BMC Genomics*, 2010, **11**, 212.
103. J. Chen, S. A. Carney, R. E. Peterson and W. Heideman, *Physiol. Genomics*, 2008, **33**, 148–158.
104. E. A. Andreasen, L. K. Mathew and R. L. Tanguay, *Toxicol. Sci.*, 2006, **92**, 254–269.
105. L. K. Mathew, S. S. Sengupta, J. Ladu, E. A. Andreasen and R. L. Tanguay, *FASEB J.*, 2008, **22**, 3087–3096.
106. C. K. Kaufman, R. M. White and L. Zon, *Nat. Protoc.*, 2009, **4**, 1422–1432.
107. W. Goessling, T. E. North and L. I. Zon, *J. Clin. Oncol.*, 2007, **25**, 2473–2479.
108. G. J. Lieschke and P. D. Currie, *Nat. Rev. Genet.*, 2007, **8**, 353–367.
109. G. W. Stuart, J. R. Vielkind, J. V. McMurray and M. Westerfield, *Development*, 1990, **109**, 577–584.

110. A. J. Udvadia and E. Linney, *Dev. Biol.*, 2003, **256**, 1–17.
111. A. Deiters and J. A. Yoder, *Zebrafish*, 2006, **3**, 415–429.
112. C. J. Mattingly, J. A. McLachlan and W. A. Toscano Jr, *Environ. Health Perspect.*, 2001, **109**, 845–849.
113. A. Hill, C. V. Howard, U. Strahle and A. Cossins, *Toxicol. Sci.*, 2003, **76**, 392–399.
114. P. Hu, M. Tian, J. Bao, G. Xing, X. Gu, X. Gao, E. Linney and Q. Zhao, *Dev. Dyn.*, 2008, **237**, 3798–3808.
115. S. Y. Yeo, M. Kim, H. S. Kim, T. L. Huh and A. B. Chitnis, *Dev. Biol.*, 2007, **301**, 555–567.
116. G. A. Molina, S. C. Watkins and M. Tsang, *BMC Dev. Biol.*, 2007, **7**, 62.
117. N. D. Lawson and B. M. Weinstein, *Dev. Biol.*, 2002, **248**, 307–318.
118. S. W. Jin, D. Beis, T. Mitchell, J. N. Chen and D. Y. Stainier, *Development*, 2005, **132**, 5199–5209.
119. Y. R. Cha and B. M. Weinstein, *Birth Defects Res., Part C*, 2007, **81**, 286–296.
120. P. A. Morcos, *Biochem. Biophys. Res. Commun.*, 2007, **358**, 521–527.
121. S. Ramachandran, B. Ruef, C. Pich and J. Sprague, *Curr. Protoc. Bioinformatics*, Unit 1.18.
122. Y. Bradford, T. Conlin, N. Dunn, D. Fashena, K. Frazer, D. G. Howe, J. Knight, P. Mani, R. Martin, S. A. Moxon, H. Paddock, C. Pich, S. Ramachandran, B. J. Ruef, L. Ruzicka, H. Bauer Schaper, K. Schaper, X. Shao, A. Singer, J. Sprague, B. Sprunger, C. Van Slyke and M. Westerfield, *Nucleic Acids Res*, 2010, **39**, D822–D829.
123. S. Henikoff, B. J. Till and L. Comai, *Plant Physiol.*, 2004, **135**, 630–636.
124. E. Wienholds, F. van Eeden, M. Kosters, J. Mudde, R. H. Plasterk and E. Cuppen, *Genome Res.*, 2003, **13**, 2700–2707.
125. E. Wienholds and R. H. Plasterk, *Methods Cell Biol.*, 2004, **77**, 69–90.
126. B. W. Draper, C. M. McCallum, J. L. Stout, A. J. Slade and C. B. Moens, *Methods Cell Biol.*, 2004, **77**, 91–112.
127. S. L. Amacher, *Briefings Funct. Genomics Proteomics*, 2008, **7**, 460–464.
128. Y. Doyon, J. M. McCammon, J. C. Miller, F. Faraji, C. Ngo, G. E. Katibah, R. Amora, T. D. Hocking, L. Zhang, E. J. Rebar, P. D. Gregory, F. D. Urnov and S. L. Amacher, *Nat. Biotechnol.*, 2008, **26**, 702–708.
129. X. Meng, M. B. Noyes, L. J. Zhu, N. D. Lawson and S. A. Wolfe, *Nat Biotechnol*, 2008, **26**, 695–701.
130. E. Genschow, H. Spielmann, G. Scholz, A. Seiler, N. Brown, A. Piersma, M. Brady, N. Clemann, H. Huuskonen, F. Paillard, S. Bremer and K. Becker, *Altern. Lab. Anim.*, 2002, **30**, 151–176.
131. W. S. Redfern, G. Waldron, M. J. Winter, P. Butler, M. Holbrook, R. Wallis and J. P. Valentin, *J. Pharmacol. Toxicol. Methods*, 2008, **58**, 110–117.
132. R. T. Peterson, B. A. Link, J. E. Dowling and S. L. Schreiber, *Proc. Natl. Acad. Sci. U. S. A.*, 2000, **97**, 12965–12969.
133. G. N. Wheeler and A. W. Brandli, *Dev. Dyn.*, 2009, **238**, 1287–1308.
134. D. S. Peal, R. T. Peterson and D. Milan, *J. Cardiovasc. Transl. Res.*, 2010, **3**, 454–460.

135. W. Alderton, S. Berghmans, P. Butler, H. Chassaing, A. Fleming, Z. Golder, F. Richards and I. Gardner, *Xenobiotica*, **40**, 547–557.
136. O. Anichtchik, V. Sallinen, N. Peitsaro and P. Panula, *J. Comp. Neurol.*, 2006, **498**, 593–610.
137. A. K. Dasmahapatra, H. L. Doucet, C. Bhattacharyya and M. J. Carvan, 3rd, *Biochem. Biophys. Res. Commun.*, 2001, **286**, 1082–1086.
138. M. J. Reimers, M. E. Hahn and R. L. Tanguay, *J. Biol. Chem.*, 2004, **279**, 38303–38312.
139. N. Lassen, T. Estey, R. L. Tanguay, A. Pappa, M. J. Reimers and V. Vasiliou, *Drug Metab. Dispos.*, 2005, **33**, 649–656.
140. S. Yasuda, A. P. Kumar, M. Y. Liu, Y. Sakakibara, M. Suiko, L. Chen and M. C. Liu, *FEBS J.*, 2005, **272**, 3828–3837.
141. M. A. Iannelli, I. Marcucci and L. Vittozzi, *Ecotoxicol. Environ. Saf.*, 1994, **28**, 172–180.
142. S. Yasuda, M. Y. Liu, Y. S. Yang, R. Snow, S. Takahashi and M. C. Liu, *Arch. Biochem. Biophys.*, 2006, **455**, 1–9.
143. S. Zok, G. Gorge, W. Kalsch and R. Nagel, *Sci. Total Environ.*, 1991, **109–110**, 411–421.
144. J. Stegeman, J. Goldstone, M. E. Jonsson and B. Woodin in *Oxidative xenobiotic metabolism in zebrafish: The cytochrome P450 gene complement, regulation and function*, American Chemical Society, Boston, MA, 2007.
145. C. L. Miranda, W. G. Chung, J. L. Wang-Buhler, T. Musafia-Jeknic, W. M. Baird and D. R. Buhler, *Aquat. Toxicol.*, 2006, **80**, 101–108.
146. J. L. Wang-Buhler, S. J. Lee, W. G. Chung, J. F. Stevens, H. P. Tseng, T. H. Hseu, C. H. Hu, M. Westerfield, Y. H. Yang, C. L. Miranda and D. R. Buhler, *Comp. Biochem. Physiol., Part C: Toxicol. Pharmacol.*, 2005, **140**, 207–219.
147. M. E. Jonsson, R. Orrego, B. R. Woodin, J. V. Goldstone and J. J. Stegeman, *Toxicol. Appl. Pharmacol.*, 2007, **221**, 29–41.
148. M. Holtta-Vuori, V. T. Salo, L. Nyberg, C. Brackmann, A. Enejder, P. Panula and E. Ikonen, *Biochem. J.*, **429**, 235–242.
149. K. Stoletov, L. Fang, S. H. Choi, K. Hartvigsen, L. F. Hansen, C. Hall, J. Pattison, J. Juliano, E. R. Miller, F. Almazan, P. Crosier, J. L. Witztum, R. L. Klemke and Y. I. Miller, *Circ. Res.*, 2009, **104**, 952–960.
150. M. Gleeson, V. Connaughton and L. S. Arneson, *Acta Diabetol.*, 2007, **44**, 157–163.
151. B. Elo, C. M. Villano, D. Govorko and L. A. White, *J. Mol. Endocrinol.*, 2007, **38**, 433–440.
152. L. Hollosi, A. Kettrup and K. W. Schramm, *J. Pharm. Biomed. Anal.*, 2004, **36**, 921–924.
153. S. Pflugmacher, C. Wiegand, K. A. Beattie, E. Krause, C. E. Steinberg and G. A. Codd, *Environ. Toxicol. Chem.*, 2001, **20**, 846–852.
154. C. Wiegand, E. Krause, C. Steinberg and S. Pflugmacher, *Ecotoxicol. Environ. Saf.*, 2001, **49**, 199–205.

155. S. Hayashi, S. Akiyama, Y. Tamaru, Y. Takeda, T. Fujiwara, K. Inoue, A. Kobayashi, S. Maegawa and E. Fukusaki, *Biochem. Biophys. Res. Commun.*, 2009, **386**, 268–272.
156. F. Busquet, R. Nagel, F. von Landenberg, S. O. Mueller, N. Huebler and T. H. Broschard, *Toxicol. Sci.*, 2008, **104**, 177–188.
157. S. Weigt, N. Huebler, T. Braunbeck, F. von Landenberg and T. H. Broschard, *Toxicology*, **275**, 36–49.
158. T. Schwerte, D. Uberbacher and B. Pelster, *J. Exp. Biol.*, 2003, **206**, 1299–1307.
159. P. Goldsmith, *Curr. Opin. Pharmacol.*, 2004, **4**, 504–512.
160. J. Y. Sire, F. Allizard, O. Babiar, J. Bourguignon and A. Quilhac, *J. Anat.*, 1997, **190**, 545–561.
161. A. Holmberg, T. Schwerte, B. Pelster and S. Holmgren, *J. Exp. Biol.*, 2004, **207**, 4085–4094.
162. S. H. Lam, S. Mathavan, Y. Tong, H. Li, R. K. Karuturi, Y. Wu, V. B. Vega, E. T. Liu and Z. Gong, *PLoS Genet.*, 2008, **4**, e1000121.
163. S. C. Neuhauss, *J. Neurobiol.*, 2003, **54**, 148–160.
164. R. Kavlock and D. Dix, *J. Environ. Sci. Health, Part C: Environ. Carcinog. Ecotoxicol. Rev.*, **13**, 197–217.
165. R. Benigni, C. Bossa, A. Giuliani and O. Tcheremenskaia, *J. Environ. Sci. Health, Part C: Environ. Carcinog. Ecotoxicol. Rev.*, **28**, 272–286.
166. D. J. Dix, K. A. Houck, M. T. Martin, A. M. Richard, R. W. Setzer and R. J. Kavlock, *Toxicol. Sci.*, 2007, **95**, 5–12.
167. R. Judson, A. Richard, D. Dix, K. Houck, F. Elloumi, M. Martin, T. Cathey, T. R. Transue, R. Spencer and M. Wolf, *Toxicol. Appl. Pharmacol.*, 2008, **233**, 7–13.
168. K. Kozak, G. Bakos, A. Hoff, E. Bennett, D. Dunican, A. Davies, D. Kelleher, A. Long and G. Csucs, *J. Biomol. Screen.*, **15**, 892–899.

CHAPTER 15

# In Vivo *Genetic Toxicology: Application to Cancer Risk Assessment*

MICHAEL J. SCHLOSSER* AND CHRISTOPHER S. FARABAUGH

WIL Research Company, 8025 Lamon Avenue, Skokie, Illinois, USA

## 15.1 Introduction

Genotoxicity studies conducted in animals are critical for determining whether a genotoxic hazard identified during *in vitro* testing will translate to a meaningful cancer risk. The more widely used *in vivo* genotoxicity assays and their relative use in regulatory testing and cancer risk assessment are listed in Table 15.1. Human cancer risk from either intentional or unintentional chemical exposure is ultimately determined from rodent cancer bioassays, after taking into account all relevant information on toxicology, exposure, biologic activity, and mechanism. Because most rodent cancer bioassays require several years and millions of dollars (US$) to complete, animal studies measuring genotoxic endpoints become early surrogates for assessing cancer risk in exposed populations. In addition, specialized *in vivo* genotoxicity studies can help define the mode of action (MoA) through which a certain chemical (or chemical class) produces tumors. Through integration of genotoxicity results with dose–response data derived from ADME (absorption, distribution, metabolism and excretion), pharmacology, toxicology and human studies, a careful and comprehensive evaluation of cancer risk can be made for the target population.

RSC Drug Discovery Series No. 12
New Horizons in Predictive Toxicology: Current Status and Application
Edited by Alan G. E. Wilson

Published by the Royal Society of Chemistry, www.rsc.org

**Table 15.1** Summary of common *in vivo* genotoxicity assays for cancer risk assessment.

| | *Hematopoietic tissue cytogenetics* | *Unscheduled DNA synthesis* | *Comet* | *Exogenous reporter gene mutation* | *Endogenous gene mutation* | *DNA adducts* |
|---|---|---|---|---|---|---|
| Relative use: | +++++ | +++ | ++++ | ++ | + | + |
| Common examples | Bone-marrow micronucleus and chromosome aberrations | Liver *ex vivo* assessment | >pH 13 elution test | Big Blue®, Muta™Mouse | *Hprt* *Pig-a*[a] | $^{32}$P Post-labeling immunoassay LC-MS/MS |
| Primary evaluation criteria | DNA damage determined by micronuclei or chromosome injury | Thymidine incorporation during DNA repair | DNA strand breaks | Phenotypic mutations in the transfected *lac* operon | Phenotypic (*Hprt*, *Pig-a*) Genotypic oncogenes random genes[a] | Chemical- and oxygen-related nucleoside base adducts |
| Regulatory guidelines | OECD 474[47] OECD 475[48] | OECD 486[101] | — | — | OECD 476[195,b] | — |
| Working group recommendations | — | — | Burlinson *et al.* 2007[105] | WHO[125] | — | Phillips *et al.* 2000[169] |

[a]Represents a new technology in toxicology.
[b]OECD 476 covers *in vitro* phenotypic measure of the *Hprt* mutation.
LC-MS/MS – liquid chromatography-tandem mass spectroscopy.

As with *in vitro* genotoxicity testing for hazard identification, genotoxicity testing in animals involves evaluating the ability of a chemical to damage DNA or alter chromosome structure or number through assessment of aberrations and mutations to genomic DNA. A mutation is a manifestation of one or more chromosomal alterations that can occur in somatic cells (most cells of the body) or germ cells (spermatozoa, ova). With somatic cells, mutations are passed to daughter cells during mitosis, while in germ cells, mutations can be passed to offspring during meiosis (see Figure 15.1).[1] Somatic cell mutations, under conditions favoring cell growth and proliferation, have the potential to induce the formation of benign or malignant tumors. With chemical-induced germ-cell mutations, changes can occur in exposed individuals that have the potential to negatively impact subsequent unexposed generations. It is important to note that chemicals that induce germ-cell mutations represent only a small subset of those chemicals that cause somatic-cell mutations. This is largely the result of natural *in vivo* barriers designed to help protect germ cells against toxicant-induced injury.[2] Although it appears that genotoxicant-induced injury to germ cells is a less likely event relative to somatic cell injury, this conclusion is based on a small database.[3] As this chapter focuses on cancer risk assessment, *in vivo* models of germ-cell injury and the assessment of risk to offspring will not be discussed here.

Underlying the basic premise for genotoxicity testing is the strong belief that by altering DNA structure or function, an increased risk of mutations will occur in somatic cells, which can predispose animals or humans to neoplastic cell growth and cancer (malignant tumors). The association between DNA damage and tumorigenesis is well established[4,5] and supported by observations of rare genetic defects in DNA repair leading to much higher risks for tumor formation in affected individuals.[6] In addition, certain DNA defects have been shown to be important in the activation of oncogenes and the inhibition of tumor-suppressor genes, both of which are associated with formation of human cancers.[7,8]

Animal genotoxicity studies, typically conducted as part of a comprehensive toxicology program, are designed to help determine whether a hazard identified during *in vitro* genotoxicity testing is highly specific for DNA injury or occurs in response to nonspecific cytotoxicity or cell death. Alternatively, genotoxicity testing in animals also allows one to identify hazards that may not be readily identified using less complex *in vitro* test systems. Ideally, *in vivo* genotoxicity studies, if designed correctly, should help identify chemicals that cause DNA damage or mutations at doses that are well tolerated and without confounding toxicities. As previously noted, knowing whether a test substance causes DNA injury and possible subsequent gene mutations can provide key information for assessing cancer risk prior to the conduct of expensive and time-consuming lifetime rodent bioassays, and provides understanding of the possible MoA by which certain chemicals produce tumors in animals and target populations.

Although not discussed in this chapter, the predictability and relevance of the chronic rodent bioassay for human cancer risk has been the subject of debate and challenge.[9–14] One major reason for the controversy is that many rodent carcinogens have been shown to produce tumors only at maximum-tolerated

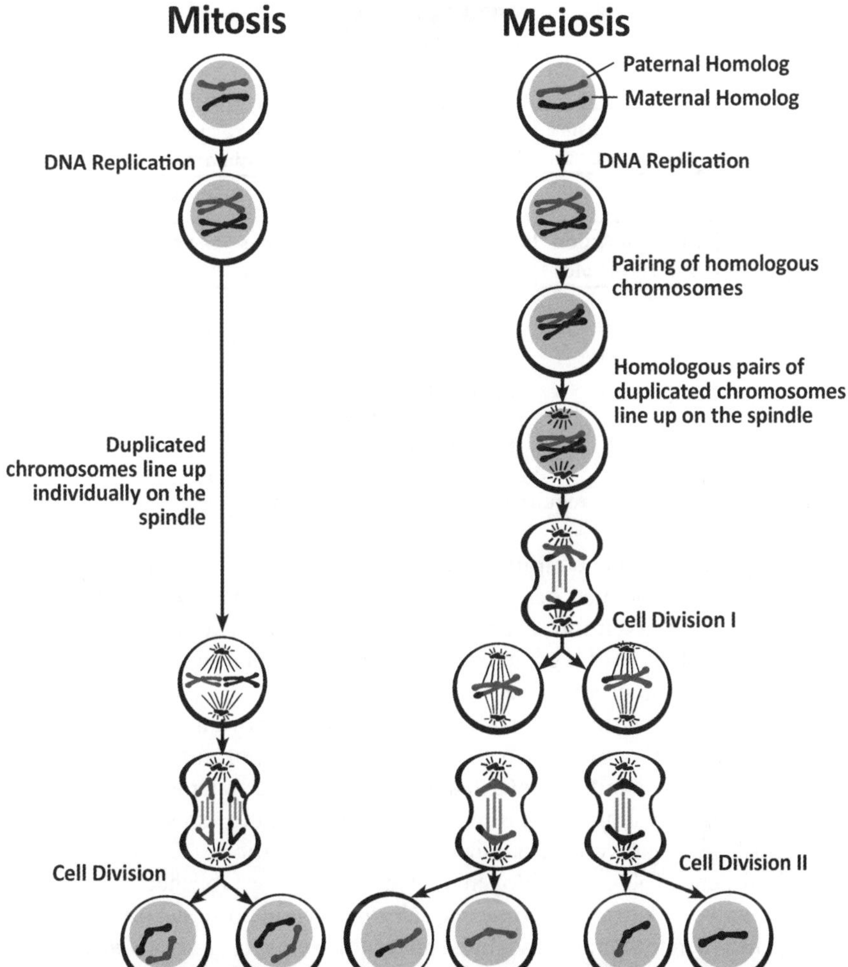


**Figure 15.1** Somatic cells divide by mitosis; metaphase cells denoted by chromosomes aligned in the center of the spindle. Meiosis has two cell divisions: 1) chromosomes decrease in number (diploid to haploid), condense, pair up, and segregate/recombine; 2) unpaired chromosomes are distributed to daughter cells. Microtubules function both to stabilize spindles and capture kinetochores, which are tri-laminar protein structures on either side of the centromeres. Described in ref. 1.

doses (MTDs), where metabolism, normal defense mechanisms, homeostasis, and/or cell turnover may be altered or compromised.

## 15.2 Hazard Identification *versus* Risk Assessment

For our purposes, hazard identification is defined as a "qualitative exercise" to identify whether a chemical should be classified as negative or positive for

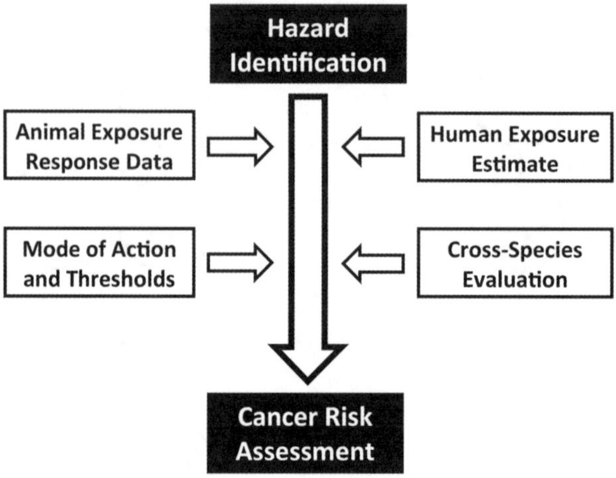


**Figure 15.2** Key factors required for cancer risk assessment.

genotoxicity under the conditions of a standardized, well-validated assay. Risk assessment is defined here as a "quantitative exercise" where all relevant scientific data are taken into account to make an informed decision about the carcinogenic potential of a chemical in the target population. Factors that can impact risk assessment are shown in Figure 15.2.

In practice, *in vivo* tests in rodents have been important for both hazard identification and risk assessment. *In vivo* testing is important to determine the relevance of positive findings revealed using *in vitro* test systems, many of which are thought to have a high rate of false positives,[15] and to assess chemicals that may yield false negative results during *in vitro* evaluation.[16] Once evidence of a potential genotoxic or carcinogenic effect has been established in an animal model (usually rodent), it becomes equally important to understand the relationship between systemic exposure and genotoxicity using both *in vitro* and *in vivo* approaches.[17,18] Animal studies allow for the collection of pharmacokinetic and target-organ data to help define the slope and shape of the exposure–response curve relative to the *in vivo* genotoxic or tumorigenic event at the target tissue. Molecular and cellular mechanistic data aid in understanding the MoA of the DNA damage and may help extrapolate the concentration required for DNA injury.[19] Information on the slope and shape of the dose–response curve from animal and cellular/molecular systems, coupled with information on chemical class, as well as a comprehensive understanding of the sensitivity, specificity, and genotoxicity assay limitations, are needed for accurate and informed risk assessment.[20]

## 15.3 Importance of Dose–Response and MoA Data

Dose–response data are extremely important in understanding the carcinogenic potential of a genotoxicant since irrelevant, high-dose effects can influence the

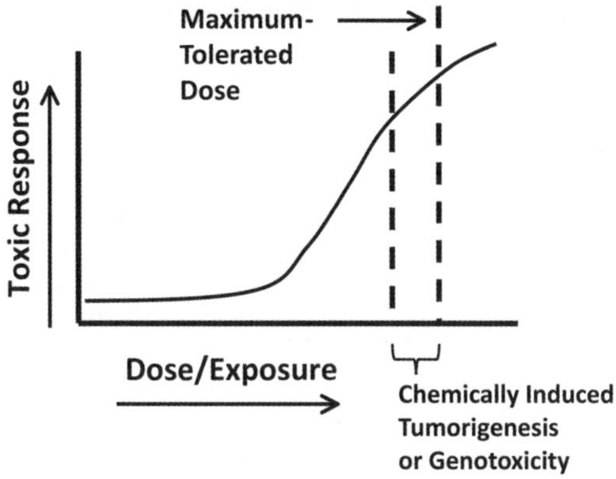


**Figure 15.3** Dose–response curve illustrating that tumorigenic or genotoxic effects seen only at or near the maximum-tolerated doses (MTD) may be secondary to high-dose effects (*e.g.*, saturation of detoxification pathways, alterations of homeostasis, cytotoxicity, inflammation, regenerative cell proliferation, *etc.*).

outcome of both carcinogenicity and genotoxicity studies conducted in animals (as illustrated in Figure 15.3). For both study types to be useful for risk assessment, dose levels, dosing regimens and systemic exposures must be compared across species in order to determine the relevance of study findings to carcinogenic potential in humans.

The MoA of a chemical carcinogen or genotoxicant is important in both hazard identification and cancer risk assessment. MoA in broad terms refers to whether a chemical suspected of being a carcinogen can be classified as genotoxic or non-genotoxic.[17,18] Non-genotoxic carcinogens are those that induce tumorigenesis through various epigenetic mechanisms, for example, 1) cell proliferation through a mitogenic action (*e.g.*, growth factors);[21] 2) cytotoxicity through regenerative cell proliferation (*e.g.*, chloroform-induced liver and kidney tumors);[22] and 3) immunosuppression by inhibiting immune-system-mediated tumor surveillance.[23] For risk assessment purposes, it is generally assumed that carcinogens that act *via* non-genotoxic mechanisms display non-linear dose–response curves, so that a no-observable-effect level (NOEL) or "threshold dose" can be identified for tumorigenesis.

## 15.3.1 Non-DNA-Reactive Genotoxicants

For chemicals that are genotoxic, DNA damage can occur through either DNA-reactive mechanisms (*e.g.*, DNA alkylating agents) or through indirect, non-DNA-reactive mechanisms.[24–26] Suspected mechanisms for some non-DNA-reactive genotoxicants are shown in Table 15.2.

From a regulatory and safety perspective, the distinction between a DNA-reactive and non-DNA-reactive MoA is important; the latter considered

**Table 15.2** Examples of non-DNA-reactive genotoxicants from refs. 19, 26 and 24.

| *Suspected mechanism* | *Chemical examples* |
|---|---|
| DNA polymerase inhibitor | Cytosine arabinoside, azidothymidine |
| Imbalance of DNA precursors | 5-Flurouracil, methotrexate |
| Inhibition of DNA repair processes | Certain kinase inhibitors |
| Topoisomerase inhibitors | Etoposide, fluoroquinolone antibiotics |
| Microtubule inhibitors | Taxol, vinblastine, colchicine |
| Sulfhydryl depletion/oxidation | Metals, diethymaleate |

needing to exceed a dose or exposure threshold (*i.e.*, concentration below which there would be no genotoxicity) to produce an effect. The threshold for a non-DNA-reactive genotoxicant is similar to the threshold considered necessary for non-genotoxic carcinogens.[27,28]

## 15.3.2 DNA-Reactive Genotoxicants

In contrast, DNA-reactive genotoxicants such as alkylating agents have been and still are considered by regulators as having no threshold and thus a linear dose–response relationship is presumed unless demonstrated otherwise by extensive animal testing.[29] The concept of a linear, no-threshold dose response for carcinogenesis has been a key (and controversial) issue in cancer risk assessment for many years, dating back to the early 1970s.[30] The no-threshold limit is basically built on the premise that carcinogenicity can occur when one base pair is altered (*e.g.*, point mutation) by one molecule ("one hit" hypothesis). The one-hit hypothesis is at odds with standard toxicological principals that involve ADME, DNA repair, immune surveillance and other detoxification mechanisms available to protect the body from toxic insult. Also, the one-hit hypothesis does not account for other mechanisms that may be required to ultimately produce tumors once an initiating DNA damage event occurs (*e.g.*, promotion, transformation, progression).

For predicting the potential of a chemical to cause cancer to humans, threshold, no-effect dose-level arguments generally become key components of risk assessment, particularly for DNA-reactive genotoxicants. Reliable biomarkers of a genotoxic response at biologically relevant chemical exposures, however, are needed to provide supportive data for the use of threshold-based risk assessments.[20] Additional data that can be useful in support of a threshold-dose level include knowledge of: 1) the background levels or spontaneous rate of DNA damage in the test system and across species in target tissues; 2) dose–response curves for DNA damage or gene mutations over a low-dose range relevant to humans; 3) DNA repair characteristics at low-exposure concentrations or doses; and 4) rate of induced cell proliferation at low doses. Figure 15.4 illustrates the basic concept for a threshold dose for a genotoxicant.

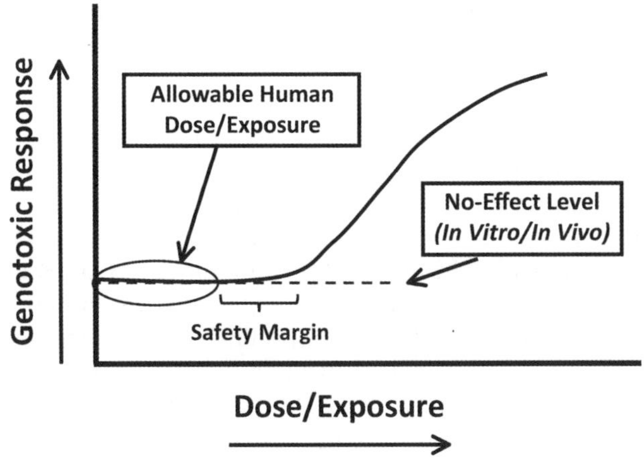


**Figure 15.4** Concept of threshold dose/exposure for genotoxicants. Allowable human exposures and safety margins determined from no-observable-effect levels and from understanding cross-species differences, mode of action, targeted human population, and risk–benefit relationship.

## 15.4 Utility of Thresholds for Genotoxicants

To help put genotoxicity data for a chemical exposure into proper perspective, there is no understating the need for collecting both *in vitro* and *in vivo* dose–response and mechanistic data, particularly for DNA-reactive genotoxicants. This helps provide the basis for evaluating the genotoxicity dose–response curve at the lower and more relevant concentrations/exposures required for risk assessment. Major efforts have been ongoing to ensure mechanistic genotoxicity data are incorporated into cancer risk assessment through development of specialized techniques to evaluate dose–response data (recent efforts are referenced).[31–33] For example, exposure levels and ADME results obtained in animal studies can be used in conjunction with MoA data obtained *in vitro* to generate threshold concentrations for assessing human cancer risk of a chemical.[19,27,28] A notable example is ethyl methanesulfonate (EMS), which was a contaminant in a pharmaceutical batch of Viracept (nelfinavir, an antiretroviral drug) at levels above the current regulatory guidelines for a genotoxicant.[29,34] EMS is a DNA-alkylating agent and well-known genotoxic and carcinogenic chemical. Extensive dose–response data have been generated to identify a no-observable-effect dose for genotoxicity using the rat bone marrow MN assay and the transgenic *lacZ* mutation Muta™Mouse assay. After considering the results of several *in vivo* studies, regulatory agencies accepted a no-observable effect threshold level for the EMS contaminant in Viracept.[29,35] It is of interest that in this case, the *in vitro* concentration–response curve accurately predicted the threshold level determined *in vivo*, hence supporting the scientific basis for using a threshold-dose level in EMS risk assessment.[36]

## 15.5 History of *In Vivo* Models for Genotoxicity Testing

Early *in vivo* genotoxicity assays traditionally focused on germ-cell mutations through visual observations of offspring. *Drosophila* (fruit fly) was the first reported species to be used as an *in vivo* model for genotoxicity testing and early studies evaluated the mutational effects of X-rays in this model.[37] Investigators at Oak Ridge National Laboratory were the first to report using rodents to study *in vivo* mutations.[38] The mouse strain developed at Oak Ridge contained recessive mutations at seven specific loci coding for visible mutations (*e.g.*, eye and coat color, ear shape). This mouse specific-locus test exposed male wild-type mice to X-rays and then mated them with known carriers of the mutant recessive genes to identify effects on germ cells. The molecular structure of DNA published in 1953 pushed forth the development of molecular techniques where the emphasis shifted from animal models to *in vitro* models of genotoxicity in the 1960s and early 1970s.[39,40]

As human cancer risk due to intentional drug/chemical exposure or unintentional environmental exposure became more apparent, Russell applied the mouse specific-locus assay to the study of chemicals.[41,42] The methodology for this assay has been since standardized and is typically classified as a male germ-cell mutation assay.[43] Today, this assay is rarely used for *in vivo* genotoxicity assessment due to the large number of mice required for statistical comparisons, the logistics of timed mating needed for the assay, the unavailability of the mouse strain, and the long study duration.

In the late 1970s, a method for evaluating mutations in embryos following administration of a chemical to pregnant mice was developed and termed the mouse spot test.[41,44] Similar to the mouse specific-locus test, mice used for this test contain recessive genes that code for hair color, but in contrast to the mouse specific-locus test, this test evaluates somatic mutations in the exposed embryos. When mutated, the wild-type gene loci are altered or lost, resulting in an increased frequency of color spots in the coat of the adult animal. The methodology for this mouse spot test has been standardized.[45] As with the mouse specific-locus test, large numbers of animals are required for statistical comparisons, the mouse strain is not readily available, and the study duration is considered excessive.[46]

## 15.6 *In Vivo* Rodent Erythrocyte Micronucleus Assay

Currently, the most widely used *in vivo* genotoxicity test is the rodent erythrocyte micronucleus (MN) test with standard, well-validated protocols available.[47–49] The experimental design aspects of the erythrocyte MN test have been evaluated, validated, and standardized through inter-laboratory efforts lead by an international expert working group formed as part of the International Workshop on Genotoxicity Tests Procedures (IWGTP).[50–52] This test is often performed as part of a genotoxicity test battery supporting clinical trials for drug candidates and for registration of new chemicals, and is specifically referenced as part of a recommended standard genotoxicity test battery in regulatory guidelines (*e.g.*, ICH).[53–55]

Micronuclei are cytoplasmic nuclear bodies formed in actively dividing cells in response to an earlier clastogenic injury (*i.e.*, structural chromosome damage) or an aneugenic event (*i.e.*, lagging or malsegregated whole chromosomes). The MN assay was originally developed in the mouse, first in bone marrow then in peripheral blood.[56,57] The rat is now widely used for the *in vivo* MN testing as it is more generally the species of choice for rodent toxicology studies; therefore, other information important for data interpretation (*e.g.*, ADME, toxicodynamics, and/or MTD levels) are usually already available for this species.

## 15.6.1 Techniques Used to Score Micronuclei

Micronuclei are typically scored in the cytoplasm of the immature erythrocyte; *i.e.*, the reticulocyte in peripheral blood and polychromatic erythrocyte (PCE) in bone marrow. There are several advantages of measuring micronuclei in immature erythrocytes (see Table 15.3).

### *15.6.1.1 Microscopy*

Micronucleated PCEs are easily evaluated microscopically in bone marrow. They occur spontaneously at low frequency (<0.5%) in animals. Microscopic evaluation is a reliable way to count micronuclei in bone marrow when using standardized techniques.[47,50] To automate bone marrow micronuclei

**Table 15.3** Attributes of the micronucleus assay in immature erythroblasts (peripheral blood reticulocytes or bone marrow polychromatic erythrocytes).

| *Attribute* | *Description* |
|---|---|
| Accessible target cell | Immature erythrocytes are formed from precursor erythroblasts, which are rapidly dividing, nucleated cells that reside in the bone marrow, a tissue well-perfused and typically reflective of circulating levels of the chemical in plasma. |
| Easily identifiable cell | Immature erythrocytes are easily identified in either bone marrow or peripheral blood of all species through their high-RNA content, presence of unique cell-surface receptors (*e.g.*, CD71+), and lack of a nucleus (extruded after final cell division). |
| Rapidly evaluated endpoint | Micronuclei are readily detected in the anuclueated reticulocytes or polychromatic erythrocytes (PCE) through the use of nuclear stains. |
| Endpoint and cell type amenable to automation | The presence of both unique cell-surface markers and anucleated cell bodies allow large numbers of either reticulocytes or PCEs to be counted and scored for micronuclei via automated techniques (*e.g.*, flow cytometry, image analysis). |
| Allows cross-species monitoring | Automation allows accurate and robust measurement of peripheral blood micronucleated reticulocytes, suitable for species with short residence times for these cells (rat, dog, monkey, human). |

evaluation *via* microscopy, imaging analysis techniques have been used following removal of nucleated cells using cellulose column separation.[58]

Although slide scoring of peripheral blood reticulocytes can be performed,[57] microscopic evaluation of bone marrow PCEs (and in the case of subchronic/chronic studies, mature erythrocytes) provides for a more robust and sensitive evaluation.[59] This is related to the higher frequencies of both non-micronucleated and micronucleated immature erythrocytes in bone marrow *versus* peripheral blood. For this reason, manual microscopic slide scoring of peripheral blood is not widely used.

#### *15.6.1.2 Flow Cytometry*

The automation afforded by flow cytometry and methods developed at Litron Laboratories (Rochester, New York) allows efficient counting of micronuclei in reticulocytes in blood utilizing the CD71+ (transferrin-receptor positive) subpopulation of erythrocytes, coupled with staining for high-RNA content to identify young reticulocytes. Using young reticulocytes lessens the influence of peripheral destruction of older micronucleated reticulocytes which are removed by the spleen.[60–64] Using this technology, tens of thousands of immature erythrocytes (10-fold higher than counted *via* microscopy) can be counted in peripheral blood within minutes,[65] overcoming the problems of manually scoring micronucleated reticulocytes in blood smears. This method has been used extensively for measuring micronucleated peripheral blood reticulocytes of mice,[62,66–69] rats,[62–65,69–71] dogs,[72] monkeys,[73] and humans.[74–77] Litron's flow cytometry method also has been applied to the erythrocyte-pure fraction from cellulose-filtered bone marrow cells.[71] Because a large number of young reticulocytes are being scored, results obtained from flow cytometry are comparable to manual microscopic scoring in bone marrow.[78] In fact, it has been shown that flow cytometry affords greater sensitivity and statistical power than manual scoring of bone marrow PCEs due to the large numbers of cells being counted.[79]

Flow cytometric analysis of peripheral blood micronuclei is acceptable to regulatory agencies if run under an appropriately validated protocol and the results are properly reported.[47,52] One important advantage of flow cytometry is that it can be applied to non-rodent laboratory species during repeat-dose studies and thus can be used to explore potential species-specific genotoxic effects (*e.g.*, potential genotoxicity of a metabolite formed only in a non-rodent species).[72,73,80]

The relationship of bone marrow PCEs to reticulocytes and their surface marker and staining characteristics are provided in Figure 15.5.

### 15.6.2 Design Considerations

As previously discussed, rats are generally considered the rodent species of choice in toxicology programs, and thus are more typically used for genotoxicity testing, since information on a chemical's tolerability and target-organ

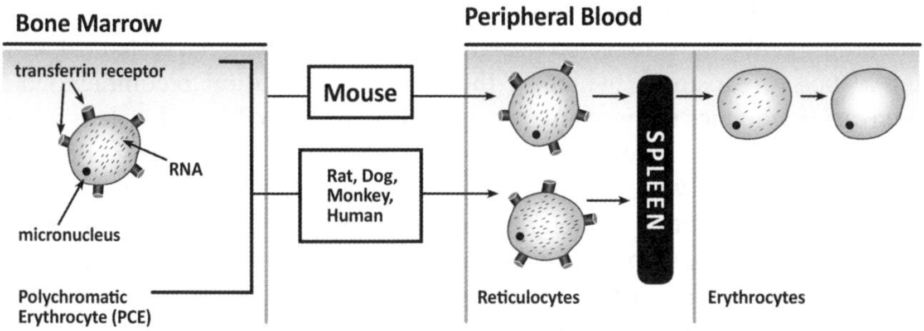


**Figure 15.5** The relationship of immature erythrocytes in bone marrow (polychromatic erythrocytes) and in peripheral blood (reticulocytes) to their surface markers (CD71-positive transferrin receptor) and cellular markers (stains for RNA and micronucleus DNA).

toxicity relative to plasma exposure and kinetics are often more readily available. Mice were initially favored for MN testing in peripheral blood, partly due to the longer residence time of micronucleated erythrocytes (one month) relative to rats, dogs, monkeys and humans.[56,81,82] However, due to automated scoring techniques, sufficient sensitivity can be obtained using peripheral blood from species other than mice.[52,72,73] When selecting a species and strain, it is important not only to consider its overall relevance to human, but also to ensure sufficient experience and historical control data are available with the scoring method to be used, as strain differences, inter-animal variability, and scoring techniques can affect the results obtained from the MN assay.[50–52,79,83–85] To ensure the MN test system is sufficiently sensitive to detect an elevation in MN, a positive control (*e.g.*, cyclophosphamide) is used in the same study; however, if there is sufficient experience by the laboratory to demonstrate competency in detecting a positive response within the dosing paradigm used, a concurrent positive control may not be necessary if sufficiently justified.

In practice, because *in vivo* MN studies are often run prior to or in parallel with definitive, repeat-dose toxicity studies, both sexes are used to ensure a robust evaluation and circumvent potential follow-up testing if unexpected sex differences are later observed. However, if no sex differences in metabolism, plasma kinetics, or toxicity of the chemical are seen, only one sex would need to be used for the *in vivo* MN assay. Previous studies have shown similar sensitivity to micronuclei induction between male and female rodents.[50]

### 15.6.3 Stand-Alone Evaluation *versus* Integration with Toxicology Study

A typical stand-alone, *in vivo* erythrocyte MN study involves 2–3 days of dosing, with bone marrow and/or blood harvested 24 h after the last dose. For measurements in bone marrow, a single dose followed by 24- and 48-h harvests can also be used. In rats tested with a variety of chemicals, blood sampling 24 h after 3 days of dosing is sufficient for determining both DNA-reactive and non-DNA-reactive genotoxicants.[51,82,83] Similarly, a wide variety of DNA-damaging agents were detected when bone marrow was harvested 24 hours after 2 days of dosing,[86] which is the minimum duration recommended by regulatory guidelines when using a single bone marrow harvest.[47] It is important to note that a 24-h bone marrow harvest after two days of dosing may not detect genotoxicity with agents requiring target tissue saturation or with delayed modes of action (*e.g.*, oligonucleotides, polymerase inhibitors); in these situations, a $\geq$3-day dosing regimen should be considered as also recommended for the testing of food ingredients.[49]

There is considerable interest in the feasibility of integrating genotoxic endpoints into repeat-dose toxicology studies.[51,82,83] In determining whether MN evaluations should be conducted in a stand-alone study or integrated into repeat-dose toxicity studies, an understanding of micronuclei formation and destruction is required. The cells targeted for chemical exposure are the bone marrow erythroblasts which extrude their nuclei as they mature. Since micronuclei formation occurs only after cell division, the expression of micronuclei is dependent on cell proliferation (*i.e.*, erythropoiesis) and peripheral destruction (splenic removal); the latter is deficient in the mouse. Therefore, factors that affect either cell-cycle kinetics in bone marrow (*e.g.*, toxicity, cytostatic agents, temperature, erythrocyte proliferation) or splenic activity (*e.g.*, toxicity, extramedullary hematopoiesis) can affect MN results. Several toxicological, pharmacological, and physiological effects can indirectly influence the expression of micronuclei to yield false positive responses (see Table 15.4).[16,24] Many of these factors are expected to be more prevalent after four weeks of dosing than after acute or short-term treatments. Short-term treatments thus allow both greater controls over toxicological variables while providing higher dose levels to be evaluated for genotoxic potential. There are, however, advantages to measuring genotoxicity endpoints as part of a two- or four-week toxicology study, particularly since good concordance between short-term and long-term MN studies has been demonstrated with a variety of genotoxicants.[83]

**Table 15.4** Chemicals positive in the *in vivo* micronucleus assay and negative in standard *in vitro* genotoxicity assays. Reviewed by Tweats *et al.*[16,24]

| *Suspected mechanism* | *Examples* |
|---|---|
| *In vivo*-specific metabolism | Urethane (CYP2E1) |
| Alterations of glucocorticoids, hypothermia | Benzene (liver and bone marrow metabolism)<br>Morphine |
| Inhibition of DNA-repair processes | Certain kinase inhibitors |
| Folate inhibition, alteration of nucleotide pool | Premetrexed (alimta®) |
| Hypothermia | Phenothiazines (*e.g.*, chlorpromazine), phenol |
| Stimulation of erythropoiesis | Erythropoietins, anoxia<br>Aniline (methemoglobinemia)<br>Anti-thrombotic agents (decrease platelets) |

### 15.6.4 Dose Setting

As with general toxicology studies, thoughtful determination in the selection of low-, mid- and high-dose levels is required for *in vivo* genotoxicity testing, taking into account ADME properties and the target hematopoietic tissue. If no pertinent toxicity data are available using the same species, strain, and route of exposure, a dose-range-finding assay should be conducted using both sexes with the same treatment regimen to be used in the MN assay. The high dose should produce some indication of toxicity to show that the test system has been "optimized" (*e.g.*, clinical signs, morbidity, bone marrow hypocellularity). In the absence of toxicity, the highest dose should be 2000 mg $kg^{-1}$ for studies $\leq$14 days, 1000 mg $kg^{-1}$ if >14 days, or the maximum feasible dose (*e.g.*, as limited by formulation).[51] Ideally, the low dose should provide exposure at, or a multiple of, the estimated human exposure.

### 15.6.5 Prediction of Rodent Carcinogenicity

Although the rodent erythrocyte MN test is specific for predicting rodent carcinogenicity (*i.e.*, low false positives), it is not a sensitive test (*i.e.*, displays high rate of false negatives). Benigni *et al.*[87] demonstrated a specificity of 75% and sensitivity of 40% (see Table 15.6), which confirmed similar predictions by other authors.[88–92] Because of this low sensitivity, follow-up testing may be considered necessary for a negative *in vivo* MN result if previous *in vitro* testing or chemical structure/class indicated, a suspected genotoxicant.

The lack of sensitivity of the MN assay for rodent carcinogenicity is partly related to the use of hematopoietic tissue, which may be unable to predict tumorigenesis in other organs/tissues. Morita *et al.* found in their retrospective analysis that the MN assay was a good predictor of rodent tumors derived from hematopoietic tissue, but as noted previously, had poor sensitivity for rodent carcinogenicity when including all tumor types.[91]

### 15.6.6 Mode of Action Information

Since micronuclei can form *via* either chromosome injury (clastogenic, DNA-reactive mechanisms) or through lagging or malsegregated whole chromosomes (aneugenic, non-DNA-reactive mechanisms), understanding the MoA will aid in risk assessment of a genotoxicant. Since aneugen-induced micronuclei contain primarily whole chromosomes, centromeres and associated kinetochore proteins should be present. To help identify aneugens, staining techniques have been used such as fluorescent *in situ* hybridization (FISH) of centromeric DNA and kinetochore analysis with "CREST" antibodies obtained from the serum of patients with the autoimmune disease syndrome termed CREST (Calcinosis, Raynaud's phenomenon, Esophageal dysmotility, Sclerodactyly and Telangiectasia). These staining techniques have been useful in identifying aneugens which display a higher proportion of centromeric signals (typically >70%) *versus* clastogens (typically <20%).[93–97] However, since these techniques are more robust for cultured cells *versus* animal tissue, particularly when compared to rat tissue, *in vitro* genotoxicity studies could provide more definitive supportive MoA data.

#### *15.6.6.1 Chromosome Aberrations*

An indirect method for understanding the origin of *in vivo* MN formation is through evaluation of bone marrow metaphase cells for chromosome aberrations.[98] This is a powerful technique for determining whether observed MN are associated with observable chromosome aberrations at the level of the nucleus. This evaluation is more rigorous than MN evaluation and can use bone marrow or peripheral blood lymphocytes harvested and cultured after *in vivo* exposure to the chemical. The *in vivo* chromosome aberration test is acceptable to regulatory agencies as an alternative to the MN assay.[53] Relative to the MN assay, fewer cells are evaluated for chromosome aberrations and the background is lower; therefore, the sensitivity of these two measures is considered equivalent for DNA-reactive genotoxicants.

## 15.7 *In Vivo* Unscheduled DNA Synthesis Assay

Historically, the *in vivo* unscheduled DNA synthesis (UDS) assay has been one of the most commonly used methods to assess DNA damage, second only to the erythrocyte MN assay in rodents. The UDS assay evaluates DNA damage indirectly through measurement of synthesis of DNA repair.[99–101] Like the MN assay, this assay has a large database of results and a well-established testing guideline.[54,55,101] The liver has been the organ of choice for the UDS assay, although there are reports of the test being applied to other tissues including colon, epidermis, nasal and tracheal epithelium, kidney, pancreas, spermatocytes, stomach and kidney.[99,100]

### 15.7.1 Summary of Assay

The primary method uses hepatocytes isolated from adult animals (usually rodents; typically rats) previously treated with the potential genotoxicant.[102] The liver is ideal for the UDS assay due to hepatocytes having: 1) a low rate of cell division and thus low background for DNA synthesis; 2) the ability to be maintained in culture; and 3) an import role in xenobiotic metabolism. DNA synthesis is evaluated in isolated hepatocytes cultured for 3–8 h with radiolabeled thymidine which incorporates into the repaired DNA. The incorporated radiolabeled thymidine is measured through autoradiography for a 7–14 day period. Grains seen on the film over the nucleus, once adjusted for background, represent areas of unscheduled DNA synthesis which are easily distinguished from nuclei undergoing cell division which display much higher numbers of grain counts.

As with other DNA damage assays, the rules of dose setting and gender selection are similar to the MN assay, particularly regarding MTD, as liver injury can greatly affect the UDS assay.[99,100] Historically, rats are sacrificed at approximately 2–4 h, as well as 14–16 h, after administration of a single dose.

### 15.7.2 Prediction of Rodent Carcinogenicity

Similar to the ability of the MN assay to predict rodent carcinogenicity, the rat liver UDS assays demonstrates a low percentage of false positives (92% specificity) and a high percentage of false negatives (44% sensitivity) (see Table 15.6).[99,103] Mathews *et al.*[103] examined published reports of 37 chemicals and found that the *in vivo* UDS assay showed 69% sensitivity and 60% specificity when predicting rodent carcinogens; however, the dataset used was limited and had a high prevalence of carcinogens.

Since the UDS assay has been used as follow-up test for evaluating chemicals that were *in vitro*-positive but negative in the *in vivo* MN assay, Kirkland and Speit assessed the sensitivity of the UDS assay for predicting rodent carcinogenicity under these conditions.[104] These authors found that only seven of 41 carcinogens that were negative or equivocal in the *in vivo* MN assay produced positive results in the liver UDS assay (sensitivity of 17%). This evaluation indicates that the liver UDS assay is not an acceptable follow-up to the *in vivo* MN assay for detecting rodent carcinogens.

The lack of sensitivity of the UDS assay is partly related to the use of the liver as the primary tissue for analysis. Although useful for orally administered compounds that are hepatic genotoxicants undergoing first-pass metabolism, the UDS assay does not appear suitable for extra-hepatic tumorigens or for other routes of administration (*e.g.*, topical, inhalation).[99] Due to the lack of sensitivity of the UDS assay for predicting rodent carcinogenicity, and the even lower sensitivity as a follow-up to a negative or inconclusive *in vivo* MN assay, this assay has fallen out of favor with regulatory scientists involved in cancer risk assessment.

### 15.7.3 Mode of Action Information

The UDS assay is useful for detecting excision repair of large regions (100 nucleotides) of DNA, which occurs following the formation of bulky adducts. However, this assay is poor at detecting DNA repair associated with smaller regions (1–10 bases) and thus is insensitive at detecting DNA injury due to single-strand breaks and oxidative damage to nucleotide bases.[99]

## 15.8 *In Vivo* Alkaline Single-Cell Gel Electrophoresis "Comet" Assay

The Comet assay evaluates the potential of a treatment to induce primary DNA damage (*i.e.*, strand breaks) in any tissue where a sufficient quantity of intact nuclei can be isolated. It is considered an alternative test to the *in vivo* liver UDS test when a second *in vivo* genotoxicity test is needed to complement the *in vivo* MN assay. As of this writing, no OECD regulatory guidance is available for the Comet assay. Although published guidelines are available,[105,106] caveats on the conduct, interpretation, and transferability of this assay from laboratory to laboratory also exist. Further validation is ongoing through international efforts led by Japanese Center for the Validation of Alternative Methods.[107] Despite the limitations of the Comet assay, it is widely accepted by international regulatory agencies as a follow-up assay to understand the relevance of an *in vitro*-positive clastogenicity result (particularly when the rodent MN test is negative), or the mode of action (MoA) of a known or suspected carcinogen. The Comet assay is currently the most feasible method to detect DNA damage in specific organs such as the stomach, kidney and bladder, organs not readily applicable to the *in vivo* micronucleus and UDS assays.[108]

### 15.8.1 Summary of Assay

Although technically known as the *in vivo* alkaline singe-cell gel electrophoresis assay, the Comet assay is named for the microscopic endpoint which resembles a comet head (core nuclear region) and tail (smaller DNA strands and/or fragments). The assay uses suspensions of single cells obtained from virtually any freshly harvested organ or tissue. These single-cell suspensions are lysed, electrophoresed on an agarose gel, and stained for DNA. The "comet" is viewed microscopically and various aspects of the comet's body and tail are quantified using various scoring techniques which can be automated. The basic assay design is shown in Figure 15.6.

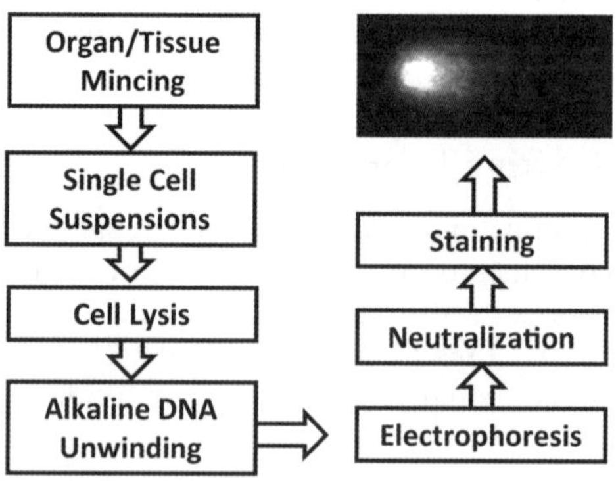


**Figure 15.6** The basic study design of the Comet assay is shown. The assay measures a broad spectrum of DNA damage, including single- and double-strand breaks. After processing the tissue and isolating nuclear DNA, the comet head (core nuclear region) and tail (smaller DNA strands and/or fragments) are quantified.

The groundwork for the Comet assay was laid in the mid-1970s.[109] The first single-cell gel electrophoresis assay was developed in the early 1980s and later modified to run under highly alkaline conditions that cause DNA to unwind and release single-strand breaks from incomplete excision repair sites.[110–112] The alkaline version of the Comet assay enhances the test's sensitivity for genotoxic agents which typically induce single-strand breaks (*versus* double-strand breaks), including those generated during nucleotide excision repair and from alkali-labile sites.

## 15.8.2 Design Considerations

Attributes of the Comet assay are listed in Table 15.5. Rats are typically used as information on ADME and toxicology is often available for this species. Since the Comet assay is currently used as a follow-up test, it is often conducted late in the genetic toxicology program using the species previously tested in the *in vivo* MN assay. In addition, information on gender differences in exposure or toxicity is usually available at this stage so decisions on whether to use one sex or both can be made.

Dose setting is similar to that for the *in vivo* MN and UDS assays in that the MTD, maximum feasible dose, or limit dose should be used. Since cytotoxicity may lead to false positive results, it is important that a clear, no-observable-effect dose level in the target tissue is included in the Comet assay.

One advantage of the Comet assay is that it is applicable to any tissue where a single-cell preparation can be obtained. The tissue for evaluation should be chosen based on the availability of historical data from structural analogs and/or from ADME and toxicology studies, if known. In the absence of information on a known target tissue, the two default tissues used have been the liver, due to this organ's first-pass metabolism capabilities, and a first-contact tissue (*e.g.*, intestine for oral administration, respiratory tract for inhalation, skin for dermal application).[113,114]

## 15.8.3 Influence of Cytotoxicity

One of the confounding factors of the Comet assay is that indirect mechanisms related to cytotoxicity (necrosis and/or apoptosis) can lead to DNA

**Table 15.5** Attributes of the Comet assay for measuring DNA damage, from refs. 113, 114, 119 and 122.

| *Advantage* | *Assay attribute* |
|---|---|
| Sensitivity | Single-cell measurement of DNA damage<br>Measures wide range of DNA damage (approximately 100 to few thousand breaks per cell) |
| Applicable to most tissues | Mitotic activity not required to detect DNA-reactive genotoxicants<br>Small number of cells required |
| Dosing duration short | DNA damage detected within 1–3 days |
| Mode of action | Allows organ-specific measurement of genotoxicity |

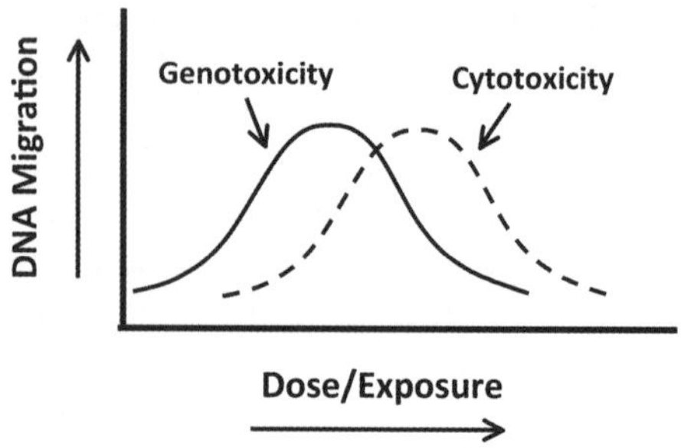


**Figure 15.7** Figure illustrates the confounding effects of target-tissue cytotoxicity in the Comet assay. Cytotoxicity leads to DNA fragmentation which can appear as a false positive in the absence of true genotoxicity or can mask genotoxicity if present. Depending on the study design and chemical being tested, target-organ cytotoxicity may occur at doses below the maximum-tolerated dose. (Courtesy of Marie Vasquez at Helix3.)

fragmentation through release of nucleases and thus produce false positive (as well as false negative) results (see Figure 15.7).[105,114–117] DNA damage related to cytotoxicity or inappropriate tissue processing can be determined by monitoring "hedgehogs" which are comets with small or non-existent heads and large, diffuse tails. Another, more accurate method of measuring DNA damage unrelated to genotoxicity is through the evaluation of low-molecular-weight (LMW) DNA fragments which are markers of early cell death measured through a neutral diffusion method.[114,115] It is important to note that cytotoxicity assessed *via* LMW DNA fragments can occur at doses below the MTD, particularly during short-term studies where evidence of cytotoxicity may not be readily apparent. During long-term Comet studies, standard histopathological and clinical chemistry evaluations are useful for evaluating organ-specific toxicity.[105,106,118] Standardization of the procedures and measurements and a standard classification scheme for cytotoxicity in the Comet assay will be needed before this assay can be confidently implemented across laboratories for routine genotoxicity testing.[119,120]

### 15.8.4 Stand-Alone Evaluation *versus* Integrated with Toxicology Study

Stand-alone studies to assess DNA damage using the Comet assay involve at least 1–3 days of consecutive dosing with sacrifice at the time of maximum chemical exposure ($T_{max}$) to optimize observing DNA damage of a potential genotoxicant, prior to significant DNA repair. Some designs have included a second sacrifice time 24 h after the last dose. There is utility in combining the Comet assay with the MN assay to enhance the robustness of the *in vivo* genotoxicity assessment while saving time and resources. This approach has been shown to provide a sensitive, efficient, and comprehensive assessment of genotoxicity in several target organs.[115,121]

As with other *in vivo* genotoxicity studies, there is considerable interest in integrating genotoxicity endpoints from the Comet assay into general repeat-dose toxicity studies. However, in contrast to acute studies, the lower doses employed in repeat-dose studies may affect the assay's ability to detect DNA damage if animal exposure was limited by species-specific toxicity not relevant to humans. In addition, during longer duration toxicity studies, where secondary effects of inflammation or other types of cell perturbations can occur after repeated administration of high doses, the potential for confounding factors increases. Despite these caveats, results obtained from a collaborative study indicated minimal differences between short-term (1–3 days) and long-term (2–4 weeks) outcomes from the rat liver Comet assay using 15 model compounds.[118] Differences observed appeared to be related to genotoxicants that had a suspected non-DNA-reactive MoA or where genotoxic metabolites may not have been at steady-state.[118] DNA-reactive chemicals are expected to be positive following both short-term and long-term administration since DNA damage is not dependent on cell division or DNA synthesis. In contrast, for some non-DNA-reactive mechanisms (*e.g.*, alterations of nucleotide pools; topoisomerase inhibition, *etc.*), DNA synthesis is required prior to DNA strand breaks and thus may require long-term dosing to manifest a response.

## 15.8.5 Prediction of Rodent Carcinogenicity

Although issues with the Comet assay exist, it has been shown to be one of the most sensitive *in vivo* genotoxicity assays currently available for predicting rodent carcinogenicity. Both high sensitivity (approximately 90%) and specificity (80%, 85%) have been reported (see Table 15.6).[104,122] When positive rodent carcinogens, either negative or equivocal in the *in vivo* MN test, are examined in the Comet assay, the sensitivity of the assay for predicting rodent carcinogenicity remains high, at 89%.[104] This indicates that the Comet assay is a good alternative when the *in vivo* MN assay is negative and further follow-up genotoxicity testing is required (*e.g.*, in the presence of an *in vitro*-only positive genotoxicity finding). It is important to note however that the Comet assay's high predictivity for rodent carcinogenicity comes from data generated primarily from one laboratory with a long history of conducting the Comet assay.[122] Since the assay procedure and evaluation criteria are not yet standardized between laboratories, particularly with respect to cytotoxicity, confounding variables affecting the interpretation of the Comet assay will remain problematic for risk assessment.

## 15.8.6 Mode of Action Information

The Comet assay is designed to detect DNA strand breaks which can be caused by both DNA-reactive and non-DNA-reactive genotoxicants. This assay is applicable to essentially any tissue where a sufficient number of cells and/or nuclei can be collected. Therefore, it allows one to investigate mechanisms of

**Table 15.6** Performance of *in vivo* genotoxicity assays in predicting rodent carcinogenicity.

| | In vivo *genotoxicity* | In vivo *rodent carcinogenicity* | | | *Predictivity* | | |
|---|---|---|---|---|---|---|---|
| In vivo *assay* | *Result* | *Carcinogen* | *Non-carcinogen* | *Total* | *Sensitivity*[a] | *Specificity*[b] | *Reference* |
| Micronucleus erythrocyte[c] | Positive | 57 | 10 | 67 | | | |
| | Negative | 86 | 30 | 116 | 40% | 75% | Benigni *et al.* 2010[87] |
| | | 143 | 40 | 183 | | | |
| Unscheduled DNA synthesis[d] | Positive | 24 | 2 | 26 | | | |
| | Negative | 31 | 22 | 53 | 44% | 92% | Matthews *et al.* 2006[103] |
| | | 55 | 24 | 79 | | | |
| Comet | Positive | 49 | 6 | 55 | | | |
| | Negative | 5 | 24 | 29 | 91% | 80% | Sasaki *et al.* 2000[122] |
| | | 54 | 30 | 84 | | | |
| Transgenic[e] | Positive | 72 | 4 | 76 | | | |
| | Negative | 20 | 9 | 29 | 78% | 69% | Lambert *et al.* 2005[99] |
| | | 92 | 13 | 105 | | | |

[a]Sensitivity is the percentage of correctly predicted rodent carcinogens; low sensitivity reflects high rate of false negatives.
[b]Specificity is the percentage of correctly predicted rodent non-carcinogens; low specificity reflects high rate of false positives.
[c]Majority of data from the analysis of micronuclei in bone marrow cells from rats and mice.
[d]Data from *in vivo*/*in vitro* rat liver assay.
[e]Majority of data from Big Blue® or Muta™Mouse assays using short-term (<4 weeks) dosing regimens.

organ-specific carcinogenicity, particularly for a compound that is negative in a standard battery of genotoxicity tests. For example, a negative Comet assay result for a carcinogen that was also negative in the Ames test and in the *in vitro* and *in vivo* micronucleus assays may provide convincing evidence for classifying a known rodent carcinogen as non-genotoxic.[123]

## 15.9 *In Vivo* Mutagenicity Assays (Transgenic Rodents)

Transgenic rodents are genetically engineered to evaluate mutational changes in any target tissue. These models possess exogenous DNA sequences integrated into the animal's genome and contained in all cells. These transgenes are used as reporter genes to detect point mutations, deletions and insertions. Like the Comet assay, transgenic rodent assays are often used when a second *in vivo* genotoxicity test is considered necessary.[104] Though these transgenic models have well-established protocols, no regulatory guidelines are available.[99,124,125] The most common *in vivo* transgenic mutation model is the Big Blue® in mice and rats and the Muta™Mouse; these are described in this section. Other transgenic models, such as the *lacZ* plasmid mouse and the *gpt* delta mouse have been used but to a lesser degree than the Big Blue® and Muta™Mouse systems.[125] In general, gene mutation assays using transgenic animals are expensive and labor intensive; this has limited their use in genotoxicity testing.

### 15.9.1 Summary of Assay

Two comprehensive reviews summarize the backgrounds of the various transgenic mutagenicity animal models.[99,125] Transgenic mutagenicity models most commonly carry exogenous reporter genes from the *lac* operon derived from *E. coli*, which normally functions to regulate synthesis of β-galactosidase. Big Blue® utilizes multiple copies of the *lacI* gene (30–40 copies for mouse and 15–20 copies for rats) within a recoverable shuttle vector on chromosome 4. The Muta™Mouse model uses about 80 copies of the *lacZ* gene within a recoverable shuttle vector on chromosome 3. The large number of copies provides a broad target for genotoxicants.

At the termination of a study, DNA is isolated from the target tissue. As with the Comet assay, care must be taken not to damage DNA during preparation, as this can affect assay performance. The *lac* genes, along with the shuttle vectors, are extracted from genomic DNA using commercial reagents, inserted into phages and then transfected into different strains of *E. coli*. The transduced bacteria are grown on agar in various selection media and mutant plaques are identified by selective growth. The selection system for Big Blue® is based on the *lacI* gene which normally suppresses the expression of the β-galactosidase gene; thus, mutant plaques will express this gene. The opposite is true for the Muta™Mouse, where mutations in *lacZ* inhibit expression of β-galactosidase. It should be noted that the background frequency for these mutants can be high relative to the signal, which may impact sensitivity.

### 15.9.2 Design Considerations

Cell proliferation in the target tissue is required to allow the DNA damage to be fixed into stable mutations.[126] Therefore, rapidly dividing cells fix the mutation more quickly than slowly dividing cells. In addition, transgenes used for mutagenicity testing are not transcriptionally active; thus, damage to these exogenous reporter genes is not readily repaired as with most endogenous genes (*e.g.*, *Hprt* gene).[127] This causes DNA damage to accumulate at the transgene relative to most endogenous genes. This can enhance the sensitivity of the assay but also lead to unstable gene vectors. Based on transgene behavior, some genotoxicants will induce strong responses after 1–5 days of consecutive dosing, whereas weak mutagens will require longer dosing. Results have shown that transgenic mutations are additive with treatments up to 90 days, while treatments longer than 90 days may lead to excessive false positives due to secondary effects related to toxicity.[126] Thus, the recommended dosing regimen is 28 days of treatment with sampling after a 3- and/or 28-day recovery period to allow adequate time for the mutations to be fixed.[124]

As with other animal genotoxicity assays, transgenic animal assays can use one gender unless sex differences in toxicity or chemical exposure exist.[124–126] In the absence of information on a known target tissue, the default tissue is either the liver or a first-contact tissue.

Since PCR-based methods are now available for assessing genomic integrity and rearrangements of the *lac* operon, genotype assays that detect the effects of clastogens and aneugens may be possible and thus may obviate the use of *E. coli* for the detection of mutations.[128]

### 15.9.3 Prediction of Rodent Carcinogenicity

Transgenic mutagenicity assays show promise in predicting rodent carcinogenicity, with good sensitivity (78%) and specificity (69%) when observed in a review of 105 chemicals (see Table 15.6).[99] It should be noted that a low number of non-carcinogens (13) were examined in this review, and that the majority of chemicals were tested in short-term treatment versus the recommended 4-week dosing period. Of the records examined, 90% were tested in the Big Blue® or Muta™Mouse assays while 10% utilized the *lacZ* plasmid mouse or the *gpt* delta assays.

Kirkland and Speit[104] reviewed rodent carcinogens tested in transgenic assays that were negative or equivocal in the *in vivo* MN assay. Seventeen of 30 carcinogens (57%) were positive in transgenic assays: lower than the Comet assay but higher than the UDS assay.[104] These data indicate that transgenic assays may be acceptable follow-ups to the *in vivo* MN assay for detecting rodent carcinogens.

### 15.9.4 Mode of Action Data

Transgenic mutagenicity assays detect carcinogens with a direct mutagenic mode of action. Mutations detected in the Big Blue® and Muta™Mouse assays include base-pair substitutions, frameshift mutations, small insertions, and small deletions. Large deletions, which cannot be incorporated into the phage-packaging system, are not detected with these assays; however, transgenic models that use plasmids as shuttle vectors can detect large deletions (*e.g., lacZ* plasmid or *gpt* delta assays).[126,129]

As with the Comet assay, any tissue can be assessed and therefore one can investigate mechanisms of organ-specific carcinogenicity. This is particularly useful for a compound that is negative in a standard battery of genotoxicity tests.

## 15.10 *In Vivo* Phenotypic Mutagenicity Assays (Endogenous Genes)

The evaluation of chemical-induced endogenous gene mutations using phenotypic measures (*e.g.*, protein product) is attractive for assessing genotoxicity, particularly MoA information. However, there are no readily available and well-validated *in vivo* mutation assays that toxicologists can use to measure endogenous gene expression or activity. Of the genes used for mutation research (*e.g., Hprt, Aprt, Tk, Dlb-1*), the most notable for use in risk assessment has been the *Hprt* gene assay which requires a labor-intensive and time-consuming recovery protocol to express the phenotype. More recently, a gene-mutation assay has been developed using cells of hematopoietic origin that carry mutations at the *Pig-a* locus. This gene is linked to the expression of glycosylphosphatidylinositol (GPI) on cell membranes which can be measured using a fluorescent-labeled antibody and flow cytometry.

### 15.10.1 *Hprt* Mutagenicity Assay

The *Hprt* assay has been used widely in research applications, but no protocol or guidance has been developed for routine genotoxicity testing. This assay employs the hypoxanthine-guanine phosphoribosyltransferase (*Hprt*) gene which is present in all tissues; however, the use of this assay is restricted to tissues which can be cultured to select mutants (*e.g.*, lymphocytes). This gene is X-linked (males and females contain one working copy) and thus a single mutation is required to affect function.[130–132]

*Hprt* mutants are determined in treated animals after isolating lymphocytes from either spleen or peripheral blood and culturing in the presence of 6-thioguanine, which is converted by *Hprt* to a cytotoxic monophosphate. Since *Hprt* mutants have no *Hprt* activity, mutant cells are resistant to the cytotoxic action of 6-thioguanine and grow in culture. The *Hprt* assay can detect point mutations, frameshift mutations, small insertions and small deletions, but does not pick up large genetic alterations. The collection of *Hprt* data is complicated by variability in mutant frequency in animals over time and with age. An advantage of this test is that it can be used to evaluate mutations across species; however, due to variability and a complicated scoring system, its use for *in vivo* evaluations has been limited.[99,131,132]

### 15.10.2 *Pig-a* Mutagenicity Assay

A promising new mutation assay that is undergoing extensive inter-laboratory testing led by Litron Laboratories is the *Pig-a* assay. The *Pig-a* (phosphatidylinositol glycan, Class A) gene is one of several genes required to form the phosphatidylinositol glycan (GPI) anchor proteins located on the surface of cells, including hematopoietic cells. As with the *Hprt* gene, the *Pig-a* gene is X-linked, so a single mutation can affect the expression of the GPI anchors. Mutations to the *Pig-a* gene can therefore be determined by examining peripheral blood erythrocytes (or other blood cells) for absence of GPI anchor.[133–135] The basis for the *Pig-a* gene mutation assay comes from research on paroxysmal nocturnal hemoglobinuria, a genetic disorder in which frame shifts, base-pair substitutions, and point mutations in the *Pig-a* gene have been associated with GPI-anchor deficiency.[133,134,136–140]

The *Pig-a* assay displays several attributes that could allow it to become the first widely used endogenous gene mutation assay (see Table 15.7). The *Pig-a* assay is able to detect genotoxic effects of extended exposures, enhancing the assay's sensitivity.[141] For example, an *N*-ethyl-*N*-nitrosourea (ENU)-induced *Pig-a* mutant phenotype in erythrocytes accumulated and persisted in rats for at least six months, indicating it is an assay capable of detecting weak mutagens with repeat administration. However, mutant additivity may be chemical- or target-cell specific as this has not been seen with other chemicals.[142]

The *Pig-a* gene's structure, function, and locus lends itself to cross-species evaluation since the gene is conserved across mammalian species of toxicological interest, including humans.[133] However, the characteristic of the GPI-anchor-deficient cells may differ between species. For example, mice erythrocytes with GPI-anchor deficiency have decreased lifespan relative to other species.[133,139,143]

The *Pig-a* assay can be performed using microliter amounts of blood. Thus, multiple blood draws can be used from the same animal over an extended

**Table 15.7** Attributes of the *Pig-a* assay in blood for measuring gene mutations, from refs. 133, 135, 138 and 140.

| *Attribute* | *Description* |
|---|---|
| Sensitive | Clonal expansion of *Pig-a* mutants in hematopoietic tissue allows accumulation of mutants; low frequency of mutants allows low background signal. |
| Rapidly evaluated endpoint | Unlike the *Hprt* assay, no *ex vivo* growth is required and results can be obtained within 48 h. |
| Endpoint and cell type amenable to automation | The presence of a fluorescence-labeled antibody to the phosphatidylinositol glycan (GPI) anchor on cell membranes allows large numbers of blood cells to be counted and scored for the absence of the GPI anchor by flow cytometry. |
| Allows cross-species monitoring | Automation and low blood volume ($<100\,\mu L$) allow accurate and robust measurements across species; allows integration into toxicology studies. |

period of time, easily enabling integration of the assay into general toxicology studies. Combining several genetic toxicology endpoints into one study may also be useful in studying the relationships between DNA damage and subsequent mutations. Since mutant cells can appear in the peripheral blood at different times depending on the cell type targeted, assaying over time provides the best opportunity to detect mutations.[133,134,142,143]

As with the *in vivo* MN assay, a limitation of the current *Pig-a* assay is the evaluation of genotoxicity in hematopoietic tissue which may not be predictive for mutagenicity in other organs/tissues where the formation of tumors are observed.

## 15.11 *In Vivo* Genotypic Mutagenicity Assays (Endogenous Genes)

Genotypic measures of mutations utilize the latest tools of molecular biology (reviewed by Shuga *et al.*[144]) to seek out and measure sequence changes in endogenous reporter genes (*e.g., Hprt*), oncogenes (*e.g.,* K-*ras*), tumor suppressor genes (*e.g., p53*), or other genes.[144] These evaluations have been useful in gaining mechanistic insight into early gene alterations related to chemically induced mutations and tumorigenesis. In addition, as some of these techniques become more automated, they could hold promise as rapid screens for studying chemically induced mutations in rodent models.

### 15.11.1 *Hprt* Gene Mutations

Mutations in the *Hprt* gene serve as a reporter or surrogate for gene mutations that can cause cancer.[145] *Hprt* is a convenient reporter gene for chemically induced mutations since it is highly conserved and can be studied in mutant cell clones obtained from peripheral blood lymphocytes (see section 15.10.1). A spectrum of mutations of the *Hprt* gene has been studied in human populations exposed to a variety of genotoxicants.[145–149] It is of interest that although the phenotypic mutational frequencies of *Hprt* increased in high-risk populations (*e.g.,* smokers, workers exposed to aromatic hydrocarbons), the genotypic mutational spectra were similar to controls, indicating that mutations due to genotoxicant exposure are similar to background mutations. Although the *Hprt* gene has provided insights on the mutational spectra in high-risk populations, its use as an endpoint in genotoxicity testing has been limited due to the difficulty of growing clones and assessing DNA sequences.

### 15.11.2 Oncogene/Tumor Suppressor Gene Mutations

Studying mutations in genes associated with tumors (*e.g.,* oncogenes) can provide information on relevant gene mutations in target tissues prior to tumor formation. For example, several studies have demonstrated an association between mutations in the H-*Ras* oncogene and tumor formation following treatment with genotoxicants.[150,151] In another example, the *p53* gene in skin showed a high frequency of a base-pair substitution following UV-B exposure; this same base substitution was prevalent in subsequently developing skin tumors.[152]

An interesting finding that has come out of research studying mutations to oncogene "hot spots" is that many mutations noted in background tumors are similar to those seen in chemically induced tumors. This observation highlights the importance of understanding the role of epigenetic mechanisms (*e.g.*, regenerative cell proliferation, apoptosis, clonal expansion) in the formation of tumors associated with known genotoxicants (reviewed by Parsons *et al.*[153]).

### 15.11.3 Random Mutations

One widely used genotypic selection assay utilizes a method based on enriching mutation sequences prior to polymerase chain reaction (PCR) amplification. One such procedure with high sensitivity is called restriction-site mutation where DNA at known mutation sites is digested prior to PCR amplification.[154] This technique had been labor-intensive and expensive, but it has recently been modified for higher throughput into a method called random mutation capture (RMC). RMC appears to be a promising tool for studying chemically induced genomic mutations.[155] The procedure allows the capture and selective sequencing of rare mutations. In contrast to transgenic mice assays that employ phenotypic selection of exogenous reporter genes (see section 15.9), the RMC assay allows direct detection of mutations in endogenous genes. Although studies with known genotoxicants and appropriate negative controls chemicals are needed to demonstrate the utility of this model, RMC could prove to be an extremely valuable tool for the future study of chemical-induced mutagenicity.

## 15.12 DNA Adducts

DNA adducts are a type of DNA damage formed through the covalent binding of reactive electrophilic chemical intermediates or oxygen-based radicals with the nucleophilic sites on nucleoside bases (*e.g.*, N7 of guanine, O8 of guanine). DNA adducts are representative of DNA-reactive genotoxicants, from simple alkyl adducts to bulky polycyclic aromatic hydrocarbon adducts. In addition, oxygen-based DNA adducts can be indicative of DNA damage caused by indirect mechanisms related to oxidative stress and lipid peroxidation. DNA adducts allow the measurement of a key event during *in vivo* genotoxicity testing at the level of the target tissue. In addition, DNA adducts can be used as biomarkers for monitoring exposure of potential genotoxicants. No formal regulatory guidance is available for the assessment of DNA adducts but several publications on the measurement and use of DNA adducts are available.[156–161]

### 15.12.1 Summary of Methods

Several techniques have been developed to detect and quantify DNA adducts; the main ones commonly used are $^{32}$P-postlabeling,[162,163] immunoassay,[164] and chromatography with tandem mass spectroscopy.[165–167] In addition, radiolabeled chemicals can be administered to animals to measure DNA-associated radioactivity.[168] All these techniques involve isolating DNA from the target tissue, hydrolyzing/digesting DNA, and then enriching and isolating DNA prior to quantitation. Although the techniques and assessment of DNA adducts are technically challenging, measuring these adducts can provide a powerful tool for monitoring exposure of the ultimate DNA-damaging metabolite in target or surrogate tissue following administration of a suspected genotoxicant.[169]

Currently, the most widely used method for studying DNA adducts is the $^{32}$P-postlabeling technique. This method is versatile, has high sensitivity and uses minimum quantities of DNA.[162,163] DNA is isolated and incubated with $^{32}$P-adenonine triphosphate (ATP) and associated enzymes to label nucleosides. DNA adducts are separated from other DNA, historically using chromatographic methods (*e.g.*, thin layer, HPLC), and measured through autoradiographic techniques. Although this technique uses radiolabeled phosphate, which limits its widespread use, its versatility allows for the measurement of a variety of DNA adduct structures.

Immunoassay procedures have been developed to measure DNA adducts, but unlike the $^{32}$P-postlabeling technique, prior knowledge of the DNA adduct structure is required to develop antibodies that are selective and sensitive. Immunoassay measurements are equally useful for both small and large adducts, and are rapid once a suitable method is developed.[164]

DNA adducts also can be quantified using classical liquid chromatography followed by tandem mass spectroscopy (LC-MS/MS) or electrochemical detection.[159,166,167] One such method ("adductome" approach) can detect multiple DNA adducts through measuring the neutral loss of 2-deoxyribose from positively ionized 2-deoxynucleoside adducts.[166] An advantage to this approach is the ability to evaluate different types of DNA adducts without the use of radiolabeled phosphate.

The methodologies for measuring DNA adducts are evolving quickly. One extremely sensitive assay for quantitating nucleoside base oxidations actually combines the three methods discussed; this assay uses an immunoaffinity isolation step followed by $^{32}$P-postlabeling and then LC-MS/MS.[159]

### 15.12.2 Interpretation

DNA adducts are of major interest as biomarkers for exposure to genotoxicants since they provide information on exposure to the ultimate reactive metabolite interacting with nucleophiles on DNA. Strong correlations between DNA adduct formation and tumor incidence have been reported for a variety of genotoxicants, especially when administered for a period of 10 days.[170] However, it is important to note that the presence of DNA adducts in a tissue does not necessarily indicate a cancer risk for that tissue. Some DNA adducts will be repaired, some un-repaired DNA adducts will interfere with replication leading to cell death, and some adducts may generate mutations.[171] The fate of DNA adducts, coupled with the background incidence of DNA adducts from diet and endogenous processes, make assessing the relevance of a DNA adduct problematic. Despite these limitations, evaluating the presence of DNA adducts in mechanistic studies for chemicals suspected of being carcinogenic may provide powerful insight into pathways by which some of these chemicals may injure DNA. For risk assessment, however, other markers of genotoxicity or carcinogenicity are required to understand the importance of a particular DNA adduct for human cancer risk.[160]

## 15.13 Toxicogenomics

Toxicogenomics refers to the measurement of endpoints allowing for the study of the complex interactions between gene expression and well-defined adverse effects (reviewed by Irwin *et al.*[172]). As applied to short-term *in vivo* studies, toxicogenomic data can help rule out a DNA-reactive MoA for known rodent hepatic carcinogens by demonstrating the presence of molecular markers associated with nongenotoxic hepatic carcinogenesis.[173–176] In addition, gene expression studies have revealed molecular profiles for genotoxic carcinogens in rats.[176,177] However, in practice, most studies using toxicogenomics to investigate the MoA of a genotoxicant have used cell-based *in vitro* systems to discriminate between DNA-reactive and non-DNA-reactive chemicals.[178–181]

Since toxicogenomics requires the use of a large number of cells for analysis, it is considered less sensitive than traditional methods (*e.g.*, micronuclei), which detect rare DNA damage events in a single cell.[181] Despite potential issues with sensitivity, toxicogenomics remains a powerful tool for understanding molecular events underlying the MoA of a genotoxicant. Until technology platforms, statistical approaches, study designs, training sets, *etc.* are standardized among laboratories, the use of toxicogenomics for cancer risk assessment will remain most appropriate for case-by-case analyses and specific to a given laboratory or platform.

## 15.14 Biomonitoring

Genotoxicity endpoints in blood and other surrogate tissues have been used successfully to monitor for carcinogenicity risk. These biomarkers allow one to bridge across species to collect information for cancer risk assessment. Biomarkers of genotoxicity are used for epidemiology research to identify relationships to exposure, occupation, lifestyle, cancer (or other diseases), and drug treatments.

### 15.14.1 Cytogenetics

Micronuclei (MN) and chromosome aberrations in human peripheral blood lymphocytes (HPBL) have been used extensively for monitoring genotoxicity in human populations.[182,183] Other measures include MN in reticulocytes,[74–77] cytogenetics in buccal epithelial cells,[184,185] and DNA damage using the Comet assay in nucleated blood cells.[186,187] Not surprisingly, studies have found associations of DNA damage with age, gender, smoking, diet, alcohol, vitamin levels, cancer chemotherapeutics, *etc.* (reviewed by Battershill *et al.*[188]). Because factors exist that can influence background levels of DNA damage, results of epidemiology studies should be viewed with caution when these variables are not properly controlled.

### 15.14.2 Mutations

As with DNA damage, mutations are another genotoxicity endpoint that can be monitored in blood. For example, *Hprt* mutation frequency has been used for monitoring human populations.[146–149,187,189] As with DNA damage endpoints, sex, smoking, age and others factors can affect the rate of *Hprt* mutations. Molecular analysis of mutations in oncogenes has also played a pivotal role in both cancer diagnosis and in developing early biomarkers of disease; however, significant challenges to implementing genomic testing routinely in the clinic still exist.[190]

### 15.14.3 Protein Adducts

Electrophilic reactive intermediates of genotoxicants not only form adducts with nucleophilic DNA, but also form adducts with nucleophilic sites on proteins (*e.g.*, cysteine). Protein adduct formation is a valuable surrogate for DNA adducts, particularly in blood where hemoglobin and albumin are abundant. Since adducts of albumin and hemoglobin are stable and have known turnover rates in blood, these protein adducts can provide a specific and sensitive measure of exposure to a genotoxicant.[191] A classic example is hemoglobin adducts of aromatic amines and nitroaromatic compounds; human epidemiology studies have shown that smokers can be easily distinguished from non-smokers through the presence of these hemoglobin adducts. Like DNA adducts, the methodologies for protein adducts can vary and are difficult; however, the information gained can provide valuable insights for studying exposures to genotoxicants.

The relationship between various cross-species measures of genotoxicity relative to the initiation and progression of carcinogenesis is shown in Figure 15.8.

## 15.15 Pharmaceuticals

### 15.15.1 *In Vivo* Genotoxicity and Cancer Prediction

For pharmaceuticals, ICH guidance allows first-in-human clinical trials in normal volunteers to begin following negative results from regulatory-acceptable

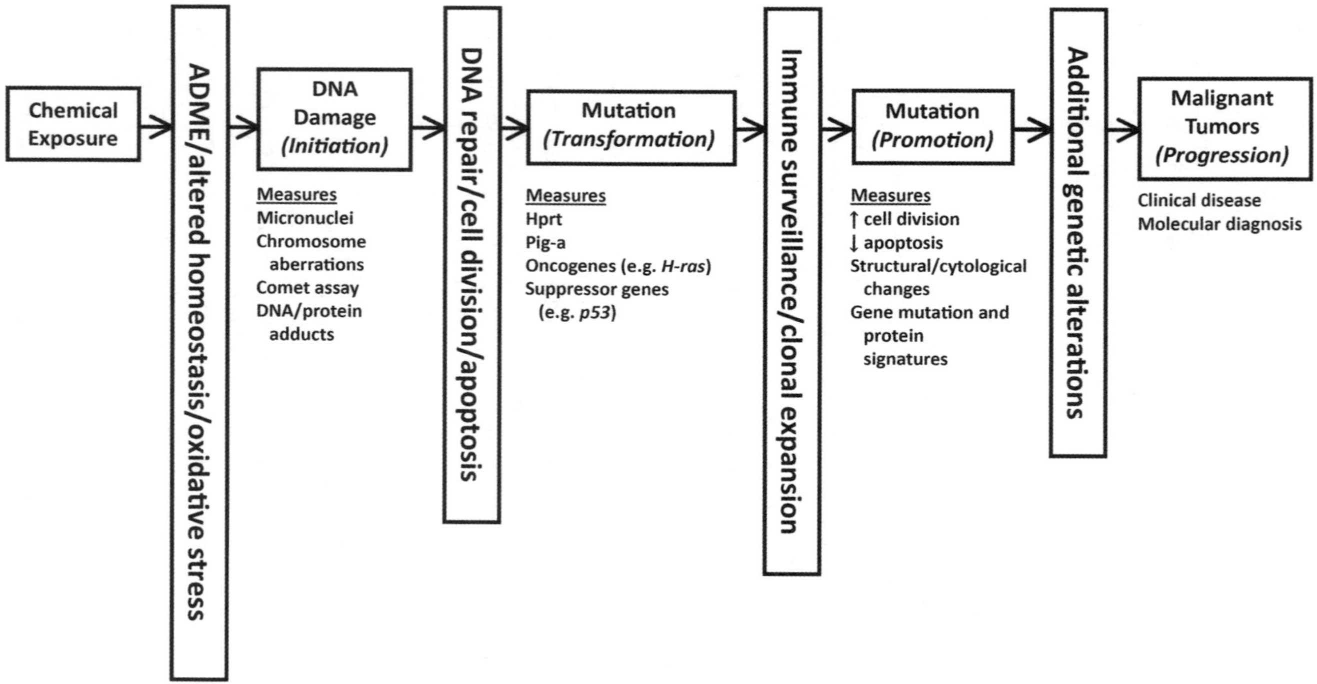


**Figure 15.8** Summary of cross-species measures and biomarkers in the evaluation of genotoxicity during the multi-stage process of carcinogenesis. The figure illustrates that accumulation of multiple genetic alterations is required to cause malignant tumors.

*in vitro* genotoxicity studies; at least one *in vivo* genotoxicity study is required to support repeat-dose clinical trials.[193] From a conservative standpoint, this practice makes sense, given the high false-positive rate of *in vitro* genotoxicity tests.[19] However, if a positive or equivocal finding occurs in the *in vitro* regulatory test battery, one or two *in vivo* genotoxicity tests may be required before starting clinical trials, potentially resulting in costly delays. Since some compound classes may actually produce false-negative results *in vitro* (*e.g.,* kinase inhibitors), a conservative recommendation has been made to conduct at least one *in vivo* genotoxicity study prior to first-in-human clinical trials.[24]

Prior to selecting a molecule for development, most pharmaceutical companies screen compounds for bacterial mutagenicity and DNA (chromosome) damage; the latter is evaluated using an *in vitro* MN screen in mammalian cells. These "Tier 1" screens are used to identify genotoxic hazards. The relationship of Tier 1 screens to Tier 2 animal genotoxicity screens and regulatory assays is illustrated for DNA damage tests in Figure 15.9.

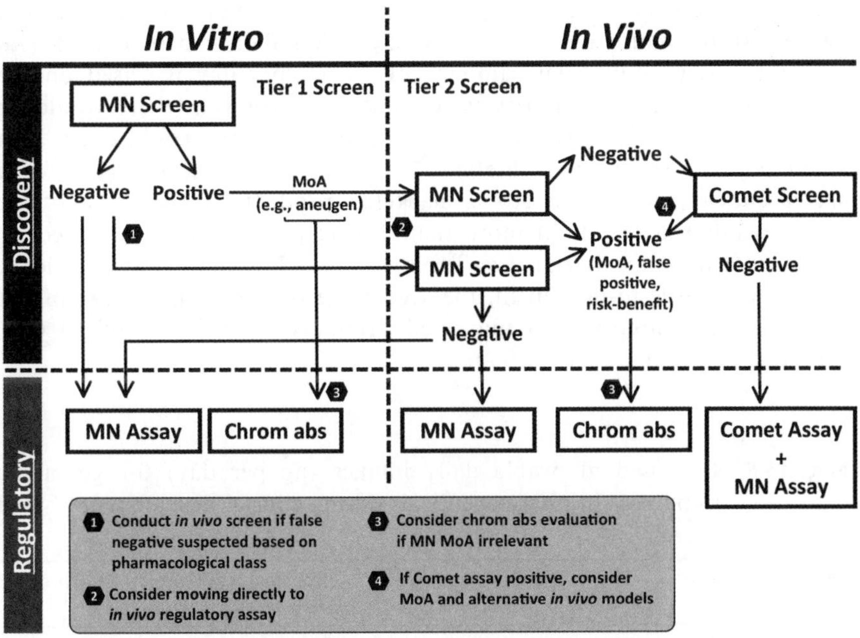


**Figure 15.9** This scheme represents one practical approach to *in vivo* genotoxicity testing used in the pharmaceutical industry for measuring DNA damage. Tier 1 *in vitro* screens are used to identify genotoxic hazards. *In vivo* studies such as the rodent erythrocyte micronucleus (MN) assay, lymphocyte chromosome aberration (chrom abs), and Comet assays can be conducted as screens in Tier 2 and/or as regulatory assays supporting clinical trials. If the *in vivo* Comet screen/assay is positive, another *in vivo* model from Table 15.1 or a go, no-go decision based on mode of action (MoA), safety margin, and risk-benefit should be considered.

This scheme represents one practical approach to *in vivo* genotoxicity testing within the pharmaceutical industry.

### 15.15.2 Risk *versus* Benefit

The assessment of cancer risk must always be balanced with the benefits of a chemical, whether it is a therapeutic drug, preservative in food, pesticide, industrial chemical or other compound. In the pharmaceutical industry, the risk-to-benefit ratio of marketed drugs can vary greatly. For example, although a standard battery of genotoxicity studies is required for supporting early-stage clinical trials with most pharmaceutical chemicals, genotoxicity studies may not be required for the registration of novel anti-cancer drugs, particularly those that have a DNA-reactive MoA (*e.g.*, doxorubicin). On the other hand, genotoxic impurities found within marketed active pharmaceutical ingredients targeted for non-life-threatening diseases, where a drug could be administered chronically (*e.g.*, anti-inflammatory agents), require a more conservative risk–benefit analysis. This analysis is defined by a European guideline limiting the daily intake of a genotoxic impurity to not more than 1.5 μg per day unless data can be collected to support a lower limit.[34] The amount of 1.5 μg per day is based on the assumption that if the impurity was a potent carcinogen, there would be about a one in 100 000 risk that an incidence of cancer would occur in a human population during a lifetime.[34] During clinical development of a pharmaceutical agent, prior to a marketed product, levels of genotoxic impurities allowed are often more than 1.5 μg per day and are based on duration of the clinical trial (see Table 15.8).[194] For industrial chemicals, where there is little-to-no benefit, the acceptable risk is often more stringent than genotoxic impurities in marketed products by a factor of 10 (*i.e.*, acceptable risk is one in 1 000 000).

**Table 15.8** Proposed allowable daily intakes (μg per day) for genotoxic impurities in pharmaceuticals during clinical development, based on ref. 194.

| *Duration of clinical exposure (months)* | *Allowable daily intake of genotoxic impurity (μg per day)*[a,b] |
|---|---|
| ≤1 | 120[c] |
| >1–3 | 40[c] |
| >3–6 | 20[c] |
| >6–12 | 10[c] |
| >12 | 1.5[d] |

[a]Allowable daily intake will be no more than 0.5% if lower than the μg per day value.
[b]Other limits may be appropriate based on risk assessment.
[c]Probability 93% of exceeding 1 in 1 000 000 cancer risk.
[d]Probability 93% of exceeding 1 in 100 000 cancer risk (same as EMEA guideline for marketed products).[34]

## 15.16 Conclusions

A considerable database related to genetic toxicology has been collected and a variety of assays applicable to laboratory animals and humans have emerged as useful for cancer risk assessment. Many of these genotoxicity models and strategies for their use are actively being evaluated by various international working groups. Despite many of the attractive features of these genotoxicity models, careful scrutiny of the expansive carcinogenicity databases reveal certain limitations, particularly in their ability to predict results from rodent carcinogenicity studies (which also have limitations in their relevance for human cancer risk).

As international collaborative efforts continue and technologies advance, improvements undoubtedly will be seen in the sensitivity and selectivity of the methods used for testing chemicals for genotoxic potential, in understanding the human relevance of positive findings, and in developing biomarkers of genotoxic exposure and subsequent effects. As well-validated, standardized genotoxicity assays become even further integrated with state-of-the-art technologies, using fundamental toxicological principles, the science of cancer risk assessment will continue to advance.

## References

1. *Molecular Biology of the Cell*, ed. A. Bruce, D. Bray, J. Lewis, M. Raff, K. Roberts and J. D. Watson, Garland Publishing, New York, 2nd edn, 1989, pp. 727–790.
2. M. D. Shelby, *Mutat. Res.*, 1996, **352**, 159–167.
3. T. M. Singer and C. L. Yauk, *Environ. Mol. Mutagen.*, 2010, **51**, 919–928.
4. J. Bartkova, Z. Horejsí, K. Koed, A. Krämer, F. Tort, K. Zieger, P. Guldberg, M. Sehested, J. M. Nesland, C. Lukas, T. Ørntoft, J. Lukas and J. Bartek, *Nature*, 2005, **434**, 864–870.
5. K. K. Khanna and S. P. Jackson, *Nat. Genet.*, 2001, **27**, 247–254.
6. S. H. Friend, R. Bernards, S. Rogelj, R. A. Weinberg, J. M. Rapaport, D. M. Albert and T. P. Dryja, *Nature*, 1986, **323**, 643–646.
7. K. M. Ryan, A. C. Phillips and K. H. Vousden, *Curr. Opin. Cell Biol.*, 2001, **13**, 332–337.
8. K. A. Nyberg, R. J. Michelson, C. W. Putnam and T. A. Weinert, *Annu. Rev. Genet.*, 2002, **36**, 617–656.
9. A. Knight, J. Bailey and J. Balcombe, *Altern. Lab. Anim.*, 2006, **34**, 29–38.
10. A. Jacobs and D. Jacobson-Kram, *Toxicol. Sci.*, 2004, **81**, 260–262.
11. M. P. Holsapple, H. C. Pitot, S. M. Cohen, A. R. Boobis, J. E. Klaunig, T. Pastoor T, V. L. Dellarco and Y. P. Dragan, *Toxicol. Sci.*, 2006, **89**, 51–56.
12. A. Jacobs, *Toxicol. Sci.*, 2005, **88**, 18–23.
13. J. S. MacDonald, *Toxicol. Sci.*, 2004, **82**, 3–8.
14. C. L. Alden, A. Lynn, A. Bourdeau, D. Morton, F. D. Sistare, V. J. Kadambi and L. Silverman, *Vet. Pathol.*, 2011, **48**, 772–784.

15. (*a*) D. J. Kirkland, M. Aardema, L. Henderson and L. Müller, *Mutat. Res.*, 2005, **584**, 1–256; (*b*) D. J. Kirkland, M. Aardema, L. Henderson and L. Müller, *Mutat. Res.*, 2005, **588**, 70.
16. D. J. Tweats, D. Blakey, R. H. Heflich, A. Jacobs, S. D. Jacobsen, T. Morita, T. Nohmi, M. R. O'Donovan, Y. F. Sasaki, T. Sofuni and R. Tice, *Mutat. Res.*, 2007, **627**, 78–91.
17. B. E. Butterworth, R. B. Conolly and K. T. Morgan, *Cancer Lett.*, 1995, **93**, 129–146.
18. K. L. Dearfield and M. M. Moore, *Environ. Mol. Mutagen.*, 2005, **46**, 236–245.
19. D. J. Kirkland, M. Aardema, N. Banduhn, P. Carmichael, R. Fautz, J. R. Meunier and S. Pfuhler, *Mutagenesis*, 2007, **22**, 161–175.
20. A. R. Boobis, G. P. Daston, R. J. Preston and S. S. Olin, *Crit. Rev. Food Sci. Nutr.*, 2009, **49**, 690–707.
21. R. Durai, W. Yang, S. Gupta, A. M. Seifalian and M. C. Winslet, *Int. J. Colorectal Dis.*, 2005, **20**, 203–220.
22. M. Andersen, D. Brusick, S. Cohen, Y. Dragan, C. Frederick, J. I. Goodman, G. Hard, B. Meek and E. J. O'Flaherty, *Toxicol. Appl. Pharmacol.*, 1998, **153**, 133–136.
23. C. K. Fraser, M. P. Brown, K. R. Diener and J. D. Hayball, *Expert Rev. Anticancer Ther.*, 2010, **10**, 917–934.
24. D. J. Tweats, D. Blakey, R. H. Heflich, A. Jacobs, S. D. Jacobsen, T. Morita, T. Nohmi, M. R. O'Donovan, Y. F. Sasaki, T. Sofuni and R. Tice, *Mutat. Res.*, 2007, **627**, 92–105.
25. V. Thybaud, M. Aardema, J. Clements, K. Dearfield, S. Galloway, M. Hayashi, D. Jacobson-Kram, D. Kirkland, J. T. MacGregor, D. Marzin, W. Ohyama, M. Schuler, H. Suzuki and E. Zeiger, *Mutat. Res.*, 2007, **627**, 41–58.
26. A. J. Olaharski, N. Gonzaludo, H. Bitter, D. Goldstein, S. Kirchner, H. Uppal and K. Kolaja, *PLoS Comput. Biol.*, 2009, **5**, 1–10.
27. L. Müller and P. Kasper, *Mutat. Res.*, 2000, **464**, 19–34.
28. D. Jacobson-Kram and A. Jacobs, *Int. J. Toxicol.*, 2005, **24**, 129–134.
29. E. Gocke and L. Müller, *Mutat. Res.*, 2009, **678**, 101–107.
30. P. J. Gehring and G. E. Blau, *J. Environ. Pathol. Toxicol.*, 1978, **1**, 163–179.
31. H. G. Neumann, *Crit. Rev. Toxicol.*, 2009, **39**, 449–461.
32. W. K. Lutz and R. W. Lutz, *Mutat. Res.*, 2009, **678**, 118–122.
33. M. Kirsch-Volders, L. Gonzalez, P. Carmichael and D. Kirkland, *Mutat. Res.*, 2009, **678**, 72–75.
34. European Medicines Agency, *Guideline CHMP/SWP/5199/02, Committee for Medicinal Products for Human Use Guideline on the Limits of Genotoxic Impurities*, EMEA, London, 2006.
35. W. K. Lutz, *Toxicol. Lett.*, 2009, **190**, 239–242.
36. S. H. Doak, G. J. Jenkins, G. E. Johnson, E. Quick, E. M. Parry and J. M. Parry, *Cancer Res.*, 2007, **67**, 3904–3911.
37. H. J. Muller, *Science,* 1927, **66**, 84–87.

38. W. L. Russell, *Cold Spring Harb. Symp. Quant. Biol.*, 1951, **16**, 327–336.
39. M. A. Bender and P. C. Gooch, *Radiat. Res.*, 1962, **16**, 44–53.
40. B. N. Ames, W. E. Durston, E. Yamasaki and F. D. Lee, *Proc. Natl. Acad. Sci. U.S.A.*, 1973, **70**, 2281–2285.
41. L. B. Russell and B. E. Matter, *Mutat. Res.*, 1980, **75**, 279–302.
42. W. L. Russell, P. B. Shelby, E. von Halle, W. Sheridan and L. Valcovic, *Mutat. Res.*, 1981, **86**, 329–354.
43. Environmental Protection Agency, *Health Effects Test Guidelines, OPPTS 870.5200 Mouse Visible Specific Locus Test*, EPA, Washington DC, 1996.
44. R. Fahrig, *Arch. Toxicol.*, 1977, **38**, 87–98.
45. Organisation for Economic Cooperation and Development, *Guideline 484: Mouse Spot Test*, OECD, Paris, 1986.
46. U. Wahnschaffe, A. Bitsch, J. Kielhorn and I. Mangelsdorf, *J. Carcinog.*, 2005, **4**, 4.
47. Organisation for Economic Cooperation and Development, *Guideline 474: Rodent Erythrocyte Micronucleus Test*, OECD, Paris, 1997.
48. Environmental Protection Agency, *Health Effects Test Guidelines OPPTS 870.5395 In Vivo Mammalian Cytogenetics Tests: Erythrocyte Micronucleus Assay*, EPA, Washington, D.C., 1996.
49. US Food and Drug Administration, *Toxicological Principles for the Safety Assessment of Food Ingredients*, FDA, Silver Spring, MD, 2000.
50. M. Hayashi, R. R. Tice, J. T. MacGregor, D. Anderson, D. H. Blakey, M. Kirsh-Volders, F. B. Oleson Jr, F. Pacchierotti, F. Romagna, H. Shimada, S. Sutou and B. Vannier, *Mutat. Res.*, 1994, **312**, 293–304.
51. M. Hayashi, J. T. MacGregor, D. G. Gatehouse, I. D. Adler, D. H. Blakey, S. D. Dertinger, G. Krishna, T. Morita, A. Russo and S. Sutou, *Environ. Mol. Mutagen.*, 2000, **35**, 234–252.
52. M. Hayashi, J. T. MacGregor, D. G. Gatehouse, D. H. Blakey, S. D. Dertinger, L. Abramsson-Zetterberg, G. Krishna, T. Morita, A. Russo, N. Asano, H. Suzuki, W. Ohyama and D. Gibson, *Mutat. Res.*, 2007, **627**, 10–30.
53. *S2B: Genotoxicity: a standard battery for genotoxicity testing for pharmaceuticals*, International Conference on Harmonisation, Geneva, Switzerland, 1997.
54. *S2A: Guidance on specific aspects of regulatory genotoxicity tests for pharmaceuticals*, International Conference on Harmonisation, Geneva, Switzerland, 1995.
55. *S2(R1): Guidance on genotoxicity testing and data interpretation for pharmaceuticals intended for human use*, International Conference on Harmonisation, Geneva, Switzerland, 2006.
56. J. A. Heddle, *Mutat. Res.*, 1973, **18**, 187–190.
57. J. T. MacGregor, C. M. Wehr and D. H. Gould, *Environ. Mutagen.*, 1980, **2**, 509–514.
58. W. Frieauff and F. Romagna, *Cell Biol. Toxicol.*, 1994, **10**, 283–289.

59. A. T. Doherty, J. E. Hayes and M. R. O'Donovan, *Environ Mol. Mutagen.*, 2010, **51**, 732.
60. M. Hayashi, Y. Kodama, T. Awogi, T. Suzuki, A. O. Asita and T. Sofuni, *Mutat. Res.*, 1992, **278**, 209–213.
61. L. Abramsson-Zetterberg, J. Grawé and G. Zetterberg, *Mutat. Res.*, 1999, **423**, 113–124.
62. G. M. Hynes, D. K. Torous, C. R. Tometsko, B. Burlinson and D. G. Gatehouse, *Mutagenesis*, 2002, **17**, 15–23.
63. D. K. Torous, S. D. Dertinger, N. E. Hall and C. R. Tometsko, *Mutat. Res.*, 2000, **465**, 91–99.
64. D. K. Torous, N. E. Hall, F. G. Murante, S. E. Gleason, C. R. Tometsko and S. D. Dertinger, *Toxicol. Sci.*, 2003, **74**, 309–314.
65. S. D. Dertinger, M. E. Bishop, J. P. McNamee, M. Hayashi, T. Suzuki, N. Asano, M. Nakajima, J. Saito, M. Moore, D. K. Torous and J. T. MacGregor, *Toxicol. Sci.*, 2006, **94**, 83–91.
66. S. D. Dertinger, D. K. Torous and K. R. Tometsko, *Mutat. Res.*, 1996, **371**, 283–292.
67. S. D. Dertinger, D. K. Torous and K. R. Tometsko, *Mutat. Res.*, 1997, **390**, 257–262.
68. D. K. Torous, S. D. Dertinger, N. E. Hall and C. R. Tometsko, *Environ. Mol. Mutagen.*, 1998, **31**, 340–344.
69. K. L. Witt, E. Livanos, G. E. Kissling, D. K. Torous, W. Caspary, R. R. Tice and L. Recio, *Mutat. Res.*, 2008, **649**, 101–113.
70. J. T. MacGregor, M. E. Bishop, J. P. McNamee, M. Hayashi, N. Asano, A. Wakata, M. Nakajima, J. Saito, A. Aidoo, M. Moore and S. D. Dertinger, *Toxicol. Sci.*, 2006, **94**, 92–107.
71. R. D. Fiedler, S. K. Weiner and M. Schuler, *Mutat. Res.*, 2010, **703**, 122–129.
72. S. B. Harper, S. D. Dertinger, M. E. Bishop, A. M. Lynch, M. Lorenzo, M. Saylor and J. T. MacGregor, *Toxicol. Sci.*, 2007, **100**, 406–414.
73. C. E. Hotchkiss, M. E. Bishop, S. D. Dertinger, W. Slikker Jr, M. Moore and J. T. MacGregor, *Toxicol. Sci.*, 2008, **102**, 352–358.
74. S. D. Dertinger, D. K. Torous, N. E. Hall, F. G. Murante, S. E. Gleason, R. K. Miller and C. R. Tometsko, *Mutat. Res.,* 2002, **515**, 3–14.
75. S. D. Dertinger, Y. Chen, R. K. Miller, K. J. Brewer, T. Smudzin, D. K. Torous, N. E. Hall, K. A. Olvany, F. G. Murante and C. R. Tometsko, *Mutat. Res.*, 2003, **542**, 77–87.
76. S. D. Dertinger, R. K. Miller, K. Brewer, T. Smudzin, D. K. Torous, D. J. Roberts, S. L. Avlasevich, S. M. Bryce, S. Sugunan and Y. Chen, *Mutat. Res.*, 2007, **626**, 111–119.
77. S. D. Dertinger, Y. Tsai, I. Nowak, O. Hyrien, H. Sun, J. C. Bemis, D. K. Torous, P. Keng, J. Palis and Y. Chen, *Mutat. Res.*, 2007, **634**, 119–125.
78. Z. Cammerer, A. Elhajouji, M. Kirsch-Volders and W. Suter, *Mutagenesis*, 2007, **22**, 129–134.
79. G. E. Kissling, S. D. Dertinger, M. Hayashi and J. T. MacGregor, *Mutat. Res.*, 2007, **634**, 235–240.

80. M. De Boeck, B. J. van der Leede, F. van Goethem, A. De Smedt, M. Steemans, A. Lampo and P. Vanparys, *Environ. Mol. Mutagen.*, 2005, **46**, 30–42.
81. W. Schmid, *Mutat. Res.*, 1975, **31**, 9–15.
82. J. T. MacGregor, J. D. Tucker, D. A. Eastmond and A. J. Wyrobek, *Environ. Mol. Mutagen.*, 1995, **25**, 328–337.
83. S. Hamada, S. Sutou, T. Morita, A. Wakata, S. Asanami, S. Hosoya, S. Ozawa, K. Kondo, M. Nakajima, H. Shimada, K. Osawa, Y. Kondo, N. Asano, S. Sato, H. Tamura, N. Yajima, R. Marshall, C. Moore, D. H. Blakey, L. M. Schechtman, J. L. Weaver, D. K. Torous, R. Proudlock, S. Ito, C. Namiki and M. Hayashi, *Environ. Mol. Mutagen.*, 2001, **37**, 93–110.
84. S. Hamada, K. Nakajima, T. Serikawa and M. Hayashi, *Mutagenesis*, 2003, **18**, 273–275.
85. J. Hayes, A. T. Doherty, D. J. Adkins, K. Oldman and M. R. O'Donovan, *Mutagenesis*, 2009, **24**, 419–424.
86. Collaborative Study Group for the Micronucleus Test, the Mammalian Mutagenesis Study Group of the Environmental Mutagen Society, Japan, *Mutat. Res.*, 1990, **234**, 205–222.
87. R. Benigni, C. Bossa and A. Worth, *Mutagenesis,* 2010, **25**, 335–341.
88. K. L. Witt, A. Knapton, C. M. Wehr, G. J. Hook, J. Mirsalis, M. D. Shelby and J. T. MacGregor, *Environ. Mol. Mutagen.*, 2000, **36**, 163–94.
89. B. S. Kim and B. H. Margolin, *Environ. Mol. Mutagen.*, 1999, **34**, 297–304.
90. E. Zeiger, *Regul. Toxicol. Pharmacol.*, 1998, **28**, 85–95.
91. (*a*) T. Morita, N. Asano, T. Awogi, Y. F. Sasaki, S. Sato, H. Shimada, S. Sutou S, T. Suzuki, A. Wakata, T. Sofuni and M. Hayashi, *Mutat. Res.*, 1997, **389**, 3–122; (*b*) T. Morita, N. Asano, T. Awogi, Y. F. Sasaki, S. Sato, H. Shimada, S. Sutou S, T. Suzuki, A. Wakata, T. Sofuni and M. Hayashi, *Mutat. Res.*, 1997, **391**, 259–267.
92. M. D. Shelby, G. L. Erexson, G. J. Hook and R. R. Tice, *Environ. Mol. Mutagen.*, 1993, **21**, 160–179.
93. M. J. Aardema, S. Albertini, P. Arni, L. M. Henderson, M. Kirsch-Volders, J. M. Mackay, A. M. Sarrif, D. A. Stringer and R. D. Taalman, *Mutat. Res.*, 1998, **410**, 3–79.
94. J. A. Heddle, M. C. Cimino, M. Hayashi, F. Romagna, M. D. Shelby, J. D. Tucker, P. Vanparys and J. T. MacGregor, *Environ. Mol. Mutagen.*, 1991, **18**, 277–291.
95. L. Migliore, L. Cocchi and R. Scarpato, *Mutagenesis*, 1996, **11**, 285–290.
96. J. M. Parry, E. M. Parry, R. Bourner, A. Doherty, S. Ellard, J. O'Donovan, B. Hoebee, J. M. de Stoppelaar, G. R. Mohn, A. Onfelt, A. Renglin, N. Schultz, C. Söderpalm-Berndes, K. G. Jensen, M. Kirsch-Volders, A. Elhajouji, P. Van Hummelen, F. Degrassi, A. Antoccia, D. Cimini, M. Izzo, C. Tanzarella, I. D. Adler, U. Kliesch, G. Schriever-Schwemmer, P. Gasser, R. Crebelli, A. Carere, C. Andreoli, R. Benigni,

P. Leopardi, F. Marcon, Z. Zinjo, A. T. Natarajan, J. J. W. A. Boei, A. Kappas, G. Voutsinas, F. E. Zarani, A. Patrinelli, F. Pachierotti, C. Tiveron and P. Hess, *Mutat. Res.*, 1996, **353**, 11–46.
97. M. Schuler, D. S. Rupa and D. A. Eastmond, *Mutat. Res.*, 1997, **392**, 81–95.
98. Organisation for Economic Cooperation and Development, *Guideline 475, Mammalian Bone Marrow Chromosome Aberration Test*, OECD, Paris, 1997.
99. I. B. Lambert, T. M. Singer, S. E. Boucher and G. R. Douglas, *Mutat. Res.*, 2005, **590**, 1280.
100. S. Madle, S. W. Dean, U. Andrae, G. Brambilla, B. Burlinson, D. J. Doolittle, C. Furihata, T. Hertner, C. A. McQueen and H. Mori, *Mutat. Res.*, 1994, **312**, 263–285.
101. Organisation for Economic Cooperation and Development, *Guideline 486, Unscheduled DNA Synthesis (UDS) Test with Mammalian Liver Cells* In Vivo, OECD, Paris, 1997.
102. J. C. Marsalis and B. E. Butterworth, *Carcinogenesis*, 1980, **1**, 621–625.
103. E. J. Matthews, N. L. Kruhlak, M. C. Cimino, R. D. Benz and J. F. Contrera, *Regul. Toxicol. Pharmacol.*, 2006, **44**, 97–110.
104. D. Kirkland and G. Speit, *Mutat. Res.*, 2008, **654**, 114–132.
105. B. Burlinson, R. R. Tice, G. Speit, E. Agurell, S. Y. Brendler-Schwaab, A. R. Collins, P. Escobar, M. Honma, T. S. Kumaravel, M. Nakajima, Y. F. Sasaki, V. Thybaud, Y. Uno, M. Vasquez and A. Hartmann, *Mutat. Res.*, 2007, **627**, 31–35.
106. C. C. Smith, D. J. Adkins, E. A. Martin and M. R. O'Donovan, *Mutagenesis*, 2008, **23**, 233–240.
107. http://jacvam.jp/en/.
108. S. Brendler-Schwaab, A. Hartmann, S. Pfuhler and G. Speit, *Mutagenesis*, 2005, **20**, 245–254.
109. P. R. Cook, I. A. Brazell and E. Jost, *J. Cell Sci.*, 1976, **22**, 303–324.
110. O. Ostling and K. J. Johanson, *Biochem. Biophys. Res. Commun.*, 1984, **123**, 291–298.
111. P. L. Olive, J. P. J Banáth and R. E. Durand, *J. Natl. Cancer Inst.*, 1990, **82**, 779–783.
112. N. P. Singh, M. T. McCoy, R. R. Tice and E. L. Schneider, *Exp. Cell Res.*, 1988, **175**, 184–191.
113. A. Hartmann, E. Agurell, C. Beevers, S. Brendler-Schwaab, B. Burlinson, P. Clay, A. Collins, A. Smith, G. Speit, V. Thybaud and R. R. Tice, *Mutagenesis*, 2003, **18**, 45–51.
114. R. R. Tice, E. Agurell, D. Anderson, B. Burlinson, A. Hartmann, H. Kobayashi, Y. Miyamae, E. Rojas, J. C. Ryu and Y. F. Sasaki, *Environ. Mol. Mutagen.*, 2000, **35**, 206–221.
115. M. Z. Vasquez, *Mutagenesis*, 2010, **25**, 187–199.
116. L. Henderson, A. Wolfreys, J. Fedyk, C. Bourner and S. Windebank, *Mutagenesis*, 1998, **13**, 89–94.

117. P. Choucroun, D. Gillet, G. Dorange, B. Sawicki and J. D. Dewitte, *Mutat. Res.*, 2001, **478**, 89–96.
118. A. Rothfuss, M. O'Donovan, M. De Boeck, D. Brault, A. Czich, L. Custer, S. Hamada, U. Plappert-Helbig, M. Hayashi, J. Howe, A. R. Kraynak, B. J. van der Leede, M. Nakajima, C. Priestley, V. Thybaud, K. Saigo, S. Sawant, J, Shi, R. Storer, M. Struwe, E. Vock and S. Galloway, *Mutat. Res.*, 2010, **702**, 40–69.
119. A. R. Collins, A. A. Oscoz, G. Brunborg, I. Gaivao, L. Giovannelli, M. Kruszewski, C. C. Smith and R. Stetina, *Mutagenesis*, 2008, **23**, 143–151.
120. T. Kumaravel, B. Vihar, S. Faux and A. Jha, *Cell Biol. Toxicol.*, 2009, **25**, 53–64.
121. L. Recio, C. Hobbs, W. Caspary and K. L. Witt, *J. Toxicol. Sci.*, 2010, **35**, 149–162.
122. Y. F. Sasaki, K. Sekihashi, F. Itumiyama, E. Nishidate, A. Saga, K. Ishida and S. Tsuda, *Crit. Rev. Toxicol.*, 2000, **30**, 629–799.
123. P. Kasper, Y. Uno, R. Mauthe, N. Asano, G. Douglas, E. Matthews, M. Moore, L. Müller, M. Nakajima, T. Singer and G. Speit, *Mutat. Res.*, 2007, **627**, 106–116.
124. V. Thybaud, S. Dean, T. Nohmic, J. de Boer, G. R. Douglas, B. W. Glickman, N. J. Gorelick, J. A. Heddle,R. H. Heflich, I. Lambert, H.-J. Martus, J. C. Mirsalis, T. Suzuki and N. Yajima, *Mutat. Res.*, 2003, **540**, 141–151.
125. International Programme on Chemical Safety, *Transgenic Animal Mutagenicity Assays (Environmental Health Criteria 233)*, World Health Organization, Geneva, Switzerland, 2006.
126. J. A. Heddle, S. Dean, T. Nohmi, M. Boerrigter, D. Casciano, G. R. Douglas, B. Glickman, N. Gorelick, J. Mirsalis, H. J. Martus, T. Skopek, V. Thybaud, K. Tindall and N. Yajima, *Environ. Mol. Mutagen.*, 2000, **35**, 253–259.
127. K. S. Tao and J. A. Heddle, *Mutagenesis*, 1994, **9**, 187–191.
128. P. S. Shwed, J. Crosthwait, G. R. Douglas and V. L. Seligy, *Mutagenesis*, 2010, **25**, 609–616.
129. B. B. Gollapudi, W. T. Stott, B. L. Yano and J. S. Bus, *Toxicol. Lett.*, 1998, **102–103**, 479–484.
130. W. Deubel, I. D. Bassukas, W. Schlereth, R. Lorenz and K. Hempel, *Mutat. Res.*, 1996, **351**, 67–77.
131. V. E. Walker, I. M. Jones, T. L. Crippen, Q. Meng, D. M. Walker, M. J. Bauer, A. A. Reilly, A. D. Tates, J. Nakamura, P. B. Upton and T. R. Skopek, *Mutat. Res.*, 1999, **431**, 371–388.
132. V. N. Dobrovolsky, T. Chen and R. H. Heflich, *Environ. Mol. Mutagen.*, 1999, **34**, 3038.
133. S. M. Bryce, J. C. Bemis and S. D. Dertinger, *Environ. Mol. Mutagen.*, 2008, **49**, 256–264.
134. S. Phonethepswath, S. M. Bryce, J. C. Bemis and S. D. Dertinger, *Mutat. Res.*, 2008, **657**, 122–126.

135. S. Phonethepswath, D. Franklin, D. K. Torous, S. M. Bryce, J. C. Bemis, S. Raja, S. Avlasevich, P. Weller, O. Hyrien, J. Palis, J. T. MacGregor and S. D. Dertinger, *Toxicol. Sci.*, 2010, **114**, 59–70.
136. M. Bessler, A. Schaefer and P. Keller, *Transfus. Med. Rev.*, 2001, **15**, 255–267.
137. W. F. Rosse and W. E. Ware, *Blood,* 1995, **86**, 3277–3286.
138. S. D. Dertinger, S. M. Bryce, S. Phonethepswath and S. L. Avlasevich, *Mutat. Res.*, 2011, **721**, 163–170.
139. V. N. Dobrovolsky, S. Y. Boctor, N. C. Twaddle, D. R. Doerge, M. E. Bishop, M. Manjanatha, T. Kimoto, D. Miura, R. H. Heflich and S. A. Ferguson, *Environ. Mol. Mutagen.*, 2010, **51**, 138–145.
140. D. Miura, V. N. Dobrovolsky, Y. Kasahara, Y. Katsuura and R. H. Heflich, *Environ. Mol. Mutagen.*, 2008, **49**, 614–621.
141. D. Miura, V. N. Dobrovolsky, T. Kimoto, Y. Kasahara and R. H. Heflich, *Mutat. Res.*, 2009, **677**, 86–92.
142. S. D. Dertinger, S. Phonethepswath, D. Franklin, P. Weller, D. K. Torous, S. M. Bryce, S. Avlasevich, J. C. Bemis, O. Hyrien, J. Palis and J. T. MacGregor, *Toxicol. Sci.*, 2010, **115**, 401–411.
143. B. Peruzzi, D. J. Araten, R. Notaro and L. Luzzatto, *Mutat. Res.*, 2010, **705**, 3–10.
144. J. Shuga, Y. Zeng, R. Novak, R. A. Mathies, P. Hainaut and M. T. Smith, *Environ. Mol. Mutagen,* 2010, **51**, 851–870.
145. R. J. Albertini, J. A. Nicklas, J. C. Fuscoe, T. R. Skopek, R. F. Branda and J. P. O'Neill, *Environ. Health Perspect.*, 1993, **99**, 135–141.
146. J. Curry, L. Karnaoukhova, G. C. Guenette and B. W. Glickman, *Genetics*, 1999, **152**, 1065–1077.
147. P. Hackman, S. M. Hou, F. Nyberg, G. Pershagen and B. Lambert, *Mutat. Res.*, 2000, **468**, 45–61.
148. B. Lambert, T. Bastlova, A. M, Osterholm and S. M. Hou, *Toxicol. Lett.*, 1995, **82–83**, 323–333.
149. P. Noori, S. Hou, I. M. Jones, C.B. Thomas and B. Lambert, *Carcinogenesis*, 2005, **26**, 1138–1151.
150. R. C. Sills, G. A. Boorman, J. E. Neal, H. L. Hong and T. R. Devereux, *IARC Sci. Publ.*, 1999, **146,** 55–86.
151. B. L. Parsons, F. A. Beland, L. S. von Tungeln, R. R. Delongchamp, P. P. Fu and R. H. Heflich, *Mol. Carcinog.*, 2005, **42**, 193–201.
152. T. L. Verkler, R. R. Delongchamp, L. H. Couch, B. J. Miller, A. Warbritton, P. W. Mellick, P. C. Howard and B. L. Parsons, *Mol. Carcinog.*, 2008, **47**, 822–834.
153. B. L. Parsons, M. B. Myers, F. Meng, Y. Wang and P. B. McKinzie, *Environ. Mol. Mutagen.*, 2010, **51**, 836–850.
154. J. M. Parry, M. Shamsher and D. O. Skibinski, *Mutagenesis*, 1990, **5**, 209–212.
155. J. H. Wright, K. L. Modjeski, J. H. Bielas, B. D. Preston, N. Fausto, L. A. Loeb and J. S. Campbell, *Nucleic Acids Res.*, 2011, **39**, e73.

156. V. Gallo, A. Khan, C. Gonzales, D. H. Phillips, B. Schoket, E. Györffy, L. Anna, K. Kovács, P. Møller, S. Loft, S. Kyrtopoulos, G. Matullo and P. Vineis, *Biomarkers*, 2008, **13**, 505–534.
157. E. Gyorffy, L. Anna, K. Kovács, P. Rudnai and B. Schoket, *Mutagenesis*, 2008, **23**, 1–18.
158. M. W. Himmelstein, P. J. Boogaard, J. Cadet, P. B. Farmer, J. H. Kim, E. A. Martin, R. Persaud and D. E. Shuker, *Crit. Rev. Toxicol.*, 2009, **39**, 679–694.
159. U. Nair, H. Bartsch and J. Nair, *Free Radic. Biol. Med.*, 2007, **43**, 1109–1120.
160. M. C. Poirier, R. M. Santella and A. Weston, *Carcinogenesis*, 2000, **21**, 353–359.
161. J. A. Swenberg, E. Fryar-Tita, Y. C. Jeong, G. Boysen, T. Starr, V. E. Walker and R. J. Albertini, *Chem. Res. Toxicol.*, 2008, **21**, 253–265.
162. D. H. Phillips, A. Hewer and V. M. Arlt, *Methods Mol. Biol.*, 2005, **291**, 3–12.
163. D. H. Phillips and V. M. Arlt, *Nat. Protoc.*, 2007, **2**, 2772–2781.
164. R. L. Divi, F. A. Beland, P. P. Fu, L. S. von Tungeln, B. Schoket, J. E. Camara, M. Ghei, N. Rothman, R. Sinha and M. C. Poirer, *Carcinogenesis,* 2002, **23**, 2043–2049.
165. I. G. Cowell, M. J. Tilb and C. A. Austin, *Mutagenesis,* 2011, **26**, 253–260.
166. R. A. Kanaly, T. Hanaoka, H. Sugimura, H. Toda, S. Matsui and T. Matsuda, *Antioxid. Redox. Signal.*, 2006, **8**, 993–1001.
167. R. Singh and P. B. Farmer, *Carcinogenesis,* 2006, **27**, 178–196.
168. H. van der Woude, G. M. Alink, B. E. van Rossum, K. Walle, H. van Steeg, T. Walle and I. M. Rietjens, *Chem. Res. Toxicol.*, 2005, **18**, 1907–1916.
169. D. H. Phillips, P. B. Farmer, F. A. Beland, R. G. Nath, M. C. Poirier, M. V. Reddy and K. W. Turteltaub, *Environ. Mol. Mutagen.*, 2000, **35**, 222–233.
170. M. Otteneder and W. K. Lutz, *Mutat. Res.*, 1999, **424**, 237–247.
171. E. R. Nestmann, D. W. Bryant and C. J. Carr, T. T. Fennell, J. E. Gallagher, N. J. Gorelick, J. A. Swenberg and G. M. Williams, *Regul. Toxicol. Pharmacol.*, 1996, **24**, 9–18.
172. R. D. Irwin, G. A. Boorman, M. L. Cunningham, A. N. Heinloth, D. E. Malarkey and R. S Paules, *Toxicol. Pathol.*, 2004, **32**, 72–83.
173. M. M. Elrick, J. A. Kramer, C. L. Alden, E. A. Blomme, R. T. Bunch, M. A. Cabonce, S. W. Curtiss, L. D. Kier, K. L. Kolaja, C. P. Rodi and D. L. Morris, *Toxicol. Pathol.*, 2005, **33**, 118–126.
174. J. A. Kramer, S. W. Curtiss, K. L. Kolaja, C. L. Alden, E. A. Blomme, W. C. Curtiss, J. C. Davila, C. J. Jackson and R. T. Bunch, *Chem. Res. Toxicol.*, 2004, **17**, 463–470.
175. C. P. Rodi, R. T. Bunch, S. W. Curtiss, L. D. Kier, M. A. Cabonce, J. C. Davila, M. D. Mitchell, C. L. Alden and D. L. Morris, *Toxicol. Pathol.*, 1999, **27**, 107–110.

176. M. D. Waters, M. Jackson and I. Lea, *Mutat. Res.*, 2010, **705**, 184–200.
177. H. Ellinger-Ziegelbauer, B. Stuart, B. Wahle, W. Bomann and H. J. Ahr, *Toxicol. Sci.*, 2004, **77**, 19–34.
178. H. Ellinger-Ziegelbauer, J. Aubrecht, J. C. Kleinjans and H. J. Ahr, *Toxicol. Lett.*, 2009, **186**, 36–44.
179. T. Hu, D. P. Gibson, G. J. Carr, S. M. Torontali, J. P. Tiesman, J. G. Chaney and M. J. Aardema, *Mutat. Res.*, 2004, **549**, 5–27.
180. A. C. Le Fevre, E. Boitier, J. P. Marchandeau, A. Sarasin and V. Thybaud, *Mutat. Res.*, 2007, **619**, 16–29.
181. R. K. Newton, M. Aardema and J. Aubrecht, *Environ. Health Perspect.*, 2004, **112**, 420–422.
182. S. Bonassi, A. Znaor, M. Ceppi, C. Lando, W. P. Chang, N. Holland, M. Kirsch-Volders, E. Zeiger, S. Ban, R. Barale, M. P. Bigatti, C. Bolognesi, A. Cebulska-Wasilewska, E. Fabianova, A. Fucic, L. Hagmar, G. Joksic, A. Martelli, L. Migliore, E. Mirkova, M. R. Scarfi, A. Zijno, H. Norppa and M. Fenech, *Carcinogenesis*, 2007, **28**, 625–631.
183. M. Fenech, N. Holland, W. P. Chang, E. Zeiger and S. Bonassi, *Mutat. Res.*, 1999, **428**, 271–283.
184. N. Holland, C. Bolognesi, M. Kirsch-Volders, S. Bonassi, E. Zeiger, S. Knasmueller and M. Fenech, *Mutat. Res.*, 2008, **659**, 93–108.
185. P. Thomas and M. Fenech, *Mutagenesis,* 2008, **23**, 57–65.
186. M. Dusinska and A. R. Collins, *Mutagenesis,* 2008, **23**, 191–205.
187. P. Vodicka, T. Tvrdik, S. Osterman-Golkar, L. Vodicková, K. Peterková, P. Soucek, J. Sarmanová, P. B. Farmer, F. Granath, B. Lambert and K. Hemminki, *Mutat. Res.*, 1999, **445**, 205–224.
188. J. M. Battershill, K. Burnett and S. Bull, *Mutagenesis,* 2008, **23**, 423–437.
189. G. Bentham, A. M. Wolfreys, Y. Liu, G. Cortopassi, M. H. Green, C. F. Arlett and J. Cole, *Mutagenesis,* 1999, **14**, 527–532.
190. P. A. Cowin, M. Anglesio, D. Etemadmoghadam and D. D. Bowtell, *Annu. Rev. Genomics Hum. Genet.*, 2010, **11**, 133–159.
191. J. Angerer, U. Ewers and M. Wilhelm, *Int. J. Hyg. Environ. Health*, 2007, **210**, 201–228.
192. G. Sabbioni and C. R. Jones, *Biomarkers*, 2002, **7**, 347–421.
193. *M3(R2): Guideline for nonclinical safety studies for the conduct of human clinical trials and marketing authorization for pharmaceuticals*, International Conference on Harmonisation, Geneva, Switzerland, 2009.
194. L. Müller, R. J. Mauthe, C. M. Riley, M. M. Andino, D. D. Antonis, C. Beels, J. DeGeorge, A. G. Knaep, D. Ellison, J. A. Fagerland, R. Frank, B. Fritschel, S. Galloway, E. Harpur, C. D. Humfrey, A. S. Jacks, N. Jagota, J. Mackinnon, G. Mohan, D. K. Ness, M. R. O'Donovan, M. D. Smith, G. Vudathala and L. Yotti, *Regul. Toxicol. Pharmacol.*, 2006, **44**, 198–211.
195. Organisation for Economic Cooperation and Development, *Guideline 476,* In Vitro *Mammalian Cell Gene Mutation Test*, OECD, Paris, 1997.

CHAPTER 16
# *Predicting Hepatotoxicity* In Vivo

TIMOTHY MAZIASZ

Allergan Inc., PO Box 19534, Irvine, CA 92612, USA

## 16.1 Introduction

Conducting clinical studies with a novel drug candidate involves a level of risk. The characterization of the toxicity profile of a new medical entity in animals prior to clinical testing is intended to mitigate this risk. Accordingly, pharmaceutical companies have invested considerable resources and technology to ensure that the potential toxicities of their drug candidates are well understood before dosing human beings. Despite best intentions and best practices, serious, and sometimes unforeseen, toxicities do occur in the clinic.

Perhaps the most difficult challenge in developing new drugs is the accurate prediction of human toxicity. Given that the vast majority of data used to accomplish this is obtained using laboratory species, this is not straightforward. The augmentation of routine non-clinical safety assessment with new assays and technologies and human tissues and cells may eventually strengthen the predictive power of non-clinical data. Until then, certain types of toxicities will continue to be problematic.

A 2002 FDA commentary acknowledged that drug-induced liver injury (DILI) and cardiotoxicity represent the major drivers for the withdrawal of marketed drugs in the US. One of the greatest needs, according to the FDA, is for improved ability to detect and predict hepatotoxicity.[1] The impact of DILI on patients can be quite severe, even with drugs that produce rare liver injury;

RSC Drug Discovery Series No. 12
New Horizons in Predictive Toxicology: Current Status and Application
Edited by Alan G. E. Wilson

Published by the Royal Society of Chemistry, www.rsc.org

historically, patients using prescription medications have suffered acute liver failure (ALF), death, liver transplantation surgery, and unresolved liver injury. The possibility of these outcomes places enormous pressure on regulators who must be certain that the hepatic safety profile of a new medical entity will not change once the drug enters wider use in a market.

DILI and hepatotoxicity are so prevalent in the literature that endeavoring to write a novel chapter on these subjects is itself a challenge. Nevertheless, this chapter will try to discuss DILI in a reasonably thorough fashion that will include the potential limitations in predicting DILI, the current strategies for hepatotoxicity screening, and some new paradigms that may help predict hepatotoxic potential for new medical entities.

Finally, while the terms DILI and hepatotoxicity are technically interchangeable, the convention used in this chapter will be to use the term DILI in reference to clinical hepatotoxicity (*i.e.*, in patients).

## 16.2 DILI with Marketed Drugs

The metrics for the occurrence of DILI associated with marketed drugs are well established: DILI is the leading cause of ALF in the US and accounts for 52% of the total ALF cases; 75% of these cases of DILI involve acetaminophen.[2] ALF secondary to DILI occurs with a nearly five-fold greater frequency than ALF caused by viral hepatitis (11% in the US), whereas viral hepatitis is the leading cause of ALF throughout the rest of the world.[2] Ninety drugs listed in the Physicians' Desk Reference are known to cause ALF and another 370 drugs are listed as possibly causing ALF; in addition, 124 drugs are contra-indicated in liver disease.[2] Among a cohort of drugs that was approved between 1975 and 1999, 45 acquired a black box warning on their label post-approval with DILI as the basis for the warning in ten cases; sixteen drugs approved during this period were subsequently withdrawn from the market, including four drugs for DILI.[3]

These estimates apply only to marketed drugs, the impact of hepatotoxicity as a factor in the attrition of drug candidates is likely to be even greater although more difficult to quantify.

## 16.3 The Liver as a Target Organ

The liver plays central roles in the physiology of intermediary metabolism, protein synthesis, digestion, hemostasis, immunity, and the detoxication and clearance of xenobiotics. The organ is particularly well adapted for its role in clearing drugs (see Table 16.1).[4,5] The anatomical blood supply of the liver includes both oxygenated arterial blood and portal blood flowing from the vasculature that drains the gastrointestinal tract. This configuration allows the liver to serve as an in-line filter and remove ingested pathogens and xenobiotics. Drugs that are absorbed can be very effectively sequestered within hepatocytes at concentrations many-fold greater than the concentration in blood. Inside the liver, drug molecules can be biotransformed by diverse enzymatic systems that

**Table 16.1** The liver as a target organ for drug-induced injury.[4,5]

| *Characteristic* | *Physiological purpose* | *Potential adverse consequence* |
|---|---|---|
| Receives blood flowing from portal circulation | Liver filters bloodborne chemicals, solutes and pathogens absorbed from the GI tract | Continuous exposure to toxicants in combination with other substances (*e.g.*, endotoxin) may predispose to organ injury |
| Hepatocellular partitioning | Hepatocytes are able to concentrate xenobiotics to concentrations many-fold greater than in blood thus hastening clearance | Concentration of xenobiotics may saturate or overwhelm hepatocellular biotransformation and/or protection mechanisms thus rendering the cells susceptible to injury |
| Biotransformation enzymes | Inactivation of xenobiotics and toxicants | Some molecules may be activated (*i.e.*, become chemically reactive) through biotransformation resulting in hepatocyte injury |
| Biliary transport | Liver can concentrate and excrete toxicants and metabolic by-products into the bile and into the GI tract | High toxicant levels in the bile may cause injury of the biliary epithelium and cessation of bile flow |

attenuate or inactivate pharmacological activity. The biliary network of the liver is an efficient and high-capacity mechanism for drug excretion that is facilitated by families of drug transporters that move both active and inactive forms of drug into bile and out of the body into the lumen of the GI tract.

Unfortunately, the liver is somewhat of a lightning rod because exposure to xenobiotics also renders this organ susceptibile to injury. In many cases, factors such as the formation of an electrophilic metabolite, accumulation of drug in the liver, or loss of hepatocellular protection (*e.g.*, depletion of glutathione) result in hepatocellular death and hepatic injury. In fact, the eventual recognition of these mechanisms enabled the first screens for predicting hepatotoxicity, *i.e.*, metabolic activation, gluathathione depletion and covalent binding.

## 16.4 Mechanisms of Hepatotoxicity

The morphological appearance of liver injury is quite variable, and typically can include any of the following: hepatocellular death (necrosis), inflammation (hepatitis), cessation of bile flow (cholestatis), or lipid accumulation (steatosis). Fibrotic change, as seen with cirrhosis of the liver, results from scarring in response to sustained hepatocellular death and marked parenchymal cell loss. All of these changes can be present in very severe forms of liver injury (see Table 16.2).

It is generally accepted that these morphological changes are each caused by a unique set of molecular events, and that each can be modeled in animals with specific hepatotoxicants. The availability of model hepatotoxicants

**Table 16.2** The primary forms of liver injury.[8,123]

| *Morphological classification* | *Key features* | *Laboratory correlates* |
|---|---|---|
| Hepatocellular injury | Focal or confluent necrosis; evidence of inflammatory and regenerative responses may be present | ALT $>2 \times$ ULN<br>ALT/ALP $\geq 5$ |
| Hepatitis | Presence of inflammatory cells | ALT $>500$ IU/L<br>Cholestatic correlates $<3 \times$ ULN |
| Steatosis | Inclusion of spherical lipid droplets in cytoplasm | Morphologic diagnosis |
| Cholestatis | Bile present in cannuliculi; bile casts may be present; bile duct proliferation may be present | ALP $>>2 \times$ ULN<br>ALT/ALP $\leq 2$<br>ALT $<300 \times$ IU/L |
| Fibrosis | Connective tissue septae radiating from portal triads | Morphologic diagnosis |
| Vascular | Occlusion of the hepatic vein; not considered an important form of drug-related toxicity for the liver | ALT$<300 \times$ IU/L<br>Cholestatic correlates $<3 \times$ ULN |

**Table 16.3** Mechanisms of hepatotoxicity.[124–128]

| *Mechanism* | *Related processes* | *Correlate(s)* |
|---|---|---|
| Electrophilic attack | Covalent binding oxidative stress plasmalemma damage | Classical hepatotoxicty potentially linked to idiosyncratic DILI |
| Mitochondrial insult | Disruption of $Ca^{2+}$ homeostasis inhibition of respiratory chain diminished ATP production | Classical hepatotoxicty potentially linked to idiosyncratic DILI |
| Oxidative stress | Reactive oxygen species generation glutathione depletion change in cell redox state | Classical hepatotoxicty potentially linked to idiosyncratic DILI |
| Bile cannulicular insult | Disruption of actin filaments transporter inhibition | Cholestasis and jaundice |
| Activation of cell-death pathways | Apoptosis & necrosis caspase activation protein kinase c activation JNK activation | Potentially linked to unpredicted DILI |

(*e.g.*, carbon tetrachloride, thioacetamide, α-naphthyl isothiocyanate, galactosamine, acetaminophen, *etc.*) has greatly facilitated the study of xenobiotic-induced liver injury in the laboratory. The outcome of this research has been a complex picture for the pathogenesis of hepatic injury that involves multiple mechanisms (see Table 16.3). This list, while short, is informative even though our understanding of the mechanisms of hepatic injury is almost certainly far from complete. First, this list accounts for the mechanistic diversity of hepatic injury, including facile mechanisms (*e.g.*, electrophile formation) and potentially more elegant mechanisms involving pharmacological disruption of cell signaling pathways (*e.g.*, kinase inhibition). Second, the variety seen with these mechanisms reflects the range of morphological changes that comprise hepatic injury. For these reasons, an arguably reasonable first approach for detecting hepatotoxic potential in drug candidates would be to screen for evidence of these activities. Although this approach would facilitate detection of classical hepatotoxic potential, not all DILI appears as straightforward.

## 16.5 Drug-Induced Liver Injury

Hepatotoxicity is not a single toxicity, but a spectrum of toxicity that ranges from very obvious and predictable to rare and poorly understood (Figure 16.1). The consequences associated with both ends of this spectrum can be quite serious, nonetheless.

### 16.5.1 Classical Hepatotoxicity

No formal definition exists for the term "classical hepatotoxicity" yet toxicologists and pathologists will intuitively understand its meaning. The term, as used here, refers to the toxicity that was initially described as "intrinsic hepatotoxicity" by Dr Hyman Zymmerman, former Professor of medicine at George Washington and Georgetown Universities, and author of *Hepatotoxicity: The Effects of Drugs and Other Chemicals on the Liver*.[6] More recently, these agents have also been referred to as "predictable hepatotoxicants".[2,7] In essence, classical hepatotoxicants produce unequivocal liver injury in animals

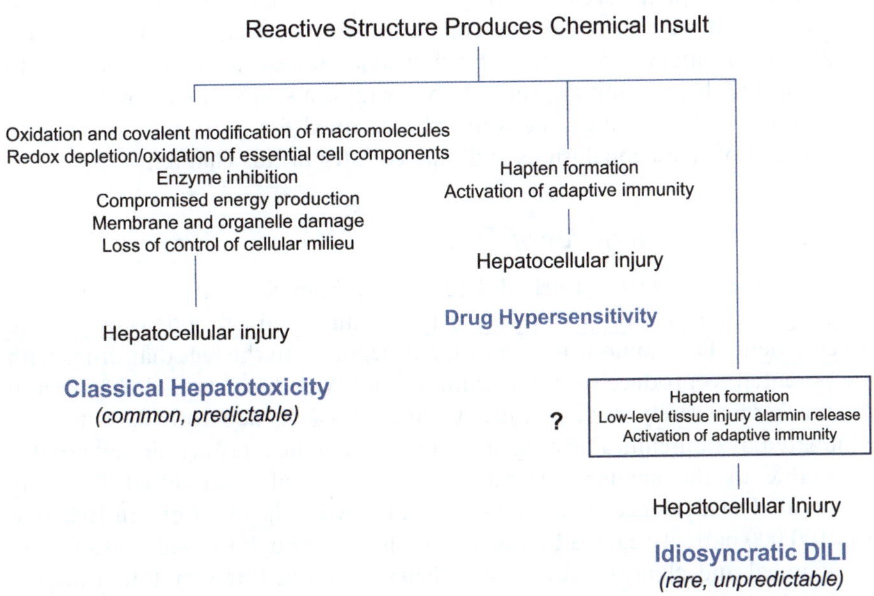


**Figure 16.1** Traditional models of hepatotoxicity.

in a dose-dependent and reproducible manner.[7] These characteristics generally extrapolate well across species, and discordances are usually explainable by species differences in biotransformation. Classical hepatotoxicants produce hepatocellular injury through the mechanisms described in Table 16.3, and not surprisingly, have historically served as the tool compounds used to study chemical-induced liver injury in the laboratory given that they produce highly reproducible and unequivocal liver injury.

Acetaminophen is a classical hepatotoxicant; it has been used as a model hepatotoxicant in countless laboratory studies and still accounts for the vast majority of the incidence of DILI in the US. Acetaminophen would almost certainly be detected with today's screening methods for hepatotoxicity, which makes this drug somewhat of a historical curiosity because classical hepatotoxicants enter clinical testing under only the most compelling risk–benefit considerations.

## 16.5.2 DILI in the Clinical Setting

DILI is observed clinically in two settings: the first is in clinical trials conducted during the development of a drug; the other is in the post-approval period with marketed drugs. DILI in the clinical setting is more complex than classical hepatotoxicity even though it was not immediately recognized by physicians as a threat to patient health. Reports of DILI increased after World War II when its incidence roughly began to parallel the rise in the number of new drugs introduced by the pharmaceutical industry.[6] An early analysis of liver injury associated with pharmaceutical drugs in patients conducted by Zimmerman produced what were then startling conclusions: First, even at a low incidence, hepatocellular injury accompanied by clinical jaundice is highly correlated with ALF. Second, hepatic injury produced by drugs is a severe disease and patients exhibiting certain harbinger signs may be destined for ALF and death.[6] The significance of these conclusions is discussed later in this chapter.

### *16.5.2.1 Characteristics of DILI*

Several features of DILI clearly differentiate it from classical hepatotoxicity.

The potential of a drug to produce DILI can remained undetected during development. The ominous nature of DILI begins with the fact that drugs with the potential to produce severe liver injury and ALF have evaded detection in pre-marketing safety assessments. Unlike classical hepatotoxicity that is eliminated by non-clinical testing or during early clinical testing, not all DILI is detectable in the smaller clinical databases typically submitted for drug approval. The incidence of severe DILI can range on the order of 1 in 10 000 to 1 in 100 000 patient-years, a frequency that is low enough to evade detection in non-clinical and clinical testing. Nonetheless, even at this very low incidence of DILI, 10% of patients will die and 50% will develop other clinical complications.[8]

There are no means of uniquely diagnosing DILI. Human liver injury is associated with morphological changes identical to those seen in laboratory animals, including necrosis, inflammatory change, cholestasis, steatosis, and vascular injury.[9] Since these changes are identical to those caused by etiologies unrelated to drugs, biopsy and liver morphology provide little value for differential diagnosis.[10] Currently, there are no validated biomarkers that are specific for DILI and traditional indicators of hepatocellular injury like transaminase activities measured in clinical chemistry panels simply confirm the presence of liver injury much like morphology. This leaves open the question of causation, which is less clear cut for the physician who is managing a DILI patient outside of a controlled clinical trial.[11]

Drugs are often not recognized as the cause of liver disease. The failure to recognize a patient complaint or illness as an adverse drug effect is a quandary that has long plagued the use of medicines. Unfortunately, this means that a particular drug can continue to adversely affect more patients until the connection is made.[12] Because of the limited diagnostic options, a diagnosis of DILI is one of exclusion requiring that all rule-outs be made.[8] In cases of rare idiosyncratic DILI, the presentation of patients with liver injury is so infrequent and sporadic that no suspicion of the drug may ever be raised.[13]

DILI is insidious. Even though it may affect a relatively small number of patients using a specific drug, DILI can be quite severe and can persist or worsen even after the drug is withdrawn.[13] The population of patients that exhibits rare but severe DILI is small and poorly characterized with regard to their risk factors for susceptibility.

### 16.5.2.2 Idiosyncratic DILI

The clinical picture of DILI is complicated by the fact that, in some cases, factors unrelated to the drug appear to play a role in the appearance of this toxicity. Drug idiosyncrasy refers to effects for which the causal basis is unknown but thought to be related to the individual.[14] Idiosyncratic toxicity is characterized by poor predictability in animal models, low frequency of occurrence and questionable relationship to dose, although some now question the latter.[14,15] Idiosyncratic DILI is a major focus in the literature on drug hepatotoxicity because its etiology is so poorly understood. Moreover, its unpredictable nature has led to the withdrawal of drugs from the market and it is estimated that idiosyncratic DILI still accounts for 13 to 17% of ALF cases in the US.[16]

It is well accepted that there are two forms of idiosyncratic DILI: an allergic type and a non-allergic type.[17,18] The clinical presentation of allergic idiosyncratic DILI includes fever, rash, eosinophilia, short latency ($\sim$1 month), presence of auto-antibodies, and rapid hepatotoxicity upon re-challenge. These features tend to be absent in the non-allergic form, which also features a much longer latency ($\geq$6 months) period during which patients can continue to receive the drug with no apparent sign of toxicity.[17] The long latency preceding non-allergic idiosyncratic DILI may reflect the involvement of intervening factors that are required for the toxicity to manifest, or could also reflect a slow developing molecular lesion.

At one time, textbooks in pharmacology and toxicology taught that the concept of drug idiosyncrasy was predicated upon unknown mechanism(s). It is safe to say that progress made in researching idiosyncratic DILI has moved our understanding further away from an "unknown mechanism" and that plausible hypotheses for this toxicity now exist. Discussions of the mechanism(s) of idiosyncratic DILI are fascinating and the brief treatise presented here does not do justice to the topic; however, since the leading hypotheses for idiosyncratic DILI are being distilled into strategies for predicting this toxicity, the following survey is warranted.

Most explanations for idiosyncratic DILI are centered on a relationship between chemical reactivity and immunological response.[16,18,19] Chemical reactivity is a fundamental mechanism for classical hepatotoxicity and molecules that are reactive or converted to reactive metabolites are usually deselected during the search for a drug candidate; one might then wonder how this mechanism might be relevant for DILI seen with marketed drugs. The answer is that the diversity in drug biotransformation potential represented by the laboratory animals and limited patient populations evaluated in the development phase represents a fraction of the diversity that exists within the human population that will be exposed during the marketing phase. Clinical databases submitted for drug approval simply are not large enough to detect the range of responses that might occur in a very large population of patients that includes individuals with unique and, perhaps rare, biotransformation phenotypes (*i.e.*, polymorphisms). Polymorphisms comprise the genetic diversity of humans and are thought to contribute to the differential susceptibility of individuals to drug toxicity.

The immunological component of idiosyncratic DILI is thought to involve activation of the adaptive immune system leading to antibody production and activation of cytotoxic T lymphocytes. As it turns out, the leading hypotheses suggest that immune activation and chemical reactivity are likely complementary events in the genesis of idiosyncratic liver injury:

Hapten Formation—Landsteiner recognized that drugs can interact with endogenous molecules to produce haptens (*i.e.*, neo-antigens) that elicit an antibody response directed at the hapten.[20] Penicillin is the premier example for the association of hapten formation and drug hypersensitivity. Hapten formation has also been proposed to explain halothane hepatitis, a rare but severe form of liver injury seen in surgical patients and anesthesiologists (estimated as 7 in 10 000 exposures).[21,22] The antibodies against liver proteins that are detected in serum of patients suffering from halothane hepatitis appear unique to halothane.[20] Some proteins that react with these antibodies are normally found in the centrilobular region of the liver, the site of halothane injury.[23,24]

Danger Hypothesis—Matzinger postulated that the immune system is keyed to "danger signals" from injured or dying cells and that activation of adaptive immunity is predicated upon some form of cell/tissue injury.[20] The controversy around this hypothesis stems from its premise that the immune system responds to chemical signals released from damaged cells and membranes (as opposed to the detection of non-self). Molecules called alarmins, when released from damaged cells and cell membranes, act to elicit an adaptive immune response; examples of alarmins include heat-shock proteins, high-mobility group box 1 proteins, and S100 proteins. In the case of idiosyncratic DILI, indolent liver injury may provide a danger signal that elicits an adaptive immune response directed at the injured tissue.[25] The danger hypothesis may be particularly relevant for hepatotoxicity arising from mitochondrial injury for which it is thought that fragments of the organelles removed by phagocytic cells of the innate immune system are processed as danger signals.[26]

Pharmacological-Interaction Model—The pharmacological-interaction model (*i.e.*, the p-i model) hypothesizes that idiosyncratic liver injury may be pharmacologic in nature. In this model, a drug or its metabolite interacts with Major Histocompatibility Complex (MHC) peptide through formation of a reversible non-covalent bond typical of receptor–ligand interactions. The formation of this bound complex is followed in close order by binding to an immunoreceptor (*e.g.*, T-cell receptor) leading to activation of the adaptive immune system.[27] Because none of the binding steps in this model require chemical reactivity, this hypothesis might account for idiosyncratic DILI observed with drugs that are not known to be bioactivated.

## 16.6 Screening for Hepatotoxicity

The ability to predict toxicity requires recognition of the signals associated with the toxic response, and the ability to then detect those signals. Our current ability to predict hepatotoxicity might be improved in several ways, including: 1) greater surveillance for and recognition of pre-monitory signals during the development phase, 2) use of new methodologies for identifying novel signals of hepatotoxicity, and 3) application of new animal models to manifest latent hepatotoxic potential.

### 16.6.1 Current Approach for the Detection of Hepatotoxicity

The fundamental approach for detecting hepatotoxicity still remains the non-clinical toxicology studies conducted in rodent and non-rodent species. Over thirty years ago, a document entitled *Guidelines for Detection of Hepatotoxicity Due to Drugs and Chemicals* summarized the outcomes of the 1978 Conference of the International Association for the Study of the Liver.[28] These guidelines provide detailed information on the design of toxicology studies, including the endpoints for measuring liver toxicity. Over the past several decades, the standard for detection of hepatotoxicity has been the empirical toxicology study conducted in accordance with standard protocols. Although simple, this approach enables detailed evaluation of drug effect through integration of clinical pathology, necropsy, microscopy, drug exposure, and mortality data.[28] The techniques used in these studies to detect liver injury are discussed in the following sections.

### 16.6.1.1 Clinical Chemistry

Clinical chemistry readouts are invaluable for signaling hepatotoxicity. In particular, the activities of aspartate and alanine aminotransferase isozymes (AST and ALT, respectively) in serum are the most commonly used indices of hepatocellular status. Their utility is predicated upon both their relatively selective (though not exclusive) localization in hepatocytes and their release into the bloodstream in response to hepatocellular insult.[29,30] Other enzymes included in typical clinical chemistry panels that also reflect hepatocellular injury are listed in Table 16.4.

While the practice of comparing circulating enzyme levels in treated and non-treated animals appears a straightforward means of detecting liver injury, most toxicologists and pathologists have encountered the scenario in which ALT values are elevated several-fold above control values only to find no concomitant morphological change.[29,30] Although the clinical chemistry data alone could be interpreted as hepatic injury, the absence of hepatocellular death or necrosis supports rationalization of the findings as evidence of increased protein synthesis or some other metabolic aberration. The interpretation of clinical chemistry data in non-clinical studies is greatly enhanced by corroboration with histopathology evaluations.

There are other nuances of clinical chemistry data that tend to complicate interpretation. The transaminases, for example, are not exclusively localized in the liver and other forms of tissue injury, like bruising and musculoskeletal trauma, can cause transaminase elevations in the complete absence of any injury to the liver.[29] Clarification of the significance of serum transaminase changes is facilitated by evaluating clustering of changes in several enzymes:[31] Thus, coordinated increases in ALT, AST and sorbitol dehydrogenase (SDH) provide an even more compelling profile for liver injury; while increased AST

**Table 16.4** Common clinical chemistry markers of liver injury.[31,32,34,129]

| *Analyte* | *Cellular locus in the liver* | *Marker* |
|---|---|---|
| Alanine aminotransferase | Cytoplasm and mitochondria | Hepatocellular injury and death |
| Aspartate aminotransferase | Cytoplasm and mitochondria | Hepatocellular injury and death |
| Sorbitol dehydrogenase | Cytoplasm | Hepatocellular injury and death |
| Glutamate dehydrogenase | Mitochondria | Hepatocellular death and necrosis |
| Lactate dehydrogenase | Mitochondria | General cell injury and death; hemolysis |
| Alkaline phosphatase | Cell and organelle membranes | Cholestasis |
| Gamma-glutamyl transpeptidase | Bile cannuliculus | Injury to the biliary tree, cholestasis |
| Bilirubin | Hepatocyte and biliary tree | Cholestasis, hepatocellular injury and death |

alone or AST with lactate dehydrogenase (LDH) correlates better with musculoskeltal injury.[31] Coordinated increases in bilirubin, alkaline phosphatase and γ-glutamyl transpeptidase provide strong evidence of biliary dysfunction or injury to the biliary tree.[32]

Interpretation of laboratory results in clinical trials can be more difficult because liver biopsy and microscopy are not routine. Transaminitis, which is characterized by increased transaminase activities unaccompanied by other laboratory changes, can be especially difficult to interpret as a potential harbinger of DILI given that up to 15% or more of patients in clinical trials exhibit episodic increases in circulating aminotransferase activity.[14] It has also been estimated that up to 4% of the population at-large exhibit increases in transaminase values while remaining totally asymptomatic.[33]

Factors unrelated to a specific drug can raise transaminase levels and provide false signals for DILI, including alcohol use, hypotension, fatty liver (associated with diet and physical condition), physical activity, and concomitant disease (hepatitis).[34] The transaminase assays, as currently applied, also do not differentiate sub-lethal hepatocellular injury from hepatocellular necrosis. It is known that cytosolic transaminase isozymes can be released into the bloodstream as a result of simple bleb formation on the hepatocellular membrane that occurs with sub-lethal injury.[30] The detection of mitochondrial enzymes in the circulation is hoped to be more dependable for gauging necrosis since complete cell lysis is thought to be required for release into the bloodstream. There are cytosolic and mitochondrial isozymes for both ALT and AST that could be leveraged for diagnosing hepatocellular necrosis if suitable clinical chemistry methodology for separating the individual isoforms were to become more amenable to use in high-throughput formats. Glutamate dehydrogenase is another mitochondrial enzyme that could be used to complement transaminase data as a potential, though un-validated, marker of hepatocellular necrosis.[30,32]

#### *16.6.1.2 Liver Function*

Clinical laboratory evaluations, such as those just discussed, are generically referred to as liver function tests (LFTs) although most do not inform about the physiological status of the liver. Patients suffering ALF with fulminant hepatic necrosis present with jaundice, encephalopathy, and coagulopathy. The pathophysiological basis for this syndrome is simply the loss of hepatic reserve needed to maintain clearance of metabolic byproducts (ammonia, cholesterol, and bilirubin) and synthesis of clotting factors.[32,34] Circulating albumin levels may be decreased secondary to diminished protein synthesis in the severely injured liver.[32,34] These endpoints collectively provide more legitimate readouts of liver function.[7]

#### *16.6.1.3 Liver Morphology*

The morphological changes that can occur with hepatic injury have already been discussed. What remains important is that while morphological changes have been historically useful for classifying hepatotoxicant action, they are not pathognomonic for drug-induced liver injury. This is a non-issue in well-controlled animal toxicology or clinical studies where other etiologies of liver injury are eliminated by design.

#### *16.6.1.4 Mitochondrial Evaluation*

Mitochondria are known targets of non-specific metabolic poisons like cyanide and rotenone, and clearly, drug-induced mitochondrial dysfunction has much broader implications for organ toxicity than liver injury alone. However, the clinical tragedy associated with fialuridine (FIAU), a thymidine-based nucleoside analog that was under development as a treatment for hepatitis B, heightened concern for liver failure resulting from mitochondrial lesions. Following the deaths of five patients and liver transplantation in two others, it was discovered that FIAU unexpectedly blocked mitochondrial replication leading to gradual mitochondrial insufficiency with failure of several organs, including the liver.[35–37] Consequently, mitochondrial evaluations have become more commonplace in candidate screening both as *in vitro* assays as well as adjunctive *ex vivo* evaluations in animal toxicology studies.[38,39]

The role of mitochondrial function in potential toxicity screening strategies is discussed in detail elsewhere in this book. However, two points are particularly relevant for liver injury. First, the mitochondrial glutathione content directly governs cellular redox state and, therefore, susceptibility to toxic insult.[39] Second, biological variability in mitochondria due to genetics, disease, senescence, *etc.* might also change an individual's susceptibility to insult by a drug.[40–42] Hepatotoxic potential may remain latent until the glutathione content in the liver becomes depleted. Glutathione depletion is not a typical background variable in a standard toxicology study because the animals are maintained with adequate nutrition and are not deliberately pre-treated with an agent that reduces glutathione levels. The relationship of mitochondrial dynamics to idiosyncractic DILI is an intriguing possibility that offers hope for the ability to identify mitochondrial variation and DILI-susceptible individuals.[43]

#### *16.6.1.5 Chemical Reactivity and Structural Alerts*

Eliminating structural reactivity is a prudent step for avoiding a variety of organ toxicities, including hepatotoxicity.[44] Current best practices for medicinal chemists who synthesize and screen drug candidates include identification of structural moieties that are reactive and can damage cells (toxicophores).[45–48] Evidence of a reactive electrophile is usually confirmed by glutathione depletion or covalent binding in the presence/absence of a metabolic activation system.[49,50] Electrophile formation *in vivo* is generally not subtle and usually is associated with some handprint of toxicity in one or more tissues that is detectable in animal toxicology studies.[51] Chemical reactivity should be scrutinized given its relationship with classical hepatotoxicity and possible relationship to idiosyncratic DILI.[52]

### 16.6.2 How Successful are the Current Approaches?

Several published analyses have evaluated the success of non-clinical safety evaluations in predicting specific human toxicities, including hepatotoxicity. As it stands, drug-induced hepatotoxicity remains one of the top reasons for failure in drug development and, at the same time, continues to be one of the most poorly predicted toxicities by non-clinical testing methodologies. These analyses evaluated toxicity-based attrition during the various stages of drug development to provide perspective on the impact of DILI in both the pre-marketing and post-marketing phases.

#### *16.6.2.1 Retrospective Analysis*

One of the first retrospective analyses was done almost one decade ago using a database consisting of approximately 150 drug candidates for each of which a human toxicity had been discovered in clinical trials.[53] The survey recorded information on the therapeutic area, the nature of the human toxicity, and the concordance of the human toxicity with the results of the respective non-clinical toxicity studies. The results showed that findings of human hepatotoxicity accounted for 55% of the decisions to terminate (*i.e.*, the trial or the candidate). Another finding of this evaluation was that DILI emerges in all phases of clinical testing: it was the basis for 27% of terminations in Phase I and accounted for 46% in Phase II. DILI was first detected as late as Phase III with four drug candidates. Perhaps one of the most interesting findings of this analysis by Olson *et al.*[53] was that human liver injury was predicted by animal toxicology studies in 17 cases as opposed to 14 cases in which the animal studies failed to predict the toxicity at all.

Recognizing that 150 molecules is a relatively small database, another report published in 2008 by the Safety Intelligence Program Board evaluated a database of 1061 active ingredients in pharmaceutical products obtained from Medline along with an additional 157 drug candidates evaluated by the European Medicines Authority.[53] Human "liver effects" were reported for 710 of 1061 drugs in the Medline compound set and for 137 of 157 drugs in the EMA set. Their analysis showed that 38% of DILI in the Medline set was unpredicted by animal studies and 51% of DILI was unpredicted in the EMA set. The outcomes of the two published reports are reasonably consistent in that they support the conclusion that non-clinical testing produces a significant rate of false negatives in predicting hepatotoxicity.

However, other analyses assert the counterpoint, *i.e.*, that those drugs withdrawn from the market for DILI did show evidence of hepatotoxicity during non-clinical testing.[55,56] This conclusion was based on a review of the data for several drugs associated with DILI, including acetaminophen, clarithromycin, telithromycin, troglitazone, trovafloxacin, bromfenac, and isoniazid. These analyses raise the possibility that our failure to recognize hepatotoxic signals in non-clinical results might be the reason for their diminished predictive power, and that our interpretation of non-clinical results might somehow require adjustment.

#### 16.6.2.2 Historical Drug Withdrawals due to Liver Injury

The list of drugs withdrawn from the market due to DILI over the past few decades is relatively small (Table 16.5). Clear correlation with therapeutic class or structure and DILI is difficult to appreciate. Assuming that it is reasonably comprehensive, this list indicates that a drug was removed from the market for hepatotoxicity about once every two years dating back over the last 30 years, with a skew in the number of withdrawals towards the last decade. If early harbinger signs went unrecognized with any of these drugs, as has been suggested, this list would be shorter simply with better execution of existing methodologies.[57,58] More controlled market entry might have also reduced the hepatotoxicity impact incurred with several of these drugs.[57] Assuming that it is unlikely that the risk of hepatotoxicity with pharmaceutical products can be completely eradicated,[57] this begs the question as to what will ultimately be viewed as success in improving our ability to predict hepatotoxicity.

## 16.7 Statement of the Problem

What might a successful scheme for predicting hepatotoxicity look like? By now, it should be abundantly clear that hepatotoxicity is a family of toxicities that includes classical hepatotoxicity, DILI encountered in clinical trials, and two forms of idiosyncratic DILI (allergic and non-allergic) that typically emerge post-marketing. Different screening paradigms would be required to eradicate or reduce the entire spectrum of hepatotoxicity.

The segments of hepatotoxicity that are typically encountered with pharmaceuticals can be categorized based on their ease of recognition (see Table 16.6). The first category is labeled "predicted" hepatotoxicity and includes the classical hepatotoxicants, which produce unequivocal evidence in animals. The decision to advance a predicted hepatotoxic drug into the clinic would require a favorable risk–benefit scenario (*e.g.*, large margin of safety or use in unmet medical need like oncology) in which this profile of hepatic safety would be tolerated. Screening for predictable hepatotoxic potential is quite effective in terms of de-selecting candidates with obvious hepatotoxic potential early in drug development.

The remaining segments of hepatotoxicity are especially problematic. The next category is "unpredicted" hepatotoxicants and includes drugs that have advanced through non-clinical testing without a signal for liver injury only to manifest DILI early in clinical testing. Unlike the idiosyncratic DILI, unpredicted DILI can be observed in initial clinical testing in patients after a few exposures to the drug; like the idiosyncratic form, this expression of DILI is also not faithfully predicted by non-clinical studies. Unpredicted hepatotoxicity probably occurs more often than expected and contributes to the undefined number of failed drug candidates that are terminated in clinical trials. The term "unpredicted" is used when the failure to predict hepatotoxicity may reflect lack of experience with the drug class or poor understanding of the target

**Table 16.5** Drugs withdrawn from the market for DILI.

| *Drug* | *Year withdrawn* | *Basis for withdrawal* | *Therapeutic target* | *Structure* |
|---|---|---|---|---|
| Benoxaprofen | 1982 | Risk of hepatotoxicity | Inflammation & pain | 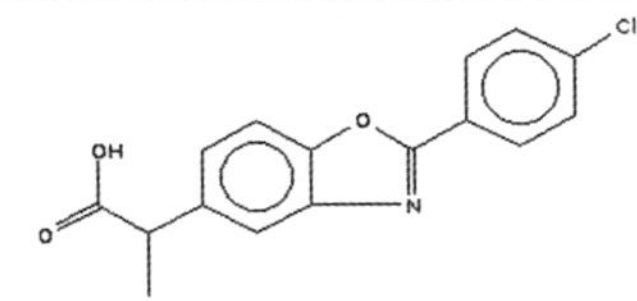 |
| Ticrynafen | 1982 | Risk of hepatitis | Diuretic & uricosuric | 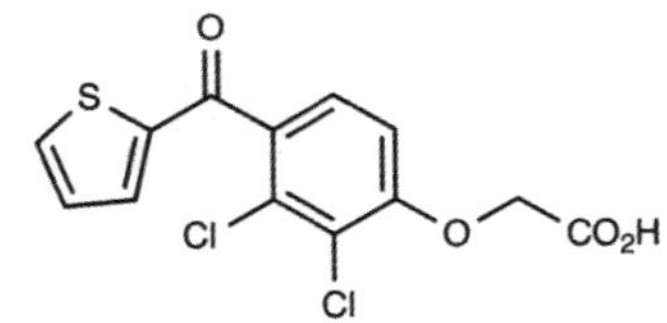 |
| Alpidem | 1996 | Rare but serious hepatotoxicity | Anti-anxiety | 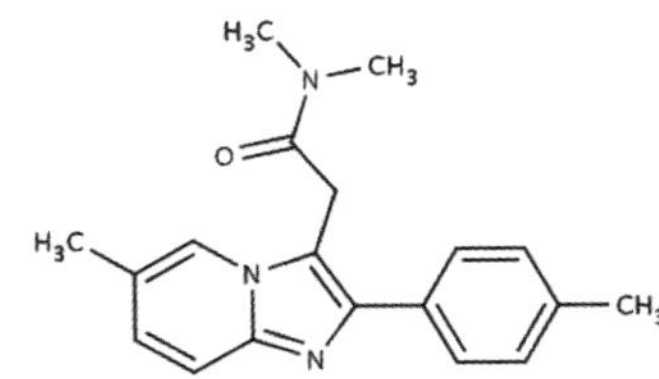 |
| Tolrestat | 1997 | Severe hepatotoxicity | Diabetes | 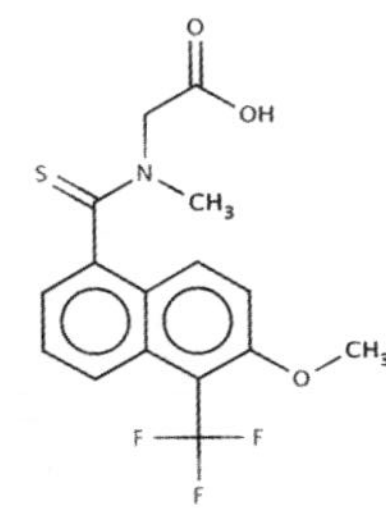 |

**Table 16.5** (*Continued*)

| *Drug* | *Year withdrawn* | *Basis for withdrawal* | *Therapeutic target* | *Structure* |
|---|---|---|---|---|
| Bromfenac | 1998 | Severe hepatotoxicity | Inflammation & pain | 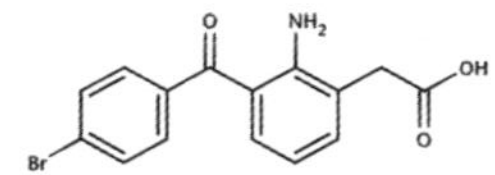 |
| Troglitazone | 2000 | Risk of hepatotoxicity | Diabetes | 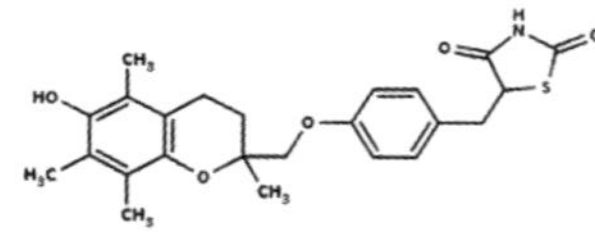 |
| Amineptine | 2000 | Risk of hepatotoxicity | Anti-depressant | 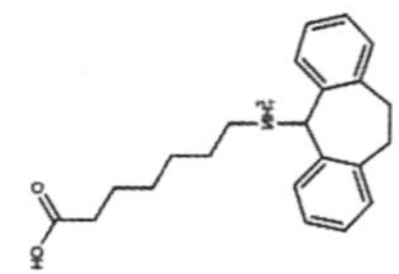 |
| Trovafloxacin | 2001 | Risk of liver failure | Anti-bacterial | 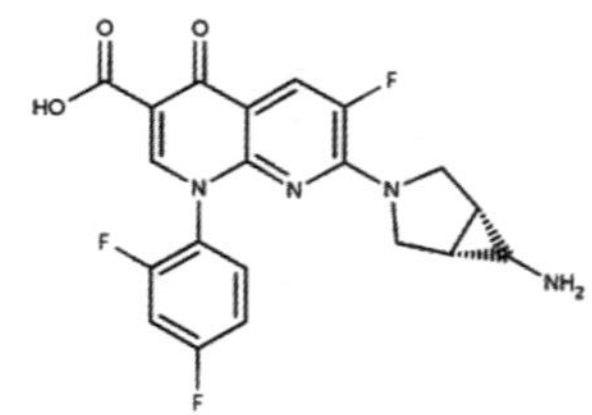 |
| Pemoline | 2005 | Risk of hepatotoxicity | Attention-deficit & hyperactivity | 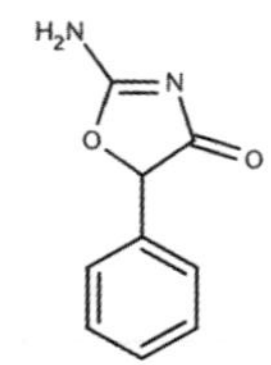 |

| | | | | |
|---|---|---|---|---|
| Ximelagatran | 2006 | Risk of hepatotoxicity | Anti-coagulant | 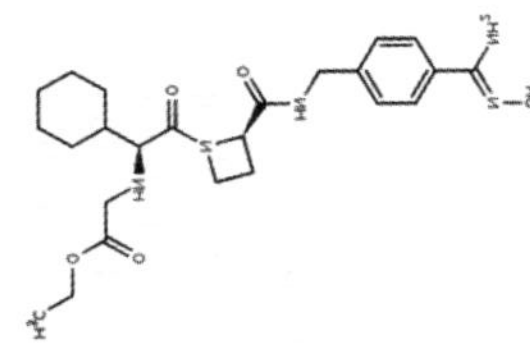 |
| Lumiracoxib | 2007–2008 | Risk of liver damage | Inflammation & pain | 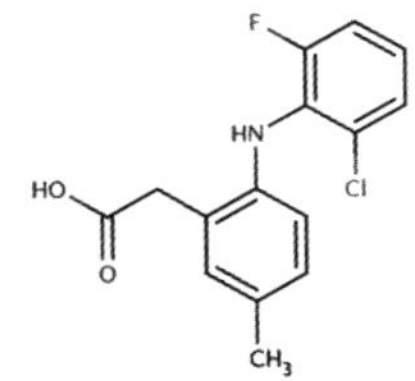 |
| Sitaxentan | 2010 | Fatal liver injury | Pulmonary hypertension | 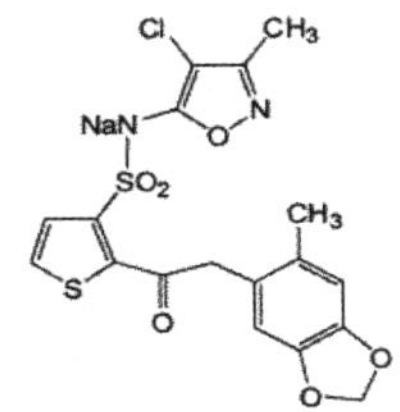 |

**Table 16.6** Hepatotoxicity in pharmaceutical development.

| | | *Stage at which hepatotoxicity is evident* | | | |
|---|---|---|---|---|---|
| *Category* | *Mechanistic basis* | *Non-clinical* | *Clinical* | *Market* | *Impact on drug candidate* |
| Predictable | Chemical reactivity of drug structure or structure of metabolite | ++ | ++ | — | Candidate is typically halted during candidate selection or in IND-enabling toxicology studies |
| Unpredicted | Therapeutic target may have unexpected relevance for human liver function | — | ++ | — | Significant contribution to drug failure during development |
| Unpredictable | Culmination of individual susceptibility, possible intervening factors, and action of the drug | — | — | ++ | Typically drives withdrawal of drug from the market |

pathway or therapeutic mechanism of action in humans. The best example is perhaps the p38 MAP kinase inhibitor programs in which several clinical candidates were halted due to transaminitis although the mechanism(s) for the human responses had not been discernible in animals.[59–61] Measures taken to safeguard patients in clinical trials make it unlikely that unpredicted DILI would progress to ALF; nonetheless, it remains a problematic outcome in drug development.

The third category includes the "unpredictable" hepatotoxicants, which are essentially the drugs that have produced idiosyncratic DILI. The term "unpredictable" is used because of the relative infrequency of idiosyncratic DILI as well as our limited mechanistic understanding challenges our ability to predict for this segment of DILI. The remainder of this chapter focuses on screening and detection strategies that will improve our ability to predict "unpredicted" and "unpredictable" hepatotoxicity. The needs are greatest for these two categories based on their impact, and also, because the current approaches and methodologies used to detect hepatotoxicity are already oriented towards the more obvious "predictable" hepatotoxicants.

## 16.8 Approaches for Better Prediction of DILI

Many of the technologies discussed here are subjects of other chapters in this book. There are definite expectations for any new technology that will be applied towards the prediction of hepatotoxicity, including: 1) elimination of false negatives in non-clinical testing (greater sensitivity), 2) reducing ambiguity of signal (enhanced recognition), and 3) greater specificity for DILI (improved diagnostic value).

### 16.8.1 Initiatives for Better Methods of Prediction

The Predictive Safety Testing Consortium was formed as part of the FDA's Critical Path Initiative. The goal of the Predictive Safety Testing Consortium is to facilitate greater success in drug development by providing new and better technologies for screening toxicity for a number of target organs, including the liver.[62] Its Hepatotoxicity Working Group is exploring many of the technologies discussed below, including biomarkers, with the goal of improved detection and recognition of DILI.

A second initiative with similar aims stems from the Liver Toxicity Biomarker Study sponsored jointly by FDA's National Center for Toxicological Research and BG Medicine, Inc. This group is focusing on delivering novel biomarkers with the goal of sharpening the ability to detect hepatotoxicity.[63]

### 16.8.2 Biomarkers

The ideal biomarker for hepatotoxicity should address the pre-stated issues concerning sensitivity, clarity and specificity, plus have utility in the non-clinical and clinical settings.[63,64] Another application of biomarkers would be the identification of individuals susceptible to DILI to better inform the physician in the selection of medication for their patient.[65]

Potential biomarkers of DILI are intended to augment the traditional clinical chemistry panels and might include both new enzyme assays and novel analytes that require non-enzymatic assays.[66,67] The target for improvement is to achieve better performance than currently possible with the serum transaminase assays. Some potential biomarkers will be well suited to screening applications (*e.g.*, glutathione-*S*-transferase-α and malate dehydrogenase), while others will be reserved for more strategic use as confirmatory procedures depending on their technical degree of difficulty or equipment requirements (*e.g.* serum F protein, mRNA, purine nucleoside phosphorylase).[68] Validation of new biomarkers for DILI will require demonstration of tissue specificity for liver, expression in both laboratory animals and humans to ensure translation, and correlation with tissue injury.

### 16.8.3 *-omics* Technologies

The promise for improving detection and characterization of hepatotoxicity using the allied fields of genomics, proteomics, and metabolomics remains under investigation. The salient feature of these technologies is the detection of toxicity measured as changes in the expression pattern of genes, proteins, and metabolites as measured in vast arrays. While systems biology remains a very intriguing branch of biological science, there is not yet enough experience to support validation of these approaches. The technical requirements of the analytical procedures may limit these technologies for use in routine screening, although it is envisioned that they may eventually become important tools for confirming and characterizing hepatotoxicity.

Toxicogenomics is perhaps the most widely used of these technologies for predicting hepatotoxicity. Toxicogenomics has been used in the pharmaceutical industry for about a decade although it has not yet been leveraged with any substantive success in breaking through the DILI-prediction barrier.[17] Some reports in the literature suggest that toxicogenomics may be useful as an adjunctive technique (*e.g.*, corroborating hepatotoxicity signals garnered from standard methodologies such as histopathology).[69,70] The FDA has stated that toxicogenomic evaluations are acceptable as adjunct data until more experience can be gained with this technique.

## 16.8.4 Identification of Sensitive Individuals

Another approach that is hoped will provide better prediction of idiosyncratic DILI is oriented to the specific traits of the individual. The characterization of genetic traits such as polymorphisms in biotransformation, immunological reactivity, and human leukocyte antigens may help to create a profile of the DILI-susceptible patient.

### *16.8.4.1 Polymorphisms in Biotransformation*

The rationale for screening chemical reactivity and reactive metabolite formation has been amply discussed in this chapter. The standard procedures in characterizing drug candidates include detailing its biotransformation products and pathways in both animals and humans. The models used to accomplish this include liver microsomes, isolated enzymes, or hepatocytes obtained from limited numbers of human donors, and therefore, provide a very limited perspective on human biotransformation.

Single nucleotide polymorphisms (SNPs) in human biotransformation pathways are well documented and are also thought to be relevant to DILI. The ramifications of SNPs for drug disposition and pharmacokinetics have become better recognized.[71] SNPs associated with glutathione-*S*-transferase gene deletions (GSTM1 and GSTT1) are correlated with increased hepatotoxicity produced by tacrine, and troglitzone in the Japanese population.[72,73] Other polymorphisms positively correlated with DILI include polymorphisms in cytochrome P450 2D6 (CYP2D6), *N*-acetyl transferase, UDP-glururonosyl transferase 1A1 (UGT1A1), and thiopurine methyltransferase 3A and 3C (TPMT 3A and 3C).[72]

### *16.8.4.2 Immunological Reactivity*

A means of identifying patients at-risk for DILI based on immunological differentiation has been of great interest, but none has met with any level of success.[74] Several early biomarker strategies for idiosyncratic DILI predicated upon detection of evidence of reactive metabolite formation in patients proved unsuccessful. As an example, the presence of drug–protein adducts in serum was hoped to predict susceptible patients, though it was discovered that this finding was not uniquely correlated with individuals who had experienced idiosyncratic DILI.[75] Another belief was that the presence of circulating anti-liver antibodies in susceptible patients would reflect haptenization; however, this approach failed to gain any traction, possibly because of its reliance on electrophoresis and its degree of difficulty.[8] Serological screening for auto-antibodies against nuclear DNA, such as those found in patients with auto-immune hepatitis, has been suggested as a screen for DILI based on the belief that the liver injury seen with the two etiologies shares a common origin.[8]

An altogether different approach made use of lymphocyte screens to detect patients at-risk for DILI. In one such method, a drug of interest was screened against a subset of T-lymphocytes that were harvested from known sensitive patients to characterize cytotoxicity. A shift in the potency for cytotoxicity was taken as evidence for the drug's potential to produce idiosyncratic hypsensitivity DILI. A slightly different variation on this theme was to characterize the sensitivity of a patient's lymphocytes to cytotoxicity produced by the reactive metabolites of diphenylhydantoin (DPH). Increased sensitivity to DPH-induced cytotoxicity was used as a barometer for patient susceptibility to DILI and was reported to correlate with patients who had experienced DILI, including several who suffered from halothane hepatitis.[76,77]

### *16.8.4.3 Human Leukocyte Antigens*

The presence of risk factors within the genetic constitution of an individual provides perhaps a more promising, if not more contemporary, means of screening susceptibility to idiosyncratic DILI. Many attempts to correlate Human Leukocyte Antigen (HLA) haplotypes with idiosyncratic DILI have been generally inconclusive because of the low power of the studies although more robustly powered studies tended to support an association of some HLA Class II haplotypes with DILI (see Table 16.7). As can also be seen in Table 16.7, certain haplotypes appear to confer protection against hepatic injury.

Some reports suggest that cytokine polymorphisms (IL-10-627*A and IL-4-509*T) associated with decreased levels of the anti-inflammatory IL-10 and increased levels of IL-4, respectively, correlate with the presence of anti-diclofenac antibodies in patients taking diclofenac.[72,74–76] These cytokines are generally thought to modulate inflammation and immunological responses; the loss of their modulatory activity may be important in the genesis of idiosyncractic DILI.

Many of the haplotypes associated with DILI are associated with auto-immune diseases such as rheumatoid arthritis, diabetes, multiple sclerosis, lupus erythamatosus, as well as infectious diseases suggesting that auto-immunity may be a risk factor for idiosyncratic DILI.

### *16.8.4.4 Human Liver Biology*

At this juncture, it must be acknowledged that a large amount of uncharted biology still exists within the realm of hepatic structure and function.

**Table 16.7** HLA haplotypes associated with DILI.[64,75,130–135]

| *Allele or haplotype* | *Correlation with DILI* | *Other pathophysiological correlations* |
|---|---|---|
| HLA-B*5701 | Flucloxacillin | Abacavir Hypersensitivity |
| HLA—DRB1*15 | Amoxicillin-Clavulanic Acid | See DRB1*1501 below |
| HLA-DQB1*06 | Amoxicillin-Clavulanic Acid, Ticlopidine | Largely protective associations, including multiple scleosis, narcolepsy, juvenile diabetes, myasthenia gravis |
| HLA-DRB1*04 | Diclofenac | Malaria, rheumatoid arthritis |
| HLA-DRB1*1501 DRB5*0101 DQB1*0602 | Amoxicillin-Clavulanic Acid | (DRB1*1501) Good pasture syndrome, juvenile rheumatoid arthritis, allergic bronchopulmonary aspergillosis, multiple sclerosis, systemic lupus erythematosus, human papillomavirus infection, Sjogren's syndrome (DRB5*0101) Multiple sclerosis (DQB1*0602) Narcolepsy |
| HLA – DQA1*0102-DQB1*0602 | Amoxicillin-Clavulanic Acid | Sensitivity to multiple sclerosis, resistance to diabetes |
| HLA-A*3303 | Ticlopidine | Post-herpetic neuralgia |
| HLA-DRB1*0701 | Ximelagatran | — |
| HLA-DQA1*02 | Ximelagatran | Diabetes, Celiac disease |
| HLA-DQB1-0201 | Isoniazid, Rifampin, Streptomycin Lapatinib | Diabetes |
| HLA-DRB1*03 | Isoniazid, Rifampin, Streptomycin | Hashimoto's disease, primary sclerosing cholangitis, myasthenia gravis, |
| HLA-DRB1*07 DRA1*0103 DRB1*13 | Associated with hepatoprotection | — |

The cellular and structural heterogeneity of the liver along with the complexity of its function rival the physiological and anatomical complexity of the brain.[78] If one makes the assumption that the complexity of an organ defines its susceptibility to toxic insult, there will almost surely be other mechanisms of hepatic injury yet to be recognized. Advances in biology are frequently a by-product of drug development, especially involving new targets. We may eventually encounter pharmacology-based hepatotoxicity if the same molecular targets active in diseases are also essential to hepatocellular viability and function.

Might the incidence of false negatives in non-clinical testing somehow reflect an erroneous assumption in the long-standing practice of predicting human response based on responses in animal livers? Extrapolation of results from animal to human liver might be limited with target-based hepatotoxicity if there is discordance between the hepatic function of the targets across species. More emphasis on basic research into the biology of the human liver is definitely warranted to help understand differences that exist with the livers of lower species to validate the practice of extrapolation with regard to hepatic safety.

### 16.8.5 Harbingers of DILI in the Clinic

Sharpening our ability to predict DILI must also include better recognition of harbinger changes in clinical trials. Retrospective analyses have shown that certain patterns of clinical laboratory data have prognostic value for predicting negative clinical outcomes and even death in patients.[79] The initial recognition of this relationship is credited to Dr Hyman Zimmerman and has been referred to as "Hy's Law".[80] His analysis showed that drug-induced hepatocellular injury and jaundice were correlated with high patient mortality; because clinical experience with DILI was minimal in the era before World War II, this observation was pivotal in helping increase physician awareness of the gravity of DILI.

Today, the broader implication of Hy's Law is that clinical safety databases in contemporary registration dossiers are scrutinized for clinical laboratory evidence of hepatocellular injury and jaundice because it is recognized that these results predict the potential for some level of severe DILI and death in a larger patient population. Harbinger evidence of DILI may not necessarily preclude approval of a drug; but, it might require additional safety studies and a risk-management plan, as well as limit the market penetration of the drug post-approval.[80] Though not formally validated, the harbinger changes central to Hy's Law were codified from experience with troglitazone (Rezulin) and bromfenac (Duract), both of which were withdrawn from the market for DILI.[80,81] Review of these clinical databases revealed that unfavorable patient outcomes were predicted when a threshold defined as $\geq$3-fold the upper limit of normal (ULN) for ALT along with $\geq$2-fold ULN for bilirubin was exceeded.[81–83] These limits have been informally referred to as the "Rezulin Rule" by some authors.[81] In the troglitazone database, an additional 2% of patients exhibited transaminitis ($\geq$3-fold the upper ULN) without concomitant changes in bilirubin, but since these changes still predicted ALF, there is also increased scrutiny of transaminitis by regulatory authorities.[84,85]

A clinical trial, for good reasons, is a relatively limited mechanism for exploring human toxicities. Despite the difficulties faced with diagnosing DILI, clinical experts generally agree that certain steps to confirm the attribution of liver injury to a drug are not warranted in a clinical trial. Biopsy procedures, in selected instances, might provide morphological corroboration of laboratory changes, but would not confirm a diagnosis of DILI or even attribution to a drug.[86] Clinicians are generally reluctant to re-challenge patients who exhibit adverse effects with a drug unless the benefit from continuing therapy is compelling.[14,87] Since DILI is a diagnosis of exclusion, re-challenge would help clarify the role of the drug in response to changes in laboratory data; however, the hazardous nature of this procedure dictates that it be done in accordance with protocol to minimize the probability of an exacerbated liver response in a potentially sensitive patient.[87]

A safer and hopefully more productive approach would be to characterize SNPs and HLA haplotype in patients who exhibit DILI as a means of growing the genetic databases for drug sensitivity. It is also possible that more might be learned about the potential for DILI with a drug by inclusion of sensitive patients into limited clinical trials. The exclusion criteria of clinical protocols preclude the entry of potentially sensitive or at-risk individuals into clinical trials, which eliminates exposure of potential sentinels of hepatotoxicity.[14] FDA guidance discussed later in this chapter suggests that the inclusion of small numbers of potentially sensitive patients in late-stage clinical trials or in a separate clinical trial with limited exposure to the drug might be useful in eliciting a DILI signal. Controlled exposure in clinical trials might make it possible to predict potentially sensitive populations even before the drug reaches its market. There is already precedence for limited exploration in sensitive patients during the drug-development process in the clinical studies that are conducted to characterize the effect of hepatic or renal disease on the pharmacokinetic profile of a drug.

## 16.9 New Paradigms for Predicting Human Hepatotoxicity

The complex nature of DILI in patients may reflect the interplay of a number of factors in the liver, in addition to the drug. The current difficulty in predicting hepatotoxicity, especially idiosyncratic DILI, might be less about technology and more about our failure to account for concomitant factors that are present in many patients.[88] This implies that results obtained with standard animal models (*i.e.*, young, healthy, genetically homogeneous animals) may be inherently limited in their ability to wholly predict hepatic safety in patients.

### 16.9.1 Rationale for a Multi-Factorial Approach

Table 16.8 illustrates why the traditional approach for studying drug effects may not be adequate to fully predict the hepatotoxicity potential of a drug used in broader patient populations. It can be seen that significant differences exist in the conditions under which laboratory species and human patients are exposed to a drug. Current safety testing approaches were originally designed as pure characterizations of the pharmacological and toxicological activity of the drug itself; but, this approach may inadvertently misrepresent the response to the drug in multivariate human beings. Consequently, it may be necessary to pay greater attention to the not-so-subtle differences that could significantly alter the toxicity profile of a drug in humans.[88]

### 16.9.2 Binary Models of Hepatotoxicity

The term, binary toxicity, is used here to describe drug toxicity that requires the presence of concomitant factor(s). This concept differs from the traditional drug–drug interaction in terms of pharmacokinetic and pharmacological outcomes. The premise is that factors such as concomitant disease, infection, inflammation, nutritional status, alcohol intake, oxidative stress, *etc.* can alter

**Table 16.8** Comparison of non-clinical and clinical models for evaluating drug toxicity.[53]

| *Variable* | *Non-clinical* | *Clinical* |
|---|---|---|
| Group size relative to potential market population | Much, much smaller | Much smaller |
| Genetic diversity | Typically use genetically in-bred strains | Highly diverse |
| Age | Adolescent to aging | Young adult to elderly |
| Background disease | None | May be present |
| Nutrition | Well maintained through diet | Variable |
| Housing | Well maintained | Variable |
| Concomitant drug exposure | Never or infrequently | Commonly |
| Dosing | Well-controlled | Dosing regularity may be variable |
| Methodologies for evaluating the liver | Invasive and comprehensive | Limited and indirect |
| Ability to establish causal relationship to drug | Very good | Possible in clinical testing phase; very challenging post-marketing |

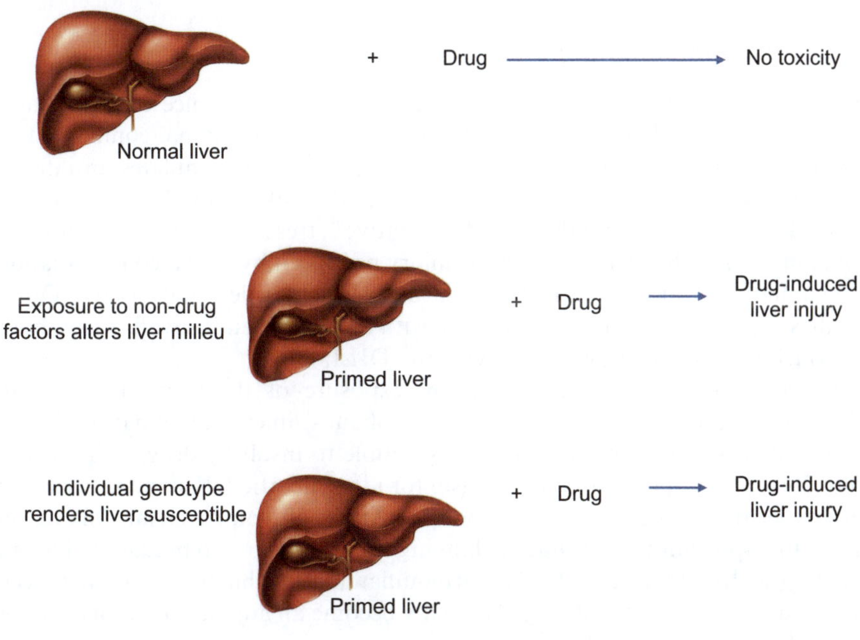


**Figure 16.2** Models of binary hepatotoxicity.

the milieu in the liver making it more susceptible to drug injury (Figure 16.2). The sensitized milieu of the liver is thought to facilitate the expression of latent hepatotoxic potential by lowering the threshold for toxicity or producing a leftward shift of the drug's dose–response curve for hepatotoxicity. Likewise, the genotype of an individual could render the liver susceptible to injury by drugs. Binary toxicity is much like the "set and setting" theory for psychoactive drugs in which the milieu, as defined by an individual's susceptibility (the set) and environmental factors (the setting), help determine the response to the drug. Following this analogy, factors other than the drug are envisioned to determine the milieu of the liver and its susceptibility to injury by the drug. Moreover, the hypothesis that idiosyncratic DILI represents the culmination of individual susceptibility, collateral factors and the action of the drug is quite consistent with the relative infrequence of this form of hepatotoxicity.

Testing for binary hepatotoxicity will require the use of new models that are quite different from the standard safety assessment models.[89] There is currently not much experience with these models and more use is needed to determine their utility. Accordingly, the information garnered with these models need not be heavily weighted in organizational or regulatory decision making, but may provide useful advisory data that could be used to establish potential correlations between the presence of external factors and drug in cases of DILI. The longer range vision would be that these models might aid in the design of limited clinical trials to confirm potentially susceptible patient populations or confirm conditions under which a particular drug should not be used.

#### *16.9.2.1 Inflammation*

The liver can mount an inflammatory response in the presence of pro-inflammatory stimuli such as lipopolysaccharide (LPS), the functional component of bacterial endotoxin found in the portal blood.[90,91] LPS stimulates an inflammatory cascade in the liver leading to increased cytokine and TNF-$\alpha$ production, kupffer cell activation, and oxidative stress.[91] With activation of inflammation in the liver, the hepatic injury produced by allyl alcohol, ethanol, acetaminophen, monocrotaline, and carbon tetrachloride is increased.[92] Other studies have also confirmed this finding with diclofenac and trovafloxacin, both of which are associated with idiosyncratic DILI.[93,94]

It has been proposed that recurrent exposure of the liver to endotoxin through the portal blood creates episodes of sub-clinical inflammation during which the organ may become more susceptible to insult by drugs.[87] This concept has been proposed as a mechanism for idiosyncratic DILI and is discussed in greater detail elsewhere in this book.[96] Although controversial, this represents an important new avenue of thinking for approaches to predicting human toxicity with animal models. The drug-inflammation binary model has been adapted to *in vitro* use and may eventually become an adjunctive evaluation for latent hepatotoxic potential.[97,98]

#### *16.9.2.2 Alcohol*

Any relationship between alcohol use and idiosycnratic DILI has been difficult to discern because of the background of severe hepatic injury seen in patients who abuse alcohol.[99] Alcohol is pro-inflammatory and does elicit an inflammatory response in the liver very similar to LPS.[100] It is possible that drug ingestion against a background of continual alcohol ingestion could support a scenario for idiosyncratic DILI through the same mechanisms discussed in section 16.9.2.1.

### *16.9.2.3 Glutathione Status*

Mechanistic research has highlighted the importance of oxidative stress, mitochondrial damage and depletion of GSH as major predictors of toxicity and cell death.[101] Intracellular glutathione protects cellular components against oxidative damage caused by xenobiotic-derived electrophiles as well as reactive oxygen species that are by-products of cellular respiration and metabolism.[102,103] Hepatocytes become vulnerable to oxidative stress under conditions in which the intracellular glutathione concentration becomes depleted, and there is ample evidence that depletion of intracellular glutathione potentiates hepatotoxicity.[103] The intracellular ratio of reduced glutathione (thiol) to oxidized glutathione (disulfide) is a major determinant of the cellular redox state, which, in turn, regulates processes critical to hepatocyte survival including protein oxidation state, cell signaling (*e.g.* kinase activity), hepatic regeneration, and apoptosis.[104]

A small, but critical, pool of GSH is maintained within mitochondria. The mitochondrial pool of glutathione is an especially critical barometer for cell survival because it is thought to regulate cell death pathways (necrosis and apoptosis) and is pivotal in preserving mitochondrial function in a milieu that includes reactive oxygen species generation by electron transport and oxidative phosphorlyation. Mitochondria cannot synthesize GSH *de novo* and must rely on anionic transporters to move GSH synthesized in the cytoplasm into the mitochondria and maintain physiologically relevant levels.[105]

There are adverse consequences for depletion or diminution of mitochondrial GSH levels.[97,106] It is known that loss of mitochondrial glutathione sensitizes hepatocytes to TNF-α-induced cell death and clearly potentiates the hepatotoxicity of acetaminophen, which itself is known to selectively decrease mitochondrial glutathione. It is not well understood whether polymorphisms exist with the multiple transporters that are thought to be involved in moving GSH into mitochondria although it is known that chronic alcohol abuse changes the fluidity of the mitochondria membranes and indirectly decreases GSH transport.[103] This appears to explain the clinical reports of accidental DILI and ALF observed after ingestion of ordinary doses of acetaminophen by persons suffering from chronic alcohol abuse.[107,108] The altered milieu of the liver under conditions of chronic alcohol exposure, and, more specifically, the glutathione content of the mitochondria effectively produce a leftward shift of the acetaminophen dose–response curve for liver injury.[109]

Experimental reagents are available for selectively diminishing the cytoplasmic and mitochondrial pools of GSH as a means of assessing latent hepatotoxicity of a drug. To date, the best clinical evidence for this scenario has been obtained with acetaminophen, a classical hepatotoxicant, and it remains unknown whether this mechanism is relevant for drugs that have produced idiosyncratic DILI. However, the scenario appears plausible just as it remains possible that continued characterization of mitochondrial genomics may uncover polymorphisms (*e.g.*, transporter) that will define DILI-susceptible individuals.

#### *16.9.2.4 Non-Alcoholic Fatty Liver Disease*

Aside from fatty liver associated with alcohol consumption, there is a high incidence of non-alcoholic fatty liver disease (NALFD) in the US.[110–111] Epidemiological studies report that patients with NALFD exhibit a four-fold increase in susceptibility to DILI.[112] Lipid accumulation within hepatocytes, a common response to ethanol, is also pro-inflammatory and patients with NAFLD do exhibit activation of genes associated with inflammation pathways.[111,113]

### 16.9.3 Hepatoprotection Mechanisms

There are hepatocellular protection mechanisms that preserve liver function in the midst of insult by xenobiotics and pathogens. An emerging hypothesis related to DILI is that inhibition of vital hepatoprotection mechanisms by a drug might enable liver injury caused by subsequent exposure to other drugs, pathogens, chemicals, alcohol, *etc.* (Figure 16.3).

Evidence for this hypothesis comes from studies of nrf-2 (Nuclear Factor [Erythroid-Related 2]-2), the transcription factor that regulates the major oxidative stress response in hepatocytes. Nrf-2 acts by binding to the antioxidant response element promoter region causing up-regulation of the genes

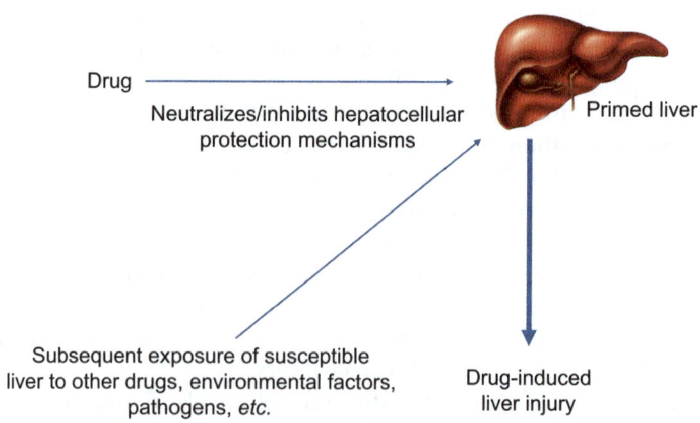


**Figure 16.3** Models of enabled hepatotoxicty.

related to anti-oxidant systems, including glutathione-*S*-transferases, quinone oxidoreductase 1, heme oxygenase-1, and γ-glutamlycytseine synthase (the rate-limiting for glutathione synthesis).[114–116] There are several lines of evidence that nrf-2 plays a role in hepatoprotection: knockout mice in which nrf-2 gene has been deleted show greater liver injury at otherwise non-toxic doses of 1-bromopropane, carbon tetrachloride, and acetaminophen.[116–119] Preservation of nrf-2 through deletion of the gene for Keap-1, a regulatory element for nrf-2 degradation, confers protection against hepatotoxicant challenge in mice.[120]

Screening for drug inhibition of hepatoprotective pathways is not yet a widespread practice, however, the ability to screen a limited set of related targets as a means of detecting inhibition of the anti-oxidant response is technologically feasible. Moreover, this screening could be done in high-throughput format as is typically used in searching for drug candidates.[117,121] Other targets possibly linked with hepatoprotection are shown in Table 16.9. Given the current direction in the search for new drugs towards inhibition of cell signaling pathways, indirect inhibition of hepatoprotection mechanisms as a downstream consequence of inhibition of a cell signaling pathway seems entirely possible.

## 16.10 Regulatory Guidance on DILI

Guidance has been provided by the major regulatory agencies to help clinical investigators studying candidate drugs better recognize hepatotoxicity. These guidance documents also share lessons learned from earlier drug failures and market withdrawals and provide prospective monitoring and recognition strategies.

### 16.10.1 Food and Drug Administration

*Guidance for Industry Drug-Induced Liver Injury: Premarketing Clinical Evaluation* (July 2009) explains how potentially severe hepatotoxicity can be detected by patterns presented in clinical chemistry changes.[109] The guidance also discusses the rule-outs that should be addressed to support a diagnosis of DILI. One interesting point relates to the practice of re-challenge to confirm the drug as the causative agent for clinical laboratory changes. The guidance discourages the practice in patients who have exhibited marked transaminase increases (> 5-fold ULN) for fear of eliciting a more severe reaction.

### 16.10.2 European Union

The European Union (EU) has issued a *Non-Clinical Guideline on Drug-Induced Hepatotoxicity* (August 2008) that provides comprehensive guidance on the detection of hepatotoxicity in non-clinical safety studies, including the use of supplemental laboratory evaluations. Many of the points presented in this

**Table 16.9** Potential hepatoprotection mechanisms.[116,136–147]

| *Target* | *Name* | *Function* | *Evidence for hepatoprotection* |
|---|---|---|---|
| Nuclear factor [erythroid related 2]-2 | Nrf-2 | Regulates major anti-oxidant response | Ablation or enhancement with genetic models modulates hepatotoxicity in several models |
| Superoxide dismutase 2 | *Sod2* | Scavenges superoxide anion formed within mitochondria thereby protecting against oxidative stress | Ablation of the gene in genetic models potentiates acetaminophen-induced liver injury |
| Inducible nitric oxide synthetase | iNOS | Inhibits apoptosis; preserves mitochondria; preserves protein structure | Small organic inhibitors of iNOS promote apoptosis in hepatocytes |
| Endothelial nitric oxide synthetase | eNOS | Preserves hepatic blood flow through sinusoids | Indirect inhibition of eNOS through phosphotidylinositol 3-kinase inhibition potentiates carbon tetrachloride-induced injury; Direct inhibition with L-NAME potentiates carbon tetrachloride-induced injury |
| Heme oxygenase-1 | HO-1 | Maintains cellular redox state through antioxidant action of biliverdin and bilirubin; carbon monoxide by-product serves to attenuate inflammation pathways | HO-1 is induced in response to hepatotoxicant-induced injury; treatment with hemin to induce HO-1 protects against injury produced by acetatminophen, carbon tetrachloride, halothane and heavy metals |
| Cyclooxygenase-2 | COX-2 | Mediates signaling for the stress response; induces heat shock protein expression | Ablation of gene with genetic model potentiates acetaminophen-induced injury |
| Sphingosine 1 phosphate | $SIP_2$ | Promotes hepatic regeneration<br>Through hepatic myofibroblast-induced matrix remodeling | Gene deletion results in reduced wound healing response post-carbon tetrachloride-induced liver injury |
| TGF-β-activated kinase 1 | TAK1 | Promotes hepatocellular homeostasis | Hepatocyte-specific TAK1-deficient mice exhibit hepatocelular death, inflammation and fibrosis |
| Signal transducer and activator of transcription-3 | STAT3 | Activated by IL-6; STAT3 promotes hepatocellular cytoprotection, liver regeneration, acute phase response, glucose homeostatis and lipid metabolism | IL-6 gene-deleted mice are more susceptible to carbon tetrachloride-induced injury and exhibit impaired hepatic regeneration |
| Early growth response-1 | Egr-1 | Immediate early gene coding for transcriptional regulator of inflammation genes involved in tissue repair | Ablation of the gene in genetic models potentiates carbon tetrachloride-induced liver injury |

chapter are discussed in this guidance, but there are some unique recommendations for cases when evidence of hepatotoxicity is observed:

1) Exploratory evaluations should be conducted to discern the nature of hepatotoxicity.
2) Non-rodent data should be evaluated based on individual animals and not mean data; any signal should be followed up with appropriate secondary studies.
3) Hepatotoxicity should be characterized with respect to dose dependency, reversibility, monitoring strategy, anticipated appearance in patients with concomitant risk factors, and any evidence of clinical relevance.
4) Hepatotoxicity detected in the non-clinical safety assessment should be discussed as a separate section in the toxicology summary.

Many of these recommendations already represent current best practices; nevertheless, some of the reaction to this draft guidance document reflected concern.[122] One of the primary concerns centered on the EU recommendation for the conduct of investigational studies in response to evidence of hepatotoxicity. Investigation of newly discovered toxicities is fairly common practice within the pharmaceutical industry; however, the specific concern is that it may not be possible to deliver definitive molecular mechanisms from exploratory studies within a time frame that is realistic for development and approval of the drug. The pharmaceutical sector also expressed concern in response to the EU's encouragement for experimentation with the novel binary models discussed earlier in this chapter on the basis that they are unvalidated models and there is relatively little experience with these systems. Finally, the pharmaceutical sector expressed the position that focus of the guidance document on non-clinical testing is unlikely to improve detection of rare idiosyncratic DILI, which is arguably true. What is clear from this guidance is that EU regulatory authorities will expect a thorough accounting of hepatic safety before a drug will be approved.

## 16.11 Conclusions

The key conclusions of this chapter are:

1) The prediction of classical hepatotoxicity poses no problem for current methodologies and approaches.
2) Better predictive insights into human hepatotoxicity will require greater investment in basic research into the biology of the human liver; especially with regard to novel targets that may have unknown hepatic function.
3) The prediction of hepatic safety will be improved with greater attention to harbinger changes in non-clinical and clinical safety results.
4) The ability to ever predict idiosyncratic DILI will require a paradigm shift in non-clinical testing and investment in the creation of databases for characterizing susceptible individuals.

# References


1. R. J. Temple and M. H. Himmel, *JAMA, J. Am. Med. Assoc.*, 2002, **287**, 2273.
2. B. Gunawan and N. Kaplowitz, *Drug Metab. Rev.,* 2004, **36**, 301.
3. K. E. Lasser, P. D. Allen, S. J. Woolhandler, D. U. Himmelstein, S. M. Wolfe and D. H. Bor, *JAMA, J. Am. Med. Assoc.*, 2002, **287**, 2215.
4. M. G. Sturgill and G. H. Lambert, *Clin. Chem.*, 1997, **43**, 1512.
5. H. Higuchi and G. J. Gores, *Curr. Mol. Med.,* 2003, **3**, 483.
6. H. J. Zimmerman, *Hepatotoxicity*, Appleton-Century-Crofts, New York, 1978.
7. V. J. Navarro and J. R. Senior, *N. Engl. J. Med.,* 2006, **354**, 731.
8. S. Verma and N. Kaplowitz, *Gut*, 2009, **58**, 1555.
9. R. J. Fontana, *Semin. Liver Dis.*, 2008, **28**, 175.
10. D. E. Kleiner, *Semin. Liver Dis.*, 2009, **29**, 364.
11. R. Ramachandran and S. Kakar, *J. Clin. Pathol.,* 2009, **62**, 481.
12. E. Bjornsson, *Semin. Liver Dis.*, 2009, **29**, 357.
13. D. N. Assis and V. J. Navarro, *Expert Opin. Drug Metab. Toxicol.,* 2009, **5**, 463.
14. M. D. Halegoua-De and V. J. Navarro, *Curr. Opin. Drug Discovery Dev.,* 2008, **11**, 53.
15. W. M. Lee and J. R. Senior, *Toxicol. Pathol.,* 2005, **33**, 155.
16. R. G. Ulrich, *Annu. Rev. Med.,* 2007, **58**, 17.
17. N. Kaplowitz, *Nat. Rev. Drug Discovery,* 2005, **4**, 489.
18. S. H. Hussaini and E. A. Farrington, *Expert Opin. Drug Saf.*, 2007, **6**, 673.
19. J. L. Walgren, M. D. Mitchell and D. C. Thompson, *Crit. Rev. Toxicol.,* 2005, **35**, 325.
20. D. J. Naisbitt, S. F. Gordon, M. Pirmohamed and B. K. Park, *Drug Saf.*, 2000, **23**, 483.
21. L. R. Pohl, J. G. Kenna, H. Satoh, D. Christ and J. L. Martin, *Drug Metab. Rev.,* 1989, **20**, 203.
22. S. Sherlock, *Gut*, 1971, **12**, 324.
23. J. L. Martin, J. G. Kenna, B. M. Martin, D. Thomassen, G. F. Reed and L. R. Pohl, *Hepatology*, 2005, **18**, 858.
24. G. C. Smith, J. G. Kenna, D. J. Harrison, D. Tew and C. R. Wolf, *Lancet*, 1993, **342**, 963.
25. J. Li and J. P. Uetrecht, in Adverse Drug Reactions, ed. J. P. Uetrecht, *Handbook of Experimental Pharmacology,* Springer, New York, 2010, vol. 196, p. 493.
26. J. P. Uetrecht, *Chem. Res. Toxicol.,* 1999, **12**, 387.
27. W. J. Pichler, *Curr. Opin. Allergy Clin. Immunol.,* 2002, **2**, 301.
28. *Guidelines for Detection of Hepatotoxicity Due to Drugs and Chemicals*, ed. C. S. Davidson, C. M. Leevy and E. C. Chamberlayne, National Institutes of Health, Washington DC, 1979.
29. D. E. Amacher, *Regul. Toxicol. Pharmacol.,* 1998, **27**, 119.
30. P. F. Solter, *Toxicol. Pathol.,* 2005, **33**, 9.

31. D. E. Amacher, *Hum. Exp. Toxicol.,* 2002, **21**, 253.
32. L. Boone, D. Meyer, P. Cusick, D. Ennulat, A. P. Bolliger, N. Everds, V. Meador, G. Elliott, D. Honor, D. Bounous and H. Jordan, *Vet. Clin. Pathol.,* 2005, **34**, 182.
33. P. T. Giboney, *Am. Fam. Physician*, 2005, **71**, 1105.
34. E. G. Giannini, R. Testa and V. Savarino, *Can. Med. Assoc. J.,* 2005, **172**, 367.
35. W. Lewis, B. J. Day and W. C. Copeland, *Nat. Rev. Drug Discovery,* 2003, **2**, 812.
36. J. M. Colacino, *Antiviral Res.,* 1996, **29**, 125.
37. R. McKenzie, M. W. Fried, R. Sallie, H. Conjeevaram, A. M. Di Bisceglie, Y. Park, B. Savarese, D. Kleiner, M. Tsokos, C. Luciano, T. Pruett, J. L. Stotka, S. E. Straus and J. H. Hoofnagle, *N. Engl. J. Med.,* 1995, **333**, 1099.
38. N. Greene and R. Naven, *Curr. Opin. Drug Discovery Dev.,* 2009, **12**, 90.
39. J. A. Dykens, L. D. Marroquin and Y. Will, *Expert Rev. Mol. Diagn.,* 2007, **7**, 161.
40. U. A. Boelsterli and P. L. Lim, *Toxicol. Appl. Pharmacol.,* 2007, **220**, 92.
41. G. Stirnimann, K. Kessebohm and B. Lauterburg, *Swiss Med. Wkly.,* 2010, **140**, 13080.
42. H. Jaeschke, *Toxicol. Sci.,* 2007, **97**, 1.
43. M. M. Ong, C. Latchoumycandane and U. A. Boelsterli, *Toxicol. Sci.,* 2007, **97**, 205.
44. A. S. Kalgutkar and J. R. Soglia, *Expert Opin. Drug Metab. Toxicol.,* 2005, **1**, 91.
45. A. S. Kalgutkar, G. Fate, M. Didiuk and J. Bauman, *Expert Rev.*, 2008, **1**, 515.
46. D. P. Williams and B. K. Park, *Drug Discovery Today*, 2003, **8**, 1044.
47. D. P. Williams and D. J. Naisbitt, *Curr. Opin. Drug Discovery Dev.,* 2002, **5**, 104.
48. G. H. Hakimelahi and G. A. Khodarahmi, *J. Iran. Chem. Soc.*, 2005, **2**, 244.
49. S. Nakayama, R. Atsumi, H. Takakusa, Y. Kobayashi, A. Kurihara, Y. Nagai, D. Nakai and O. Okazaki, *Drug Metab. Dispos.,* 2009, **37**, 1970.
50. T. Usui, M. Mise, T. Hashizume, M. Yabuki and S. Komuro, *Drug Metab. Dispos.,* 2009, **37**, 2383.
51. D. P. Williams, *Toxicology*, 2006, **226**, 1.
52. J. Uetrecht, *Drug Metab. Rev.,* 2006, **38**, 745.
53. H. Olson, G. Betton, D. Robinson, K. Thomas, A. Monro, G. Kolaja, P. Lilly, J. Sanders, G. Sipes, W. Bracken, M. Dorato, D. K. Van, P. Smith, B. Berger and A. Heller, *Regul. Toxicol. Pharmacol.,* 2000, **32**, 56.
54. S. Spanhaak, D. Cook, J. Barnes and J. Reynolds, *Species Concordance for Liver Injury*, Biowisdom Ltd, Cambridge, UK, 2008.
55. T. S. Peters, *Toxicol. Pathol.,* 2005, **33**, 146.
56. C. Alden, J. Lin and P. Smith, *Preclinica*, 2003, 27.
57. R. J. Andrade and M. I. Lucena, *Rev. Esp. Enferm. Dig.,* 2001, **93**, 48.

58. P. B. Watkins, *Toxicol. Pathol.,* 2005, **33**, 1.
59. D. M. Goldstein and T. Gabriel, *Curr. Top. Med. Chem.,* 2005, **5**, 1017.
60. M. C. Genovese, *Arthritis Rheum.,* 2009, **60**, 317.
61. S. E. Sweeney and G. S. Firestein, *Ann. Rheum. Dis.,* 2006, **65**, iii83.
62. J. Woodcock and R. Woosley, *Annu. Rev. Med.,* 2008, **59**, 1.
63. R. N. McBurney, W. M. Hines, L. S. Von Tungeln, L. K. Schnackenberg, R. D. Beger, C. L. Moland, T. Han, J. C. Fuscoe, C. W. Chang, J. J. Chen, Z. Su, X. H. Fan, W. Tong, S. A. Booth, R. Balasubramanian, P. L. Courchesne, J. M. Campbell, A. Graber, Y. Guo, P. J. Juhasz, T. Y. Li, M. D. Lynch, N. M. Morel, T. N. Plasterer, E. J. Takach, C. Zeng and F. A. Beland, *Toxicol. Pathol.,* 2009, **37**, 52.
64. S. Amur, F. W. Frueh, L. J. Lesko and S. M. Huang, *Biomarkers Med.,* 2008, **2**, 305.
65. P. B. Watkins, *Semin. Liver Dis.*, 2009, **29**, 393.
66. M. Miyamoto, M. Yanai, S. Ookubo, N. Awasaki, K. Takami and R. Imai, *Toxicol. Sci.,* 2008, **106**, 538.
67. S. Lacour, J. C. Gautier, M. Pallardy and R. Roberts, *Cancer Biomarkers,* 2005, **1**, 29.
68. J. Ozer, M. Ratner, M. Shaw, W. Bailey and S. Schomaker, *Toxicology,* 2008, **245**, 194.
69. W. R. Foster, S. J. Chen, A. He, A. Truong, V. Bhaskaran, D. M. Nelson, D. M. Dambach, L. D. Lehman-McKeeman and B. D. Car, *Toxicol. Pathol.,* 2007, **35**, 621.
70. A. N. Heinloth, G. A. Boorman, J. F. Foley, N. D. Flagler and R. S. Paules, *Toxicol. Pathol.,* 2007, **35**, 276.
71. S. J. Gardiner and E. J. Begg, *Pharmacol. Rev.,* 2006, **58**, 521.
72. D. A. Katz, B. Murray, A. Bhathena and L. Sahelijo, *Nat. Rev. Drug Discovery,* 2008, **7**, 293.
73. M. I. Lucena, R. J. Andrade, C. Martinez, E. Ulzurrun, E. Garcia-Martin, Y. Borraz, M. C. Fernandez, M. Romero-Gomez, A. Castiella, R. Planas, J. Costa, S. Anzola and J. A. Agundez, *Hepatology*, 2008, **48**, 588.
74. C. Ju, *Curr. Opin. Drug Discovery Dev.,* 2005, **8**, 38.
75. R. J. Andrade, M. Robles, E. Ulzurrun and M. I. Lucena, *Pharmacogenomics,* 2009, **10**, 1467.
76. Y. Huang, *Pers. Med.*, 2010, **7**, 5.
77. G. Farrell, D. Prendergast and M. Murray, *N. Engl. J. Med.,* 1985, **313**, 1310.
78. D. E. Malarkey, K. Johnson, L. Ryan, G. Boorman and R. R. Maronpot, *Toxicol. Pathol.,* 2005, **33**, 27.
79. J. R. Senior, *Pharmacoepidemiol. Drug Saf.*, 2006, **15**, 235.
80. R. Temple, *Pharmacoepidemiol. Drug Saf.*, 2006, **15**, 241.
81. J. H. Lewis, *Pharmacoepidemiol. Drug Saf.*, 2006, **15**, 221.
82. J. R. Senior, *Clin. Pharmacol. Ther.,* 2009, **85**, 331.
83. E. Bjornsson, *Clin. Pharmacol. Ther.,* 2006, **79**, 521.
84. L. Goldkind and L. Laine, *Pharmacoepidemiol. Drug Saf.*, 2006, **15**, 213.

85. Y. L. Lin, H. D. Chern and M. L. Chu, *Drug Inf. J.*, 2003, **37**, 155.
86. R. J. Andrade, M. Robles, A. Fernandez-Castaner, S. Lopez-Ortega, M. C. Lopez-Vega and M. I. Lucena, *World J. Gastroenterol.,* 2007, **13**, 329.
87. R. J. Andrade, M. Robles and M. I. Lucena, *Expert. Opin. Drug Saf.*, 2009, **8**, 709.
88. S. Russmann, G. A. Kullak-Ublick and I. Grattagliano, *Curr. Med. Chem.,* 2009, **16**, 3041.
89. J. Uetrecht, *AAPS J.,* 2005, **7**, E914.
90. F. Tacke, T. Luedde and C. Trautwein, *Clin. Rev. Allergy Immunol.,* 2009, **36**, 4.
91. G. L. Su, *Am. J. Physiol. Gastrointest. Liver Physiol.*, 2002, **283**, G256.
92. F. F. Tukov, J. F. Maddox, D. E. Amacher, W. F. Bobrowski, R. A. Roth and P. E. Ganey, *Toxicol. in Vitro*, 2006, **20**, 1488.
93. X. Deng, M. J. Liguori, E. M. Sparkenbaugh, J. F. Waring, E. A. Blomme, P. E. Ganey and R. A. Roth, *J. Pharmacol. Exp. Ther.,* 2008, **327**, 634.
94. P. J. Shaw, P. E. Ganey and R. A. Roth, *J. Pharmacol. Exp. Ther.,* 2009, **328**, 62.
95. P. E. Ganey, J. P. Luyendyk, J. F. Maddox and R. A. Roth, *Chem.–Biol. Interact.,* 2004, **150**, 35.
96. R. A. Roth and P. E. Ganey, *J. Pharmacol. Exp. Ther.,* 2010, **332**, 692.
97. I. Grattagliano, P. Portincasa, V. O. Palmieri and G. Palasciano, *Ann. Hepatol.,* 2002, **1**, 162.
98. B. D. Cosgrove, B. M. King, M. A. Hasan, L. G. Alexopoulos, P. A. Farazi, B. S. Hendriks, L. G. Griffith, P. K. Sorger, B. Tidor, J. J. Xu and D. A. Lauffenburger, *Toxicol. Appl. Pharmacol.,* 2009, **237**, 317.
99. T. Mahl and J. O'Grady, *Fast Facts: Liver Disorders*, Health Press Limited, Oxford, 006.
100. P. Mandrekar and G. Szabo, *J. Hepatol.,* 2009, **50**, 1258.
101. J. J. Xu, P. V. Henstock, M. C. Dunn, A. R. Smith, J. R. Chabot and D. de Graaf, *Toxicol. Sci.,* 2008, **105**, 97.
102. J. C. Fernandez-Checa and N. Kaplowitz, *Toxicol. Appl. Pharmacol.,* 2005, **204**, 263.
103. J. C. Fernandez-Checa, N. Kaplowitz, C. Garcia-Ruiz, A. Colell, M. Miranda, M. Mari, E. Ardite and A. Morales, *Am. J. Physiol.*, 1997, **273**, G7.
104. D. Han, N. Hanawa, B. Saberi and N. Kaplowitz, *Am. J. Physiol. Gastrointest. Liver Physiol.*, 2006, **291**, G1.
105. L. H. Lash, *Chem.–Biol. Interact.,* 2006, **163**, 54.
106. J. M. Jimenez-Lopez, D. Wu and A. I. Cederbaum, *Toxicol. in Vitro*, 2008, **22**, 106.
107. H. Licht, L. B. Seeff and H. J. Zimmerman, *Ann. Intern. Med.,* 1980, **92**, 511.
108. G. G. Gyamlani and C. R. Parikh, *Crit. Care*, 2002, **6**, 155.
109. C. J. McClain, J. P. Kromhout, F. J. Peterson and J. L. Holtzman, *JAMA, J. Am. Med. Assoc.*, 1980, **244**, 251.

110. A. S. Dabhi, K. J. Brahmbhatt, T. P. Pandya, P. B. Thorat and M. C. Shah, *J. Indian Acad. of Clin. Med.*, 2008, **9**, 36.
111. D. Preiss and N. Sattar, *Clin. Sci.*, 2008, **115**, 141.
112. G. Tarantino, P. Conca, V. Basile, A. Gentile, D. Capone, G. Polichetti and E. Leo, *Hepatol. Res.*, 2007, **37**, 410.
113. D. Greco, A. Kotronen, J. Westerbacka, O. Puig, P. Arkkila, T. Kiviluoto, S. Laitinen, M. Kolak, R. M. Fisher, A. Hamsten, P. Auvinen and H. Yki-Jarvinen, *Am. J. Physiol. Gastrointest. Liver Physiol.*, 2008, **294**, G1281.
114. D. D. Zhang, *Drug Metab. Rev.*, 2006, **38**, 769.
115. S. Numazawa and T. Yoshida, *J. Toxicol. Sci.*, 2004, **29**, 81.
116. L. M. Aleksunes and J. E. Manautou, *Toxicol. Pathol.*, 2007, **35**, 459.
117. S. O. Simmons, C. Y. Fan and R. Ramabhadran, *Toxicol. Sci.*, 2009, **111**, 202.
118. F. Liu, S. Ichihara, W. M. Valentine, K. Itoh, M. Yamamoto, M. S. Sheik, J. Kitoh and G. Ichihara, *Toxicol. Sci.*, 2010, **115**, 596.
119. W. Xu, C. Hellerbrand, U. A. Kohler, P. Bugnon, Y. W. Kan, S. Werner and T. A. Beyer, *Lab. Invest.*, 2008, **88**, 1068.
120. A. Enomoto, K. Itoh, E. Nagayoshi, J. Haruta, T. Kimura, T. O'Connor, T. Harada and M. Yamamoto, *Toxicol. Sci.*, 2001, **59**, 169.
121. H. Takakusa, H. Masumoto, A. Mitsuru, O. Okazaki and K. Sudo, *Drug Metab. Dispos.*, 2008, **36**, 816.
122. B. Hughes, *Nat. Rev. Drug Discovery*, 2008, **7**, 719.
123. W. M. Lee, *N. Engl. J. Med.*, 2003, **349**, 474.
124. I. Grattagliano, P. Portincasa, V. O. Palmieri and G. Palasciano, *Ann. Hepatol.*, 2002, **1**, 162.
125. J. M. Cullen, *Toxicol. Pathol.*, 2005, **33**, 6.
126. H. Jaeschke, G. J. Gores, A. I. Cederbaum, J. A. Hinson, D. Pessayre and J. J. Lemasters, *Toxicol. Sci.*, 2002, **65**, 166.
127. D. Han, M. Shinohara, M. D. Ybanez, B. Saberi and N. Kaplowitz, in Adverse Drug Reactions, ed. J. P. Uetrecht, *Handbook of Experimental Pharmacology*, Springer, New York, 2010, vol. 196, p. 267.
128. H. Jaeschke, *Toxicol. Sci.*, 2006, **89**, 31.
129. D. R. Dufour, J. A. Lott, F. S. Nolte, D. R. Gretch, R. S. Koff and L. B. Seeff, *Clin. Chem.*, 2000, **46**, 2050.
130. G. Liss and J. H. Lewis, *Expert. Opin. Drug Metab. Toxicol.*, 2009, **5**, 843.
131. D. M. Altmann, D. Sansom and S. G. Marsh, *Immunol. Today*, 1991, **12**, 267.
132. J. Klein and A. Sato, *N. Engl. J. Med.*, 2000, **343**, 782.
133. N. Chalasani and E. Bjornsson, *Gastroenterology*, 2010, **138**, 2246.
134. R. A. Wilke, D. W. Lin, D. M. Roden, P. B. Watkins, D. Flockhart, I. Zineh, K. M. Giacomini and R. M. Krauss, *Nat. Rev. Drug Discovery*, 2007, **6**, 904.
135. K. Pachkoria, M. I. Lucena, M. Molokhia, R. Cueto, A. S. Carballo, A. Carvajal and R. J. Andrade, *Curr. Drug Saf.*, 2007, **2**, 97.

136. Y. Wang, Y. Vodovotz, P. K. Kim, R. Zamora and T. R. Billiar, *Ann. N. Y. Acad. Sci.*, 2002, **962**, 415.
137. S. Inokuchi, T. Aoyama, K. Miura, C. H. Osterreicher, Y. Kodama, K. Miyai, S. Akira, D. A. Brenner and E. Seki, *Proc. Natl. Acad. Sci., U. S. A.*, 2010, **107**, 844.
138. V. Serriere-Lanneau, F. Teixeira-Clerc, L. Y. Li, M. Schippers, W. de Wries, B. Julien, J. Tran-Van-Nhieu, S. Manin, K. Poelstra, J. Chun, S. Carpentier, T. Levade, A. Mallat and S. Lotersztajn, *FASEB J.*, 2007, **21**, 2005.
139. B. Gao, *Cell. Mol. Immunol.*, 2005, **2**, 92.
140. S. Haga, K. Terui, H. Q. Zhang, S. Enosawa, W. Ogawa, H. Inoue, T. Okuyama, K. Takeda, S. Akira, T. Ogino, K. Irani and M. Ozaki, *J. Clin. Invest.*, 2003, **112**, 989.
141. A. Moh, Y. Iwamoto, G. X. Chai, S. S. Zhang, A. Kano, D. D. Yang, W. Zhang, J. Wang, J. J. Jacoby, B. Gao, R. A. Flavell and X. Y. Fu, *Lab. Invest.*, 2007, **87**, 1018.
142. H. Liu, C. Subramony and M. Nowicki, *Pediatr. Res.*, 2008, **63**, 613.
143. H. Ikeda, Y. Kume, K. Tejima, T. Tomiya, T. Nishikawa, N. Watanabe, N. Ohtomo, M. Arai, C. Arai, M. Omata, K. Fujiwara and Y. Yatomi, *Am. J. Physiol. Gastrointest. Liver Physiol.*, 2007, **293**, G911.
144. K. Fujimoto, K. Kumagai, K. Ito, S. Arakawa, Y. Ando, S. Oda, T. Yamoto and S. Manabe, *Toxicol. Pathol.*, 2009, **37**, 193.
145. T. P. Reilly, J. N. Brady, M. R. Marchick, M. Bourdi, J. W. George, M. F. Radonovich, C. A. Pise-Masison and L. R. Pohl, *Chem. Res. Toxicol.*, 2001, **14**, 1620.
146. M. T. Pritchard, J. I. Cohen, S. Roychowdhury, B. T. Pratt and L. E. Nagy, *J. Hepatol.*, 2010, **53**, 655.
147. E. O. Farombi and Y. J. Surh, *J. Biochem. Mol. Biol.*, 2006, **39**, 479.

CHAPTER 17

# Immunotoxicity Testing

THOMAS T. KAWABATA,* SANDRA CASINGHINO, MARK COLLINGE, CRIS KAMPERSCHROER AND JESSICA WHRITENOUR

Pfizer Inc., Drug Safety Research and Development, Groton, CT 06340, USA

## 17.1 Introduction

Immunotoxicology is the study of suppression or enhancement of the immune response by chemicals or drugs. Suppression of the immune response may result in decreased host resistance to pathogens or tumors. Immune enhancement or stimulation may result in the release of cytokines (cytokine release syndrome, CRS) or the development of autoimmune diseases. Immunotoxicology also includes the study of hypersensitivity reactions which are triggered by immune- and non-immune-mediated responses against chemicals or drugs.

This chapter will focus on immunotoxicity testing of drugs, both small molecular entities and biopharmaceuticals, but many of the approaches described may be applicable to non-drug chemicals. There are several reviews and book chapters available that describe many of the more commonly used assays.[1–3] In the future, we expect to see an increase in assays that can better bridge non-clinical findings to human risk. In addition, with the development of immunomodulatory agents against novel targets, many of which are biologicals and require testing in non-human primates (NHP), more sophisticated methods will be needed to assess unwanted immune modulation (*e.g.*, off-target effects or super-pharmacology). To this end, this chapter will focus on *in vitro* assays that utilize human cells. In addition, a section on

RSC Drug Discovery Series No. 12
New Horizons in Predictive Toxicology: Current Status and Application
Edited by Alan G. E. Wilson

Published by the Royal Society of Chemistry, www.rsc.org

*ex vivo* T-cell assays that can be used in conjunction with standard toxicity studies will be included. For this chapter, it is assumed that the reader has some understanding of basic immunology concepts. These basic concepts are needed to understand the different types of assays. More in-depth immunology background information will be provided to understand the specific assays covered in this chapter.

## 17.2 Developing Immunotoxicity Testing Strategies

For those toxicologists with a limited background in immunotoxicology, the development of an immunotoxicity testing strategy (which assays to use and when they should be used during the drug development process) can be a daunting task. This is attributed to the wide variety of assays available and a number of factors that must be considered, including the mechanism of action, planned clinical dosing regimens (acute *vs.* chronic) and potential impact of immunotoxicity in relation to the indication and current standard of care. In general, most immunotoxicology studies are designed on a case-by-case basis but follow the principles recommended in the ICH S8 guidance on "Immunotoxicity Testing of Human Pharmaceuticals".[4] Although the scope of the ICH S8 guidance is focused on small molecule drugs that are not intended to modulate the immune response, many of the principles are applicable to biologicals and drugs designed to be immunomodulators.

The first critical step in developing an immunotoxicology testing strategy is to determine whether testing is needed and if so, to determine if testing would involve assays beyond the typical endpoints included in standard toxicology studies (*e.g.*, hematology, thymus and spleen weights, histopathology of lymphoid organs). The decision involves taking into consideration several different factors such as: 1) findings from standard toxicity studies (*e.g.*, hematology, organ weights, histopathology), 2) pharmacological properties of the drug, 3) the intended patient population, 4) structural similarities to known immunomodulators, 5) the disposition of the drug (*e.g.*, in macrophages), and 6) clinical information that may suggest alterations to the immune system.

All of the gathered information is collectively evaluated and weighed to determine if there is a cause for concern. If there is sufficient cause for concern, additional immunotoxicity testing should be considered. The immunotoxicity testing strategy that one uses should be based on all data obtained. The field of immunology has been moving rapidly and there is a dizzying array of assays to choose from. Some assays simply quantify immune cells. Others are more complex functional assays that measure responses to foreign antigens or pathogens *in vitro* or *in vivo*. To help better understand the types of assays and their application, it is important to first understand the different ways that these assays may be classified. Three general classification schemes will be discussed, based on the type of immune response, the experimental design, or the number of different cell types involved.

# 17.3 Classification of Approaches for Immunotoxicity Tests

## 17.3.1 Classification According to the Type of Immune Response

Immunotoxicologists most often classify assays according the type of cell or function that is being measured. This classification scheme is divided into two major categories of immune responses: innate and adaptive. The innate immune system is the first line of defense that provides a quick response. This response involves the complement system, macrophages, neutrophils, natural killer T-cells (NKT) cells and natural killer (NK) cells. The adaptive immune response is divided into two subcategories: humoral and cell-mediated immunity. Humoral immunity involves the development of antigen-specific antibodies by B-cells which assist in the clearance of the antigen. Cell-mediated immunity involves the development of T-cell responses which leads to the killing of target cells. This occurs by the secretion of various cytokines and chemokines which leads to the recruitment and activation of other cell types involved in killing the invading organism.

Assays that evaluate innate and adaptive immune responses are usually classified according to the cell type and/or function involved. The following are the more common types of methods that immunotoxicologists use to assess innate and adaptive immunity (Table 17.1). There are several limitations to this classification scheme. The scheme does not directly apply to some types of

**Table 17.1** Classification scheme of immunotoxicity assays based on innate and adaptive immune responses.

| *Cell types* | *Function being measured* | *Assay description* |
|---|---|---|
| *Innate* | | |
| Macrophages, neutrophils, NK cells | Not applicable | Relative cell numbers in peripheral blood or tissues by hematology analysis/cytometry and/or histopathology |
| Monocytes, neutrophils | Phagocytosis | Ability to phagocytize beads or bioparticles |
| Neutrophils | Oxidative burst | Production of oxygen radicals following activation |
| NK cells | Killing | Killing target cells or cytokine production |
| *Adaptive* | | |
| B- and T-cells | Not applicable | Relative cell numbers in peripheral blood or tissues by cytometry or standard histopathology |
| B- or T-cells | Mitogen responses | Ability of B- and/or T-cells to respond and proliferate *in vitro* upon stimulation with a mitogen |
| B- and T-cell and APC | TDAR | Amount of antibody or antibody secreting cells produced upon *in vivo* immunization of test species administered test article |

NK: natural killer; APC: antigen presenting cell; TDAR: T-dependent antibody response.

hypersensitivity-like reactions (*e.g.*, pseudoallergic reactions or CRS) or to the situation in which cells of the innate and adaptive immune responses both contribute to the adaptive immune response (*e.g.*, T-dependent antibody response in which macrophages or dendritic cells act as antigen presenting cells).

### 17.3.2 Classification According to the Experimental Design

An alternative way to classify immunotoxicity assays is based on general experimental design (Table 17.2). By classifying assays in this manner, one may be able to better envision how they are used in the general scheme of immunotoxicity testing. This classification is based on drug-exposure schemes (*in vivo* or *in vitro*), whether a challenge is included and if the challenge is *in vitro* or *in vivo*. As shown in Table 17.2, there are five general types of assays. Type 1 assays are the most often used since they are required for most standard toxicity studies and can be easily built into toxicology studies. These involve drug treatment of animals with subsequent evaluation of lymphoid tissues,

**Table 17.2** Classification scheme of immunotoxicity assays according to experimental design.

| *Assay type* | *Drug exposure* | *Challenge exposure* | *Examples* |
|---|---|---|---|
| 1 | *In vivo* | None | Lymphoid organ weights and histopathology.<br>Hematology and lymphocyte subset analysis (immunophenotyping) by flow cytometry.<br>Measuring cytokines or complement fragments in serum/plasma. |
| 2 | *In vivo* | *In vivo* | T-Dependent antibody response (TDAR): immunization of rats with keyhole limpet hemocyanin (KLH) or another antigen and antigen-specific IgM and IgG are measured in serum by ELISA.<br>Delayed-type hypersensitivity response: immunize rats with antigen and several weeks later, challenge with an intradermal injection of antigen in the ear. Measure ear swelling (edema) 1–3 days after the challenge. |
| 3 | *In vivo* | *In vivo* | Mitogen stimulation assay: monkey blood lymphocytes are incubated *in vitro* with concanavalin A. Proliferative or cytokine response of the activated lymphocytes is measured.<br>Natural killer cell assay: spleen cells from rats are incubated with tumor cells *in vitro*. Natural killer cell activity is measured by the ability to lyse tumor cells. |
| 4 | *In vitro* | *In vitro* | Mishell–Dutton assay: spleen cells from mice are incubated with test drug and sheep red blood cells. The number of cells that produce sheep specific IgM antibody is measured. |
| 5 | *In vitro* | None | Cytokine release assay: incubation of a monoclonal antibody against a receptor on lymphocytes. Measure cytokines released into the supernatant. |

measuring numbers of cells within lymphocyte subsets or measuring cytokine levels in blood. They do not involve antigen or pathogen challenge.

Type 2 assays involve drug treatment of animals with an *in vivo* challenge phase. Examples include the T-dependent antibody response (TDAR) and the delayed-type hypersensitivity (DTH) response. More details on the TDAR are discussed below. Type 3 assays are also commonly called "*ex vivo*" assays that involve obtaining cells from drug-treated animals, challenging the cells with antigen or mitogens *in vitro* and then measuring the response of the cells. Examples provided are concanavalin A (ConA) responses and NK cell killing of tumor cells.

Type 4 assays involve *in vitro* drug exposure and *in vitro* challenge. A good example of this assay is the Mishell–Dutton assay in which primary antibody responses of mouse spleen cells are generated *in vitro* against sheep red blood cells. These assays are useful for compound screening due to the lower requirement of bulk compound needed and the higher throughput compared to *in vivo* studies. These assays can also be helpful to better understand the mechanism of immunotoxicity. Type 5 assays involve *in vitro* exposure to drug and measuring a response without antigen challenge. These assays evaluate the ability of the drug to stimulate an immune response. An example is the cytokine release assay in which drugs such as monoclonal antibodies are evaluated for their ability to stimulate cytokine production and release.

### 17.3.3 Classification Based on the Number of Cell Types Involved

Another way that immunotoxicologists categorize assays is in regards to the number of cell types that are required to ultimately generate a response. An example of an assay that requires several different cell types is the TDAR. Antigen immunization results in antigen processing and presentation by dendritic cells or macrophages. Antigen presentation and co-stimulation result in T-cell activation. Activated T-cells produce cytokines that can help antigen-activated B-cells to proliferate and differentiate to antibody-producing cells. Thus, if a drug has an effect on any one of the cell types, the antibody response will be altered. These types of "holistic" assays are primarily used to screen for immunotoxicity and therefore the TDAR is one of the key assays recommended in the ICH S8 guidance document.[4] On the other hand, there are also other types of assays that specifically evaluate the function of one type of cell. Examples of these "cell-specific" assays include the NK cell assay and anti-CD3 stimulation of T-cells. These assays are more commonly used to assess the affect of drugs on a specific cell type, and are sometimes considered second-tier assays that are used to investigate a specific cause for concern based on data from initial immunotoxicity studies. They are also often used in determining mechanism of action.

Historically, the more commonly used immunotoxicity tests are Type 1 and 2 assays since they can be incorporated into standard toxicity studies.

**Table 17.3** Classification scheme of the assays presented in this chapter.

| *Assay* | *Immune response* | *Design* | *Holistic/specific* |
|---|---|---|---|
| Pseudoallergic | Not applicable | *In vitro*/none | Specific |
| Complement | Innate | *In vitro*/none | Specific |
| Cytokine release | Not applicable | *In vitro*/none | Specific |
| HuLA | Adaptive/innate | *In vitro*/*in vitro* | Holistic |
| 3D Cultures | Adaptive/innate | *In vitro*/*in vitro* | Holistic |
| T-Cell response | Adaptive/innate | *In vivo*/*in vitro*; *in vitro*/*in vitro* | Holistic |

To evaluate specific effects on the immune system and to evaluate mechanism, Type 3–5 assays have been used. This chapter will focus on new or improved *in vitro* assays for immunotoxicity testing. First, testing approaches for pseudoallergic reactions (direct mast-cell activation and complement activation) and CRS will be discussed. These hypersensitivity-like reactions and associated assays do not require antigen challenge. Second, the other assays will focus on testing the effects of drug on secondary immune responses with *in vitro* antigen challenge. This includes the human lymphocyte activation (HuLA) assay, 3D culture systems and T-cell assays. Table 17.3 lists these assays and how they fit into the three classification schemes.

# 17.4 Hypersensitivity Reactions

## 17.4.1 Background

Hypersensitivity has been defined as "a response observed by exposure to a stimulus at a dose that is tolerated in normal subjects".[5] However, in practice, the term hypersensitivity is more broadly used to describe a wide variety of adverse drug reactions including anaphylaxis, infusion reactions, cytokine release syndrome, delayed-type cutaneous reactions, and pseudoallergy. Although each of these falls under the category of drug hypersensitivity and in some cases may present with a similar clinical picture, the mechanisms driving the pathogenesis of the responses can be quite different.

In the broadest terms, hypersensitivity responses can be categorized based on mechanism, that is, whether the observed reaction is immune-mediated or not (Figure 17.1). In immune-mediated hypersensitivity responses, antigen-specific components of the immune system (antibodies, T-cells) drive the response. For example, in the case of anaphylaxis, the cross-linking of drug-specific IgE on the surface of mast cells or basophils leads to cellular degranulation and subsequent severe (and sometimes life-threatening) biological effects such as hypotension, urticaria, bronchospasm, nausea, and erythema. Delayed-type drug hypersensitivity responses (typically manifested in the form of a skin rash) can also be attributed to the generation of an immune response against the drug. In this case, hapten formation due to the generation of reactive metabolites or direct interaction of the drug with endogenous proteins can lead to T-cell sensitization. The idiosyncratic nature of immune-mediated

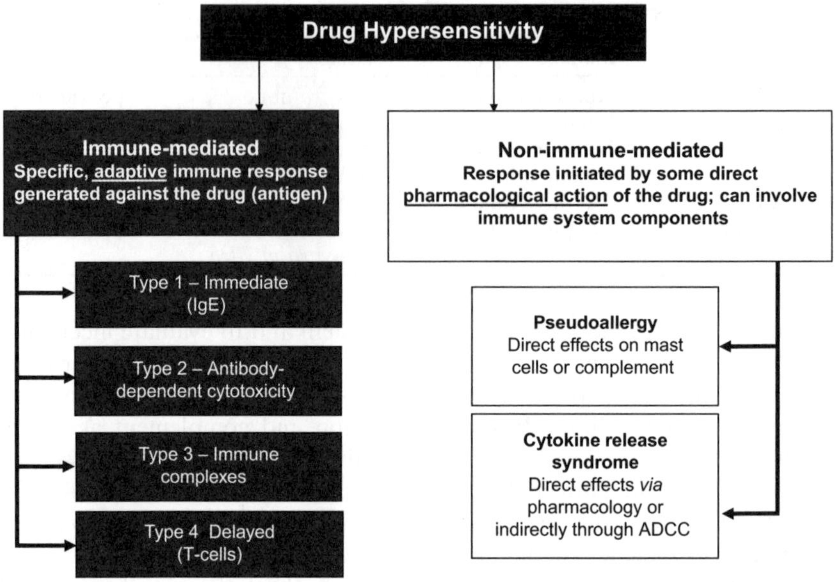


**Figure 17.1** Drug hypersensitivity classification scheme.

hypersensitivity responses coupled with the lack of full understanding behind individual susceptibility factors and the absence of animal models, make predicting this category of hypersensitivity responses difficult.

Non-immune mediated reactions are not caused by an immunological mechanism (*e.g.*, drug-specific IgE or T-cells) (Figure 17.1). These reactions most often occur with the first dose of intravenously administered drugs with an onset of minutes to a few hours after administration and with transient symptoms (lasting hours to one day) similar to those observed for IgE-mediated reactions. Non-immune-mediated reactions can be generally subcategorized according to mechanism and include pseudoallergy (or anaphylactoid) and CRS (Figure 17.1). The term, "infusion reaction" is also commonly used to describe immune and non-immune hypersensitivity reactions that occur soon after intravenous administration. This section will focus on pseudoallergic reactions; CRS will be discussed in more detail later in this chapter.

Pseudoallergic reactions are clinically indistinguishable from IgE-mediated hypersensitivity reactions since both (in most cases) appear to be due to the widespread activation and degranulation of mast cells and/or basophils. However, these reactions can be differentiated based on the mechanism by which the cellular degranulation occurs. In the case of pseudoallergy, drugs activate mast cells and/or basophils either directly or indirectly in an IgE-independent fashion. This activation may occur due to drug-induced osmotic stress, binding of drug to G-protein-coupled receptors on mast cells, and/or activation of the complement cascade, resulting in the release of the anaphylatoxins C3a and C5a.[6–9] Aside from effects on mast-cells/basophils, other mechanisms of pseudoallergy include drug-induced alterations in eicosanoid synthesis (*e.g.*, aspirin) and/or disruptions in bradykinin synthesis and metabolism (*e.g.*, contaminated heparin, angiotensin-converting enzyme inhibitors).[10,11]

## 17.4.2 Pseudoallergic Reactions

### *17.4.2.1 Direct Stimulation of Mast Cells*

Mast cells are located in tissues throughout the body and mature into populations with functional and biochemical phenotypes specific for the anatomical area in which they are located.[12,13] In contrast, basophils are mainly found in the circulation. Both cell types express the high-affinity IgE receptor (FcεRI) and contain cytoplasmic granules where preformed mediators such as histamine, proteases, and some cytokines are stored and released from the cell *via* exocytosis upon stimulation.[12,14] In addition, these cells can also release newly synthesized mediators such as prostaglandins and additional cytokines in response to activation. The normal physiological role for mast cells and basophils is believed to be in acute, IgE-dependent hypersensitivity responses, which help to provide immunity against some pathogens, especially parasites. However, inappropriate, uncontrolled activation of these cells (as occurs in a pseudoallergic response) can have severe consequences. Therefore, non-clinical methods to reliably predict such responses are needed.

Pseudoallergic responses appear to be pharmacologically related as evidenced by the following observations: responses are usually observed with the first dose and are typically dose-dependent and transient; subsequent responses are not observed in the absence of a secondary exposure; and there is no escalation in the severity of the response with additional exposure. Thus, the possibility exists that predictive models for pseudoallergy can be successfully developed. *In vitro* and *in vivo* models have been used to evaluate compounds for their potential to induce mast cell degranulation. Measurements of histamine release as an indicator of cellular degranulation are most frequently reported, although studies have looked at the release of other mediators stored in mast cell granules such as tryptase, serotonin, cytokines, and platelet-activating factor.[15–17] With regard to histamine measurements, older studies have utilized fluorometric or radioenzymatic methods, whereas more recent studies have taken advantage of commercial histamine enzyme-linked immunosorbent assay (ELISA) kits that are available for both cell culture and biological fluid sample types. The ELISA kits come in a 96-well format and are relatively simple to perform, however cost may be a concern if a large number of samples require analysis.

*In vitro* studies using primary human mast cells as well as mast cells isolated from a variety of species have demonstrated the ability to detect histamine release following exposure to non-immunological stimuli.[9,18–20] Although the use of these *in vitro* models has demonstrated the success for evaluating drug-induced mast cell degranulation, several limitations exist that must be kept in mind when interpreting data. For example, the tissue source of the mast cells (skin, lung, peritoneum), cell-isolation procedures and culture conditions (presence or absence of serum proteins, calcium) can all affect the response. Also important are the differences in species sensitivity to a particular stimulus.

Mast cell lines including the rat basophilic leukemia and human LAD2 and HMC-1 lines have been established and used for investigating drug-induced mast-cell degranulation.[21] However, the extent of the similarities (or dissimilarities) to mature tissue mast cells is not yet fully known, thus questioning the usefulness of these models for predicting human responses.[22,23]

Histamine release from basophils has also been used as a tool for evaluating activation of this cell type.[24] This has mainly been done as a diagnostic test after an anaphylactic or pseudoallergic response has been observed in the clinic. However, the time and technical restraints of this method have limited the widespread usage of basophils for developing a predictive assay for pseudoallergic reactions.

The *in vitro* differentiation of human progenitor cells to generate mast-cell cultures has been reported.[25] As in the case of the human cell lines, the functional similarities of these differentiated cell populations to that of mature tissue mast cells may not be fully appreciated. Moreover, in the context of pseudoallergy, the usefulness of human progenitor-derived mast cells has not been extensively explored. Recently, an *in vitro* model using human $CD34^+$ hematopoietic stem cell-derived mast cells has been investigated as a tool for predicting pseudoallergic responses.[26] Data from these studies have demonstrated the sensitivity of this model for detecting mast cell degranulation (measured by histamine release) induced by compounds known to produce pseudoallergic reactions in humans (*e.g.*, morphine, tubocurarine). While this approach has demonstrated promising results, further validation and determination of the specificity and sensitivity of the response need to be completed. One major limitation of this model is the assumption of a direct effect of the drug on the mast cell, as opposed to an indirect effect resulting from complement activation or some other mechanism. Thus, as with any *in vitro* system, one must interpret the data in the context of the *in vivo* study data. All in all, successful development of this model may prove to be a useful, and desperately needed, tool for predicting pseudoallergic drug responses in humans.

### *17.4.2.2 Complement Activation*

The complement system is a vital component of a host's innate immune response against infection and is composed of about thirty proteins, many of which are enzymes. Activation of complement triggers a tightly regulated cascade of events that culminates in inflammation and destruction or removal of the offending organisms. This cascade contributes to pathogen resistance using several mechanisms. Complement facilitates phagocytosis of organisms through opsonization or induces inflammation by producing anaphylatoxins and thereby stimulating recruitment of immune cells to the site of infection. Also, several complement proteins are capable of combining to form the membrane-attack complex (MAC), which inserts into bacterial cell membranes, forms a pore and results in lysis of the organism. Complement system proteins also enhance B-cell responses to antigens and contribute to the clearance of damaging large antigen–antibody complexes.

The complement cascade proceeds by three intertwined pathways, namely the classical, alternative and lectin pathways. The classical pathway is initiated by the binding of the complement protein C1 to antigen–antibody complexes. These complexes can be host antibodies bound to proteins on pathogen surfaces, or circulating soluble immune complexes, such as those found in patients with autoimmune diseases like systemic lupus erythematosus. The alternative pathway is triggered when complement protein C3b is deposited on the surface of an organism or of a biomaterial. The lectin pathway is activated when mannose residues on organisms bind mannan-binding lectin on host cells.[27] The role of complement in innate immunity and the complement activation scheme are reviewed elsewhere.[28]

Excessive systemic complement activation can lead to pseudoallergic reactions. Complement fragments are known to stimulate the degranulation of mast cells and the release of various components such as histamine. Various drugs or vehicles that are administered intravenously are known to produce pseudoallergic reactions through complement activation. These vehicles or drug-delivery systems may appear as danger signals to the host and interact with complement system proteins, triggering the cascade. Complement can be activated by nanoparticles (carbon nanotubes),[29,30] liposomes,[31,32] Cremophor EL and radio-contrast media.[6] Complement-activation measurements have been shown to correlate with clinical symptoms in patients receiving liposomal doxorubicin,[33] suggesting that *in vitro* screening assays for complement activation may be predictive.

Biological therapeutics such as antibodies and oligonucleotides have induced serious side-effects associated with complement activation. For example, OKT3 is an antibody therapeutic used to prevent and treat transplanted organ rejection. Serious respiratory side-effects correlated with complement activation, although causality was not proven. The mechanism of complement activation was hypothesized to involve OKT3-coated T-lymphocytes.[34] Rituximab, used to treat non-Hodgkin's lymphoma, induced complement activation in some patients. This activation correlated with the severity of side-effects, as well as with the level of circulating B-cells at the start of infusion, leading to a proposal that the mechanism involved the interaction of rituximab with B-cells.[35] In a Phase I trial, the antisense phosphorothionate oligonucleotide therapeutic, ISIS 5132, induced serious adverse events in patients with advanced cancer. Dose-dependent complement activation by the drug was demonstrated. Oligonucleotides with phosphorothionate backbones were previously shown to activate complement in non-human primate studies.[36,37]

It should also be noted that complement activation is a major pathway for some types of immune-mediated Type III-like hypersensitivity reactions.

For example, the administration of monoclonal antibody drugs may lead to the generation of circulating anti-drug IgG antibodies. With subsequent administration of drug, anti-drug antibodies form immune complexes with the drug, and may lead to systemic complement activation, resulting in symptoms similar to pseudoallergic and immune-mediated IgE reactions.

The potential for severe clinical adverse events, and the speed and intensity of the response to danger signals, provide the rationale for the necessity of complement-activation testing of human serum with novel drug substances such as biological therapeutics and drug-delivery vehicles during preclinical evaluation. In addition, if there is a suspected risk for complement activation, preliminary *in vitro* studies using serum from the toxicity test species may be advisable to prevent significant toxicities during toxicology studies. In addition, if direct complement activation is suspected in toxicity studies, *in vitro* complement activation assays may be used to investigate potential mechanisms. In general, the design of the *in vitro* complement activation assay is relatively simple. Human serum or serum from species used for toxicity studies is incubated with the test article for at least 30 min. As activation occurs, complement fragments accumulate in serum or plasma, and can be measured by several methods as described below.

The preferred and easiest method to measure complement activation is by ELISAs specific for individual complement fragments. Several of the activated fragments can be assayed using commercial kit formats for human samples. Commonly measured fragments are C3a des-Arg (arginine is immediately cleaved from C3a upon activation to the more stable form C3a des-Arg), C5a and sC5b-9 (soluble form of MAC). Measurement of Bb and C4d can determine whether complement activation is occurring by the alternative or classical pathways, respectively (Figure 17.2). Alternatively, the fragments can be assayed by Western blot if the appropriate antibodies are available. Fortunately, many of the anti-human complement antibodies also cross-react with cynomolgus and rhesus macaque complement fragments (C3a des-Arg, sC5b-9, Bb, C4d). On the other hand, antibodies to individual human complement fragments do not generally react with rodent or canine complement fragments. Although there are commercially available antibodies to the unactivated parent complement protein, C3, for rodents and canines, these cannot be used to measure complement activation by ELISA, since they are not specific for the activation fragments.

When immunoassays for complement fragments are not available, alternative assays such as the hemolytic assay may be used. The hemolytic assay, commonly known as the CH50 assay, measures complement consumption and has been widely used for many years. This assay uses IgG-coated sheep red blood cells (SRBC), which are lysed by the MAC. The quantity of lysed SRBC, which is measured spectrophotometrically, is proportional to the amount of complement in the original sample. The advantages of the hemolytic assay are that the assay does not require expensive reagents and works for multiple species without a need for species-specific antibodies. However, this assay is limited by low sensitivity (measures complement consumption rather than

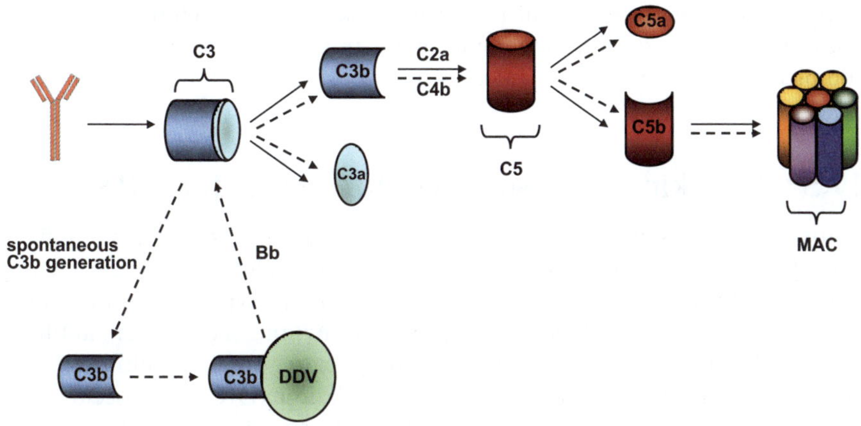


**Figure 17.2** Activation of the complement pathways by biotherapeutics and drug-delivery vehicles. Therapeutic antibodies may trigger the classical pathway (solid arrows) resulting in the cleavage of complement protein C3 into C3a (anaphylatoxin) and C3b. C3b subsequently interacts with other complement proteins (C2a and C4b) to form an enzyme that cleaves C5 into C5a (anaphylatoxin) and C5b. C3b is constitutively cleaved from C3 at low levels through hydrolysis. C3b binds to some drug-delivery vehicles (DDV), then interacts with complement protein Bb, triggering the alternative pathway (dashed arrows), and like the classical pathway, results in cleavage of C5. C5b from both pathways initiates the formation of the membrane attack complex (MAC). Anaphylatoxins, C3a and C5a, have potent biological activity and can lead to severe adverse clinical events.

generation of complement fragments), potential assay interference by drug-delivery vehicles and the use of SRBC which have a short shelf life and may vary from lot-to-lot.[38]

Another approach involves indirectly measuring complement activation by thromboxane B2 (TXB2) generation *in vivo*. This approach may be useful for examining the effects of a test article on complement activation in rats and dogs. *In vivo*, complement activation fragments induce thromboxane A2 (TXA2) production by platelets. TXA2 is labile and is quickly converted to the more stable TXB2. Increases in TXB2 levels are therefore an indirect indication of the amount of complement activation.[29] Availability of a commercial ELISA kit for TXB2 and the ability to be used with multiple species are the advantages of this assay, but there are several limitations: the measurement of complement activation is indirect, stress to the animals can induce TXB2, platelets may be activated directly by the test material and results between animals can be variable. Additional work is needed to determine if this is a viable alternative to measuring complement activation fragments.

Ongoing development of new biotherapeutics and nanoscale drug-delivery platforms is driving the need for non-clinical complement activation testing. Determination of the mechanisms by which these therapeutics interact with complement proteins is critical to designing safe and efficacious drugs. Antibody reagents for rat and dog complement fragments are needed to test for complement activation in toxicology studies.

## 17.5 Cytokine Release Assay to Predict for CRS

Cytokine release syndrome (CRS) or "cytokine storm" is a systemic inflammatory immune response characterized by a variety of symptoms including headache, chills, fever, nausea, vomiting, myalgia and hypotension. In extreme cases, such as the cytokine storm produced by the monoclonal antibody TGN1412,[39] tissue and organ damage, pulmonary cellular infiltrates, renal failure, and disseminated intravascular coagulation (DIC) may occur. CRS occurs primarily on first infusion with biopharmaceutical drugs and is associated with systemic increases in pro-inflammatory cytokines including TNF-α, IFN-γ and IL-6. This production of cytokines may be the result of intended pharmacology or indirect antibody dependent cellular cytotoxicity (ADCC).

A number of therapeutic monoclonal antibodies (mAbs) are known to cause CRS[40] including OKT3 (muromonab-anti-CD3),[41–43] anti-CD52 (alemtuzumab; CAMPATH-1H)[44,45] and anti-CD20 (rituximab).[46] A comprehensive review of antibodies associated with CRS has recently been published[47] and will not be discussed in detail here. While TGN1412 was not the first therapeutic mAb to be associated with CRS, it is perhaps the most high-profile case and has significantly raised the importance of non-clinical predictive testing for CRS. During clinical testing of TGN1412, six healthy male volunteers developed symptoms consistent with CRS.[39] TGN1412 is an anti-CD28 superagonist antibody, capable of activating T-cells without the need for prior engagement of the T-cell receptor (TCR). A number of *in vivo* preclinical toxicity studies in rodent and NHP models, as well as *in vitro* testing with human cells were performed. However, these failed to predict CRS upon first-dose administration in humans.[40]

These *in vitro* experiments included presenting TGN1412 to human peripheral blood mononuclear cells (PBMC) either alone or cross-linked *via* its Fc portion in solution. Subsequently it was found that TGN1412 only stimulated pro-inflammatory cytokine release *in vitro* if appropriately presented to human PBMCs either by immobilization of antibody onto tissue culture plastic, or added to PBMCs that were co-cultured with endothelial cells.[48,49]

The proposed mechanisms for occurrence of CRS include direct pharmacological effects on immune cells which may involve direct binding of an antibody to its target on immune cells (*e.g.*, muromonab-CD3 and TGN1412) or direct stimulation through toll-like receptors (*e.g.*, LPS, oligonucleotides). Cytokine release may also be mediated by ADCC (*e.g.*, CAMPATH-1H, rituximab).[44,45] This is often an intended, indirect mechanism for several mAb that are targeted to kill certain tumors. The mAb will first bind to its target on the tumor cells. Natural killer cells will then bind to the Fc region of the antibodies (primarily IgG1 antibodies) *via* their Fc receptors (CD16).

This leads to the activation of NK cells and release of cytokines such as interferon-γ and TNF-α. Thus the tumor burden with first administration may determine the severity of ADCC-related cytokine release.

The Committee for Medicinal Products for Human use (CHMP) guidelines[50] on strategies to identify and mitigate risks for first-in-human (FIH) clinical trials note that when planning a FIH clinical trial, sponsors and investigators should identify all risk factors and apply appropriate risk mitigation strategies. Cytokine release is identified as one such risk factor, and regulatory agencies have subsequently requested sponsors to assess whether biologic therapeutics are capable of eliciting *in vitro* cytokine release.[48,51] However, there is no consensus on the preferred methods or how results should be interpreted, but that this should be considered on a case-by-case basis.[51] It has been recommended that the selected assay design should be mechanism-based and may need to be modified to best fit the mechanism.[52] There are several factors to consider in selecting the best assay design, such as assay format, the use of whole blood or PBMCs, and the types of cytokine to measure.

There are two general assay formats that are commonly used: the soluble- and solid-phase assays. The soluble-phase assays involve incubating human whole blood or PBMCs with the test drug for 4–24 h. The cells are pelleted and the supernatant is collected for cytokine analysis by standard immunoassay methods (ELISA or multiplex beads or plates). The solid-phase assays use the dry-coat method developed by Stebbings and co-workers.[48] For this method, the test biological therapeutic is added as a solution into polystyrene or polypropylene 96-well plates and air dried. As an alternative, anti-Fc antibody is dry-coated on the plates and is used to bind and capture the test mAb, *via* its Fc region. This method was found to be as effective as the direct dry-coating approach. Cell culture media, PBMCs and test article are added and incubated for 4–24 h. Cell culture supernatant is collected and analyzed for cytokines. Controls for these assays include vehicle or media control as negative controls, and the addition of anti-CD3 as a positive control.

The solid-phase assay format was developed in response to the TGN1412 incident. The soluble-phase method was not able to replicate cytokine release *in vitro*. However, the solid-phase method produced a robust response.[48] The ability of TGN1412 to induce cytokine release only when immobilized suggests that this process permits some form of cross-linking, allowing TGN1412 to be presented to CD28 in a manner similar to the *in vivo* situation. In contrast to TGN1412, anti-CD3 antibodies are able to stimulate in either the soluble- or solid-phase formats.

For mAbs that are of the IgG1 subclass, ADCC may be a concern. Appropriate testing formats to predict cytokine release or severity of the cytokine release have not been adequately developed. *In vitro* assays for ADCC can be developed but the translation of these findings to FIH clinical trials has not been established. While it has been noted that immobilization of antibodies often generates more robust responses, assay formats that include immobilization may not be appropriate for mAbs that mediate their effects through Fc-receptors (ADCC). There is also concern that the Fc region of the dry-coated

IgG1 antibody may cross-link macrophages or NK cells and stimulate cytokine release, producing an artifact of the assay rather than a real mechanism for cytokine release *in vivo*.

Another factor to consider for assay design is the use of whole blood or PBMCs. In general, PBMCs produce greater cytokine release than whole blood in these assays. This may be due to a number of factors, including decreased interference of red blood cells binding to the target, initial activation or priming of the cells during the isolation procedure, or removal of molecules that normally down-regulate cytokine release which are present in whole blood.[52] While PBMCs may give a more robust response, they may lack critical factors present in whole blood, for example complement or other soluble mediators.

The specific types of cytokines chosen to analyze should at least include TNF-α, IL-6 and IFN-γ. Other pro-inflammatory cytokines (*e.g.*, IL-1, IL-8) may also be measured but are likely to parallel production of TNF-α, IL-6 and IFN-γ. For NK-mediated ADCC reactions and for T-cell-mediated reactions, it is expected that TNF-α and IFN-γ will be released. Macrophage activation would result in IL-6 and TNF-α release. The panel of cytokines measured should ultimately be based on possible targets and the types of cytokines produced. In general, a very large panel of cytokines is not necessarily needed since there is significant co-regulation of synthesis of cytokines.

Cytokine release assays are best used for hazard identification[52] but may also be useful to provide data on the potential mechanism for CRS in human. Drugs ranging from small molecules to large biologics may benefit from CRAs but products which target membrane- bound antigens and receptors of immune cells, rather than soluble molecules, potentially pose the biggest risk.[52] The current state of the science is not adequate to allow specific recommendations on the most appropriate CRA format for different targets and mechanisms of action. It is also not possible with current assays to define a threshold or limit for cytokine release above which would there would be a cause for concern for CRS in humans.[52] In some cases cytokine release due to ADCC or an intended pharmacologic effect may be an expected effect. For these situations, extrapolating the *in vitro* findings to what may happen *in vivo* would be difficult with current assays. At best, it may be possible to rank different compounds to minimize undesired effects. There is consensus[52] that a positive result in a CRA would not necessarily be a reason to stop development of a program, but should be used in risk–benefit management through risk-mitigation strategies for FIH studies. However, one of the key challenges is to ensure that a negative *in vitro* CRA can reliably be used to make assumptions about human risk.

Despite these challenges, the CRA should be helpful in predicting the potential to trigger CRS in humans and the clinical consequences. However, the failure of the pre-clinical testing of TGN1412 to predict toxicity in man provides an excellent example which highlights the need for better *in vitro* methods for prediction of CRS. Several companies developing mAbs are actively using the CRA and will continue to improve upon the method to meet their needs.

## 17.6 Human Lymphocyte Activation (HuLA) Assay

As described in the introduction to this chapter, *in vitro* assays using human immune cells are being developed to enhance the translation of non-clinical findings to humans. The *in vivo* TDAR assay is a widely used approach for assessing drug-induced immunotoxicity. The response generated with this method relies upon the functional coordination between antigen processing and presentation by antigen-presenting cells, and B- and T-cells to generate antibody-secreting cells. A drug-induced suppression of a TDAR may trigger additional testing to determine specifically which cell type(s) is being targeted by the drug. Although the TDAR assay is currently recommended in guidance documents for drugs that may pose a risk for immunotoxicity,[4] there are several drawbacks that limit the routine use of the assay for standard immunotoxicity assessment. For example, the need for satellite animals increases the overall numbers of animals as well as the quantity of drug required to run such a study. In addition, although the TDAR assay has been shown to be sensitive to known immunosuppressants,[53] the extrapolation of results from pre-clinical species to human risk assessment may not always be clear cut.

*In vitro* assays that require less drug than *in vivo* methods have also been developed. One such example is the Mishell–Dutton assay that evaluates primary or secondary antibody responses of rodent spleen cells to sheep red blood cells (a T-dependent antigen).[54] Although animal numbers and drug requirements are not considered limitations for this assay, the use of rodent cells raises some concerns about the translatability of the response. Furthermore, this method has proven to produce variable responses both within and between different laboratories.

The development of an *in vitro* assay that addresses many of the limitations of the aforementioned methods was recently published.[55] The HuLA assay, like the TDAR, is capable of assessing both the innate (antigen-presentation) and adaptive (T- and B-cell responsiveness) immune response in one assay system. The HuLA assay is performed *in vitro* using human cells, which addresses the concerns of translatability, drug requirement, and animal usage that limit the widespread usage of other available methods. Briefly, the HuLA assay uses fresh or frozen human PBMCs from flu-vaccinated individuals and evaluates the proliferation of these cells when stimulated *in vitro* with the flu antigen. Inhibition of cell proliferation against the flu antigen when treated with a test compound suggests an impairment of the immune response. The sensitivity of the HuLA assay to known immunosuppressive drugs with different mechanisms of action (rapamycin, cyclosporine, methotrexate, mycophenolate and dexamethasone) was recently demonstrated.[55] The $IC_{50}$ values of these compounds in the HuLA assay were similar to their respective target therapeutic exposure ranges.

The benefits of the HuLA assay include the low amount of drug required, the use of human cells, medium throughput, a high signal-to-noise proliferative response, and the simplicity of the assay endpoints. Moreover, other endpoints may be evaluated based on the specific question being asked of the assay. Such endpoints may include measuring the production of flu-specific antibody secreting cells, cytokine secretion and the identification of the specific cell types that proliferate in response to antigen (determined by flow cytometry). Although the sensitivity of the HuLA assay was demonstrated across multiple individual human donors, the ability of other labs to replicate these data is needed in order to confirm the robustness of the assay between labs.

The HuLA assay may be used to help rank the relative immunosuppressive properties of different compounds early in the discovery phase so that the best compound may be selected for clinical development. It may also be used to determine potential off-target effects on the immune system. For example, if a drug being developed targets macrophage function to inhibit inflammation, the HuLA assay may help determine if the desired pharmacologic effect translates into decreased adaptive immune responses. As another example, if signals from standard toxicity assays suggest potential immunotoxicity (*e.g.*, decreased circulating lymphocytes, lymphocyte depletion in the spleen or lymph nodes), the HuLA assay may be a relatively simple way to help determine potential risk in humans.

### 17.6.1 Three-dimensional Immune Cell Cultures

Along the lines of the HuLA assay described above, one of the approaches to assess the effects of drugs on human immune function is through the use of an *in vitro* assay that uses multiple human cell types (holistic) to mimic complex immune processes. This is necessary since many of the immune responses require complex interactions of many types of cells, such as monocytes, macrophages, dendritic cells and T- and B-lymphocytes. The HuLA assay addresses these needs but is considered a two-dimensional (2D) tissue culture assay system. Other 2D systems include simple mitogen-response assays using PBMC or *in vitro* T-cell systems described in the following section. These are considered 2D since cells are added to culture wells and are not similar to lymphoid organs with a three-dimensional (3D) structure. The HuLA assay and the antigen-specific T-cell assays evaluate secondary (recall) responses to antigen. Two-dimensional cultures of human PBMC are unable to generate primary immune responses *in vitro*. So why is it important to also evaluate primary immune responses? Since the processes and cell types involved in secondary immune responses differ from primary responses, certain drugs may not alter secondary response but may inhibit primary responses. In addition, the ability to generate a primary immune response *in vitro* may help determine potential immunogenicity or allergenicity of low-molecular-weight drugs or biologicals. A 3D system may also enhance the predictivity of assays for immunostimulatory drugs (*e.g.*, CRA), especially for drugs that target receptors on leukocyte subsets that may not be present in PBMCs. Therefore, more complex *in vitro* systems comprised of more types of cells that better mimic lymphoid organs are needed. Systems that can more completely represent the complexity of the human immune system could lead to improvements in the accuracy of immunotoxicology prediction and reduce the number of animals needed for toxicology studies.

Three-dimensional *in vitro* systems may address these needs by providing additional cell types and a more natural architecture that is critical to mimic the lymph node *in vivo*. These cultures would also contain dendritic cells (DC) that are needed for antigen presentation and/or stromal epithelial cells that provide support for lymphocyte development and differentiation, and contribute to the architecture of the lymph node. In the HuLA assay and the *in vitro* secondary T-cell assays, antigen presentation to T-cells most likely is mediated by macrophages and B-cells for the recall response. However, with primary immune responses, DC may be needed for antigen presentation. Several 3D systems have been or are being developed. These systems contain biomaterial scaffolds which support cell attachment and migration of immune cells, resulting in more physiologically relevant cell-to-cell interactions.

The MIMIC® system was designed to evaluate the immunogenicity of novel vaccines (primary immune responses) in humans to help select the best clinical candidates for development. This system is composed of several components, a peripheral tissue equivalent (PTE) and a lymphoid tissue equivalent (LTE), designed to simulate the innate immune response and the adaptive immune response, respectively. The PTE contains a collagen matrix, endothelial cells and whole blood or PBMCs (Figure 17.3). Monocytes enter the matrix and differentiate into DC without exogenously added cytokines. The LTE is comprised of activated DC (derived from the PTE), as well as lymphocytes, and is capable of producing activated T-cells, antibodies and cytokines, mimicking lymph node function.[56] Several immunomodulators have been tested in this system and responses of the MIMIC® system have agreed well with the known *in vivo* biological activities of the immunomodulators. For example, Toll-like receptor (TLR) agonists, poly I:C, lipopolysaccharide, Gardiquimod and CpG, known activators of immune cells, induced cytokine and chemokine production and promoted DC differentiation and maturation in PTE.[57] Known immunosuppressive agents such as cyclosporine A, methotrexate and dexamethasone, all inhibited MIMIC® activity.[56] The MIMIC® system has been used to elicit *in vitro* antigen-specific antibody responses to tetanus[58,59] and influenza,[56] using cells from vaccinated individuals, indicating functional recall responses. Primary immune responses to vaccines and keyhole limpet hemocyanin (KLH) have also been demonstrated. MIMIC® cultures composed of naïve cells significantly increased IgG production when exposed to a seasonal influenza vaccine,[56] and IgM production when exposed to KLH.[60]

A human lymph node micro-organoid model has been developed by ProBioGen and contains PBMCs and DCs that have been seeded in agarose and cultured in disposable miniaturized bioreactors for up to 30 days. This long-term culture system allows repeated drug exposure. In this model, human monocytes are differentiated into mature DCs using cytokines and growth factors followed by exposure to antigen. The cellular immune response to antigen is measured by

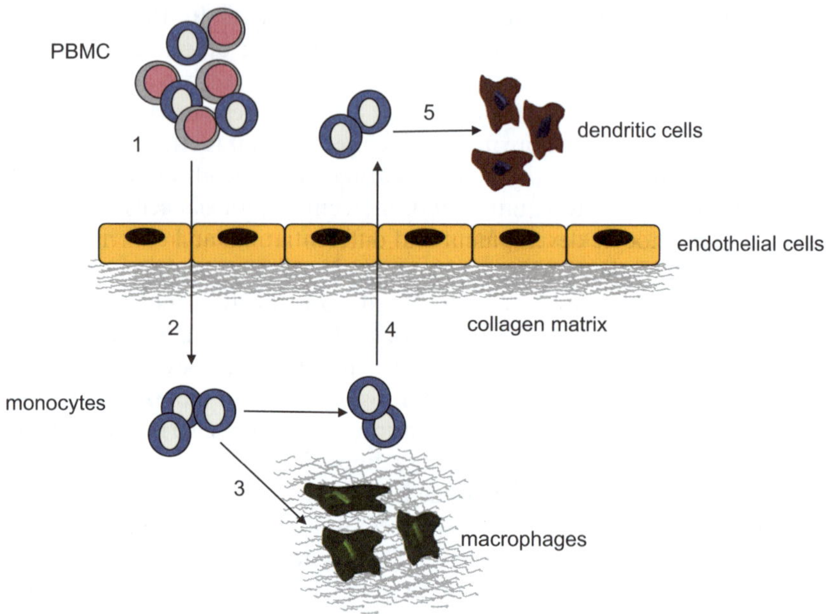


**Figure 17.3** Three-dimensional immune construct. PBMCs are added to a confluent layer of endothelial cells grown on a collagen matrix (1). Monocytes migrate through the endothelial cells into the collagen (2). The monocytes differentiate into macrophages which remain in the collagen layer (3) or migrate back through the endothelial layer (4) where they differentiate into dendritic cells (5), remarkably without the addition of exogenous cytokines.

cytokine analysis while humoral immunity is verified by B-cell activation, plasma-cell formation and secretion of IgM and IgG antibodies.[61] In this model, LPS increases cytokine release[61] and dexamethasone decreases cytokine release,[62] reflecting their natural immune-modulating activities. Primary immune responses to the hepatitis A vaccine (Havrix) were demonstrated by increased IL-2 release and production of hepatitis-A-specific IgM.

Xenogeneic thymic organoids have been produced by seeding carbon matrices with murine thymic stroma and human-bone-marrow-derived hematopoetic progenitor cells. After 14 days in culture, 62% of the cells in the organoid were T-lymphocytes, and both $CD4^+$ (T-helper-cells) and $CD8^+$ (cytotoxic T-cells) cells were identified. The T-lymphocytes were shown to be functional since they responded to both mitogenic and antigenic stimulation.[63] This system can potentially be used to generate human T-cells for drug toxicity testing.

Nichols *et al.*[64] developed a bone marrow analog by seeding human stromal and hematopoetic stem cells into a unique scaffold that mimicked the structural topology of the natural bone marrow matrix. This system was capable of generating functional B-cells, as evidenced by expression of key signal proteins, presence of immunoglobulin class switching and production of antigen-specific antibodies.[64]

While great progress has been made toward addressing the complexity of the human immune response through the use of 3D architecture and the inclusion of multiple cell types, more refinements and development of additional systems are needed. The 3D culture technology is still in its infancy and at present several limitations exist. These include having a low-throughput format, as well as high cost due to technical complexity and requirement of a highly skilled work force. Future technological advances are needed to overcome these limitations. Recent advancements include engineering of human lymph vessels aimed at improving lymphoid 3D models,[65] increasing assay throughput by use of a chip-based multi-micro-organoid culture system[66] and development of artificial spleens in rodents that someday may be applicable to create human *in vitro* spleen culture systems.[67,68] Most importantly, the relevance of 3D culture technology remains unproven, and only after additional studies have been conducted, will the ability of these *in vitro* assays to predict human immunotoxicology be determined.

## 17.7 *In Vitro* T-Cell Assays

T-Cells play a key role in adaptive immune responses and altered T-cell functions may lead to increased infections and neoplasm. Unexpected effects of drugs on T-cells could impact the development of drugs and put patients at risk, if appropriate risk-management approaches are not used during clinical trials. In order to address these concerns, we need methods to predict the effects of drugs on T-cells. In addition to evaluating the number of T-cells and T-cell subsets there is a need to measure T-cell function and the number of T-cells which are capable of responding to specific stimuli (mitogens or antigen).

The decision to perform testing for T-cell function, like immunotoxicology testing in general, is made on a case-by-case basis (ICH S8). There are certain findings in toxicology studies that would alert an investigator to a potential effect on T-cells. For example, alterations in thymus weight or histology and/or substantial changes in lymphocyte numbers would suggest T-cell effects. Increased infections in toxicity studies, may also suggest effects on T-cells depending the type of infection observed. T-cell assays may also be included in the toxicity testing paradigm if there is concern based on the known pharmacology of the test article.

T-Cell function in the whole animal can be measured using a delayed-type hypersensitivity response (Type 2 assay). Animals are treated with test compound, immunized with an antigen (or may already be immunized to environmental antigens) and challenged with the antigen by the intradermal route. Twenty four to 48 hours later the immune response is measured in the skin by evaluating swelling and/or cellular infiltrate. This assay is challenging to conduct and is difficult to incorporate into standard toxicity studies. Satellite groups or stand-alone studies are needed. An alternative is the use of *ex vivo*

Type 3 assays in which animals are treated with test article, immune cells are collected and the T-cell responses to mitogens or antigens are evaluated *in vitro*. These types of assays can be readily incorporated into toxicity studies. With non-rodent studies (*e.g.*, non-human primates and dogs), blood samples may be collected over the course of the toxicity study. These assays may also be modified for Type 4 assays. This would involve culturing cells from untreated animals with mitogen or antigen along with test article and then measuring T-cell responses.

This section will focus on Type 3 *ex vivo* T-cell assays. To understand these assays, the following overview of T-cell biology is provided. In general, there are two major T-cell subsets, CD4 and CD8 T-cells. The control of intracellular infections and tumor growth depends heavily on the functions of cytotoxic CD8 T-cells. CD8 T-cells protect the host from intracellular infections and tumor growth by directly recognizing cells bearing foreign antigen and killing them. CD8 T-cells recognize infected cells or tumor cells as foreign through binding of the T-cell receptor (TCR) to small peptides derived from foreign proteins that are presented on the cell surface by major histocompatibility (MHC) class I molecules. This recognition of peptide-MHC complexes (along with co-stimulatory signals) activates CD8 T-cells to become cytotoxic T-lymphocytes (CTL) capable of killing antigen-bearing target cells (*e.g.*, tumor cells, virus-infected cells).[69,70] CD4 T-cells, also known as T-helper (Th) cells, are thought of as the conductors of the immune response since they can influence the functions of nearly all immune cell types. Their TCRs recognize foreign antigens presented by MHC class II molecules on the surface of cells, typically professional antigen-presenting cells (APC) like dendritic cells and macrophages. Naïve CD4 T-cells can differentiate into various helper T-cell (Th) subpopulations upon antigen recognition depending on the environment in which they are stimulated—these include but are not limited to Th1, Th2, Th17, follicular helper T-cells (Tfh), and regulatory T-cells (Treg).[71–74] These different Th subsets can have a range of different functions mediated by either cytokine secretion or expression of cell surface molecules. Th-derived cytokines can shape the immune response as it develops, and can mean the difference between health and disease by balancing protective immunity *versus* pathology or immune suppression *versus* autoimmunity.

In the past, T-cell responses have most often been measured *in vitro* or *ex vivo* by stimulating mixed cultures of cells with mitogens, superantigens, or other reagents known to activate T-cells regardless of TCR specificity (collectively termed as "mitogens"). Examples include concanavalin A (ConA), phytohemagglutinin (PHA), staphylococcal enterotoxin B (SEB), pokeweed mitogen, phorbol myristate acetate (PMA) plus ionomycin, and anti-CD3 antibody with or without anti-CD28 antibody. After stimulation, responses are typically detected by measuring either bulk proliferation or by measuring cytokines secreted into the supernatant.[75–78] These methods have the advantage that they are relatively inexpensive and easy to use, often work in multiple species, and generate responses from a large proportion of T-cells that are easily detected. While these methods are useful for probing general T-cell responsiveness, they can be generally less sensitive to known immunosuppressive drugs and their mechanisms of T-cell activation are generally different from biological recognition of foreign antigens. Additionally, they cannot be used for measuring responses against specific pathogens of concern.

Measuring *in vitro* antigen-specific T-cell responses may better reflect T-cell function *in vivo*. In general, these assays involve incubating antigen and immune cells (from PBMCs or lymphoid organs) from animals or individuals that already have been exposed to that specific antigen in the past. The immune response generated *in vitro* is a secondary response and is mediated by memory T-cells. This is the approach used for the HuLA assay described above (Type 4 assay). Another approach is to evaluate secondary immune responses to pathogens such as latent infections (*e.g.*, herpes viruses) for which the test animal will have already developed a T-cell response. The antigen used for these *in vitro* assays may be purified or recombinant proteins, synthetic peptides, killed pathogens or cell lysates from pathogen-infected cells. For toxicity studies, the animals may be immunized before the start of the dosing phase or during the dosing phase of the study (primary immune response). Immune cells are then collected from these animals for *ex vivo* evaluation.

Antigen-specific T-cell responses may be measured by evaluating cell proliferation or cytokines in culture supernatants as described for the mitogen responses. However, more current methods are able to measure T-cell responses on an individual cell basis. These methods are able to provide more information about effects on specific function and leukocyte subsets. The more commonly used assays include the enzyme-linked immunosorbant spot (ELISPOT) assay, intracellular cytokine staining (ICS), and peptide–MHC multimer staining. ELISPOT is used to detect factors like cytokines that are secreted by stimulated T-cells and enumerates cells secreting the factor. The cytokine most commonly measured is IFN-$\gamma$ but ELISPOT has been used to detect many different cytokines secreted by T-cells. Other molecules, like perforin or granzymes secreted by CTL during granule exocytosis, can also be measured using ELISPOT.[79] The advantage to ELISPOT is that it can detect very low frequencies of responding T-cells.[80]

The major drawback of the ELISPOT is that it does not provide phenotypic information on the responding cells (*e.g.*, CD4 *vs.* CD8 T-cells). The ICS method enumerates cells that produce cytokines in response to an antigenic stimulus but can also provide phenotypic information about the responding cells. ICS measures cytokines produced by stimulated T-cells, but cytokine is detected inside cells after stimulation of T-cells in the presence of intracellular transport inhibitors. The cytokine is detected using flow cytometry, allowing for staining of other markers to determine the phenotype of responding cells.[81] A drawback to ICS is that it requires specialized training and sophisticated equipment and is difficult to standardize across different laboratories. An additional consideration for cytokine-based readouts is that antigen-specific cells can only be detected if they produce the cytokines tested.

To determine the number of antigen-specific T-cells irrespective of function, soluble recombinant peptide–MHC complexes can be used. Because of the relatively low affinity of the TCR for peptide–MHC complexes, the peptide–MHC molecules must be multimerized (typically as tetramers or pentamers) to gain enough avidity to be useful as a staining reagent.[82] Stable multimers of MHC class II are also available, although they are technically more difficult to produce than those with MHC class I due to issues of stability.[83] For staining, peptide–MHC multimers are usually conjugated to fluorescent molecules so they can be visualized using flow cytometry, which allows them to be combined with ICS and any number of other staining reagents to detect phenotypic properties of T-cells. Thus, if for example you are interested in determining the effect of a test drug on the number of CD8 T-cells that are specific for cytomegalovirus (CMV), class I multimers containing peptides of CMV can be used to determine the absolute number of CMV-specific CD8 T-cells. In addition, markers associated with T-cell activation (CD25, CD69, CD40 ligand, 4-1BB and many others), markers of proliferation (Ki-67), markers that identify degranulating CTL or NK cells (CD107a), or markers that identify specific T-cell subsets or T-cell functions can be used to further characterize the CMV-specific T-cells. Due to the large amount of information that can be determined at the single-cell level, flow cytometry is an extremely powerful tool for measuring antigen-induced T-cell responses, and its use is now widespread in academic and industry settings.[81]

In summary, *in vitro* T-cell responses can be measured using *ex vivo* Type 3 assays. These assays may have broader use than the delayed-type hypersensitivity response assay (Type 2 assay). However, there are several limitations when compared to Type 2 assays. Immune responses are often measured in peripheral blood and these cell types may not reflect the response of the entire immune system. In addition, numbers of circulating leukocyte subpopulations are known to fluctuate with stress (*e.g.*, during dosing and blood collection). If PBMCs are used, drug will be removed during the processing of the cells from blood. Thus, drug is not present during the *in vitro* activation of the PBMCs by mitogen and antigen. For drugs that inhibit lymphocyte activation or antigen presentation that occurs during the culture period of the assay, *ex vivo* responses to mitogens or antigens will not be altered. This is an important point since most *ex vivo* assays do not work optimally in whole blood and PBMCs are needed.

To produce T-cell responses in culture, *ex vivo* Type 3 T-cell assays use two general stimuli: mitogens and specific antigens. There are a number of pros and cons to be considered when determining if mitogens or antigen-specific T-cell assays should be used (Table 17.4). The major benefit of the antigen-specific T-cell response is its greater relevance to true immune response to pathogens, which may make it more sensitive to immunosuppression than mitogen-induced T-cell responses. On the other hand, antigens of interest must be known and it must be possible to generate either protein or peptide antigens for assays. In addition, individual peptide epitopes are restricted by specific MHC alleles, some of which may be at low frequencies in a given population, yet

**Table 17.4** Pros and cons of measuring T-cell responses to antigens or mitogens.

| *Antigen-specific T-cell response* | *Mitogen-induced T-cell response* |
|---|---|
| **Pros** | **Pros** |
| Measures T-cell responses in relevant biological context | Stimulating reagents easily obtained and inexpensive |
| Can monitor T-cell immunity against pathogens of concern | Stimulating reagents effective in multiple species |
| May be more sensitive to immunosuppression | Responses large and easily detected |
| **Cons** | **Cons** |
| Frequency of responders is often low, making responses difficult to detect | Mechanisms of T-cell activation generally not biologically relevant |
| Must know antigen of interest and have a source of peptide or protein antigen | Cannot measure T-cell responses against specific pathogens |
| Need to do MHC typing of subjects if defined peptide epitopes are used | Do not generally provide information at the single-cell level |
| Information on epitopes and MHC not available in some species (*e.g.*, rat, dog) | |

MHC: Major histocompatibility complex.

MHC typing is not always practical or even feasible. Also, reagents for more sophisticated methods are often not available for some species used for toxicology, such as dog or rat. This has limited the use of such methods for general immunotoxicology evaluations during drug development.

## 17.8 Conclusions

A portion of this chapter focused on the growing use of human cells for *in vitro* immunotoxicity assays. The major advantage of using human cells is the greater translation to human risk. Additionally, many of the reagents such as monoclonal antibodies and cytokines for these assays are already commercially available. There are also several challenges and limitations of these *in vitro* assays. One of the primary concerns is with donor-to-donor variability. Depending on the assay and cell type, the differences observed could be significant. Thus, several donors need to be evaluated when developing and validating the assays as well as during the actual testing of the drug. Another challenge is the translation of exposure levels that have an effect *in vitro* to what may occur at similar exposure levels *in vivo*. For these approaches, as more experience is gained, we may be able to get around some of these issues and further expand our repertoire of testing methods.

This chapter also focused on the use of *ex vivo* assays to monitor T-cell function from animals in toxicity studies. These assays may be used more in the future since they can readily be incorporated into the design of most toxicity studies and responses may be followed over the course of the study. It is expected that in the future, methods to monitor antigen-specific T-cell responses in toxicity studies may be further expanded using novel antigens and in multiple species. In addition, reagents for these assays in various toxicology species may be more readily available.

## References


1. *Immunotoxicity Testing: Methods and Protocols*, ed. R. R. Dietert, Humana Press, New York City, 2009.
2. *Immuntoxicology Strategies for Pharmaceutical Safety Assessment*, ed. D. B. Herzyk and L. Jeanine, John Wiley & Sons, New York, 2008.
3. *Methods in Immunotoxicology*, ed. G. R. D. Burleson, H. Jack and A. E. Munson, Wiley-Liss, New York, 1995.
4. Department of Health and Human Services, *Federal Register*, 2006, **71**, 19193–19194.
5. S. G. Johansson, J. O. Hourihane, J. Bousquet, C. Bruijnzeel-Koomen, S. Dreborg, T. Haahtela, M. L. Kowalski, N. Mygind, J. Ring, P. van Cauwenberge, M. van Hage-Hamsten and B. Wuthrich, *Allergy*, 2001, **56**, 813–824.
6. J. Szebeni, *Toxicology*, 2005, **216**, 106–121.
7. K. E. Barke and L. B. Hough, *Life Sci.*, 1993, **53**, 1391–1399.
8. M. Mousli, C. Bronner, Y. Landry, J. Bockaert and B. Rouot, *FEBS Lett.*, 1990, **259**, 260–262.
9. K. Mori, C. Maru, K. Takasuna and K. Furuhama, *Eur. J. Pharmacol.*, 2000, **394**, 51–55.
10. E. A. Berkes, *Clin. Rev. Allergy Immunol.*, 2003, **24**, 137–148.
11. L. B. Schwartz, *N. Engl. J. Med.*, 2008, **358**, 2505–2509.
12. L. B. Schwartz, *Curr. Opin. Immunol.*, 1994, **6**, 91–97.
13. S. J. Galli, J. Kalesnikoff, M. A. Grimbaldeston, A. M. Piliponsky, C. M. Williams and M. Tsai, *Annu. Rev. Immunol.*, 2005, **23**, 749–786.
14. S. J. Galli, J. R. Gordon and B. K. Wershil, *Curr. Opin. Immunol.*, 1991, **3**, 865–872.
15. M. Veien, F. Szlam, J. T. Holden, K. Yamaguchi, D. D. Denson and J. H. Levy, *Anesthesiology*, 2000, **92**, 1074–1081.
16. P. Vadas, M. Gold, B. Perelman, G. M. Liss, G. Lack, T. Blyth, F. E. Simons, K. J. Simons, D. Cass and J. Yeung, *N. Engl. J. Med.*, 2008, **358**, 28–35.
17. A. D. Hogan and L. B. Schwartz, *Methods*, 1997, **13**, 43–52.
18. D. C. Morrison, J. F. Roser, B. J. Curry, P. M. Henson and R. J. Ulevitch, *Inflammation*, 1978, **3**, 7–25.
19. K. Mori, C. Maru and K. Takasuna, *J. Pharm. Pharmacol.*, 2000, **52**, 577–584.
20. J. M. Hermens, J. M. Ebertz, J. M. Hanifin and C. A. Hirshman, *Anesthesiology*, 1985, **62**, 124–129.
21. M. Kulka, C. H. Sheen, B. P. Tancowny, L. C. Grammer and R. P. Schleimer, *Immunology*, 2008, **123**, 398–410.

22. S. Guhl, M. Babina, A. Neou, T. Zuberbier and M. Artuc, *Exp. Dermatol.*, 2010, **19**, 845–847.
23. K. M. Carroll, E. M. Carey and B. A. Helm, *J. Chromatogr., B: Anal. Technol. Biomed. Life Sci.*, 2002, **771**, 289–301.
24. H. Nishi, S. Nishimura, M. Higashiura, N. Ikeya, H. Ohta, T. Tsuji, M. Nishimura, S. Ohnishi and H. Higashi, *J. Immunol. Methods*, 2000, **240**, 39–46.
25. M. Holm, H. B. Andersen, T. E. Hetland, C. Dahl, H. J. Hoffmann, S. Junker and P. O. Schiotz, *J. Immunol. Methods*, 2008, **336**, 213–221.
26. K. Haskell, J. Whritenour, C. Donahue, W. Blake, T. Wolfram, L. He, T. Kawabata and M. Thiede, *J. Immunol.*, 2010, **184**, 86.3.
27. R. Coico and G. Sunshine, *Immunology: a short course*, John Wiley & Sons, Hoboken, NJ, 6th edn, 2009.
28. D. Ricklin, G. Hajishengallis, K. Yang and J. D. Lambris, *Nat. Immunol.*, 2010, **11**, 785–797.
29. I. Hamad, A. Christy Hunter, K. J. Rutt, Z. Liu, H. Dai and S. Moein Moghimi, *Mol. Immunol.*, 2008, **45**, 3797–3803.
30. C. Salvador-Morales, E. Flahaut, E. Sim, J. Sloan, M. L. Green and R. B. Sim, *Mol. Immunol.*, 2006, **43**, 193–201.
31. J. Szebeni, L. Baranyi, S. Savay, J. Milosevits, R. Bunger, P. Laverman, J. M. Metselaar, G. Storm, A. Chanan-Khan, L. Liebes, F. M. Muggia, R. Cohen, Y. Barenholz and C. R. Alving, *J. Liposome Res.*, 2002, **12**, 165–172.
32. S. M. Moghimi, A. J. Andersen, S. H. Hashemi, B. Lettiero, D. Ahmadvand, A. C. Hunter, T. L. Andresen, I. Hamad and J. Szebeni, *J. Control. Release*, 2010, **146**, 175–181.
33. A. Chanan-Khan, J. Szebeni, S. Savay, L. Liebes, N. M. Rafique, C. R. Alving and F. M. Muggia, *Ann. Oncol.*, 2003, **14**, 1430–1437.
34. M. H. Raasveld, F. J. Bemelman, P. T. Schellekens, F. N. van Diepen, A. van Dongen, E. A. van Royen, C. E. Hack and I. J. ten Berge, *Kidney Int.*, 1993, **43**, 1140–1149.
35. L. E. van der Kolk, A. J. Grillo-Lopez, J. W. Baars, C. E. Hack and M. H. van Oers, *Br. J. Haematol.*, 2001, **115**, 807–811.
36. R. Advani, B. L. Lum, G. A. Fisher, J. Halsey, R. S. Geary, J. T. Holmlund, T. J. Kwoh, F. A. Dorr and B. I. Sikic, *Invest. New Drugs*, 2005, **23**, 467–477.
37. C. M. Rudin, J. Holmlund, G. F. Fleming, S. Mani, W. M. Stadler, P. Schumm, B. P. Monia, J. F. Johnston, R. Geary, R. Z. Yu, T. J. Kwoh, F. A. Dorr and M. J. Ratain, *Clin. Cancer Res.*, 2001, **7**, 1214–1220.
38. J. Szebeni, L. Baranyi, S. Savay, J. Milosevits, M. Bodo, R. Bunger and C. R. Alving, *Methods Enzymol.*, 2003, **373**, 136–154.
39. G. Suntharalingam, M. R. Perry, S. Ward, S. J. Brett, A. Castello-Cortes, M. D. Brunner and N. Panoskaltsis, *N. Engl. J. Med.*, 2006, **355**, 1018–1028.
40. M. Wing, *J. Immunotoxicol.*, 2008, **5**, 11–15.

41. D. Abramowicz, L. Schandene, M. Goldman, A. Crusiaux, P. Vereerstraeten, L. De Pauw, J. Wybran, P. Kinnaert, E. Dupont and C. Toussaint, *Transplantation*, 1989, **47**, 606–608.
42. R. S. Gaston, M. H. Deierhoi, T. Patterson, E. Prasthofer, B. A. Julian, W. H. Barber, D. A. Laskow, A. G. Diethelm and J. J. Curtis, *Kidney Int.*, 1991, **39**, 141–148.
43. C. Sgro, *Toxicology*, 1995, **105**, 23–29.
44. M. G. Wing, T. Moreau, J. Greenwood, R. M. Smith, G. Hale, J. Isaacs, H. Waldmann, P. J. Lachmann and A. Compston, *J. Clin. Invest.*, 1996, **98**, 2819–2826.
45. M. G. Wing, H. Waldmann, J. Isaacs, D. A. Compston and G. Hale, *Ther. Immunol.*, 1995, **2**, 183–190.
46. U. Winkler, M. Jensen, O. Manzke, H. Schulz, V. Diehl and A. Engert, *Blood*, 1999, **94**, 2217–2224.
47. P. J. Bugelski, R. Achuthanandam, R. J. Capocasale, G. Treacy and E. Bouman-Thio, *Expert Rev. Clin. Immunol.*, 2009, **5**, 499–521.
48. R. Stebbings, L. Findlay, C. Edwards, D. Eastwood, C. Bird, D. North, Y. Mistry, P. Dilger, E. Liefooghe, I. Cludts, B. Fox, G. Tarrant, J. Robinson, T. Meager, C. Dolman, S. J. Thorpe, A. Bristow, M. Wadhwa, R. Thorpe and S. Poole, *J. Immunol.*, 2007, **179**, 3325–3331.
49. R. Stebbings, S. Poole and R. Thorpe, *Curr. Opin. Biotechnol.*, 2009, **20**, 673–677.
50. The Committee for Medicinal Products for Human Use Guidelines, European Medicines Agency, London, 2007.
51. C. J. Horvath and M. N. Milton, *Toxicol. Pathol.*, 2009, **37**, 372–383.
52. J. M. Vidal, T. T. Kawabata, R. Thorpe, B. Silva-Lima, K. Cederbrant, S. Poole, J. Mueller-Berghaus, M. Pallardy and J. W. Van der Laan, *Cytokine*, 2010, **51**, 213–215.
53. M. I. Luster, D. G. Pait, C. Portier, G. J. Rosenthal, D. R. Germolec, C. E. Comment, A. E. Munson, K. White and P. Pollock, *Toxicol. Lett.*, 1992, **64–65**, 71–78.
54. R. I. Mishell and R. W. Dutton, *Science*, 1966, **153**, 1004–1006.
55. M. Collinge, S. H. Cole, P. A. Schneider, C. B. Donovan, C. Kamperschroer and T. T. Kawabata, *J. Immunotoxicol.*, 2010, **7**, 357–366.
56. http://www.vaxdesign.com/.
57. Y. Ma, L. Poisson, G. Sanchez-Schmitz, S. Pawar, C. Qu, G. J. Randolph, W. L. Warren, E. M. Mishkin and R. G. Higbee, *Immunology*, 2010, **130**, 374–387.
58. B. C. Schanen and D. R. Drake III, *J. Immunol. Methods*, 2008, **335**, 53–64.
59. A. M. Byers, T. M. Tapia, E. R. Sassano and V. Wittman, *Biologicals*, 2009, **37**, 148–151.
60. W. L. Warren, H. Fahlenkamp, R. Higbee, A. Kachurin, C. Li, M. Nguyen, R. Parkhill, G. Sanchez-Schmitz, D. J. Irvine, G. J. Randolph, N. Hacohen, B. Torbett, Inventors; Assigned to VaxDesign Corp., Orlando, FL, USA, *United States Pat.*, US 7,855,074, 2010.
61. C. Giese, A. Lubitz, C. D. Demmler, J. Reuschel, K. Bergner and U. Marx, *J. Biotechnol.*, 2010, **148**, 38–45.

62. C. Giese, C. D. Demmler, R. Ammer, S. Hartmann, A. Lubitz, L. Miller, R. Muller and U. Marx, *Artif. Organs*, 2006, **30**, 803–808.
63. M. C. Poznansky, R. H. Evans, R. B. Foxall, I. T. Olszak, A. H. Piascik, K. E. Hartman, C. Brander, T. H. Meyer, M. J. Pykett, K. T. Chabner, S. A. Kalams, M. Rosenzweig and D. T. Scadden, *Nat. Biotechnol.*, 2000, **18**, 729–734.
64. J. E. Nichols, J. Cortiella, J. Lee, J. A. Niles, M. Cuddihy, S. Wang, J. Bielitzki, A. Cantu, R. Mlcak, E. Valdivia, R. Yancy, M. L. McClure and N. A. Kotov, *Biomaterials*, 2009, **30**, 1071–1079.
65. T. Hitchcock and L. Niklason, *Ann. N. Y. Acad. Sci.*, 2008, **1131**, 44–49.
66. F. Sonntag, N. Schilling, K. Mader, M. Gruchow, U. Klotzbach, G. Lindner, R. Horland, I. Wagner, R. Lauster, S. Howitz, S. Hoffmann and U. Marx, *J. Biotechnol.*, 2010, **148**, 70–75.
67. T. C. Grikscheit, F. G. Sala, J. Ogilvie, K. A. Bower, E. R. Ochoa, E. Alsberg, D. Mooney and J. P. Vacanti, *J. Surg. Res.*, 2008, **149**, 214–218.
68. S. H. Glanville, V. Bekiaris, E. J. Jenkinson, P. J. Lane, G. Anderson and D. R. Withers, *Eur. J. Immunol.*, 2009, **39**, 280–289.
69. M. Barry and R. C. Bleackley, *Nat. Rev. Immunol.*, 2002, **2**, 401–409.
70. M. R. Jenkins and G. M. Griffiths, *Curr. Opin. Immunol.*, 2010, **22**, 308–313.
71. K. M. Murphy and B. Stockinger, *Nat. Immunol.*, 2010, **11**, 674–680.
72. N. Fazilleau, L. J. McHeyzer-Williams, H. Rosen and M. G. McHeyzer-Williams, *Nat. Immunol.*, 2009, **10**, 375–384.
73. D. A. Vignali, L. W. Collison and C. J. Workman, *Nat. Rev. Immunol.*, 2008, **8**, 523–532.
74. C. T. Weaver, R. D. Hatton, P. R. Mangan and L. E. Harrington, *Annu. Rev. Immunol.*, 2007, **25**, 821–852.
75. M. J. Barten, S. Dhein, H. Chang, H. B. Bittner, A. Tarnok, A. Rahmel, F. W. Mohr and J. F. Gummert, *J. Immunol. Methods*, 2003, **283**, 99–114.
76. M. Carfi, A. Gennari, I. Malerba, E. Corsini, M. Pallardy, R. Pieters, H. Van Loveren, H. W. Vohr, T. Hartung and L. Gribaldo, *Toxicology*, 2007, **229**, 11–22.
77. F. J. Dumont, M. J. Staruch, S. L. Koprak, M. R. Melino and N. H. Sigal, *J. Immunol.*, 1990, **144**, 251–258.
78. H. Lebrec, R. Roger, C. Blot, G. R. Burleson, C. Bohuon and M. Pallardy, *Toxicology*, 1995, **96**, 147–156.
79. A. Malyguine, S. Strobl, L. Zaritskaya, M. Baseler and K. Shafer-Weaver, *Adv. Exp. Med. Biol.*, 2007, **601**, 273–284.
80. M. McCutcheon, N. Wehner, A. Wensky, M. Kushner, S. Doan, L. Hsiao, P. Calabresi, T. Ha, T. V. Tran, K. M. Tate, J. Winkelhake and E. G. Spack, *J. Immunol. Methods*, 1997, **210**, 149–166.
81. D. L. Bolton and M. Roederer, *Expert Rev. Vaccines*, 2009, **8**, 779–789.
82. J. D. Altman, P. A. Moss, P. J. Goulder, D. H. Barouch, M. G. McHeyzer-Williams, J. I. Bell, A. J. McMichael and M. M. Davis, *Science*, 1996, **274**, 94–96.
83. E. A. James, R. LaFond, I. Durinovic-Bello and W. Kwok, *J. Vis. Exp.*, 2009, DOI: 10.3791/1167.

CHAPTER 18

# In Vitro *Developmental Models and Their Applications in Teratology Research*

KAREN AUGUSTINE-RAUCH,* JULIETA M. PANZICA-KELLY AND CINDY X. ZHANG

Bristol–Myers Squibb, Discovery Toxicology Group, 311 Pennington-Hopewell Road, Pennington, NJ 08534, USA

## 18.1 Introduction

Although research in mechanisms of normal and abnormal development has been active throughout the last century, the tragedy of thalidomide in the late 1950s led to substantial growth of the field and establishment of the Teratology Society in the 1960s. In these early years, the research focused on characterizing teratogenicity of substances in whole-animal models. However as teratogenic agents were identified and characterized, a need for *in vitro* systems became evident. This chapter provides an overview of various developmental model systems and how they have been applied to study mechanisms underlying normal and abnormal development. In addition, generation of developmental toxicology screens is described with an emphasis on how high-throughput strategies are currently being integrated. By no means does the content cover all of the critical advances that occurred over the last few decades but attempts to reflect vignettes of notable advances that have contributed to the current state of the science with an emphasis on advancements that have been beneficial for characterizing/optimizing safety profiles of chemicals in a more rapid, cost-effective manner.

RSC Drug Discovery Series No. 12
New Horizons in Predictive Toxicology: Current Status and Application
Edited by Alan G. E. Wilson

Published by the Royal Society of Chemistry, www.rsc.org

## 18.2 An Overview of Developmental Model Systems

Between 1960s and 1980s, developmental model systems were extensively studied and culture conditions were optimized. These included whole-embryo culture and tissue grafting techniques to study mechanisms of development, as well as the development of cell-based assays like the rodent midbrain and limb bud micromass assays and the embryonic stem cell test (EST) to assess the embryotoxic potential of chemicals.

### 18.2.1 Whole-Embryo Culture Models

#### *18.2.1.1 Mammalian Embryo Culture (Rodent and Rabbit)*

Rodent whole-embryo culture techniques were established about two decades after avian embryo culture when Denis New published a successful method for culturing rat postimplantation embryos from gestation day nine to gestation day 11 (the period of major organogenesis)[1] (Figure 18.1). Unlike other attempts to grow rodent embryos, New's technique incorporated the use of rotating bottles which simulated growth *in vivo*. About a year later, Sadler modified New's technique to culture post-implantation mouse embryos.[2] These

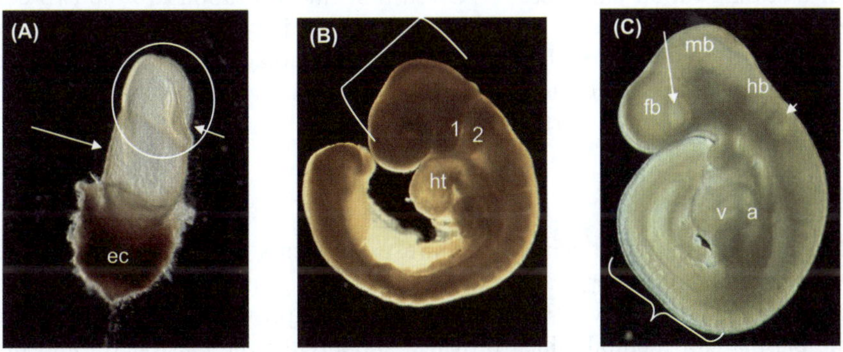


**Figure 18.1** Representative developmental stages of cultured rodent embryos. A) Mouse or rat embryos are entered into culture at the early neurulation stage. The embryo (circled) is beginning neurulation with the headfold (small arrow) present. In culture, the embryo is prepared so that it remains within the amniotic sac which is surrounded by the intact visceral yolk sac (large arrow) and attached to the ectoplacental cone (ec). B) At approximately 24 h in culture, the neural folds are undergoing closure and other organogenesis is underway. The primitive brain (bracket), two pharyngeal arches (1 and 2) and heart are apparent. C) Mid organogenesis-stage rat embryo at 44 h in culture. Brain development has advanced to discern three vesicles (the forebrain (fb), midbrain (mb) and hindbrain (hb). The primitive eye (optic placode; large arrow) and inner ear (otic placode; small arrow) can be discerned. Cardiac looping has completed and the primitive chambers of the heart and outflow track are apparent (v: ventricle; a: atrium). Axial formation is underway with approximately 20–25 pairs of somites formed by this stage (bracket).

two techniques served as the foundation of rodent whole-embryo culture and are still being used today in many laboratories around the world. Throughout the years, rodent whole-embryo culture was a key technique used in identifying the fate of the three germ layers into the different cells of the body. For example, Rosa Beddington developed a technique similar to the original Rosenquist chick thymidine technique in which she injected donor mouse embryos with thymidine, then excised and injected these cells into similarly staged mouse embryos. The cells were then followed by radioautographic analysis to determine their differentiation path.[3] By using this technique, Beddington established that anterior embryonic ectoderm gives rise to definitive surface ectoderm and neuroectoderm, that distal embryonic ectoderm gives rise to gut endoderm, notochord and mesodermal derivatives including somites, and that posterior ectoderm gives rise to both embryonic and extraembryonic mesodermal tissues.[3,4] Rodent whole-embryo culture was not only essential in the discovery of mechanisms of early embryonic development as described above, but it has also been instrumental in testing and correctly identifying the teratogenic potential of various chemicals[5–8] and in the establishment of developmental toxicology assays that are currently being used in industrial safety testing today.[9] In recent years, techniques have been established for culturing rabbit embryos *in vitro*[10] as well as a morphological scoring system for assessing rabbit embryos.[11,12] Given that rat and rabbit are the two conventional test species used in regulatory teratogenicity evaluation, the respective *in vitro* systems could potentially work as adjacent screens to enhance predictivity power for correctly identifying compounds that have teratogenic properties distinct to a particular species.

#### *18.2.1.2 Chick*

The earliest reports of embryo culture experiments go back to 1912 when McWhorter and Whipple succeeded in culturing primitive streak-stage chick embryos.[13] By the early 1930s, the method was improved by the adaptation of the plasma clot method which provided support for the blastoderm and promoted intact embryo development. However, when these embryos were compared to embryos developing in the egg, it was found that their embryonic axis was often stunted.[14] Thereafter, the plasma clot method was later replaced by a combination of agar with egg albumen[15,16] or egg-yolk dialysate,[17] but neither of these seemed to improve embryo development *in vitro*. By 1955, Denis New developed a chick-embryo culture technique that consisted of dissecting the blastoderm with its own vitelline membrane and stretching it around a glass ring placed on a watch glass. Egg albumen was then added underneath the membrane to supply the nutrients required for appropriate embryonic growth. It turned out that the use of the vitelline membrane along with the egg albumen promoted the expansion of the embryonic axis at the same pace as in the egg.[18,19] Although many adaptations to this method have been published,[20–22] New's technique was the foundation of the chick-embryo culture method that is still in use today. From that point forward, chick-embryo culture was used by many investigators to study mechanisms of early embryonic development. Unlike other whole-embryo models, the chick embryos are flat, which facilitates the tissue to be manipulated for cellular microinjection, bead implants or tissue-grafting studies. For example, in the late 1960s and early 1970s, Rosenquist published a number of fate-mapping experiments in which he labeled hypoblasts of donor embryos with thymidine, and excised and transplanted these grafts to the epiblast, primitive streak, or endoderm-mesoderm (hypoblast) layers of similarly staged embryos. The movement of the labeled cells were tracked by radioautographic analysis to determine the fate of the three germ layers; ectoderm, mesoderm and endoderm.[23] By applying this method in chick embryos, Rosenquist explored the origin and migration of limb-bud epithelium and mesenchyme, as well as the origin and movement of nephrogenic, cardiogenic, hepatogenic, pre-gut and pre-lung cells.[24,25] By the early 1980s, Rosenquist used this same technique to study the origin and migration of neural crest cells.[26] In the mid-to-late 1980s, fate-mapping experiments became more popular with the development of the quail/chick chimera technique in which specific regions of the chick are substituted with nuclear stained quail counterparts. The quail nuclear marker facilitates visualization of cell migration making it easy to build fate maps. This technique provided some explanations of how specific malformations may be manifested. For example, fate mapping of the prosencephalic neural plate and neural folds, as well as migration of neural crest cells provided an explanation of how interruption of these processes may cause neuronal and facial malformations in humans.[27] Similar approaches were used by Margaret Kirby and colleagues in the early 1990s in a seminal study that identified that the endocardial cushions of the cardiac outflow track were populated by a population of neural crest originating in the hindbrain.[28] This study unraveled the riddle that perplexed teratologists for years related to why so many teratogenic syndromes included a combination of craniofacial and cardiac/great vessel malformations. Currently, the chick-embryo model is not commonly used in safety assessment of chemicals. This is likely due to the low sample number that can be evaluated in an experiment, but for mechanistic studies, the model has unique attributes, such as for assessing limb development and the relative ease for manipulating and tracking specific cell populations *in vitro*. Today it remains a critical mechanistic model and has been utilized to characterize target pharmacology and teratogenic impact of compounds which will be described in the final section of this chapter.

#### *18.2.1.3 Zebrafish*

Zebrafish were first explored by Joseph Streisinger as a developmental model system in the 1980s. Prior to zebrafish, Medaka were commonly used in ecotoxicity testing and developmental biology studies. Although both species of fish exhibit developmental processes similar to mammalian development, the zebrafish develop more quickly and the embryos maintain transparency into the larva stage, facilitating detailed evaluation of structures and organ systems. Furthermore, the entire zebrafish genome has recently been sequenced.[29]

As early as the 1980s, zebrafish quickly became a versatile model for developmental genetics research and have supported seminal work associated with manipulation of the genome and subsequent evaluation of phenotype that led to advances in transgenic animal models. Such studies included development of *in vitro* fertilization techniques in zebrafish that produced haploid embryo development and the generation of homozygous mutant lines of fish.[30] Researchers later adapted mutagenesis strategies to the zebrafish and established *N*-ethyl-*N*-nitrosourea (ENU)-based mutagenesis to generate zebrafish mutants, of which phenotypic changes could be readily mapped to genotype, leading to thousands of characterized mutants.[31,32] In recent years, antisense strategies were found to work well in zebrafish embryos as a loss-of-function approach. In these studies, morpholino antisense oligonucleotides are injected into the yolk for uptake into the embryo proper and have been found to inhibit translational expression of selected targets.[33] With prudent sequence selection and the use of appropriate controls, this approach has been valuable for gene functional characterization and mechanistic studies.[34]

The zebrafish embryo-larva is of considerable interest for generation of an *in vitro* teratogenicity assay. The zebrafish-embryo model has been evaluated with a metabolic activation system (rat liver microsomes) to demonstrate cyclophosphamide and ethanol-based teratogenicity could be detected with the zebrafish model following metabolic activation by the microsomes.[35] Additional progress has been made in developing zebrafish teratogenicity assays and will be described in detail in the next section.

#### 18.2.1.4 Frog

Frog embryos have been used extensively for evaluating mechanisms of early development. In particular, research with early frog embryos were crucial in functional characterization of the Organizer and early developmental processes establishing the body plan (reviewed by De Robertis,[36,37]). Frog embryos are relatively easy to obtain and are easy to culture and manipulate. Like rodents and zebrafish, the genome for at least one frog species has been characterized and the model is conducive for gene manipulation including transgenic models and transcriptional knockdown treatments. Along with zebrafish, the frog model also presents some unique advantages for manipulating gene expression as the embryos from both species are conducive to gain-of-function applications using mRNA injections or expression vectors. Because frog development includes metamorphosis, the model has also been studied for its utility in studying post-natal development, particularly in regard to hormonal regulation.[38–40] In particular, the frog presents similar hormonal regulation of the hypothalmic-pituitary-thyroid axis and has presented utility as a bioassay for identifying chemicals that disrupt thyroid function.[40] A well-studied teratogenicity assay that uses the frog embryo model is called FETAX (Frog Embryo Toxicity Assay-*Xenopus*). Frog embryos are cultured through 48 or 96 h post fertilization in the presence of the test compound.[41] The assay presents good predictivity power, with 83% general concordance in correct classification of mammalian *in vivo* teratogens and non-teratogens out of a test set of 35 compounds. Furthermore the assay had a 67% success rate in correct prediction of types of mammalian malformations associated with the teratogens.[42,43] However, like zebrafish, the non-mammalian nature of the system as well as the aqueous culture environment could be a drawback for routine testing of novel pharmaceutical compounds.

## 18.2.2 Cell Culture Models

### *18.2.2.1 Rat Micromass*

The rat micromass assay is a five-day assay where primary cultures of midbrain or limb bud cells are harvested from mid-gestation embryos and treated *in vitro* with test compounds.[9,44] The midbrain or limb bud micromass cultures are stained with specific dyes to identify differentiating cells. Hematoxylin has been traditionally used for marking midbrain cells undergoing neuronal differentiation whereas alcian blue is used to identify foci from limb buds that are undergoing cartilaginous differentiation. The concentration at which each compound inhibits the formation of differentiated foci by 50% of the control value ($IC_{50}$) is determined. A micromass developmental toxicity screen has been developed and validated by the European Centre for the Validation of Alternative Methods (ECVAM) and will be discussed in next section of this chapter.

### *18.2.2.2 Mouse Embryonic Stem-Cell Applications*

The mouse D3 embryonic stem cell line is one of the most characterized and widely used stem-cell models. In the presence of Leukemia Inhibitory Factor (LIF), the cells can be cultured in the pluripotent state. Cellular differentiation occurs when LIF is removed from the culture. When the cells are grown in conditions promoting aggregation, such as in the hanging drop culture or in low-adherence flasks, the differentiating cells are prompted to form "embryoid bodies". Embryoid bodies are clusters of differentiating cells that undergo differentiation into cells of the three germ layers. The cells can be manipulated with various culture techniques or with growth factors to differentiate into cardiac, neuronal, hematopoietic and osteoblastic lineages.

The EST was developed as a cell-based developmental toxicity screen in the early 1990s. It is a 10-day assay, where the stem cells are cultured as hanging drops to initiate differentiation into embryoid bodies. The embryoid bodies (EBs) are evaluated on day 10 of culture for the presence of beating myocardiocytes.[45,46] Compounds are assessed for their potential to inhibit beating cardiomyocyte formation in a population of EBs (typically 24 EBs per test concentration) against the NIH3T3 $EC_{50}$ value. This assay was further validated by ECVAM and is discussed in detail in the next section of the chapter.

## 18.3 Applications of *In Vitro* Models in Developmental Toxicology Screens

### 18.3.1 Background

*In vitro* developmental toxicology screens have been developed and improved over the past few decades in support of the three Rs perspective (**reduction** of the number of animals used, **refinement** of techniques and procedures to reduce pain and distress, and **replacement** of animal with non-animal techniques) (reviewed by W. M. S. Russell and R. L. Burch[47]). ECVAM performed an extensive intra-laboratory validation of a number of *in vitro* teratogenicity assays. The purpose of the validation was to assess general concordance and provide guidance on which assays could be considered for inclusion in regulatory testing in the EU.[48,49] The validation effort was made to support the EU REACH (Registration, Evaluation and Authorization of Chemicals) system for the safety testing and risk assessment of chemicals in replacement of *in vivo* toxicology studies.[50] The ECVAM validation project evaluated three rodent-based developmental toxicity assays including the mouse embryonic stem-cell test, the rat micromass assay, and the rat whole embryo culture assay. A review of these assays and strategies to improve their throughput are summarized in this section.

#### *18.3.1.1 Rat Whole-Embryo Culture Assay*

ECVAM developed a novel rat whole-embryo culture (rWEC) assay for classifying teratogenic potential of compounds. In this assay, compounds are initially characterized for cytotoxicity by treatment along a concentration range in NIH3T3 cells. The concentration that caused 50% loss in viability ($EC_{50}$) was determined and used in the assay prediction model for classifying teratogenic potential. In the model, the NIH3T3 $EC_{50}$ represents a surrogate value for adult toxicity. The concentration identified to cause developmental toxicity is determined by assessing the compound in the rat whole-embryo culture model. Neurulating embryos were treated with various concentrations of test compounds and after two days of culture, the gestation day 11 embryos were assessed and scored for growth/developmental staging parameters using the Brown and Fabro morphological score system to determine a Total Morphological Score (TMS).[51] To support the ECVAM validation effort, a statistical prediction model was developed by incorporating both TMS and NIH3T3 $EC_{50}$ values. The concordance in correct classification of *in vivo* teratogens and non-teratogens was 80%, which was the most robust outcome amongst the three developmental toxicology assays evaluated.[48]

A primary advantage of the rat WEC assay is that it represents a whole-organismal model system in one of the most commonly used test species for *in vivo* developmental toxicity study. Therefore, it reduces the use of animal numbers required for toxicological testing. The *in vitro* WEC assay also provides well-controlled experimental conditions and the embryos can be easily manipulated during the culture period and for evaluating specific properties of test compounds.

The limitations of the WEC assay include the relatively short embryo culture duration limited in the first 2–3 days during the organogenesis period. Although the critical window of sensitivity of many teratogens may cover within this period, the insult may not manifest morphologically until a later time in embryonic development.[52–54] Lack of maternal–embryo interactions or maternal influences during drug testing is another limit that this *in vitro* assay can not overcome comparing to *in vivo* studies.

Even though the WEC assay presented the highest concordance among all ECVAM-validated assays, the assay is labor intensive because of the cytotoxicity evaluation required in a surrogate cell line, the relatively large series of test concentrations required, and the extensive morphological score assessment. Therefore, the WEC assay is relatively low throughput with only 1–2 compounds capable of being assessed subsequent to obtaining the NIH3T3 $EC_{50}$ value.

Efforts have been undertaken to further abbreviate the assay by reducing test concentrations and morphological endpoints to improve throughput and reduce animal use. The abbreviated WEC assay uses a new score system called the 'Dysmorphological Score system' which quantitates morphological integrity of structures and organ systems. This enables more subtle or selective effects to be discerned in contrast to the TMS method.[55]

To support the abbreviated rWEC assay, a statistical prediction model has been built on the data generated from assessing 63 test compounds with known *in vivo* teratogenicity properties. By using Linear Discriminant analysis and Recursive Partitioning analysis, a prediction model was established with only one test concentration (1 μM) and just three morphological endpoints (spinal cord, heart, and number of somites) required for classification of teratogenic potential. After cross-validation, the overall error rate is 24% with 76% cumulative concordance. The screening throughput is increased from 1–2 compounds to up to 14 compounds per week.[56]

### *18.3.1.2 Rat Micromass Assay*

The rat limb bud micromass assay was also validated by ECVAM. As mentioned previously, limb buds are harvested from gestational day-12 embryos and the disassociated cells are cultured for 5 days and treated with test compounds. The cultured tissues are stained with alcian blue to identify foci that are undergoing cartilaginous differentiation. The concentration at which each compound inhibits the formation of differentiated foci by 50% of the control value ($IC_{50}$) is determined. The rat limb bud micromass assay was assessed in the ECVAM validation project supported by a predictive statistical model and determined to have fairly good concordance (70%) in correct classification of *in vivo* teratogens and non-teratogens.[48,49] The limb bud micromass assay has potential to be conducive for high-throughput screening platforms given the relative ease of dissecting mid-gestation limbs and the substantial cell numbers produced for seeding plates. Fluorescent-labeled protein markers of neuronal and chondrocytic differentiation endpoints have also been explored for high-throughput screening and provided similar concordance metrics (unpublished data). Outside of the manual work involved in tissue harvest, micromass certainly has the potential to be developed as a high-throughput screening platform. However, there has been more emphasis on developing high-throughput screening assays using embryonic stem cells. This is in part due to 1) superior results of the validation of the embryonic stem-cell test (EST) with a 78% total concordance, 2) no animals are used to support the assay, and 3) all aspects of the culture and assay can be conducted by automated means.[48–58]

#### *18.3.1.3 Mouse Embryonic Stem-Cell Test and Refined Assays*

The traditional mouse embryonic stem cell test (EST) is a 10-day assay in which murine D3 embryonic stem cells are cultured with test compounds in hanging drops to initiate differentiation into embryoid bodies (Ebs). By the end of the 10-day culture, morphologic evaluation of each EB for the presence of beating cardiomyocytes is assessed and an $ID_{50}$ is calculated (the test concentration in which 50% of differentiation into cardiomyocytes is inhibited).[59,60] Furthermore, the prediction model for the EST requires determining the compound's $IC_{50}$ in ES and NIH3T3 cells. ECVAM validated the EST assay and found it to be 78% concordant in correct classification of *in vivo* teratogens and non-teratogens.[48]

The advantages of using the EST are to eliminate animal use, reduce the costs associated with *in vivo* animal testing, and potentially automate the assay. However, this assay has some limits and there are areas that need to be improved for higher efficiency. For example, it is difficult to differentiate weak and non-teratogens.[61] Also, the hanging-drop culture and counting beating cardiomyocytes are both very labor intensive and time consuming. Therefore, a number of laboratories have made efforts to shorten the duration of the EST, as well as to enhance the assay throughput capabilities in the past few years.

Efforts are continuing to streamline the EST so that the assay could be outfitted for high-throughput screening. Improvements in culture protocols have enabled EB formation in low-adherence plates, without the manual manipulation required in conducting hanging-drop cultures. Various investigators are focused on identifying molecular endpoints, fluorescent cell sorting (FACS) and critical windows of differentiation, with the intent to shorten the assay duration as well as enhance predictivity.[62–64] One approach to improve throughput is incorporating molecular endpoints associated with pluripotency, gastrulation, and differentiation. Success in identifying gene expression changes in EBs that reflect specific cell types or organ systems affected by certain teratogens has been reported.[65–67]

In a similar fashion, we have developed a molecular-based stem cell assay (MESCA) using the murine D3 cell line. The selection of the target genes were based on published literature information as well as data from microarray analysis focused on functional relevance in early embryonic development.

The target gene expression panel was designed to represent pluripotency and also included differentiation markers associated with primitive germ layer determination or hematopoietic, vascular, neuronal or craniofacial cell lineages. Gene expression profiles were analyzed from the EBs treated with known teratogens and non teratogens. An example of preliminary work from this study is illustrated (Figure 18.2). In this experiment, a series of non-teratogens and teratogens were evaluated for transcriptional response over the 10-day culture period to determine whether there were particular culture days, targets, and compound concentrations that could delineate a teratogenic signal. The peak concentration that maintained 100% viability in a preliminary cytotoxicity evaluation was selected as the high concentration and a series of lower concentrations were selected along a log increment. The respective transcriptional responses of ascorbic acid (non-teratogen) and valproic acid (a teratogen) are illustrated (Figure 18.2). With statistical algorithms now in place, the MESCA assay is able to provide good concordance in correctly classifying teratogens and non-teratogens using a streamlined assay duration and study design.

### *18.3.1.4 Zebrafish Teratogenicity Assays*

There is increasing interest in establishing a developmental toxicity assay using the zebrafish embryo-larva model. The simplicity of maintaining and breeding the adults as well as their rapid organogenesis makes zebrafish an ideal model for developmental toxicity screens with high-throughput potential.

A number of laboratories have studied the zebrafish embryo-larva as a model for developmental toxicology assessment and have worked individually in assessing this assay. Various investigators met at the first workshop on '*In Vitro* Developmental Toxicology Assays' sponsored by the Health and Environmental Science Institute (reviewed by Chapin *et al.*[68]). At the time, there were few publications describing these studies and the positive and negative attributes of the zebrafish assay. However, recently, we have described a zebrafish teratogenicity assay using de-chorinated zebrafish embryos[69] (Figure 18.3). Preliminary evaluation of 30 pharmaceutical compounds with this assay yielded promising results with approximately 87% total concordance and < 15% error rate in misclassification of *in vivo* teratogens and non-teratogens.[69] However, the act of a delicate enzymatic treatment, manual removal of the chorion and labor-intensive morphological score procedure do not render the current assay conducive to an automated platform for high-throughput screening.

Acting in the form of a consortium and using the basic framework of the dechorinated assay, a number of pharmaceutical and biotechnology companies are evaluating a chorion-on assay with the intent to streamline the protocol and make it more conducive to high-throughput screening.[70] Approximately 60 compounds will be evaluated in multiple zebrafish strains by various laboratories with the results anticipated to be published in the near future. The goals

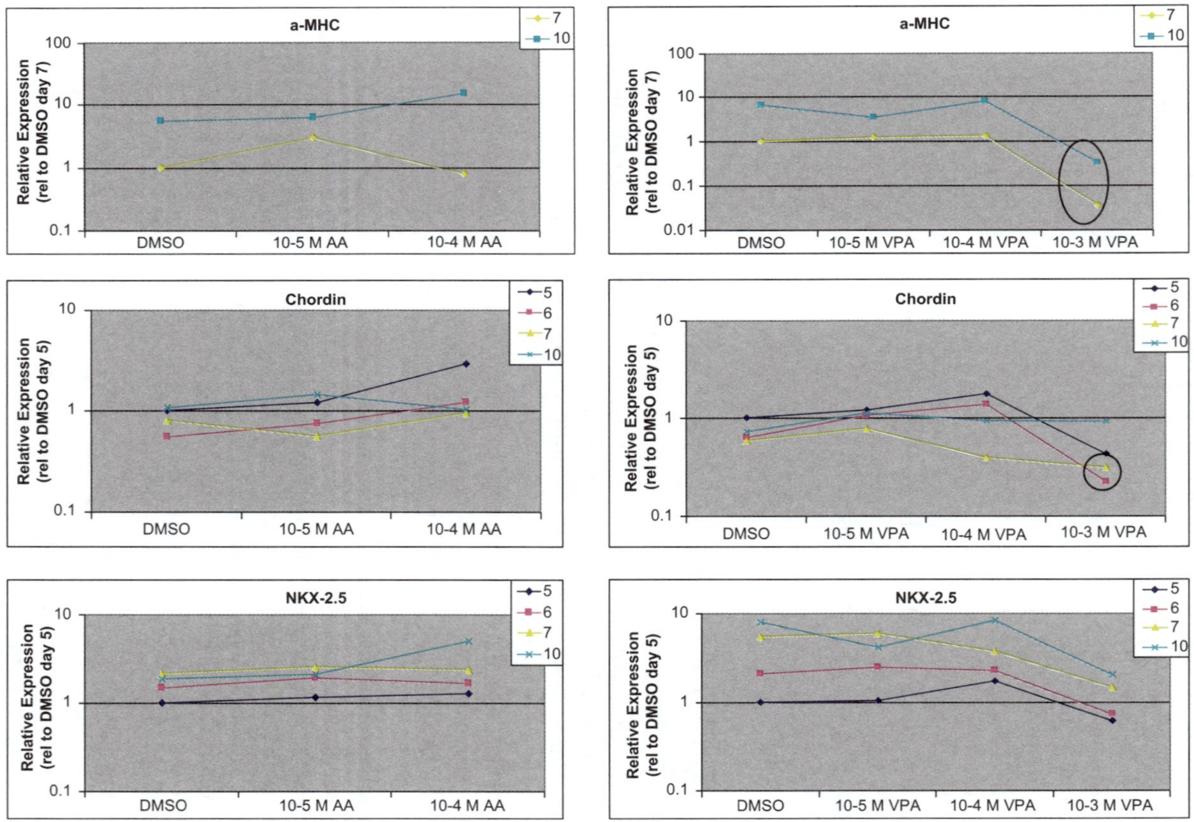


**Figure 18.2** Time-course evaluation of several differentiation markers in embryoid bodies and respective response to a non-teratogen and teratogen. Differences in transcriptional response of the differentiation markers were compared following exposure of embryoid bodies to ascorbic acid (AA, a non-teratogen) and valproic acid (VPA, a teratogen). The DMSO vehicle control was used as a reference to normalize relative change in expression over the time course. The results of this experiment suggested some transcriptional change could be detected with valproic acid treatment and the changes could be discerned at earlier time points (day 7 or earlier). Circled: endpoints with approximately $\geq$ 50% inhibition in transcriptional expression.

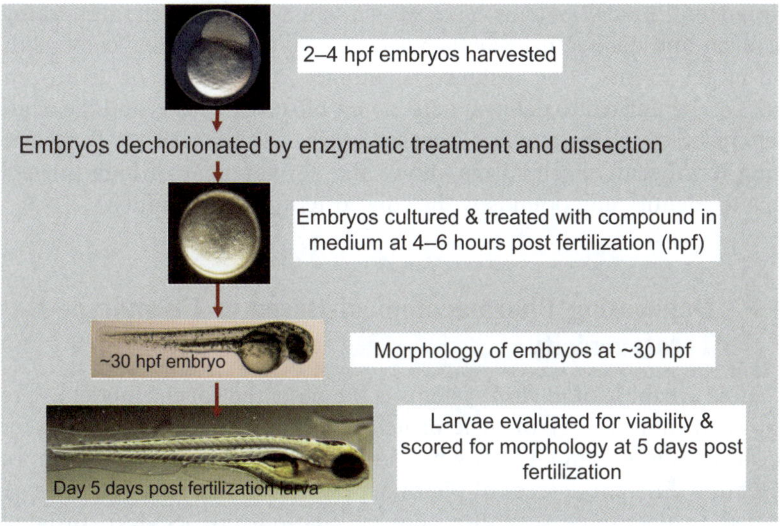


**Figure 18.3** Representative developmental stages and steps associated with the dechorinated zebrafish teratogenicity assay.

of this consortium are to share current assay experiences and results, assess variability between laboratories and wild-type strains, establish a harmonized protocol, and develop a statistical predication model to support the assay using fewer morphological endpoints. If these goals are successfully met, the assay will be higher throughput with potential for automation. The major obstacle in integrating the zebrafish assay into a high-throughput platform is the morphological assessment. A breakthrough in an automated platform for zebrafish manipulation and imaging was reported recently.[71] Functional attributes of this system include automated fish larvae loading with placement in correct orientation for imaging, high-speed confocal imaging, and laser manipulation for superficial and deep-organ imaging. With this automated screening system available, the feasibility of a high-throughput zebrafish screening platform is promising in the near future.

## 18.4 Applications of Developmental Models in Mechanistic Studies

In cases where a compound produces a direct teratogenic insult to the embryo-fetus that is unrelated to changes in maternal status, two potential origins of teratogenicity exist. One origin is directly related to the drug target, where developmental processes are altered by the intended pharmacology. This occurs because many drug targets are proteins that have essential biological functions in the embryo-fetus. The other origin is related to the chemical structure, where the compound has altered the function of an unintended "off-target". *In vitro* developmental model systems have shown value in characterizing teratogenic mechanism and delineating whether it occurs by pharmacologically mediated or off-target events. For instance, combined application of teratogenicity screens can be utilized to delineate on- *versus* off-target effects and the degree of conservation of adverse effect across species (Figure 18.4). Furthermore, defining teratogenic mechanisms allows the development of high-throughput screens to identify compounds with reduced teratogenic liability.

### 18.4.1 Delineating Pharmacological-Based or Chemotype-Based Teratogenicity

A valuable attribute of *in vitro* systems is the potential for the model to present a change in morphology or gene/protein expression indicative of the teratogenic insult. Once a model provides such sensitivity, additional compounds representing different degrees of pharmacology or structural similarities can be evaluated to determine structure–activity relationships (SARs). Insight into SARs could make it feasible for a chemist to re-design the compound to lose teratogenic properties and maintain pharmacologic potency. Such studies can be elegantly simple. For instance, we have developed a morphological score system for the mid-gestation rat embryo as well as for the day-5 post fertilization zebrafish larva that can be used for such purposes.[55,73] Both score systems use a similar numerical system, with similar criteria for severity and nomenclature to enable zebrafish and rodent assays to be used interchangeably or exclusively depending upon the issue at hand. This approach was used to assess the SAR of a potent skeletal teratogen, the 5HT1B/D inverse agonist, SB-236057, against a battery of compounds. These compounds included individual side-groups and the compound's structural core along with compounds of the related chemotype series or distinct structures but potent target pharmacology. A selected concentration causing SB-236057 teratogenicity *in vitro* and *in vivo* (maternal AUC) was used thereafter for screening purposes to enhance throughput. The rat whole-embryo culture model was used since the model presented similar malformations to those that were produced *in vivo* (axial malformations) and the compound was a definitive rat teratogen. Therefore, a tailored assay was generated that compared somite morphology and caudal extension scores benchmarked against the dysmorphology scores of SB-236057 at a biologically relevant concentration (Figure 18.5). By this approach, approximately 50 compounds were evaluated over a few weeks of WEC screening. Results from this study suggested that the intended pharmacology of SB-236057 was not causing the malformations. The basis appeared to be related to chemical structure and was refined to a spiropiperdine moiety that caused the teratogenicity in this chemotype series.[74]

Extensive SAR evaluation has also conducted on valproic acid (VPA). This work has included both *in vivo* and *in vitro* studies with VPA and structural analogues to better characterize how chemical structure relates to anti-seizure activities, teratogenicity and ability to inhibit proliferation and HIV infection

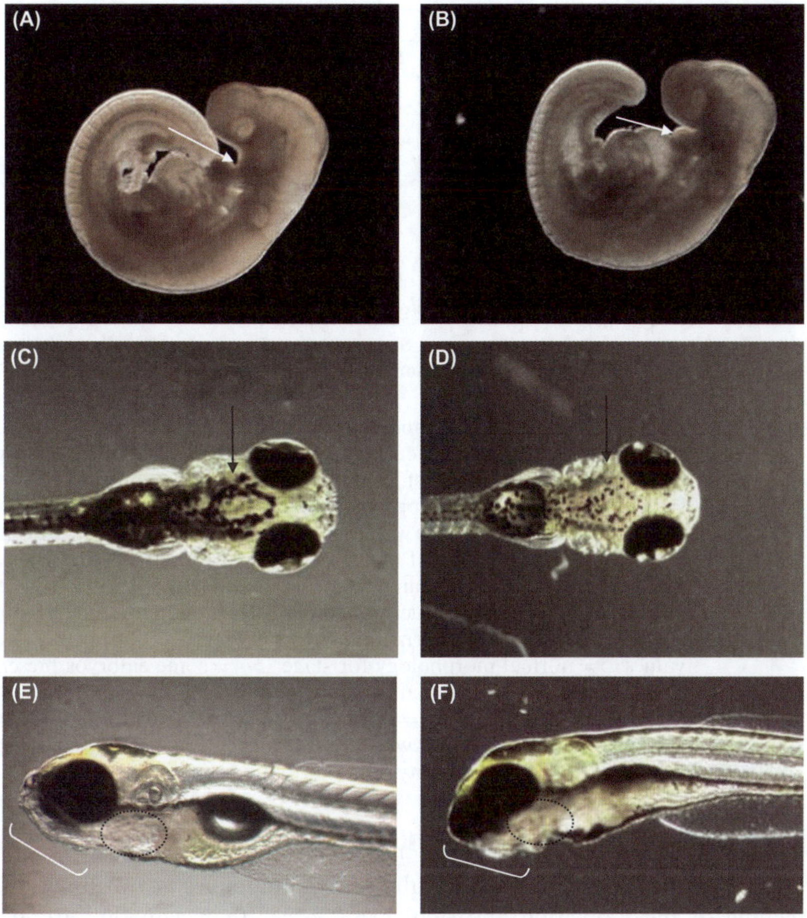


**Figure 18.4** Neural crest-derived malformations from elevation of oxysterols in cultured rat and zebrafish embryos. A study was conducted to examine whether elevation of oxysterols would lead to malformations similar to those reported in Insig 1/2 double-mutant knockout mice. The Insig 1/2 double knockouts present elevated oxysterol levels and possess structural malformations of various crest-associated craniofacial structures, including the palate, face, brain, middle and inner ear.[72] In these studies rat and zebrafish embryos were treated with an endogenous oxysterol, 22(*R*)-hydroxycholesterol, and a series of synthetic oxysterols. 22(*R*)-Hydrooxycholesterol and some of the synthetic oxysterols produced similar craniofacial malformations to those reported in the Insig 1/2 double knockout mouse. A) Day-11 cultured rat embryo with normal morphology. B) Oxysterol-treated rat embryo presenting first pharyngeal arch defects. The arrow points to abnormal oral grove caused by deficiency in primitive maxilla region of the first pharyngeal arch. C) Dorsal view of 5 dpf zebrafish presenting a normal amount and distribution of pigmented melanocytes which are derived from neural crest (arrow). D) Oxysterol-treated zebrafish larva presenting a reduced number of melanocytes (arrow). E) Lateral view of a 5dpf zebrafish larva presenting normal craniofacial morphology (bracket: lower jaw; circle: pharyngeal arches). F) Oxysterol-treated zebrafish larva presenting severe malformations/deficiency of the lower jaw (bracket) and pharyngeal arches (circle).

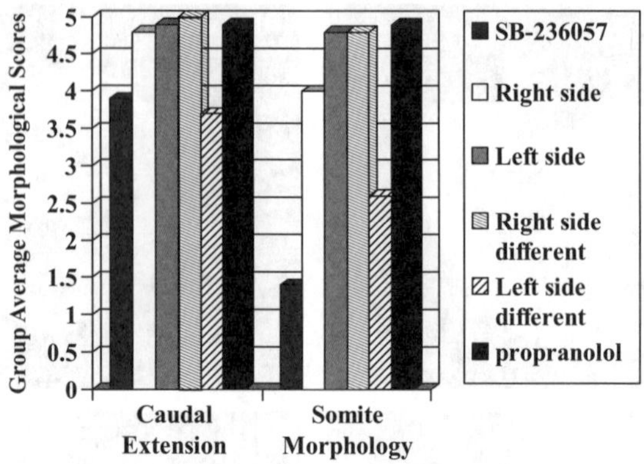


**Figure 18.5** Relationships between compound structure and axial malformations. In this study rat embryos were cultured with a known axial-skeletal teratogen, SB-236057, and a series of chemical moieties that contributed to the structure of SB-236057. Propranolol, a compound with similar pharmacology but distinct structure was also included to facilitate the investigation of SARs. Relative effects of the compounds on somite development and axial extension were compared and revealed that the teratogenicity was related to the SB-236057 structure and that alterations to the moieties on the right-side rescued axial formation. Morphological group average score values: 5 = normal morphology for stage; >4 = some embryos presented subtle anomalies or mild malformations but overall the group was within the range of normal; ≤4 = various embryos with malformations were identified within the group with lower group average score values representing an increase in severity of malformations and incidence.

(reviewed by Terbach and Williams[75]). SAR evaluation provided insight on teratogenic moieties. For instance, evaluation of analogues *in vivo* showed that branching of the α-position and side-chains larger than a methyl group are attributed to teratogenicity whereas substitution of the α-position hydrogen abolishes teratogenicity.[76,77] Increased understanding of pharmacological activity of VPA on essential functions in embryo-fetal development (*e.g.*, Class I and II Histone Deactylase inhibition, alteration of folate metabolism, and activation of PPAR delta receptors) may be linked to a complex array of teratogenic mechanisms.[78,79] Advances in cell-based assays, such as use of F9 teratocarcioma cell lines led to informative SAR data on VPA teratogenic mechanisms, allowing identification of offending structural motifs.[79] Such characterization raises the possibility of identifying novel analogues with less teratogenic liability.

### 18.4.2 Off-Target Teratogenicity: Advances in Identifying the Teratogenic Target

Developing strategies that characterize small molecule–protein interactions provides valuable opportunities in both drug discovery and toxicology. In recent years, such approaches have identified unintended "off-targets" of drugs causing teratogenicity. *In vitro* models have played a critical role in such studies. Furthermore, an ultimate strategy of these approaches is to utilize a high-throughput platform. To this end, either a cell-based or biochemical protein-binding assay could be designed to detect binding affinity to undesirable off-target proteins, enabling identification of new molecules that maintain desirable pharmacology without off-target activity. Three examples are provided to describe approaches which have integrated small-molecule protein binding strategies and *in vitro* developmental model systems to identify putative off-targets.

### *18.4.2.1 SB-236057 and Phage Display*

SB-236057 is a 5Ht1B/D inverse agonist that was found to be an axial-skeletal teratogen in rats, mice and rabbits. A combination of phage display and rat whole-embryo culture was useful in identifying a putative off-target. Phage display uses bacteriophage libraries that contain random sequences of peptides (such as 7 or 12-peptide-long configurations). These peptide sequences are expressed on a specific region of the coat of the phage. Bacteriophage are incubated over a substrate that is bound to a "bait" such as an antibody, epitope or small molecule. Through a series of incubations and washes called "biopanning", phage with binding affinity to the bait will remain bound and can be eluted and the peptide can be identified by sequencing (reviewed by Taipa[80]). In this study, a biotinylated form of SB-236057 was synthesized to bind to strepavidin-coated plates for biopanning. A bacteriophage library containing random sequences of peptides in 12-mer confirmations was used and a series of nucleotide sequences were identified. These sequences included one that had 100% homology to the rat enhancer of split 1 gene (rESP1), which was speculated to be involved in Notch signaling. Subsequent studies in rat whole-embryo culture demonstrated rESP1 expression to be similar to molecular oscillators involved in Notch signaling and somite formation, where it was expressed in paraxial mesoderm that would give rise to somites, with expression ceasing at the edge of the most-recently formed somite (Figure 18.6).[74] Evidence for rESP1 being a potential teratogenic target for SB-236057 was further demonstrated by similarity of axial and somite malformations produced in cultured rat embryos treated with SB-236057 or rESP1 antisense oligonucleotides (Figure 18.6).[74] Currently, advances in proteomic technology, protein sequencing and computational biology increase the promise of using phage-display approaches for characterizing small molecule–protein interactions. This is because peptide sequences can now be evaluated on the level of protein conformation against drug targets and other targets and assessed for similarity in putative binding pockets.

### *18.4.2.2 Homocysteine and Pharmacology Assays*

Maternal elevation in homocysteine levels is a well-established risk factor for embryotoxicity or congenital malformations, particularly neural tube defects.

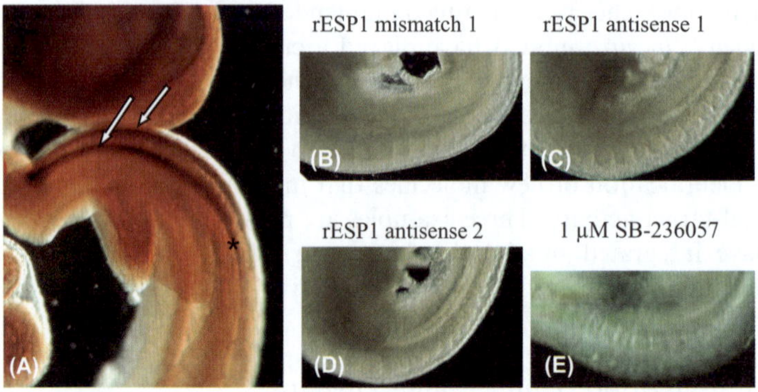


**Figure 18.6** Evaluation of putative off-target expression and function in rodent embryos. Mechanistic evaluations of SB-236057 led to rat enhancer of split 1 (rESP1) as a potential off-target candidate for teratogenicity. rESP1 expression was characterized in the organogenesis-stage rat embryo and identified to be expressed in the paraxial mesoderm (arrows) that gives rise to the somites A). B) A series of rat whole-embryo culture studies were conducted to compare effects of attenuating rESP1 expression with morpholino antisense treatments to SB-236057 treatments on somite and caudal morphology. Effects of these treatments are illustrated in plates B–E and provided further support that rESP1 was the putative target of SB-236057 teratogenicity. Reproduced from ref. 74 with permission. Copyright John Wiley and Sons, 2004.

The exact mechanism remains unknown but elevated homocysteine is theorized to be the result of faulty folate metabolism because folate supplementation significantly reduces the risk of malformed babies born to women presenting elevated homocysteine levels. Homocysteine has also been implicated to act directly as a teratogen (reviewed by Brauer and Tierney[81]). Pharmacology studies have shown that homocysteine may act as a ligand for the *N*-methyl-D-aspartate (NMDA) receptors, a class of ion-channel receptors gated by glutamate and glycine involved in regulating calcium entry into the cell.[82,83] NMDA receptors are important in survival and migration of neurons and are expressed in the neural tube and neural crest.

On the NMDA receptor, homocysteine acts as an agonist and a partial agonist at the glutamate and glycine sites, respectively. The chick embryo provided great utility for evaluating teratogenic properties of compounds with NMDA pharmacology (reviewed by Brauer and Tierney[81]). Various NMDA channel blockers produced craniofacial malformations and neural tube defects similar to those produced with homocysteine treatment in chick-embryo culture. Glycine gate-specific antagonists also produce these effects but at less potency, suggesting that homocysteine may interact more broadly as a channel blocker. Furthermore, homocysteine co-administration with glycine or glutamate ameliorated the teratogenic effects.

The results of these studies provide a thoughtful characterization of a potential teratogenic target of homocysteine, and possibly folate deficiency.

Given the relevance of the NMDA receptor as a potential drug target, such studies show how a receptor can be pharmacologically manipulated, and what types of mediation may or may not impact teratogenic liability.

### *18.4.2.3 Thalidomide*

Understanding the target and mechanism underlying thalidomide teratogenicity has mystified researchers for 50 years. Recently, a study that combined state-of-the-art affinity purification methods identified a potential protein target for thalidomide that was further validated as a potential target of teratogenicity using the zebrafish and chick-embryo models.[84] Ferrite glycidyl methacrylate (FG) beads were conjugated with a carboxylic thalidomide derivative, FR259625, and used in protein affinity purification of various cell extracts from human cell lines such as HeLa.[84,85] Two polypetides were purified and identified as cereblon (CBRN) and damaged DNA binding protein 1 (DDB1). Further co-immunoprecipitation studies with thalidomide-bound beads and histidine-tagged CBRN and DDB1, identified DDB1 to precipitate only when CBRN protein was also present, suggesting thalidomide directly interacted with CBRN, and CBRN was bound to other proteins like DDB1 in a complex.

Zebrafish- and chick-embryo culture were used in this study to validate CBRN as the teratogenic target for thalidomide. Thalidomide administration to zebrafish embryos suppressed otic placode size in 30-h post-fertilization (hpf) embryos and pectoral fin abnormalities were identified by 48 hpf. Expression of the zebrafish orthologue, zCBRN, was inhibited by morpholino antisense and produced similar malformations and these effects were rescued when zCBRN mRNA was co-injected with the antisense.

Chick-embryo culture was used as model to complete the validation of CBRN as a teratogenic target for thalidomide, as the compound is a confirmed teratogen in chicken as well as humans and rabbits. Thalidomide exposure *in vitro* caused forelimb deletions at a high incidence, which was associated with chick CBRN directly interacting with thalidomide and also binding to DDB1. Over-expression of a drug-binding-deficient form of CBRN in cultured chick limbs made them resistant to thalidomide teratogenicity.

The results of these investigations shed new light on a potential target (conserved across species) and mechanism for thalidomide teratogenicity. This work has opened potential opportunities for researchers to develop new analogues of thalidomide that may maintain efficacy for treating sleep disorders, leprosy and multiple myleoma but lack teratogenic liability.

## 18.5 Conclusions

A multitude of developmental model systems are available to researchers for conducting teratology research. This chapter described several models widely used by researchers and their applications pertaining to screening compounds for teratogenic potential and evaluating mechanisms of teratogenicity. Much has been accomplished in recent years related to integration of these assays into automated platforms. With such approaches in place, high-throughput screening will likely enhance optimization of the pharmaceutical pipeline for reduced teratogenic potential and better safeguard employees and the public with production of safer chemicals that could be encountered in the workplace or by consumers. Hopefully, recent results with VPA and thalidomide demonstrate the potential to develop safer, efficacious analogues of teratogenic compounds.

## References


1. D. A. New, *Biol. Rev. Camb. Philos. Soc.,* 1978, **53**, 81–122.
2. T. W. Sadler, *J. Embryol. Exp. Morphol.,* 1979, **49**, 17–25.
3. S. P. Beddington, *J. Embryol. Exp. Morphol.*, 1981, **64**, 87–104.
4. R. S. Beddington, *J. Embryol. Exp. Morphol.*, 1982, **69**, 265–285.
5. B. P. Schmid, E. Goulding, K. Kitchin and M. K. Sanyal, *Toxicology*, 1981, **22**, 235–243.
6. T. W. Sadler, W. E. Horton and C. W. Warner, *Teratog. Carcinog. Mutagen.*, 1982, **2**, 243–253.
7. B. P. Schmid, A. Trippmacher and A. Bianchi, *Dev. Toxicol. Environ. Sci.*, 1983, **11**, 563–566.
8. L. Cicurel and B. Schmid, *Experientia* 1988, **44**, 833–840.
9. A. H. Piersma, *Toxicol. Lett.*, 2004, **149**, 147–153.
10. R. H. Foote and E. W. Carney, *Reprod. Toxicol.*, 2000, **14**, 477–493.
11. J. A. Pitt and E. W. Carney, *Teratology*, 1999, **59**, 102–109.
12. J. A. Pitt and E. W. Carney, *Teratology*, 1999, **59**, 88–101.
13. J. E. McWhorter and A. O. Whipple, *Anat. Rec.*, 1912, **6**, 121–139.
14. C. H. Waddington, *Philos. Trans. R. Soc., B*, 1932, **221**, 179–230.
15. N. T. Spratt Jr, *J. Exp. Zool.*, 1947, **106**, 345–365.
16. N. T. Spratt Jr, *Science*, 1947, **106**, 452.
17. N. T. Spratt Jr and H. Haas, *J. Exp. Zool.*, 1960, **144**, 139–147.
18. D. A. New, *J. Embryol. Exp. Morphol.*, 1959, **7**, 146–164.
19. D. A. New, *J. Embryol. Exp. Morphol.*, 1955, **3**, 326–331.
20. L. F. Jaffe and C. D. Stern, *Science*, 1979, **206**, 569–571.
21. W. Seidl, *Folia Morphol.*, 1977, **25**, 43–45.
22. P. Kucera and M. B. Burnand, *Teratog. Carcinog. Mutagen.*, 1987, **7**, 427–447.
23. G. C. Rosenquist, *Carn. Contrib. Embryol.*, 1966, **262**, 31–110.
24. G. C. Rosenquist, *Dev. Biol.*, 1970, **22**, 461–475.
25. G. C. Rosenquist, *J. Embryol. Exp. Morphol.*, 1971, **25**, 85–96.
26. G. C. Rosenquist, *Dev. Biol.*, 1981, **87**, 201–211.
27. G. F. Couly and N. M. Le Douarin, *Dev. Biol.*, 1987, **120**, 198–214.
28. M. L. Kirby, T. F. Gale and D. E. Stewart, *Science*, 1983, **220**, 1059–1061.
29. K. Jekosch, *Methods Cell. Biol.*, 2004, **77**, 225–239.
30. G. Streisinger, C. Walker, N. Dower, D. Knauber and F. Singer, *Nature*, 1981, **291**, 293–296.

31. W. Driever, L. Solnica-Krezel, A. F. Schier, S. C. Neuhauss, J. Malicki, D. L. Stemple, D. Y. Stainier, F. Zwartkruis, S. Abdelilah, Z. Rangini, J. Belak and C. Boggs, *Development*, 1996, **123**, 37–46.
32. P. Haffter and C. Nusslein-Volhard, *Int. J. Dev. Biol.*, 1996, **40**, 221–227.
33. S. C. Ekker, *Yeast*, 2000, **17**, 302–306.
34. D. R. Corey and J. M. Abrams, *Genome Biol.*, 2001, **2**, reviews1015.
35. F. Busquet, R. Nagel, F. von Landenberg, S. O. Mueller, N. Huebler and T. H. Broschard, *Toxicol. Sci.*, 2008, **104**, 177–188.
36. E. M. De Robertis and H. Kuroda, *Annu. Rev. Cell Dev. Biol.*, 2004, **20**, 285–308.
37. E. M. De Robertis, *Mech. Dev.*, 2009, **126**, 925–941.
38. J. R. Tata, *Biochem. Soc. Symp.*, 1996, **62**, 123–136.
39. J. R. Tata, *Mol. Cell Endocrinol.*, 2006, **246**, 10–20.
40. D. J. Fort, S. Degitz, J. Tietge and L. W. Touart, *Crit. Rev. Toxicol.*, 2007, **37**, 117–161.
41. M. O. Song, D. J. Fort, D. L. McLaughlin, R. L. Rogers, J. H. Thomas, B. O. Buzzard, A. M. Noll and N. K. Myers, *Drug Chem. Toxicol.*, 2003, **26**, 177–189.
42. D. J. Fort, P. D. Guiney, J. A. Weeks, J. H. Thomas, R. L. Rogers, A. M. Noll and C. D. Spaulding, *Toxicol. Sci.*, 2004, **81**, 454–466.
43. D. J. Fort, R. L. Rogers, J. H. Thomas, B. O. Buzzard, A. M. Noll and C. D. Spaulding, *J. Appl. Toxicol.*, 2004, **24**, 443–457.
44. O. P. Flint, *J. Cell Sci.*, 1983, **61**, 247–262.
45. D. R. Newall and K. E. Beedles, *Toxicol. in Vitro*, 1994, **8**, 697–701.
46. D. R. Newall and K. E. Beedles, *Toxicol. in Vitro*, 1996, **10**, 229–240.
47. W. M. S. Russell and R. L. Burch, *The Principles of Humane Experimental Technique*, Universities Federation for Animal Welfare, London, 1958.
48. E. Genschow H. Spielmann, G. Scholz, A. Seiler, N. Brown, A. Piersma, M. Brady, N. Clemann, H. Huuskonen, F. Paillard, S. Bremer and K. Becker, *Altern. Lab. Anim.*, 2002, **30**, 151–176.
49. H. Spielmann and M. Liebsch, *Toxicol. in Vitro*, 2001, **15**, 585–590.
50. W. Lilienblum W. Dekant, H. Foth, T. Gebel, J. G. Hengstler, R. Kahl, P. J. Kramer, H. Schweinfurth and K. M. Wollin, *Arch. Toxicol.*, 2008, **82**, 211–236.
51. N. A. Brown and S. Fabro, *Teratology*, 1981, **24**, 65–78.
52. H. Asada, Y. Kawamura, K. Maruyama, H. Kume, R. G. Ding, N. Kanbara, H. Kuzume, M. Sanbo, T. Yagi and K. Obata, *Proc. Natl. Acad. Sci. U. S. A.*, 1997, **94**, 6496–6499.
53. S. Spence, C. Anderson, M. Cukierski and D. Patrick, *Reprod. Toxicol.*, 1999, **13**, 15–29.
54. K. A. Treinen, C. Louden, M. J. Dennis and P. J. Wier, *Teratology*, 1999, **59**, 51–59.
55. C. X. Zhang, T. L. Danberry, M. A. Jacobs and K. A. Augustine-Rauch, *Birth Defects Res., Part B*, 2010, **89**, 485–492.
56. C. X. Zhang, J. C. Cao, J. Panzica-Kelly, D. S. Stock and K. A. Augustine-Rauch, *Birth Defects Res., Part A*, 2010, **88**, 361.

57. K. A. Augustine-Rauch, *Curr. Drug. Metab.*, 2008, **9**, 971–977.
58. K. A. Augustine-Rauch, C. X. Zhang and J. M. Panzica-Kelly, *Birth Defects Res., Part C*, 2010, **90**, 87–98.
59. H. Spielmann, *Toxicol. Appl. Pharmacol.*, 2005, **207**, S375–S380.
60. H. Spielmann, I. Pohl, B. Doering, M. Liebsch and F. Moldenhauer, *In Vitro Toxicol.*, 1997, **10**, 119–127.
61. E. Genschow, H. Spielmann, G. Scholz, I. Pohl, A. Seiler, N. Clemann, S. Bremer and K. Becker, *Altern. Lab. Anim.*, 2004, **32**, 209–244.
62. R. Buesen, A. Visan, E. Genschow, B. Slawik, H. Spielmann and A. Seiler, *Altex,* 2004, **21**, 15–22.
63. R. Buesen, E. Genschow, B. Slawik, A. Visan, H. Spielmann, A. Luch and A. Seiler, *Toxicol. Sci.*, 2009, **108**, 389–400.
64. A. Seiler, A. Visan, R. Buesen, E. Genschow and H. Spielmann, *Reprod. Toxicol.*, 2004, **18**, 231–240.
65. N. I. zur Nieden, G. Kempka and H. J. Ahr, *Toxicol. Appl. Pharmacol.*, 2004, **194**, 257–269.
66. M. Festag, C. Sehner, P. Steinberg and B. Viertel, *Toxicol. in Vitro*, 2007, **21**, 1619–1630.
67. D. A. van Dartel, J. L. Pennings, P. J. Hendriksen, F. J. van Schooten and A. H. Piersma, *Reprod. Toxicol.*, 2009, **27**, 93–102.
68. R. Chapin, K. Augustine-Rauch, B. Beyer, G. Daston, R. Finnell, T. Flynn, S. Hunter, P. Mirkes, K. S. O'Shea, A. Piersma, D. Sandler, P. Vanparys and G. Van Maele-Fabry, *Birth Defects Res., Part B*, 2008, **83**, 446–456.
69. K. C. Brannen, J. M. Panzica-Kelly, T. L. Danberry and K. A. Augustine-Rauch, *Birth Defects Res., Part B*, 2010, **89**, 66–77.
70. K. Augustine-Rauch, C. X. Zhang and J. M. Panzica-Kelly, *Birth Defects Res., Part C*, 2010, **90**, 87–98.
71. C. Pardo-Martin, T. Y. Chang, B. K. Koo, C. L. Gilleland, S. C. Wasserman and M. F. Yanik, *Nat. Methods*, 2010, **7**, 634–636.
72. L. J. Engelking, B. M. Evers, J. A. Richardson, J. L. Goldstein, M. S. Brown and G. Liang, *J. Clin. Invest.*, 2006, **116**, 2356–2365.
73. J. Panzica-Kelly, C. X. Zhang, T. L. Danberry, A. Flood, J. DeLan, K. C. Brannen and K. Augustine-Rauch, *Birth Defects Res., Part B*, 2010, **83**, 1–14.
74. K. A. Augustine-Rauch, Q. J. Zhang, J. L. Leonard, A. Chadderton, M. J. Welsh, H. K. Rami, M. Thompson, L. Gaster and P. J. Wier, *Birth Defects Res., Part A*, 2004, **70**, 789–807.
76. (*a*) N. Terbach and R. S. Williams, *Biochem. Soc. Trans.*, 2009, **37**, 1126–1132; (*b*) M. G. Narotsky, E. Z. Francis and R. J. Kavlock, *Fundam. Appl. Toxicol.*, 1994, **22**, 251–265.
77. U. Bojic, K. Ehlers, U. Ellerbeck, C. L. Bacon, E. O'Driscoll, C. O'Connell, V. Berezin, A. Kawa, E. Lepekhin, E. Bock, C. M. Regan and H. Nau, *Eur. J. Pharmacol.*, 1998, **354**, 289–299.
78. D. Eikel, A. Lampen and H. Nau, *Chem. Res. Toxicol.*, 2006, **19**, 272–278.
79. U. Werling, S. Siehler, M. Litfin, H. Nau and M. Gottlicher, *Mol. Pharmacol.*, 2001, **59**, 1269–1276.

80. M. A. Taipa, *Comb. Chem. High Throughput Screening*, 2008, **11**, 325–335.
81. P. R. Brauer and B. J. Tierney, *Curr. Pharm. Des.*, 2004, **10**, 2719–2732.
82. W. K. Kim and Y. S. Pae, *Neurosci. Lett.*, 1996, **216**, 117–120.
83. S. A. Lipton, W. K. Kim, Y. B. Choi, S. Kumar, D. M. D'Emilia, P. V. Rayudu, D. R. Arnelle and J. S. Stamler, *Proc. Natl. Acad. Sci. U. S. A.*, 1997, **94**, 5923–5928.
84. T. Ito, H. Ando, T. Suzuki, T. Ogura, K. Hotta, Y. Imamura, Y. Yamaguchi and H. Handa, *Science*, **327**, 1345–1350.
85. K. Nishio, Y. Masaike, M. Ikeda, H. Narimatsu, N. Gokon, S. Tsubouchi, M. Hatakeyama, S. Sakamoto, N. Hanyu, A. Sandhu, H. Kawaguchi, M. Abe and H. Handa, *Colloids Surf., B*, 2008, **64**, 162–169.

CHAPTER 19

# *Role and Status of Bridging Biomarkers in Predictive Toxicology*

WILLIAM B. MATTES

PharmPoint Consulting, 17014 Hersperger Lane, Poolesville, MD 20837, USA

## 19.1 Introduction: Prediction and Bridging Biomarkers

*Predict*: to declare or tell in advance; prophesy; foretell: to predict the weather; to predict the fall of a civilization.[†]
*Predict*: to declare or indicate in advance; especially: foretell on the basis of observation, experience, or scientific reason.[‡]

The key questions as one considers *Predictive Toxicology* are: "What are we trying to predict?" and "based on what data?" Clearly we are predicting toxicology, and not the weather, but exactly what toxicology? Using data from an *in vitro* cell system to predict the potential of a chemical for eliciting an adverse reaction in an extremely small percentage of the human population might be viewed as a tall order; it is a very different task from that of using the same data to predict the potential of the chemical to induce histopathological liver lesions in a large percentage of exposed rats, particularly if primary rat hepatocytes are used in the cell system. Of course, the question of what data the prediction is

[†] dictionary.com
[‡] Merriam–Webster dictionary

RSC Drug Discovery Series No. 12
New Horizons in Predictive Toxicology: Current Status and Application
Edited by Alan G. E. Wilson

Published by the Royal Society of Chemistry, www.rsc.org

based on must consider what doses and/or exposures are used in the experimental system and anticipated in the predicted system. What data the prediction is based on also considers the endpoints measured in the experimental system and the measurement of toxicity in the predicted system.

In terms of the data used for prediction, it is relevant to consider the definition of a biomarker. The importance of this definition is such that a Working Group crafted one for publication. A biological marker, or biomarker is "a characteristic that is objectively measured and evaluated as an indicator of normal biologic or pathogenic processes or pharmacological responses to a therapeutic intervention".[1] It should be noted that this definition is broad and can extend to endpoints measured *in vitro*, *in silico* calculations, multivariate "signatures", and perhaps even histopathology. Thus, almost all of the topics in this book cover biomarkers and their role in predictive toxicology. For the purposes of narrowing its scope, this chapter will focus on biomarkers that are simple endpoints used in animal and clinical studies, such as serum enzyme measurements (*e.g.*, glutamate dehydrogenase[2]), protein molecules (*e.g.*, urinary albumin[3]), signaling molecules (*e.g.*, cytokines[4,5]), small-molecule metabolites (*e.g.*, urinary taurine[6] or serum ophthalmate[7]), *etc.* Such biomarkers might be described as translational, accessible biomarkers or "bridging" biomarkers to underscore their capability of being measured without sacrificing the subject, a characteristic considered important for human use.

The adjective "bridging" applied to a biomarker underscores its ability to connect the results obtained in one system with those obtained in another. That ability can play several key roles in extending and confirming the results and utility of a predictive model system. Thus, such biomarkers can 1) confirm a prediction of a model system, 2) examine predictions across species, 3) allow clinical monitoring of predictions, and 4) allow qualification of a predictive model system. Obviously, these are only slightly different aspects of the same concept, that of extending the prediction from model to target systems and, in the process, affirming the use of the model. An assumed (but actually hypothetical) basis for these roles is that the biological function and response of the bridging biomarker is fundamentally the same in different systems. This assumption (*i.e.*, hypothesis) should certainly be reconsidered if differences between systems in the response of the biomarker present themselves, but in many cases, such as for a leakage biomarker, the basis of the response is clearly similar across systems. Nonetheless, to illustrate the roles bridging biomarkers can play several examples will be given and the ways they have used to support predictive systems.

## 19.2 Examples

### 19.2.1 Alanine aminotransferase

Alanine aminotransferase (ALT) (formerly called serum glutamate pyruvate transaminase or SGPT) is a 55 kDa enzyme expressed mostly in liver. It is released from hepatocytes when they are damaged or necrotic, and increases in its activity may be easily measured in serum following hepatic injury.[8] While it is not the only serum marker of liver injury,[6,8,9] and recent studies have suggested that measuring ALT isoenzymes may offer more discrimination of liver damage,[10] over several decades serum ALT measurements have become the standard in clinical practice for assessing human liver disease or injury.[11,12] Importantly, it may be used to assess liver disease and injury in rats,[6,13,14] mice,[15,16] dogs[17,18] and monkeys.[18] As such, it provides an important tool to correlate findings between species. Given this capability, it is surprising that it has not seen wider use in assessing hepatotoxicity in *in vitro* systems. ALT release into the medium has been used to assess the merits of hepatocyte suspensions[19] and spheroid cultures[20] in assessing ethionine and methotrexate hepatotoxicity relative to assessments in primary hepatocyte cultures. In both cases the *in vitro* results could be compared to the known effects of these toxicants on serum ALT levels following *in vivo* treatments. These comparisons effectively allowed "qualification" of the model systems, *i.e.*, evaluation of their ability to model *in vivo* responses.

### 19.2.2 Troponin

Cardiac troponin T (cTnT), coded by the TNNT2 gene in humans, is a 37 kDa subunit of the troponin complex that, together with the I and C subunits, regulates the force and velocity of cardiac muscle contraction.[21,22] As these are cardiac-specific proteins, their release into serum was explored in the early 1990s for the detection of myocardial injury in patients.[21,23] Unfortunately, a full appreciation of the role and specificity of cTnT as a biomarker for cardiac damage in both clinical and animal use was complicated by the disparate performances of the many different assays developed.[21–24] However, critical evaluation and standardization of the available assays for humans[25,26] and pre-clinical species[22,27] have led to a comfort level in using cTnT as a reliable biomarker of cardiac injury. Importantly, assays have been compared in dogs, rats and mice,[28] and the value of this biomarker, as compared to that of other markers of cardiotoxicity, in a larger number of pre-clinical species has been affirmed.[29] It is worth noting, however, that while serum cTnT levels do reflect drug-induced cardiac damage as assessed by histopathology, their peak occurs at times following dosing that precede those where microscopic lesions are evident.[22,30] Indeed, there is evidence that serum troponin levels may be increased by treatments with cardiotoxic agents at doses that do not elicit histopathological findings,[31] suggesting an exquisite sensitivity. Altogether, cardiac troponin offers a truly translational (*i.e.*, bridging) biomarker of treatment-induced cardiac injury,[29,31] allowing confirmation and/or examination in a second species of experimental results found in any given animal model.

Importantly, from the standpoint of predictive toxicology, troponin release can be monitored from *in vitro* systems.[32] Thus, Andersson and colleagues demonstrated the utility of human embryonic stem cell-derived cardiomyocytes as a screen for cardiotoxins. Such cells released cardiac troponin T into the medium following treatment with doxorubicin in a fashion similar to the release from damaged heart tissue of cardiac troponin T into serum following doxorubicin treatment of humans, dogs and rats.[22] Cardiac troponin T release, in this case, qualifies the use of the assay, but could also be used in a forward fashion to confirm in animal models observations made in the *in vitro* system.

### 19.2.3 Kidney Injury Molecule 1

Kidney injury molecule 1 (coded for by the HVARC gene) was discovered as a transcript with increased expression in rat kidney tissue following ischemic injury.[33] A human homolog was cloned and subsequently homologs have been found in most mammalian species.[34] Both the mRNA for this cell membrane glycoprotein and its protein product are increased after ischemia/reperfusion injury in rat kidney tissue[33] and in human kidney biopsies from patients with acute tubular necrosis.[35] Furthermore, in both rats[36] and humans[35] the external domain of kidney injury molecule 1 (KIM-1) is shed from the cell surface and released into urine after kidney injury.

Drug-induced kidney injury is a serious concern in drug development,[37] and a key strategy is to develop technologies that can be applied throughout the drug-development cycle to detect and monitor kidney injury. On the other hand, acute kidney injury (AKI) is a serious concern in medical practice, often as a result of antibiotic treatment or use of imaging agents.[34] Diagnosis of AKI by serum creatinine is complicated by that biomarker's insensitivity as a true measure of injury, hence for both drug development and clinical practice there is great interest in new biomarkers that are more sensitive and specific in their detection and diagnosis of kidney injury, ideally before major compromises to renal function have occurred. Numerous studies have shown urinary levels of KIM-1 to be a sensitive indicator of kidney injury in both pre-clinical models and clinical experience,[34,38,39] including injury induced by a wide variety of drugs and chemicals in rats; in addition, Vaidya and coworkers have shown urinary KIM-1 levels increased in patients treated with the nephrotoxic anti-tumor agent *cis*-platin.[40] Finally, a body of collaborative work qualifying KIM-1 for use in standard pre-clinical safety assessment studies has shown its ability to outperform standard clinical chemistry measures of nephrotoxicity.[41]

The fact that KIM-1 responds to injury at the levels of mRNA expression, protein expression, and even extracellular release lends its use as a bridging biomarker that can correlate results obtained not only with various animal studies but also with *in vitro* models. To explore this possibility Rached and coworkers examine the mRNA levels of KIM-1 and several other nephrotoxicity biomarkers in NRK-52E cells treated with the kidney proximal tubule toxin ochratoxin A.[42] Even though this line was derived from proximal tubule epithelium, minimally cytotoxic doses of ochratoxin failed to elicit mRNA responses for the various biomarkers, and the mRNA for KIM-1 was undetectable by real-time quantitative PCR. The results suggested that this *in vitro* system may be lacking certain factors, such as culture or treatment conditions, that would facilitate its faithful modeling of *in vivo* nephrotoxicity. In this case the bridging biomarker provides valuable insight into the *in vitro* model system and its predictivity.

### 19.2.4 Flow Cytometric Micronucleus Test

The safety assessment of chemicals and drugs almost always includes an evaluation of the compound's ability to induce genetic damage in a model system. This evaluation of genetic toxicology is motivated by the understanding that genetic abnormalities can underlie birth defects, inherited syndromes and neoplasia, and that many chemicals that can cause genetic damage in model systems can also enhance tumor rates in rodent models of carcinogenesis. Chemicals can cause genetic abnormalities by many different mechanisms[43] and consequently assessment of a chemical's potential for genetic toxicity requires tests that are based on those different mechanisms. While a myriad of test systems have been examined over the last half century,[43,44] current regulatory guidelines suggest a battery of only one or two *in vitro* tests and one *in vivo* test.[45,46]

Of the *in vivo* tests for genotoxicity available, the one most commonly used to support first-in-human studies by the pharmaceutical industry is the bone marrow micronucleus test.[45] This test makes use of the fact that one outcome of chromosome damage may be chromosome fragments that were not incorporated into a daughter nucleus at mitosis. Historically the test was conducted by microscopically examining polychromatic (immature) erythrocytes from bone marrow of rats or mice and counting these fragments. In the last two decades a flow-cytometry-based analysis has been developed to monitor micronuclei in peripheral blood reticulocytes.[47] It is based on parallel labeling of DNA and the transferrin receptor (TFRC, CD71), the latter to identify immature reticulocytes. Not only is this assay well established for rats,[48] it has been applied to peripheral blood from dogs,[49] monkeys,[50] and humans.[51] It has been accepted for use in studies regulated by health authorities[52] and its use in standard 28-day rat studies is being considered.[53]

The traditional, microscopy-based micronucleus test was also adapted for *in vitro* use with cell lines, as a rapid screen for genotoxicity.[54] Not surprisingly, flow cytometric analysis, as applied to this *in vitro* model, can greatly enhance the throughput of the *in vitro* assay.[55] All in all, flow cytometric analysis of micronuclei is a model of a true bridging biomarker and its assay, as it can be applied in a predictive *in vitro* screen and later used to confirm results in a variety of species and even clinical settings. This biomarker serves as an example of the power and potential of intentionally developing tools that can link predictive models with *in vivo* models and ultimately human experience.

## 19.3 Discovery of Bridging Biomarkers

Biomarker discovery has been greatly accelerated through the use of -omics technologies, where hundreds to thousands of analytes or endpoints in a biological system are interrogated simultaneously in response to a perturbation.

As an example, KIM-1 was identified by Representational Difference Analysis (RDA) as an mRNA transcript up-regulated in rat kidney tissue after ischemic injury.[33] Other studies using microarray analysis of kidney tissue from rats treated with various nephrotoxins also identified KIM-1 as an up-regulated transcript.[56] Subsequent studies showed that the ectodomain of the KIM-1 protein was shed from cells, and as such, serves as a urinary marker of kidney injury in humans and rats.[35,39] Nonetheless, the initial focus on KIM-1 as a biomarker was on the mRNA transcript, with subsequent confirmation of the ectodomain biomarker as translational (*i.e.*, cross-species) and accessible.

Searfoss and co-workers describe a different approach to bridging biomarker discovery using -omics technology.[57] Investigating the gastrointestinal toxicity caused by a functional γ-secretase inhibitor (FGSI) in rats, they used microarray analysis to identify transcripts up-regulated in the ileum of treated animals. However, they mined their transcript data specifically for genes whose protein products are secreted from the cell. They identified the serine protease adipsin as a gene whose product is secreted and whose mRNA is up-regulated by FGSI treatment before the onset of histological lesions, a finding confirmed using PCR. Using an anti-adipsin antibody these authors showed that elevated levels of the protein could be identified in feces early after the initiation of treatment. Furthermore they also demonstrate that adipsin mRNA is up-regulated by FGSI treatment in cultured cell models, thus affording a true bridging biomarker for connection *in vitro* predictive models to *in vivo* confirmation. Their strategy thus moves quickly from a global -omics survey to candidates for accessible, and potentially bridging, biomarkers. Given the availability of databases of secreted proteins[58–60] and the ability to search UniProt/SwissProt for secreted proteins,[61] moving from global transcriptional profiles to potentially accessible biomarkers seems a logical approach.

On the other hand, global profiling of proteomic changes in accessible fluids, such as blood, under conditions of toxicity can serve as a direct and powerful means of identifying safety biomarkers.[62] As an example, Amacher and co-workers used two-dimensional gel electrophoresis to examine the serum proteome of rats treated with four compounds having different hepatotoxic modes of action. Careful analysis of the temporal response of protein changes and other factors yielded 19 proteins as possible biomarkers for altered liver function, including paraoxonase (PON1), malate dehydrogenase (MDH), purine nucleoside phosphorylase (PNP), and $\alpha_1$-macroglobulin.[63] By the very nature of the discovery approach these are accessible biomarkers and they are being explored further for their general utility and translatability as biomarkers of liver injury.[9]

A third global profiling approach, metabonomics, examines the spectrum of small-molecule changes in response to an environmental change.[64] Using this approach two groups have screened the "metabolome" for potential biomarkers of phospholipidosis, characterized histologically as intracellular vacuoles and biochemically as an excessive accumulation of intracellular phospholipids. This condition can be elicited by a wide variety of compounds, but generally those described as cationic amphiphilic drugs (CADs).[65] Using metabonomics,

Mortuza and coworkers identified di-docosahexaenoyl (C22:6)-bis(monoacylglycerol) phosphate (BMP) as elevated in liver, lung, lymphocytes and serum of rats treated with the CAD amiodarone.[66] Baronas and coworkers extended this observation with metabonomics to urine of rats treated with amidarone or two other phospholipidosis-inducing drugs.[67] In a similar fashion, Soga and coworkers examined the metabolite changes in livers of mice treated with hepatotoxic doses of acetaminophen.[7] They identified increases in ophthalmate as a clear result of the treatment and correlated with glutathione depletion. In confirming the presence of elevated ophthalmate in serum they suggest this small molecule as a biomarker of hepatotoxic oxidative stress. As with the proteomic examination of serum, these studies result in a direct discovery of an accessible biomarker, leaving only the development of a robust assay and confirmation of its translatability across species and to *in vitro* models as the final steps in establishing a true bridging biomarker.

## 19.4 Future Possibilities

### 19.4.1 Unmet Bridging Biomarker Needs

As noted earlier, several toxicities such as phospholipidosis, are observed preclinically by standard histopathology, but lack true bridging biomarkers that can link the pre-clinical finding to either *in vitro* predictive models or clinical studies. Hepatotoxicity remains a problematic area where ALT levels are preclinically not always correlative with histopathology, and clinically often seen transiently elevated.[68] Many new biomarkers of liver toxicity are being explored[9] and it remains to be seen which, if any, may serve to bridge models of hepatotoxicity. Testicular toxicity also presents serious challenges,[69,70] with only a few potential biomarkers such as serum inhibin B.[71] A recent study using metabonomic analysis and EGME-treated rats suggests a number of small-molecule candidate biomarkers in serum and urine, but the applicability of these to other testicular toxicants and models remains to be determined.[72] Likewise, teratogenicity represents an adverse event that currently is only evaluated through morphology. Various studies such as those of Kultima and co-workers have explored global transcript profiling to identify potential gene expression changes indicative of teratogenicity, but have not pursued the potential for any of the expressed proteins to serve as biomarkers (although one, LGALS1, is known to be a secreted peptide).[73] Clearly, the field of safety bridging biomarker discovery and qualification offers many areas for further work.

### 19.4.2 Blood mRNA

While global transcript profiling of tissue responses to toxicant treatment has been a mainstay of toxicogenomics, mRNA changes in whole blood have recently been shown to have promise as biomarkers of response. The technology for obtaining transcriptomic profiles from whole blood has been optimized[74,75] and several studies have shown that such profiles can distinguish control from hepatotoxicant-treated rats.[76,77] Surprisingly, these profiles can be replicated in humans treated with non-toxic doses of hepatotoxicants[76,78,79] strongly suggesting translatability. Finally, Miyamoto and coworkers have shown that cell-free mRNAs in rat blood can also serve as markers of liver-specific toxicity.[80] Thus transcriptomic-based biomarkers in accessible fluids may offer unique possibilities for improved monitoring of target-organ toxicities.

### 19.4.3 Cytokines

Yet another opportunity for biomarker discovery comes with the development of technologies that simultaneously measure levels of multiple cytokines.[81–83] Given the importance of immune system signaling in biological responses to environmental changes, it is not surprising that cytokine profiling is pursued as potential source of safety biomarkers.[5,84] As with any biomarker, the robustness of a cytokine response is a critical consideration, although these molecules by their very nature have short half-lives and are not tissue-specific.[84]

### 19.4.4 Metabonomics

While mentioned earlier in this chapter, it should be noted that as the technology applied to metabolic profiling improves, along with tools for analysis[85] and approaches to comparing results across platforms,[86] the application of this safety biomarker discovery approach will undoubtedly increase.[87] Already multiple metabonomic databases[88,89] allow metabolite profiling data to be considered in context, and several recent studies[72,90–93] point to the potential for rapidly screening for and identifying biomarkers in accessible fluids. That the technology can be readily applied to any biological model is compelling, although the cross-species applicability of any given biomarker must be determined on a case-by-case basis. Nonetheless, small-molecule biomarkers remain an attractive potential tool for comparing observations in predictive models of toxicity with pre-clinical and clinical studies.

## 19.5 Conclusions

Bridging biomarkers play a key role in fully empowering predictive models by allowing confirmation of predictions, comparisons across species (including humans) and ultimately qualification of the model. All too often these tools are considered secondary to the development of model systems, yet their consideration and application in the early stages of model development can provide the basis for confidence in the model and its results. Given the array of technologies available for discovery and implementation of such biomarkers, embracing them should not be considered a distraction, but an integral part of predictive toxicology.

## References


1. B. D. W. Group, *Clin. Pharmacol. Ther.*, 2001, **69**, 89.
2. P. J. O'Brien, M. R. Slaughter, S. R. Polley and K. Kramer, *Lab. Anim.*, 2002, **36**, 313.
3. Y. Yu, H. Jin, D. Holder, J. S. Ozer, S. Villarreal, P. Shughrue, S. Shi, D. J. Figueroa, H. Clouse, M. Su, N. Muniappa, S. P. Troth, W. Bailey, J. Seng, A. G. Aslamkhan, D. Thudium, F. D. Sistare and D. L. Gerhold, *Nat. Biotechnol.*, 2010, **28**, 470.
4. G. N. Dietsch, C. R. Dipalma, R. J. Eyre, T. Q. Pham, K. M. Poole, N. B. Pefaur, W. D. Welch, E. Trueblood, W. D. Kerns and S. T. Kanaly, *Toxicol. Pathol.*, 2006, **34**, 39.
5. S. Lacour, J. C. Gautier, M. Pallardy and R. Roberts, *Cancer Biomark.*, 2005, **1**, 29.
6. D. E. Amacher, *Hum. Exp. Toxicol.*, 2002, **21**, 253.
7. T. Soga, R. Baran, M. Suematsu, Y. Ueno, S. Ikeda, T. Sakurakawa, Y. Kakazu, T. Ishikawa, M. Robert, T. Nishioka and M. Tomita, *J. Biol. Chem.*, 2006, **281**, 16768.
8. J. J. Reichling and M. M. Kaplan, *Dig. Dis. Sci.*, 1988, **33**, 1601.
9. J. Ozer, M. Ratner, M. Shaw, W. Bailey and S. Schomaker, *Toxicology*, 2008, **245**, 194.
10. R. Z. Yang, S. Park, W. J. Reagan, R. Goldstein, S. Zhong, M. Lawton, F. Rajamohan, K. Qian, L. Liu and D. W. Gong, *Hepatology*, 2009, **49**, 598.
11. W. R. Kim, S. L. Flamm, A. M. Di Bisceglie and H. C. Bodenheimer, *Hepatology*, 2008, **47**, 1363.
12. H. J. Zimmerman, *Hepatotoxicity: The Adverse Effects of Drugs and Other Chemicals on the Liver*, Lippincott Williams & Wilkins, Philadelphia, 2nd edn, 1999.
13. B. L. Copple, C. M. Rondelli, J. F. Maddox, N. C. Hoglen, P. E. Ganey and R. A. Roth, *Toxicol. Sci.*, 2004, **77**, 172.
14. G. B. Corcoran and B. K. Wong, *J. Pharmacol. Exp. Ther.*, 1987, **241**, 921.
15. J. S. Gujral, T. R. Knight, A. Farhood, M. L. Bajt and H. Jaeschke, *Toxicol. Sci.*, 2002, **67**, 322.
16. D. P. Williams, C. Garcia-Allan, G. Hanton, J. L. LeNet, J. P. Provost, P. Brain, R. Walsh, G. I. Johnston, D. A. Smith and B. K. Park, *Chem. Res. Toxicol.*, 2004, **17**, 1551.
17. C. L. Gaskill, L. M. Miller, J. S. Mattoon, W. E. Hoffmann, S. A. Burton, H. C. Gelens, S. L. Ihle, J. B. Miller, D. H. Shaw and A. E. Cribb, *Vet. Pathol.*, 2005, **42**, 147.
18. R. L. Hall and N. E. Everds, *Toxicol. Pathol.*, 2003, **31**, 6.
19. C. J. Waterfield, C. Westmoreland, D. S. Asker, J. C. Murdock, E. George and J. A. Timbrell, *Arch. Toxicol.*, 1998, **72**, 588.
20. T. M. Walker, P. C. Rhodes and C. Westmoreland, *Toxicol. in Vitro*, 2000, **14**, 475.
21. Y. Sato, T. Kita, Y. Takatsu and T. Kimura, *Heart*, 2004, **90**, 1110.

22. K. B. Wallace, E. Hausner, E. Herman, G. D. Holt, J. T. MacGregor, A. L. Metz, E. Murphy, I. Y. Rosenblum, F. D. Sistare and M. J. York, *Toxicol. Pathol.*, 2004, **32**, 106.
23. O. Hetland and K. Dickstein, *Clin. Chem.*, 1998, **44**, 1430.
24. F. S. Apple, H. E. Quist and M. M. Murakami, *Arch. Pathol. Lab. Med.*, 2004, **128**, 430.
25. F. S. Apple, *Toxicol. Pathol.*, 2006, **34**, 91.
26. F. S. Apple, *Clin. Chem.*, 2009, **55**, 1303.
27. F. S. Apple, M. M. Murakami, R. Ler, D. Walker and M. York, *Clin. Chem.*, 2008, **54**, 1982.
28. P. J. O'Brien, D. E. Smith, T. J. Knechtel, M. A. Marchak, I. Pruimboom-Brees, D. J. Brees, D. P. Spratt, F. J. Archer, P. Butler, A. N. Potter, J. P. Provost, J. Richard, P. A. Snyder and W. J. Reagan, *Lab. Anim.*, 2006, **40**, 153.
29. P. J. O'Brien, *Toxicology*, 2008, **245**, 206.
30. M. York, C. Scudamore, S. Brady, C. Chen, S. Wilson, M. Curtis, G. Evans, W. Griffiths, M. Whayman, T. Williams and J. Turton, *Toxicol. Pathol.*, 2007, **35**, 606.
31. B. R. Berridge, S. Pettit, D. B. Walker, A. S. Jaffe, A. E. Schultze, E. Herman, W. J. Reagan, S. E. Lipshultz, F. S. Apple and M. J. York, *Am. Heart J.*, 2009, **158**, 21.
32. H. Andersson, B. Kagedal and C. F. Mandenius, *Anal. Bioanal. Chem.*, 2010, **398**, 1395.
33. T. Ichimura, J. V. Bonventre, V. Bailly, H. Wei, C. A. Hession, R. L. Cate and M. Sanicola, *J. Biol. Chem.*, 1998, **273**, 4135.
34. V. S. Vaidya, M. A. Ferguson and J. V. Bonventre, *Annu. Rev. Pharmacol. Toxicol.*, 2008, **48**, 463.
35. W. K. Han, V. Bailly, R. Abichandani, R. Thadhani and J. V. Bonventre, *Kidney Int.*, 2002, **62**, 237.
36. V. S. Vaidya, V. Ramirez, T. Ichimura, N. A. Bobadilla and J. V. Bonventre, *Am. J. Physiol. Renal. Physiol.*, 2006, **290**, F517.
37. F. Dieterle, E. Marrer, E. Suzuki, O. Grenet, A. Cordier and J. Vonderscher, *Curr. Opin. Drug Discovery Devel.*, 2008, **11**, 60.
38. V. S. Vaidya, S. S. Waikar, M. A. Ferguson, F. B. Collings, K. Sunderland, C. Gioules, G. Bradwin, R. Matsouaka, R. A. Betensky, G. C. Curhan and J. V. Bonventre, *Clin. Transl. Sci.*, 2008, **1**, 200.
39. T. Ichimura, C. C. Hung, S. A. Yang, J. L. Stevens and J. V. Bonventre, *Am. J. Physiol. Renal Physiol.*, 2004, **286**, F552.
40. V. S. Vaidya, G. M. Ford, S. S. Waikar, Y. Wang, M. B. Clement, V. Ramirez, W. E. Glaab, S. P. Troth, F. D. Sistare, W. C. Prozialeck, J. R. Edwards, N. A. Bobadilla, S. C. Mefferd and J. V. Bonventre, *Kidney Int.*, 2009, **76**, 108.
41. V. S. Vaidya, J. S. Ozer, F. Dieterle, F. B. Collings, V. Ramirez, S. Troth, N. Muniappa, D. Thudium, D. Gerhold, D. J. Holder, N. A. Bobadilla, E. Marrer, E. Perentes, A. Cordier, J. Vonderscher, G. Maurer, P. L. Goering, F. D. Sistare and J. V. Bonventre, *Nat. Biotechnol.*, 2010, **28**, 478.

42. E. Rached, D. Hoffmann, K. Blumbach, K. Weber, W. Dekant and A. Mally, *Toxicol. Sci.*, 2008, **103**, 371.
43. R. J. Preston and G. R. Hoffman, in *Casarett and Doull's Toxicology*, ed. C. D. Klaassen, McGraw-Hill, New York, 7th edn, 2008, p. 381.
44. E. Zeiger, *Environ. Mol. Mutagen.*, 2010, **51**, 781.
45. P. Baldrick, *Regul. Toxicol. Pharmacol.*, 2008, **51**, 237.
46. *SR(R1): Technical requirements for registration of pharmaceuticals for human use*, International Conference on Harmonisation, Geneva, Switzerland, 2008.
47. S. D. Dertinger, M. E. Bishop, J. P. McNamee, M. Hayashi, T. Suzuki, N. Asano, M. Nakajima, J. Saito, M. Moore, D. K. Torous and J. T. Macgregor, *Toxicol. Sci.*, 2006, **94**, 83.
48. J. T. MacGregor, M. E. Bishop, J. P. McNamee, M. Hayashi, N. Asano, A. Wakata, M. Nakajima, J. Saito, A. Aidoo, M. M. Moore and S. D. Dertinger, *Toxicol. Sci.*, 2006, **94**, 92.
49. S. B. Harper, S. D. Dertinger, M. E. Bishop, A. M. Lynch, M. Lorenzo, M. Saylor and J. T. MacGregor, *Toxicol. Sci.*, 2007, **100**, 406.
50. C. E. Hotchkiss, M. E. Bishop, S. D. Dertinger, W. Slikker Jr., M. M. Moore and J. T. Macgregor, *Toxicol. Sci.*, 2008, **102**, 352.
51. S. D. Dertinger, R. K. Miller, K. Brewer, T. Smudzin, D. K. Torous, D. J. Roberts, S. L. Avlasevich, S. M. Bryce, S. Sugunan and Y. Chen, *Mutat. Res.*, 2007, **626**, 111.
52. M. Hayashi, J. T. MacGregor, D. G. Gatehouse, D. H. Blakey, S. D. Dertinger, L. Abramsson-Zetterberg, G. Krishna, T. Morita, A. Russo, N. Asano, H. Suzuki, W. Ohyama and D. Gibson, *Mutat. Res.*, 2007, **627**, 10.
53. S. D. Dertinger, S. Phonethepswath, D. Franklin, P. Weller, D. K. Torous, S. M. Bryce, S. Avlasevich, J. C. Bemis, O. Hyrien, J. Palis and J. T. MacGregor, *Toxicol. Sci.*, 2010, **115**, 401.
54. B. M. Miller, E. Pujadas and E. Gocke, *Environ. Mol. Mutagen.*, 1995, **26**, 240.
55. J. Shi, R. Bezabhie and A. Szkudlinska, *Mutagenesis*, 2010, **25**, 33.
56. R. P. Amin, A. E. Vickers, F. Sistare, K. L. Thompson, R. J. Roman, M. Lawton, J. Kramer, H. K. Hamadeh, J. Collins, S. Grissom, L. Bennett, C. J. Tucker, S. Wild, C. Kind, V. Oreffo, J. W. Davis II, S. Curtiss, J. M. Naciff, M. Cunningham, R. Tennant, J. Stevens, B. Car, T. A. Bertram and C. A. Afshari, *Environ. Health Perspect.*, 2004, **112**, 465.
57. G. H. Searfoss, W. H. Jordan, D. O. Calligaro, E. J. Galbreath, L. M. Schirtzinger, B. R. Berridge, H. Gao, M. A. Higgins, P. C. May and T. P. Ryan, *J. Biol. Chem.*, 2003, **278**, 46107.
58. H. F. Clark, A. L. Gurney, E. Abaya, K. Baker, D. Baldwin, J. Brush, J. Chen, B. Chow, C. Chui, C. Crowley, B. Currell, B. Deuel, P. Dowd, D. Eaton, J. Foster, C. Grimaldi, Q. Gu, P. E. Hass, S. Heldens, A. Huang, H. S. Kim, L. Klimowski, Y. Jin, S. Johnson, J. Lee, L. Lewis, D. Liao, M. Mark, E. Robbie, C. Sanchez, J. Schoenfeld, S. Seshagiri, L. Simmons, J. Singh, V. Smith, J. Stinson, A. Vagts, R. Vandlen, C. Watanabe,

D. Wieand, K. Woods, M. H. Xie, D. Yansura, S. Yi, G. Yu, J. Yuan, M. Zhang, Z. Zhang, A. Goddard, W. I. Wood, P. Godowski and A. Gray, *Genome Res.*, 2003, **13**, 2265.

59. Y. Chen, Y. Zhang, Y. Yin, G. Gao, S. Li, Y. Jiang, X. Gu and J. Luo, *Nucleic Acids Res.*, 2005, **33**, D169.
60. S. M. Grimmond, K. C. Miranda, Z. Yuan, M. J. Davis, D. A. Hume, K. Yagi, N. Tominaga, H. Bono, Y. Hayashizaki, Y. Okazaki and R. D. Teasdale, *Genome Res.*, 2003, **13**, 1350.
61. *Nucleic Acids Res.*, 2009, **37**, D169.
62. D. E. Amacher, *Toxicol. Appl. Pharmacol.*, 2010, **245**, 134.
63. D. E. Amacher, R. Adler, A. Herath and R. R. Townsend, *Clin. Chem.*, 2005, **51**, 1796.
64. D. G. Robertson, *Toxicol. Sci.*, 2005, **85**, 809.
65. W. H. Halliwell, *Toxicol. Pathol.*, 1997, **25**, 53.
66. G. B. Mortuza, W. A. Neville, J. Delaney, C. J. Waterfield and P. Camilleri, *Biochim. Biophys. Acta*, 2003, **1631**, 136.
67. E. T. Baronas, J. W. Lee, C. Alden and F. Y. Hsieh, *Toxicol. Appl. Pharmacol.*, 2007, **218**, 72.
68. P. B. Watkins, N. Kaplowitz, J. T. Slattery, C. R. Colonese, S. V. Colucci, P. W. Stewart and S. C. Harris, *JAMA, J. Am. Med. Assoc.*, 2006, **296**, 87.
69. P. Y. Muller and F. Dieterle, *Expert Opin. Drug Metab. Toxicol.*, 2009, **5**, 1023.
70. P. M. D. Foster, in *Toxicology: The Basic Science of Poisons*, ed. C. D. Klaassen, McGraw Hill, New York, 7th edn, 2008, p. 761.
71. J. Stewart and K. J. Turner, *Cancer Biomark.*, 2005, **1**, 75.
72. M. Takei, Y. Ando, W. Saitoh, T. Tanimoto, N. Kiyosawa, S. Manabe, A. Sanbuissho, O. Okazaki, H. Iwabuchi, T. Yamoto, K. P. Adam, J. E. Weiel, J. A. Ryals, M. V. Milburn and L. Guo, *Toxicol. Sci.*, 2010, **118**, 643.
73. K. Kultima, A. M. Nystrom, B. Scholz, A. L. Gustafson, L. Dencker and M. Stigson, *Environ. Health Perspect.*, 2004, **112**, 1225.
74. Z. Tian, N. Palmer, P. Schmid, H. Yao, M. Galdzicki, B. Berger, E. Wu and I. S. Kohane, *PLoS One*, 2009, **4**, e5157.
75. K. Vartanian, R. Slottke, T. Johnstone, A. Casale, S. R. Planck, D. Choi, J. R. Smith, J. T. Rosenbaum and C. A. Harrington, *BMC Genomics*, 2009, **10**, 2.
76. P. R. Bushel, A. N. Heinloth, J. Li, L. Huang, J. W. Chou, G. A. Boorman, D. E. Malarkey, C. D. Houle, S. M. Ward, R. E. Wilson, R. D. Fannin, M. W. Russo, P. B. Watkins, R. W. Tennant and R. S. Paules, *Proc. Natl. Acad. Sci. U. S. A.*, 2007, **104**, 18211.
77. J. Huang, W. Shi, J. Zhang, J. W. Chou, R. S. Paules, K. Gerrish, J. Li, J. Luo, R. D. Wolfinger, W. Bao, T. M. Chu, Y. Nikolsky, T. Nikolskaya, D. Dosymbekov, M. O. Tsyganova, L. Shi, X. Fan, J. C. Corton, M. Chen, Y. Cheng, W. Tong, H. Fang and P. R. Bushel, *Pharmacogenomics J.*, 2010, **10**, 267.

78. D. M. van Leeuwen, R. W. Gottschalk, G. Schoeters, N. A. van Larebeke, V. Nelen, W. F. Baeyens, J. C. Kleinjans and J. H. van Delft, *Environ. Health Perspect.*, 2008, **116**, 1519.
79. R. D. Fannin, M. Russo, T. M. O'Connell, K. Gerrish, J. H. Winnike, J. Macdonald, J. Newton, S. Malik, S. O. Sieber, J. Parker, R. Shah, T. Zhou, P. B. Watkins and R. S. Paules, *Hepatology*, 2010, **51**, 227.
80. M. Miyamoto, M. Yanai, S. Ookubo, N. Awasaki, K. Takami and R. Imai, *Toxicol. Sci.*, 2008, **106**, 538.
81. W. de Jager, H. te Velthuis, B. J. Prakken, W. Kuis and G. T. Rijkers, *Clin. Diagn. Lab. Immunol.*, 2003, **10**, 133.
82. C. A. Ray, R. R. Bowsher, W. C. Smith, V. Devanarayan, M. B. Willey, J. T. Brandt and R. A. Dean, *J. Pharm. Biomed. Anal.*, 2005, **36**, 1037.
83. S. X. Leng, J. E. McElhaney, J. D. Walston, D. Xie, N. S. Fedarko and G. A. Kuchel, *J. Gerontol., Ser. A*, 2008, **63**, 879.
84. J. M. Tarrant, *Toxicol. Sci.*, 2010, **117**, 4.
85. A. Kaever, T. Lingner, K. Feussner, C. Gobel, I. Feussner and P. Meinicke, *BMC Bioinf.*, 2009, **10**, 92.
86. H. Redestig, M. Kusano, A. Fukushima, F. Matsuda, K. Saito and M. Arita, *BMC Bioinf.*, 2010, **11**, 214.
87. C. J. Clarke and J. N. Haselden, *Toxicol. Pathol.*, 2008, **36**, 140.
88. B. van Ravenzwaay, G. C. Cunha, E. Leibold, R. Looser, W. Mellert, A. Prokoudine, T. Walk and J. Wiemer, *Toxicol. Lett.*, 2007, **172**, 21.
89. E. P. Go, *J. Neuroimmune. Pharmacol.*, 2010, **5**, 18.
90. K. J. Boudonck, M. W. Mitchell, L. Nemet, L. Keresztes, A. Nyska, D. Shinar and M. Rosenstock, *Toxicol. Pathol.*, 2009, **37**, 280.
91. C. L. Waterman, R. A. Currie, L. A. Cottrell, J. Dow, J. Wright, C. J. Waterfield and J. L. Griffin, *BMC Genomics*, 2010, **11**, 9.
92. R. D. Beger, J. Sun and L. K. Schnackenberg, *Toxicol. Appl. Pharmacol.*, 2010, **243**, 154.
93. T. M. O'Connell and P. B. Watkins, *Clin. Pharmacol. Ther.*, 2010, **88**, 394.

CHAPTER 20

# Renal Toxicity

K. NASIR M. KHAN,[a] GORDON C. HARD*[b] AND ZAHER A. RADI[c]

[a] Pfizer, Worldwide R&D, Drug Safety Research and Development, Groton, CT 06340, USA; [b] Private Consultant, 203 Paku Drive, Tairua 3508, New Zealand; [c] Pfizer, Worldwide R&D, Drug Safety Research and Development, Cambridge, MA 02140, USA

## 20.1 Introduction: Overview of Basic Principles in Prediction of Renal Toxicity

The kidney is a common target organ of toxicity related to occupational and accidental exposure to chemicals or as a result of exposure to drugs and imaging agents. In fact, the kidney receives more blood flow per gram of tissue than any other organ. Thus in pre-clinical safety studies where test articles are used at very large dosages, nephrotoxicity is a common finding occurring from both specific and non-specific mechanisms. A systematic approach therefore is needed to assess the potential renal effects, first by using standard toxicity and pathology endpoints in general toxicology studies and then refining the risk assessment by designing specific mechanistic studies and by the application of advanced molecular techniques. When translating pre-clinical data to humans, further consideration should be given to age, gender, and species-related differences in general responses to renal toxicants.

This chapter provides an overview of the utilization of basic principles of renal anatomy, physiology, and biomarkers to aid in predicting nephrotoxic responses. Additionally, a concise review is provided on the *in vivo* and *in vitro* models of nephrotoxicity, application of emerging technologies and utilization

RSC Drug Discovery Series No. 12
New Horizons in Predictive Toxicology: Current Status and Application
Edited by Alan G. E. Wilson

Published by the Royal Society of Chemistry, www.rsc.org

of novel renal biomarkers to predict renal injury. Rodents are used in a majority of discussions as these are the most frequently used animal species in nephrotoxicity assessments.

### 20.1.1 Anatomic Considerations

The rate of maturity of nephron components and associated growth factors can be different in fetal, neonatal, and adult kidneys which in turn can affect the susceptibility to, and the mechanisms involved in, nephrotoxicity by the same agent. In mammals, embryonic development of the permanent kidney (metanephros) begins when the tip of the mesonephric duct (Wolffian duct), known as the ureteric bud, invades the undifferentiated mesenchyme. The ureteric bud and metanephric mesenchyme induce each other during kidney development. Nephrogenesis is completed during the perinatal period in most mammalian species. The branching ureteric duct reaches the outer cortex approximately 12 weeks before full-term birth in humans. This period is roughly equivalent to day 15 of gestation in rodents. In humans, nephron formation completes prior to birth, with up to 60% of the nephrons developing in the third trimester, while in monkeys nephrogenesis is complete at birth. In rats, nephrogenesis ends by the eigth postnatal day, while in mice nephrogenesis completes before birth. In dogs, nephrogenesis is not complete until three weeks after birth, after which renal growth occurs by a 2–3 fold increase in tubular volume and a moderate increase in glomerular volume. Changes in glomerular and tubular growth in the dog are essentially complete by approximately two months of age.

The relative corticomedullary width, number of nephrons per kidney, and the organization of medulla can vary among different species (Table 20.1), which may also contribute to differential susceptibility to nephrotoxicants. Inter-species comparison of renal structure and function is summarized in Table 20.1. The light microscopic and ultrastructural characteristics of the nephron can be subdivided into the following functional units: glomerulus, proximal convoluted tubule, *pars recta*, loop of Henle, thick ascending tubule, juxtaglomerular apparatus, the distal convoluted tubule, the collecting ducts, and interstitium. A brief overview of microanatomy of kidney is discussed below.

The basic functional unit of kidney is the nephron. The glomerulus or renal corpuscle represents the filtering unit for blood through which the plasma filtrate is derived in the first part of the uriniferous space (Figures 20.1 and 20.2). Filtration is influenced by glomerular hydrostatic pressure and oncotic pressure of the filtrate. Any pathophysiologic process that interferes with the structural integrity and function of the glomerulus can result in abnormal loss of protein in the urine, predominantly albumin. The number of nephrons varies from species to species (Table 20.1) and this can have an impact on the development of renal pathologies. For example, F344 rat strain is shown to be more vulnerable to development of progressive kidney damage due to the relatively low nephron number.[1] Spontaneously hypertensive rats (SHR) have

**Table 20.1** Comparative renal structure and function, data taken from ref. 5.

| *Renal characteristic* | *Rat* | *Dog* | *Monkey* | *Man* |
|---|---|---|---|---|
| Body weight (kg) | 0.24 | 9.1 | 3.8 | 70 |
| Kidney weight (g) | 0.75 | 31 | 9 | 157 |
| Renal organization | Unipapillary | Unipapillary | Unipapillary | Multipapillary |
| Medullary structure | Complex | Simple | Simple | Simple |
| Nephrons (per g body weight) | 128 | 45 | 49 | 16 |
| Number of nephrons (thousands) | 30 | 340–490 | 103–123 | 300–1100 |
| Glomeruli radius (μm) | 61 | 90 | 83 | 100 |
| Proximal tubule length (mm) | 12 | 20 | — | 16 |
| Tubule radius (μm) | 29 | 33 | — | 36 |
| Long loops (%) | 28 | 100 | — | 14 |
| Medullary thickness (relative) | 5.8 | 4.3 | — | 3.0 |
| Maximum osmolality (mOsmol $kg^{-1}$) | 2610 | 2610 | 1900 | 1400 |
| Inulin clearance (mL $min^{-1}$ $kg^{-1}$) | 6.0 | 4.3 | 1.9 | 2.0 |
| Maximal GFR (mL $min^{-1}$ $m^2$) | 35 | 104 | — | 75 |

GFR = glomerular filtration rate.
— Data not available.

10–25% fewer nephrons than their normotensive counterparts. Exposure to the antibiotic, gentamicin, induces a lower nephron number. Similarly, environmental factors, such as dietary restriction in fetal growth, can affect the number of glomeruli. Light microscopic evaluation of 2 to 4 μm thick sections is optimal to get an accurate assessment of glomerular cellularity and its size. Glomeruli of short-looped nephrons are approximately 20% smaller in cross-sectional diameter than long-looped (juxtamedullary) nephrons.

Proximal tubules begin at the urinary pole of the glomerulus and consist of an initial convoluted portion, the proximal convoluted tubules (PCTs). The vast majority of structural subunits in the cortex represent PCTs (Figure 20.1). The PCT and *pars recta* are qualitatively differentiated from the remainder of the nephron and collecting duct by their lumenal brush border. Ultrastructurally, endocytotic vesicles, lysosomes, phagolysosomes, endoplasmic reticulum, Golgi apparatus, and mitochondria are prominent in PCTs. This prominent endocytic-lysosomal apparatus of PCTs is responsible for the re-absorption and degradation of albumin and proteins filtered by the glomerulus. The *pars recta* or straight portion of the proximal tubule of the juxtamedullary nephron is located in the outer stripe of the medulla (Figure 20.1). *Pars recta* of short-looped nephrons are found within the medullary rays or within the outer stripe. Differentiation between PCT and *pars recta* has significant functional and toxicologic relevance. The proximal tubule morphologically is divided into three segments ($S_1$, $S_2$, and $S_3$) in rat, rabbit, mouse, and the rhesus monkey.

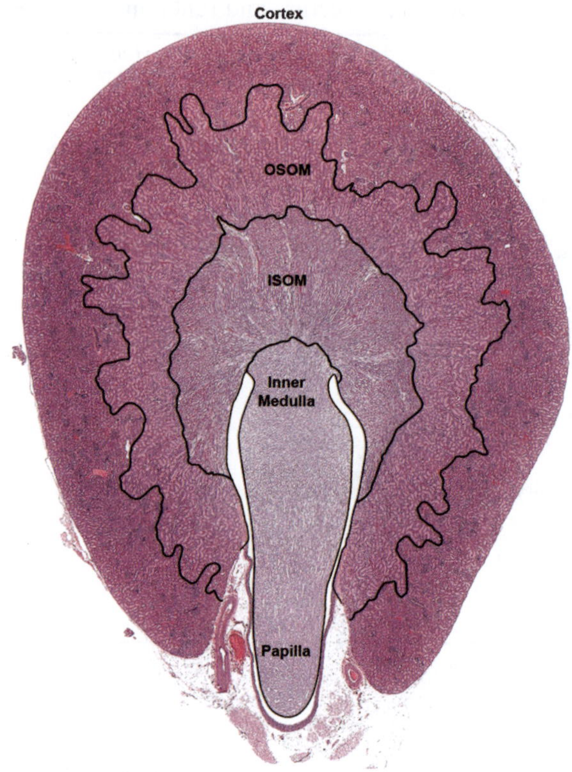


**Figure 20.1** Sub-gross anatomical regions of the rat kidney. ISOM = Inner Stripe of Outer Medulla; OSOM = Outer Stripe of Outer Medulla. Hematoxylin and eosin stain.

Only the PCT and *pars recta* have been positively identified in the normal human kidney. The $S_1$, segment is short, connecting with the glomerular filtration space. Cells of this segment have the highest rate of oxidative metabolism in the kidney. The $S_2$ segment represents the vast majority of the PCT and extends a short distance into the *pars recta*. The vast majority of the *pars recta* consist of the $S_3$ segment. The transition from the proximal tubule to the descending thin limb of loop of Henle is abrupt and marks the boundary between the outer and inner stripes of the outer medulla. This transition, which is of pathologic relevance, occurs at the junction of inner and outer stripe. The inner stripe of the outer zone of the medulla consists of Henle's loops, thick ascending tubules (thick ascending segment or straight portion of the distal tubule), and collecting ducts. The inner zone of the medulla consists of Henle's loops and collecting ducts.

The distal tubule is comprised of three structurally distinct segments, the thick ascending limb of loop of Henle (TAL), the macula densa, and the distal convoluted tubule (DCT). TAL is found in the outer zone of the medulla and in

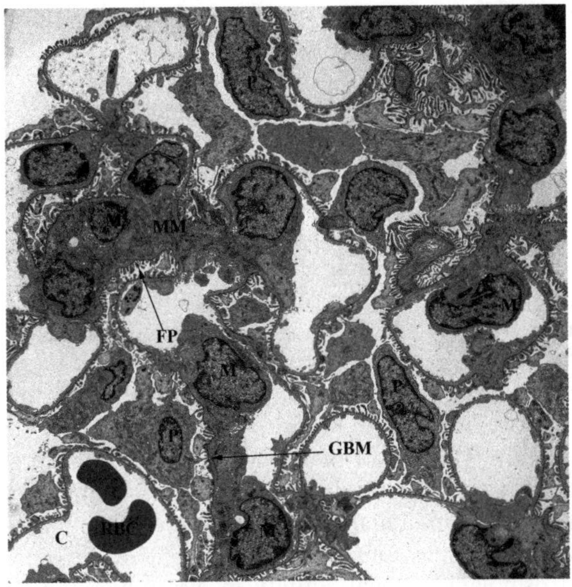


**Figure 20.2** Electron micrograph of glomerulus of the cynomolgus monkey kidney. C = Capillary loop lumen; FP = Foot Processes; P = Podocyte; GBM = Glomerular Basement Membrane; M = Mesangial cell; MM = Mesangial Matrix; RBC = Erythrocyte (image courtesy of Dr Xiantang Li, Pfizer).

the cortex, ending near its own glomerulus, just past the macula densa. In the rat and rabbit, the cortical TAL extends beyond the vicinity of the macula densa and forms an abrupt transition with the DCT. Although significant ultrastructural heterogeneity occurs at various levels of the thick ascending tubule, no relevant toxicologic correlate has been described. The juxtaglomerular apparatus (JGA) is located at the vascular pole of the glomerulus, where a portion of the distal nephron comes into contact with its parent glomerulus. The main components of JGA are the macula densa of the thick ascending limb, the renin-producing granular cells of the afferent arteriole, and the extraglomerular mesangial cell (*lacis* or Goormaghtigh cells). The macula densa is a specialized region of the TAL adjacent to the hilum of the glomerulus.

The DCT begins at a variable distance beyond the macula densa and extends to the connecting tubule that connects the nephron with the collecting duct. The connecting tubule is well defined in rabbits but not in rat, mouse or human kidney. The collecting duct extends from the connecting segment in the cortex through the outer and inner medulla to the tip of the papilla. Collecting ducts progressively anastomose from cortex to papilla. In the papilla, collecting ducts form the ducts of Bellini, which empty into the pelvis. The cortex in the rat consists of 7% interstitium by volume, of which only 3% represent the interstitial cells. In contrast, the amount of interstitium in the medulla continuously increases toward the tip of the papilla, reaching up to 29% by volume.

The interstitium of the papilla consists of mucopolysaccharides and three cell types: stellate cell, monocyte, and pericyte. The proportion of interstitium in the inner medulla increases with age and ischemia.

### 20.1.2 Physiological Considerations

The primary functions of kidneys can be divided into four major categories: 1) control of the body's fluid and electrolytes, 2) elaboration of hormones, 3) excretion of the waste products of metabolism, and 4) selected metabolic activities. Nitrogenous waste products consisting of urea, creatinine, and ammonia are excreted in the urine; thus any significant alterations in renal function are manifested in retention of these waste products in the body.

The kidneys play a major role in the control of fluid and electrolyte composition of the body. The size of the body fluid compartment and total body water are kept remarkably constant by control of fluid osmolality through control of thirst centers and renal sodium and water excretion. Sodium and its attendant anions contribute approximately 90–95% of the osmotic activity of the body fluid osmolality. Renal activity in electrolyte and fluid balance is mediated by modulation of the glomerular filtration rate (GFR), adrenergic nerve activity, antidiuretic hormone (ADH), aldosterone, and natriuretic hormones. Re-absorption of NaC1 accounts for most of the energy expenditure in the kidney. Normal renal function is predicated on adequate perfusion (pressure and volume). The kidneys typically receive 25% of the cardiac output. However, only about 10% of oxygen consumption occurs in the kidneys. Approximately 85% of renal flow can be associated with cortex, 14% with outer medulla, and 1% with inner medulla, reflecting heterogeneity in intrarenal flow distribution. GFR is the basic determinant in urine formation and a key measurement of kidney function. Discrimination in GFR for larger molecules occurs based on molecular size, configuration, and charge. Transport of cationic molecules is facilitated, whereas that of anionic molecules is restricted. Vascular resistance varies within the kidney so renal blood flow remains constant (autoregulation) over a wide range of systolic pressures from 90 to 220 mm Hg. Neural regulation of renal blood flow is minimal in the normal steady state.

The proximal tubule represents the site of re-absorption of the most sodium. Regardless of body needs, obligatory water re-absorption occurs. This water re-absorption is passive, accompanying active re-absorption of solutes. Sodium is transported passively in the TAL, but actively elsewhere in the distal nephron, and is dependent on body needs with responsiveness to aldosterone. Active transport of sodium is mediated by $Na^+$–$K^+$–ATPase (sodium pump) in the basolateral cell surface membranes. An osmotic gradient is established and maintained by selective permeability in the loops of Henle and passive diffusion in the vasa recta. The ability of the kidneys to concentrate urine is dependent on the gradient of increasing interstitial osmolality running from the outer medulla to the tip of the papilla created by the countercurrent system.

Chloride is actively transported in the thick ascending tubules. Regulation of body needs for facultative re-absorption of water is controlled by ADH. Permeability to water is low in the absence of ADH in the distal nephron. The potassium ion is the principal intracellular electrolyte. Potassium excretion is also influenced by hormonal control (aldosterone) in the distal nephron. The kidney is responsible for controlling the concentration of potassium in the body. The proximal tubule is the site of approximately 70% of potassium re-absorption. A marked decrease in urinary potassium clearance does not occur until body potassium stores are depleted by 20–40%. An increase in potassium load, however results in a prompt rise in urinary potassium clearance.

The kidney may be regarded as a primary or secondary organ for the generation of various hormones and growth factors such as erythropoietin, renin, prostaglandins, and various growth factors. In addition, the kidney is a site of degradation of hormones, such as insulin and aldosterone and is also responsible for the production of the active form of vitamin D derived from vitamin $D_3$ under the influence of parathyroid hormone. Erythropoietin (EPO) which stimulates erythrocytes production is largely produced by renal cortical peritubular interstitial cells. Several intracellular pathways involved in EPO effects include JAK-2 and Akt (protein kinase) phosphorylation and NF-κB transcription factor. Renin is produced within juxtaglomerular cells (JG) after processing and cleavage of prorenin, which is produced in the liver. Reduced renal perfusion pressure and hyponatremia are the primary stimuli for renin release from JG cells. In addition, renin release is influenced by the sympathetic nervous system and angiotensin II (AII), ADH, endothelin, and prostaglandins. Renin activates angiotensin II, which causes secretion of aldosterone by the adrenal cortical zona glomerulosa. The net effect is systemic vasoconstriction, intrarenal vasoconstriction, and increased aldosterone release. The effect of aldosterone is predominantly on the distal tubular network, affecting an increase in sodium re-absorption in exchange for potassium.

Many metabolic activities and the transport of various products take place in the kidney. A wide variety of organic acids existing as anions, both endogenous products of catabolism and exogenous substrates are transported by the proximal convoluted tubule. Of the amino acids in the glomerular filtrate, 99% are actively re-absorbed. This occurs within the first millimetre past the glomerulus in the dog and human; different transport systems are responsible for transport of neutral, acidic, and glycine shared amino acids. Proteins of a size up to that of albumin or slightly larger enter urine in the glomerular filtrate. Protein re-absorption is thought of as a low-affinity, high-capacity, and low-specificity process. Filtered proteins bind to the brush border then are taken up by endocytosis. Transport of proteins is affected by size, charge and configuration. For example, cationic albumin is re-absorbed in a five-fold greater amount than anionic albumin. The female rat re-absorbs more labeled protein and then degrades the re-absorbed protein more rapidly than the male in the same unit of time.

Regulation of acid–base balance is a very important function of the kidney. The kidneys regulate hydrogen ion concentration by three mechanisms

1) re-absorption of filtered bicarbonate, 2) secretion of titratable acid, and 3) secretion of ammonia. In the dog, 85% of bicarbonate re-absorption takes place in the proximal tubule. In tubular cells, hydrogen ions are produced by hydration of carbon dioxide. These hydrogen ions are secreted into the tubular lumen in exchange for a sodium ions, leaving sodium and bicarbonate ions behind within the cell. Buffers in the tubular lumen accept the hydrogen ions, passing down the nephron as a titratable acid.

### 20.1.3 Pathologic Considerations

Nephrotoxicity can be categorized based on (i) morphologic presentation of lesions or (ii) mechanism of renal injury.[2]

#### *20.1.3.1 Morphologic Features of Nephrotoxicity*

Drugs and chemicals can have direct toxic effects on cells of the renal vasculature, tubules and glomeruli, and/or induce inflammation of the renal interstitium, leading to acute intrinsic renal failure. Morphologic presentation of nephrotoxicity at the cellular level can occur as necrosis, apoptosis, or hyperplasia.[2,3] In necrosis, loss of cell volume homeostasis resulting in swelling of plasma and organelle membranes leads to rupture and dissolution of organized cell structure. Necrotic cells are typically enlarged and less intensely eosinophilic than normal. In apoptosis, condensation of the cytoplasm and nuclei is followed by cell fragmentation and formation of apoptotic bodies. Increased apoptosis can be recognized in histology sections by increased tissue replication rate in the absence of hyperplasia, by terminal deoxynucleotidyl transferase (TdT) nick end-labeling (TUNEL) or by demonstration of increased apoptotic cells in urine or urineferous spaces. In addition, expression levels of messenger RNA (mRNA) and protein of apoptosis-related genes such as bax, bcl-2, cytochrome *c*, caspase-9, and caspase-3 can be used in nephrotoxicity assessment.[4]

Increased apoptosis occurs in the steady-state kinetics of healthy adult tissue. Apoptosis plays an important role in nephron development in fetal kidney and in tubular repair following renal insult. Accelerated apoptosis has been defined as a pivotal feature in renal toxicity such as observed in fumonisin-induced injury in rats. Numerous toxicants (heavy metals, drugs and naturally occurring toxins) have been implicated to trigger or block the intracellular processes resulting in abnormal regulation of apoptosis mediating a wide range of pathologic consequences ranging from renal agenesis to neoplasia. Renal cellular hyperplasia can be an immediate repair response to tubular necrosis with intact basement membranes or can be a chronic response to long-term exposure to xenobiotics including neoplasm development in some cases.

The microscopic lesions of nephrotoxicity in the glomerulus can simply manifest as thickening of basement membranes or can include inflammatory cell infiltrates. The non-inflammatory glomerular disease is characterized by thickening of capillary wall and basement membranes with or without an increase in the number of cells in the glomerulus (membranoproliferative and membranous nephropathy, respectively). Membranous nephropathy can be caused by immune complex deposition in the glomerular tuft which is seen after repeated dosing with biological products. Electron microscopy, immunofluorescence, and special histochemical stains such as PAS (periodic acid Schiff), trichrome and silver stains can be used to further characterize the glomerular changes. It is important to note that, unlike humans, renal glomeular deposition of immune complexes by itself without evidence of an inflammatory response in non-human primates does not necessarily imply a disease state. Cell proliferation is the hallmark of an inflamed glomerulus, termed glomerulonephritis and is sometimes seen following treatment with immunosuppressive agents. If the proliferating cell is mesangial, the process is designated mesangioproliferative glomerulonephritis. If neutrophils are increased in the tuft, the process is designated exudative glomerulonephritis. Postinfectious glomerulonephritis (*e.g.*, post-streptococcal glomerulonephritis) is an example of exudative glomerulonephritis which can stem from an immunologic phenomenon.

### *20.1.3.2 Mechanistic Approach to Nephrotoxicity*

Mechanisms with which xenobiotics can elicit renal injury are summarized in Table 20.2 and are further discussed below. Consideration of these potential mechanisms can help employ appropriate *in vivo* and *in vitro* tools and selection of relevant biomarkers in refining the risk assessment or in monitoring the progression of nephrotoxicity.

**Direct Effect on Cells and Their Functions.** Nephrotoxicity due to direct perturbation of cellular or subcellular organelle function occurs most commonly in the highly metabolically active PCTs and less so the distal tubules and collecting ducts. The injury can be related to accumulation of xenobiotics or their metabolites in subcellular organelles *e.g.*, aminoglycoside antibiotic lysosomal overload. Lysosomal overload of gentamicin and phospholipid membranes results in compromised lysosomal membrane integrity. Lysosomal enzyme leakage occurs as a consequence and possibly explains cell necrosis as

**Table 20.2** Potential mechanisms of nephrotoxicity by xenobiotics.

| *No* | *Mechanism* |
|---|---|
| 1 | Direct effect on cells and their functions |
| 2 | Injury *via* reactive intermediates or oxidative stress |
| 3 | Effects on endogenous or nutritive substrate |
| 4 | Effects on renal hemodynamics |
| 5 | Elicitation of immune-mediated injury |
| 6 | Obstructive nephropathy |
| 7 | Exacerbation of spontaneous age-related nephropathy |
| 8 | Induction of renal neoplasia |

the overt manifestation of toxicity. Heavy metals typically accumulate in the kidney, liver, bone and brain. The injury in the kidney typically involves the PCT. The common examples of heavy metals resulting in direct cellular toxicity in the kidney include cadmium, mercury, manganese, and lead.

**Injury *via* Reactive Intermediates or Oxidative Stress.** Xenobiotic-metabolizing enzymes, including cytochrome P450-dependent mixed-function oxidases, are present in the kidney.[5] Mixed-function oxidase activity occurs primarily in the *pars recta* or $P_2$ segment in the rat. Cytochrome P450 content of the kidney is only 10–20% of liver content; however, at the cell level, the concentrations in the cells of the *pars recta* in the outer stripe are comparable to hepatocytes. Thus, the outer stripe is typically the primary site for xenobiotics injury *via* metabolic activation. It is in these cells then that cytochrome P450 and mixed functions oxidases catalyze reactions to produce a more readily excretable form of the parent xenobiotic. Xenobiotic injury *via* the β-lyase pathway is also preferentially expressed in the outer stripe. The renal clearance mechanism of the test article should be evaluated if nephrotoxicity is observed in *in vivo* toxicity studies. Several xenobiotics require transport as an organic ion to initiate cell injury such as cephalosporin antibiotics, citrinin, mercuric anion and cysteine conjugates. The organic ion transporter present at all levels in proximal tubules may play an important role in renal toxicity. Organic anion transport is presumed to be involved in the transport of important proximal tubule nutrient substrates such as succinate. *p*-Aminohippuric acid (PAH) represents a model organic anion in the study of this transporter. Transport of PAH is inhibited by organic anions such as probenecid and penicillin. PAH and probenecid have been demonstrated to reduce toxicity of drugs requiring transport as an organic anion in mechanistic studies. Mepiperphenidol, quinine, and quinidine have been used as inhibitors of organic base transporters.

**Effects on Endogenous or Nutritive Substrate.** Examples of nephrotoxicity from perturbation of endogenous or nutritive substrates include phosphate toxicity, iron toxicity, zinc toxicity, osmotic nephrosis, oxalate nephrosis, inducible alpha2u-globulin nephropathy syndrome, light-chain nephropathy, amino acid toxicity, synthetic-diet-induced nephrocalcinosis, myoglobin nephropathy, and hemoglobin nephropathy.[2]

**Effects on Renal Hemodynamics.** Therapeutic agents such as non-steroidal anti-inflammatory drugs (NSAIDs) can result in renal injury through reduced blood flow to the kidney.[6] Acute renal failure is the most common form of NSAID-related renal toxicity in humans caused by a hemodynamic effect due to loss of counter-regulatory prostaglandins (PGs).[7,8] Conditions that may reduce actual or effective circulation volume, *e.g.*, plasma volume contraction (hemorrhage, salt loss, hypoalbuminemia), congestive heart failure, cirrhosis and ascites, cause a homeostatic increase in vasoconstrictors including norepinephrine and angiotensin II. Vasodilatory effects of PGs at the afferent arteriole counterbalance this vasoconstrictor effect to maintain GFR and renal perfusion.[8] In the rat kidney subjected to ischemia, and then re-perfused, necrosis occurs in PCTs, invariably accompanied by medullary congestion, which is most marked in the outer stripe. This tubular injury appears after periods of ischemia as short as 15 min. The shorter the period of ischemia, the longer the re-perfusion interval required before necrotic cells can be visualized in this model. With slightly longer periods of ischemia (45 to 60 min) and re-perfusion (up to 24 h), necrosis appears in PCTs; but the *pars recta* is most prominently affected. Distribution of proximal tubule necrosis in ischemia-reflow injury has features in common with a pattern produced by hypoxia, as well as by mitochondrial toxins such as mercury. Prolonged ischemia (over 2 h) results in infarction. Prolonged ischemia induced by temporary clamping of the renal artery results in cortical infarction, whereas occlusion of venous return results in medullary infarction. Obstruction of the arcuate artery results in a wedge-shaped cortical necrosis.[2] Changes in renal perfusion pressure can cause alterations in regional cortical distribution of blood flow. Chronic decreased perfusion pressure as may be seen in hemorrhagic hypotension and renal artery stenosis leads to increased blood flow to the inner cortex in comparison to the outer cortex.[9] This can result in necrosis preferentially in the outer cortex. Prostaglandins play an important role in intracortical redistribution of renal blood flow (RBF) during reduced perfusion pressure resulting in increased blood flow to the inner cortex.

**Elicitation of Immune-Mediated Injury.** Immune-mediated kidney injury accounts for most forms of primary glomerular disease in humans while drug-associated immune-mediated kidney injury represents an important differential etiologic diagnosis in all renal diseases in humans. An occasional industrial or environmental chemical has also been implicated by association in development of immune-mediated kidney disease. Immune-mediated renal toxicity can appear as interstitial inflammation characterized by infiltration of lymphocytes, monocytes, eosinophils and plasma cells within the interstitium, active urinary sediment with pyuria and/or white blood cell casts, eosinophiluria, hematuria, and mild to moderate proteinuria. This type of renal disease has been seen with a variety of drugs in humans including penicillin, methicillin ampicillin, rifampin, sulfonamides, thiazides, cimetidine, phenytoin, allopurinol, cephalosporins, cytosine arabinoside, furosemide, interferon, NSAIDs, ciprofloxacin, clarithromycin, telithromycin, pantoprazole, omeprazole, and atazanavir.[10] The drug-associated immune-mediated kidney injury in humans depends on host factor variability for expression, as well as interaction with pre-existing disease. Immune-mediated kidney injury in animals represents an important consideration in establishing causality of spontaneous disease especially in diseased animal models. In routine toxicology studies primary immune-mediated renal toxicity is rare; however, recently there has been greater recognition of immune-mediated renal toxicity in non-human primates and rarely in rodents when given protein therapeutics over long periods of time. The mechanisms may involve deposition of systemically circulating immune complexes or immune complexes formed *in situ* comprising anti-drug antibody (ADA) with or without the elicitation of glomerular or interstitial inflammation. It should be noted that there is light microscopic (LM), electron microscopic (EM) and/or immunohistochemistry (IHC) evidence of glomerular immune complexes in clinically normal cynomolgus monkeys which may significantly increase following treatment with protein therapeutics.

**Obstructive Nephropathy.** Obstructive nephropathy is a relatively common condition in animals and humans.[5,10] It is classified according to the degree, duration, and site of the urinary tract obstruction. Obstruction can occur anywhere from the level of renal tubules to the urethral meatus. In the adult human kidney, approximately two litres of urine flows through the renal papilla daily. Any obstruction to this unidirectional flow can lead to build up of urine flow and pressure affecting renal functions. Urinary symptoms may or may not occur along with changes in urine output. Mild episodes of polyuria may alternate with periods of oliguria or occasionally anuria. A complete obstruction of short duration results in profound alterations in renal hemodynamics and glomerular filtration with minimal anatomic changes. The causes of obstructive nephropathy may be intra- or extra-renal and may be congenital or acquired.[6] Among acquired intra-renal causes, accumulation of drugs and chemicals[11] in the urinary tract is an important condition especially in susceptible populations. Intra-renal obstruction occurs secondary to accumulation of poorly soluble materials within the tubules such as following high dosages of xemilofiban, naproxen, methotrexate, acyclovir, and triamterene. NSAIDs and analgesics can lead to ureteral obstruction as a result of papillary necrosis.[12] Uric acid crystal deposition can occur with acid urine usually after cancer chemotherapy with alkylating agents and the risk of its development is related directly to the plasma uric acid concentrations.

**Exacerbation of Spontaneous Age-related Nephropathy.** Familiarity with spontaneous renal pathologies in laboratory animals and in animal models of renal disease is essential for the establishment of the nature and cause of renal damage by xenobiotics because the most minimal expression of nephrotoxicity may occur simply as a slight exacerbation of the severity of a spontaneous lesion which may mask or mimic a toxicologic response. Chronic progressive nephropathy (CPN) is a spontaneous disease of laboratory rats that represents a significant confounder for interpretation of renal histology in toxicology studies.[13,14] Rodent CPN is characterized by basophilic tubules with conspicuously thickened basement membranes, tubules in the medulla (and later cortex also) filled or dilated with hyaline proteinaceous casts, and with time, glomerulosclerosis. The disease progresses relentlessly, at least in rats of the Sprague–Dawley and F344 strains, from a solitary affected tubule in the earliest stage, to formation of multiple foci, ultimately involving the whole kidney when death occurs through chronic renal failure. Despite extensive laboratory experience with CPN over many decades, the cause of this spontaneous disease process remains unknown. Its incidence and severity are mainly influenced by diet and hormones. Reducing or increasing protein in the diet decreases or enhances CPN, respectively, while caloric restriction is the most effective dietary manipulation for reducing the incidence and severity of CPN through the life stages of a rat.[2,15] Male gender is a primary risk factor for developing CPN, this male sex predisposition having been linked to the presence of androgen rather than to an absence of estrogen.[16] CPN is a confounding factor in both sub-chronic toxicity studies and chronic bioassays because these basophilic lesions have to be discriminated from chemically-induced toxicity and some chemicals are capable of exacerbating the severity of CPN in a dose-related fashion. Furthermore, advanced CPN itself appears to be a risk factor for the development of a marginal increase in renal tubule tumors.[17,18] This means that chemicals exacerbating CPN as their only renal effect can appear spuriously to be causing a dose-related increase in renal tubule tumors in two-year bioassays.

**Induction of Renal Neoplasia.** Nephrotoxicity with drugs and chemicals can manifest itself as a proliferative lesion. The renal tumor that is the most relevant to humans with respect to risk assessment is of tubule origin, termed renal tubule tumor in rodents, and renal cell carcinoma in humans. Nephroblastoma has been induced in rats only by genotoxic chemicals and mostly by direct-acting nitrosoureas administered transplacentally.[19] Nephroblastomas have not been induced by any chemical tested in the National Toxicology Program (NTP), NIH, carcinogenicity bioassays. Current knowledge of chemical renal carcinogenesis has its foundations in early work in developing chemical induction models of renal cancer, and studying tumor pathogenesis. For renal tubule tumors, these earlier models employed genotoxic carcinogens such as *N*-nitrosomorpholine,[20] *N*-nitrosodimethylamine,[21,22] *N*-(4′-fluoro-4-biphenylyl)acetamide,[23] and *N*-ethyl-*N*-hydroxyethylnitrosamine.[24] These various studies provided evidence that renal tubule tumor is preceded by a stage of tubule alteration involving hyperplasia of the lining epithelium. It is now generally accepted that this alteration, known as atypical tubule hyperplasia, is a precursor of, and on a continuum with, renal tubule adenoma and carcinoma.[25–28] It has also been shown recently that atypical tubule hyperplasia has the morphological characteristics of an expansile lesion.[29,30] Foci are surrounded peripherally, at least partially, by attenuated fibroblasts and/or capillaries, and they have a high DNA-synthesis labeling rate, indicating that the lesion is expanding in size, on the pathway to becoming an adenoma. Consequently, induction of foci of atypical tubule hyperplasia by a chemical in a truncated bioassay predicts that the test chemical is a renal carcinogen. Based on the evidence accumulating from studies with chemical agents, Hard[31,32] proposed a list of mechanisms by which chemicals were believed to produce, or be associated with, an increase in renal tumors in the rodent. This mechanistic approach was later used to analyze and categorize the chemicals in the NTP database.[33] The possible mechanisms of xenobiotic-induced carcinogenesis are summarized in Table 20.3. These include direct or indirect

**Table 20.3** Demonstrated mechanisms of renal carcinogenesis by xenobiotics.

| *No* | *Mechanism* |
|---|---|
| 1 | Direct DNA reactivity |
| 2 | Indirect DNA reactivity exemplified by oxidative stress pathways |
| 3 | Multiphase bioactivation usually involving glutathione conjugation in liver and subsequent enzymatic activation in kidney |
| 4 | Direct cytotoxicity stimulating a sustained regenerative response |
| 5 | Indirect degenerative/regenerative response associated with perturbation of a physiological process, such as lysosomal digestions nephropathy |
| 6 | Association with exacerbation of spontaneous CPN |

DNA reactivity, multiphase bioactivation usually involving glutathione conjugation in liver and subsequent enzymatic activation in kidney, direct or indirect cell damage stimulating a sustained regenerative response, or association with exacerbation of CPN. Renal carcinogenesis associated with direct or indirect cytotoxicity and CPN involves non-genotoxic chemicals.

While a clear understanding of the molecular pathogenesis of chemically-induced renal tubule tumors remains elusive, the group of Dr O. Hino in Japan has explored the field of spontaneous renal tumor development by studying the molecular biology responsible for the Eker rat tumor. Eker rat renal tumor is a dominantly inherited familial cancer syndrome of the Long–Evans strain, in which the homozygous condition is lethal *in utero*, but the heterozygous state leads to a 100% renal tubule tumor incidence within 12 months of age.[34] The Hino group has shown that this syndrome is associated with a mutation of the rat homolog of the tuberous sclerosis 2 (Tsc 2) gene located on rat chromosome 19q.[35–37] Because Tsc 2 functions as a tumor suppressor gene, this mutation results in the high incidence of renal tubule tumors. Renal cell cancer is an important tumor in humans, and appears to be increasing in incidence on a global basis.[38] This increase is associated with both the more widespread use of diagnostic imaging and increasing prevalence of established risk factors, cigarette smoking, obesity, and hypertension.[39] Because of its metastatic potential, this tumor imposes a serious socioeconomic burden worldwide.[40] Orthotopic models of heterotransplanted human renal carcinoma cells in nude mice can be used to provide further understanding of the molecular pathogenesis of renal cell cancer in humans, and to test the effectiveness of new chemotherapeutic or biological modifying agents for tumor treatment.[41] In the past decade there has also been some interest invested in developing transgenic models of cancer for these purposes. A high percentage (60–70%) of renal cell cancer is associated with mutations or hypermethylation of the von Hippel–Lindau (*VHL*) gene located on chromosome 3p25.[42] Development of a transgenic mouse model of renal cell cancer by inactivation of the *VHL* gene therefore seemed plausible. However, conditional inactivation of this tumor suppressor gene in mice resulted in production of renal cysts only, and not renal cancer.[43] A transgenic mouse deficient in metallothionein (MT) genes has been investigated in the context of metals that are carcinogenic for the kidney.[44,45]

MT is a low-molecular-weight protein that avidly binds metals and appears to sequester these toxic agents into a non-toxic form, sometimes as intra-nuclear inclusion bodies, as is the case with lead in rat kidney.[46] MTs are particularly important in kidney where the major forms are MT-I and MT-II.[46] Lead salts are potent renal carcinogens in the rat, and have been judged probable carcinogens for humans.[47] Lead acetate administered to MT-I/II knockout mice induced higher incidences of renal tubule cancers and precursor hyperplasias than the insensitive wild-type mouse.[44] However, treatment of these genetically altered mice with another metallic renal carcinogen, nickel subsulfide, produced no difference in cancer outcome between the MT-null mice and the wild-type.[45]

## 20.1.4 Age, Gender, and Species Considerations

Potential effects of age, gender, and species-related differences in anatomy and physiology should be thoroughly considered in translating preclinical toxicity data to humans.[5] Drug response in patients of various ages including children and the elderly are common, often leading to challenges in optimizing dosages and duration of use. For example, developmental changes in renal function can dramatically alter the plasma clearance of compounds with extensive renal elimination and thus can enhance renal and systemic toxicity of these drugs.[48] Because of the challenges presented for pediatric clinical trials, attention has turned to the supportive pre-clinical data that accompany clinical trials. It has been recognized that there are circumstances where the existing toxicology studies in adult animals may need to be supplemented by added investigation using juvenile animals. However, the juvenile animal data can only be useful to guide safety of the pediatric human population if evaluated in the most appropriate species at the most relevant age considering the comparability of the specific organ system development in question coupled with the disease indication, existing toxicological data and the likely route of human exposure.[48] The interspecies differences in renal structure and function are summarized in Table 20.1 and age, gender, and species considerations in predicting nephrotoxic responses are summarized in Table 20.4.

Age-related renal damage contributes significantly to abnormalities in GFR and tubular function resulting in different susceptibility of the aged population to nephrotoxic response as compared to neonates, juveniles, and young adults. In rats, GFR gradually decreases with age, and by 18 months, the GFR is decreased to approximately 68% of its rate compared to young adults. These age-related changes are manifested in decreased urine output, decreased sodium excretion, increased blood urea nitrogen (BUN), and proteinuria. Proteinuria along with urinary loss of albumin is evident as early as six months of age.[2] In dogs, there is a gradual increase in GFR in the first three weeks post-natally. This increase in GFR is primarily the result of continuing glomerular differentiation in the outer cortical region. With progressive nephron loss in older dogs, there are decreases in GFR, similar to those in rats. In humans, before 34 weeks of gestational age, the functional demands on the fetal kidney are

**Table 20.4** Species, age, and gender considerations in predicting nephrotoxic responses, modified from ref. 5.

| *Variable* | *Contributing factors* |
|---|---|
| Species | Renal anatomy and physiology<br>CYP450 polymorphisms<br>Renal enzyme presence and distribution (*e.g.*, cyclooxygenase, β-lyase)<br>Specific protein production (*e.g.*, α2u-g) |
| Age | Alterations in renal mass, nephron number, and function<br>Changes in tissue glutathione concentrations<br>Altered responsiveness to vasoactive mediators and hormones<br>Altered renal cytokine profile<br>Age-related spontaneous syndromes (*e.g.*, CPN) |
| Gender | Hormonal status<br>Variations in xenobiotic metabolism by glutathione conjugation and differences in CYP450 polymorphisms<br>Specific protein production (*e.g.*, α2u-g)<br>Differences in GFR<br>Variations in responsiveness to vasoactive mediators |

minimal, but these increase dramatically in the last part of the third trimester and with birth. While the adult kidney receives 20–25% of the cardiac output, the human fetal kidney receives only 4%, which increases to 10% by the end of the first post-natal week. Renal function in neonates remains different from that of adults, and GFR and RBF corrected for body size are not comparable to adult values until the child is 12 months old. GFR gradually increases until adolescence, where it is maintained at adult levels. After the age of 40 in humans, there is a progressive decrease in renal function, which is primarily the result of progressive loss of renal mass and nephron number.

Changes in tubular function, similar to GFR, occur with age and are important in age-dependent differences in susceptibility to nephrotoxicity *e.g.*, aminoglycosides and vancomycin.[5] Fetuses and neonates have inefficient urine concentrating ability, both as a result of short proximal tubules and inefficient tubular transport. The tubular function in human kidney reaches adult capacity by 18 months of age and rat kidney by six weeks of age. While the impaired tubular transport capacity of the neonate is generally of no clinical significance, it may be more vulnerable to disease than GFR. The neonatal renal tubular function for the transport of organic ions is low and so is the accumulation of nephrotoxic substances into the proximal tubular epithelial cells. Increased kidney : body volume in neonates is also believed to reduce the nephrotoxic susceptibility of neonates to xenobiotics. Therefore, neonates are generally less likely to have drug-induced nephrotoxicity. Examples of specific compounds, in which adults have a higher risk of nephrotoxicity than neonates, include aminoglycosides, vancomycin, cadmium, cisplatin, and acetaminophen.

Tubular transport efficiency is greatly reduced in the aged kidney as a result of progressive nephron loss, decreased mitochondrial function, and reduced numbers of proximal tubular ion transporters. Rats also develop age-related changes in normal tubular transport function. This is characterized by progressive decreases in urinary concentrating ability and decreased chloride, calcium, and potassium retention. Defects in tubular transport with increasing age are demonstrated by decreases in PAH uptake by proximal tubular cells. Between the ages of 12 and 27 months, there is a 40% decrease in active renal tubular transport in rats. Changes in tubular transport function are also evident as 5–10% decreases in urine osmolality in rats as early as six months of age. Similar to rats and humans, age-related differences in tubular function are noted in dogs. Renal tubular function in dogs does not reach adult levels until after one to two months of age, as evidenced by reduced renal amino acid reabsorption in puppies as compared to adult dogs. With age, dogs develop reductions in urinary concentrating capacity.

## 20.2 Application of Predictive Methodologies to Assess Renal Toxicity

Routine methodologies comprising standard biomarkers in blood and urine followed by gross and microscopic pathology are considered appropriately sensitive in standard preclinical toxicity testing. Once nephrotoxicity potential is recognized, additional *in vitro*, *ex vivo*, or specialized *in vivo* studies can be done to gain further understanding of the mechanisms of toxicity or to screen a subsequent library of test articles if availability of enough test material limits assessment in standard toxicology studies.[2] Methodologies of potential use in predictive renal toxicity are summarized in Table 20.5.

### 20.2.1 *In Vivo* Approaches

Combination of standard general toxicology studies and specialized *in vivo* models with focus on renal hemodynamics, renal clearance, and renal disease models are commonly used to gain insights into the potential mechanisms of nephrotoxicity. The important aspects of renal evaluation are discussed below.

#### *20.2.1.1 Assessments in General Toxicology Studies*

At the end of drug-exposure period in a general toxicology study, the minimum assessments to determine nephrotoxicity can include standard clinical chemistry screens with BUN and serum creatinine (sCr), along with electrolytes, urinary excretion of protein and electrolytes, urinalysis (with volume, specific gravity, and microscopic sediment evaluations), absolute and relative kidney weight determination, and gross and microscopic examination of the kidney tissue.

For accurate assessment of urinary biomarkers, it is essential to collect urine specimens of good quality over a 16–24 h period ideally in metabolism cages on cold packs. Historical control data from the testing facility can help to distinguish subtle drug-induced effects from background and in assessing individual animal variability. In rats, renal function tests may become more variable

**Table 20.5** Methodologies of potential use in predictive renal toxicity.

| *Assessment* | *Potential methodologies* |
|---|---|
| Morphology | Routine histology, histochemistry & special stains |
| | Immunofluorescence microscopy (IF) |
| | Morphometric image analysis |
| | Electron microscopy |
| | Urinary sediment |
| | Magnetic resonance imaging (MRI) |
| | Computed tomography (CT) |
| Molecular pathology | Immunohistochemistry (IHC) |
| | *In situ* hybridization (ISH) |
| | Reverse transcriptase-polymerase chain reaction (RT-PCR), Western blotting, and immunoprecipitation |
| | Tissue and antibody microchip arrays |
| | Laser capture microscopy (LCM) |
| | Laser scanning cytometry (LSC) |
| Renal blood flow | PAH clearance (RPF clearance) |
| | Transabdominal renal Doppler ultrasonography |
| | Transcutaneous ultrasonography |
| | Regional localization of microsphere beads |
| Glomerular filtration | Endogenous creatinine clearance |
| | Inulin clearance |
| | Radioactive iothalamate clearance |
| | MRI |
| Serum and urine analyses | Standard and novel biomarkers |
| | Electrolytes |
| Stones, casts, and crystals | Computed tomography |
| | Routine microscopy |
| | Analytical electron microscopy |
| | Proton nuclear magnetic resonance imaging spectroscopy (PNMR) |
| | Infra-red and Raman spectroscopy |
| | Time-of-flight secondary ion mass spectroscopy (TOF-SIMS) |
| Sophisticated technologies | Proteomoics |
| | Metabonomics |
| | Toxicogenomics |
| | High-resolution two-dimensional gel electrophoresis |
| | Liquid chromatography-mass spectrometry (LC-MS) |
| | Gas chromatography-mass spectrometry (GC/MS) |
| | Isotope-coded affinity tags |
| | Surface-enhanced laser desorption/ionization-time-of-flight-mass spectrometry (SELDI-TOF-MS) |

due to development of spontaneous age-related CPN as early as 12 weeks of age. Rats with nephropathy may show increases in kidney weights; increased urinary excretion of protein and calcium; decreased urinary excretion of sodium, chloride, and *N*-acetyl-β-(D)-glucosaminidase (NAG); decreased creatinine clearance; increased serum levels of BUN, sCr, sodium, and chloride; and decreased serum levels of albumin.

Histopathology is generally recognized as the single most appropriate screen for evidence of renal injury. For routine microscopic examination, immersion fixation in 10% neutral buffered formalin of a single longitudinal section of the left and transverse section of the right kidney represents a practical approach in allowing thorough examination of all elements within the kidney. An unambiguous descriptive terminology in describing microscopic lesions *versus* using traditional diagnostic concepts can improve the risk assessment process. Reprocessing with plastic embedding, sectioning at 1 μm, and staining with Lee's hematoxylin provides sub-topographical identification of the lesion site.

Perfusion fixation optimally prepares the kidney for the examination of luminal surfaces, for IHC, or for EM evaluation. Perfusion fixation can induce cytoplasmic vacuolar artifacts, which cannot be differentiated from hydropic phagolysosomal swelling. Additionally, glutaraldehyde can interfere with special stains such as the Mallory Heidenhain. Specimens for ultra-structural evaluation to determine the organellar target should be selected to include one or two affected animals from the earliest time point and lowest affected dose group and one or two animals from the next period time point, in addition to appropriate controls. Renal epithelial cell counts in urine or apoptotic cells in tissue sections can be a more sensitive indicator of increased apoptosis than routine light microscopy, and should be included in analyses if warranted. Typically, after examination of the sections by light microscopy, the earliest time points of observed effect and the lowest dose exerting this effect are identified, establishing the sub-topographical target.

### *20.2.1.2 Assessments in Purposely Designed Mechanistic Studies*

In general, specialized studies may be designed to gain further understanding of injury at the sub-cellular level, to explore structure–activity relationships, to search for sensitive predictors of nephrotoxic events and to refine the risk assessment based on potential mechanisms of toxicity. The approach for refined assessment of renal damage can include animal models of disease including transgenic or knockout models and specially designed time– and dose–response studies complemented with detailed morphologic, ultra-structural, biochemical, and functional assessments. Table 20.6 summarizes common *in vivo* animal disease models of nephrotoxicity. Initial studies are designed to confirm organelle targets, to establish the relationships between renal lesions and biochemical or functional perturbations, to differentiate pre-renal and post-renal injury from the primary renal insult, and to search for early biomarkers of the injury process. The next phase of assessment is to conduct time– and dose–response studies using sufficiently high dosages that will manifest in acute injury. There is a risk that, by increasing the dosage to develop an acute model, new or different types of injury may occur. However, models requiring weeks to months of exposure may be impractical for a rapid assessment of the source of the renal damage. Time intervals for sacrifice in the acute injury model to establish the time response could include one, three, five, and seven days after initiation of treatment. Sub-chronic studies with sequential interim evaluation may be needed to explore the relationship between acute/sub-acute lesions and sub-chronic/chronic lesions.

**Table 20.6** *In vivo* models of nephrotoxicity.

| *Model* | *Potential applications* | *Potential endpoints* | *Examples of toxicants studied* | *References* |
|---|---|---|---|---|
| Eker rat | Chemically induced nephrocarcinogenicity | Pathology, DNA damage | Hydroquinone | 141 |
| Chemical induction models of renal cancer | Renal tumor pathogenesis | Pathology, DNA damage | *N*-nitrosomorpholine, *N*-nitrosodimethylamine, *N*-(4′-fluoro-4-biphenylyl)acetamide, *N*-ethyl-*N*-hydroxyethyl nitrosamine | 20–24 |
| MT-I and MT-II knockout mice | Renal carcinogenic mechanism of metals | Molecular pathology | Lead | 44, 45 |
| Models of toxicity of renal medulla | Pathology and physiology of renal papilla | Histopathology, molecular expression profiles | Indomethacin, 2-bromoethanamine hydrobromide | 12 |
| Spontaneously hypertensive rat (SHR) | Radiocontrast renal failure | Renal function and histopathology | Diatrizoate meglumine sodium | 142 |
| Spontaneously hypertensive rat (SHR) | Chemically induced nephrotoxicity | Renal function and histopathology | Cyclosporine | 143 |
| Models of acute renal failure | Chemically induced acute renal failure | Renal function and pathology | Aminoglycosides, cisplatin | 144, 145 |
| Diabetic nephropathy | Chemically induced nephropathy | Renal function and pathology | Streptozotocin | 146 |

Once the appropriate analyses have been conducted in the time– and dose–response models, a mechanistic hypothesis can be developed and studies designed that will utilize the morphologic or biochemical biomarkers that indicate the onset of renal injury. This is based on the concept that the earliest and most sensitive indicators of perturbation will lead to the discovery of the primary mechanism of injury in contrast to the aftermath of the injury. Upon confirmation of a sensitive specific biomarker, the mechanistic hypothesis can be tested by experimental manipulation designed to modify the toxic response. Objective quantitation of the biomarker by automated image analysis provides an important tool for improving the sensitivity, reliability, and efficiency of the evaluation. Examples include: quantitation of mitotic figures in specially stained sections, identification of the segment of the nephron unit undergoing hypertrophy, and quantitation of hyaline-droplet response in specially stained sections.

Response to demand for altered function on an entire organ basis can be studied by extirpation of one kidney for increased demand or surgical implantation of a kidney for decreased demand. Compensatory hypertrophy occurs in the kidney after extirpation of the contralateral kidney. Hypertrophy is recognized by an increase in the volume of the cortex without an increase in nephron number, primarily involving PCTs, with some increase in glomerular volume. Measurement of the cross-sectional area of PCTs parallels functional adaptation measurements more precisely than does organ weight. The PCT response primarily represents hypertrophy with only slight hyperplasia.

Quantitative contribution of each kidney to the glomerular filtration rate in a rat with an implanted third kidney can be assessed using technetium-labelled diethylenetriamine pentaacetate (Tc-DTPA) scanning. Total GFR is unaltered because of compensatory atrophy with 15% reduction in weight and 30–40% reduction of GFR, with no change in glomerular numbers in each of the native kidneys. The implanted kidney loses 20% of its nephrons as a consequence of surgery; thus, its GFR is 20% less than the native kidney. Several stimuli are recognized as causes of renal hypertrophy, including administration of increased protein, amino acids, urea, or NaCl. Testosterone treatment, adrenocorticotropic hormone-mediated hyperadrenocorticism, and diabetes mellitus also cause renal hypertrophy. Xenobiotics metabolized by the kidney can cause renal enlargement, presumably through adaptive increase in metabolizing-enzyme synthesis activity. Biochemically, compensatory hypertrophy leads to an increase in the RNA : DNA ratio. In contrast, this change in RNA : DNA ratio apparently does not occur in renal parenchyma undergoing tissue repair. Serum factors seem to be involved in the stimulation of compensatory renal growth.

Some examples of xenobiotic-induced animal models for human disease include: liquoid for disseminated intravascular coagulation, polyvinyl alcohol for mesangial microgranulomas, maleic acid for tubular proteinuria, 2-amino-4,5-diphenylthiazole for renal polycystic disease, and hydralazine for lupus erythematosus.[2]

### *20.2.1.3* In vivo *Prediction of Renal Carcinogenic Potential*

The two-year chronic bioassay conducted in rodents has been the in-life strategy for determining the carcinogenic potential of drugs, industrial chemicals, agrochemicals, and food-related substances for over four decades. This *in vivo* assay took its origin from the 1940s and 1950s,[49] and in terms of general principles and approach, has changed little in the intervening years. However, an understanding of the various mechanisms underlying the development of chemically associated cancer has increased markedly, often stimulated by carcinogenicity bioassay results. In particular, the accumulation of knowledge is on key, often histopathological, events occurring on a causal pathway leading to cancer in target organs during sub-chronic phases of study, which are now referred to as modes-of-action (MoA). Relevant to the kidney, these MoA include evidence of cytotoxicity and increased cell proliferation. For the kidney, some of the MoA, such as hyaline-droplet nephropathy due to chemical binding to the protein alpha2u-globulin (α2u-g), are rodent-specific and have been judged not relevant to humans by regulatory and authoritative bodies.[50,51] In fact, α2u-g nephropathy is a male-rat-specific phenomenon because this specific protein occurs only in the rat, and is synthesized in significant amounts only in the liver of male rats.[3,52]

Because of the long duration and expense of the two-year rodent bioassay, and increasing concern regarding its relevance to human carcinogenic risk for non DNA-reactive chemicals, there have been numerous calls for a modified *in vivo* test. The latest is the suggestion by Cohen[53] that an enhanced 90-day toxicity study would be sufficient for identifying carcinogens relevant to humans. The new approach involves a short-term screen, in which the *in vivo* segment would rely on organ weight evaluation and histopathology including a labeling assay for cell proliferation. Such an approach might be applicable to kidney, as suggested by analyses of Boobis *et al.*[54] (see below), but would require rigorous validation to determine false-positive/false-negative rates.

The International Life Sciences Institute (ILSI) Health and Environmental Sciences Institute (HESI), Washington, DC, recently funded an investigation to test the hypothesis that key events predictive of later development of cancer can be detected in studies of shorter duration than two years. In addressing this issue Boobis *et al.*[54] conducted a retrospective analysis of 16 chemicals that had been tested for both carcinogenicity and sub-chronic toxicity by the NTP, focusing on three organ systems, one of which was kidney. Five of the 16 chemicals had produced renal tubule tumors in the two-year studies and four of these were associated with histopathological alterations in the respective 13-week toxicity studies. The histologic findings included hyaline-droplet accumulation (anthraquinone, decalin), apoptosis (fumonisin), regeneration (benzophenone, decalin, fumonisin), or exacerbated CPN in the case of anthraquinone. In addition, all five chemicals (as cited above and including methyleugenol) were associated with the non-specific finding of increased kidney weight, both absolute and relative, at 13 weeks. The combination of kidney weight and histopathologic change at 13 weeks for this series of chemicals identified all of the renal carcinogens. However, there were also false positives in this analysis as some chemicals that did not produce renal tumors after two years were associated with renal lesions or organ weight increase at 13 weeks. Boobis *et al.*[54] concluded that 13-week studies using conventional endpoints were not adequate to identify all non-genotoxic chemicals with the potential to produce tumors by two years. Additional endpoints, such as bromodeoxyuridine (BrdU) labeling for cell turnover or a measure of apoptosis were suggested as possible complements to the routine evaluation.[54]

Subsequently, Travlos *et al.*[55] reported on the occurrence of CPN in 13-week NTP studies, and the predictiveness of CPN exacerbation by test chemicals for renal tubule tumors in carcinogenicity bioassays of those chemicals. In this investigation, a series of 43 NTP 13-week toxicity studies were histopathologically re-evaluated for incidence and severity of CPN, involving a diverse range of chemicals. The effect of diet on chemical exacerbation of CPN was also assessed, as approximately half of the studies involved feeding high protein NIH-07 and the other half, low-protein NTP-2000. The severity of CPN was graded on an extended scale that recognized the earliest stages of this disease process. Although NTP diet was associated with a lower CPN severity range than NIH-07, it did not eliminate the early stages, as the incidence of CPN across all studies, involving 1090 male rats of around 4–5 months of age, was 100%. Furthermore, one third of the chemicals exacerbated CPN at 13 weeks, irrespective of diet type. Of the 43 chemicals for which 13-week studies were re-evaluated, 24 also had two-year carcinogenicity bioassays. In all cases where there was a statistically significant increase in renal tubule tumors at two years (seven chemicals), CPN had been exacerbated by the chemical at 13 weeks, and that early CPN exacerbation had predicted renal tumor outcome with 100% sensitivity and 88% specificity.[55]

Several caveats need to be considered in assessing the significance of this interesting finding. The number of chemicals associated with renal tumors was relatively low, at seven. Of those seven chemicals, over half (four) had produced hyaline-droplet nephropathy at 13 weeks. Hyaline-droplet nephropathy is known to be accompanied by CPN exacerbation,[3] and this association may have influenced the finding of a correlation between CPN exacerbation and renal tumor outcome. In addition, it is possible that this was a male-rat-specific finding as female rats were not included in the study.[55] In any case, the predictiveness demonstrated in this investigation would not be of relevance to humans. In terms of the biology of rat CPN and the combination and pattern of histological changes, there is no form of human nephropathy that represents a counterpart of CPN.[15] As a potential MoA in rodents, CPN exacerbation is therefore not relevant for species extrapolation in human cancer risk assessment.

### 20.2.2 Renal Function Assessments

Tests that can be employed in assessing renal functions are summarized in Table 20.5. Several functional parameters become routine in the time– and dose–response studies, including renal clearance. By definition, renal clearance is a measure of the volume of plasma completely freed of a given substance per unit time by the kidney. Thus, renal clearance is the ratio of the renal excretion rate of the substance to its concentration in the plasma. Routine tests include inulin and PAH clearances for determination of GFR and renal plasma flow (RPF), respectively. Additional methods include creatinine clearance, renal flow probes, regional localization of microsphere beads, and imaging techniques CT, ultrasonography (US), nuclear scintigraphy, and magnetic resonance imaging (MRI). Creatinine clearance (CrCl) is the volume of blood plasma that is cleared of creatinine per unit time and is a useful measure for approximating the GFR. CrCl involves a 16–24 h urine collection to measure creatinine excretion and is often used for the evaluation of renal toxicity.

Several renal blood flow (RBF) techniques are readily available in laboratory animal facilities these days. Transabdominal renal Doppler ultrasonography is a primary modality for assessing RBF. With this technique, two-dimensional scanning of the main renal arteries is followed by analysis of renal artery velocities by Doppler.[56] Transcutaneous ultrasonography is well established as a diagnostic tool for detecting abnormal RBF patterns in many disease states.[56] A transesophageal echocardiography (TEE) probe can image the renal vasculature during surgery.[56] Intra-renal distribution of RBF within and between the renal cortex and medulla is based on studies using radioactive gases. Intrarenal localization of microspheres represents regional RBF within the kidney. Intrarenal localization of microspheres can be determined by injecting radioactive microspheres into the central circulation and it is presumed that the microspheres are distributed to and within organs proportional to blood flow. The organs are removed and dissected, and radioactivity is counted. CT is used to detect calcified kidney stones. In addition, CT has been used in renal densitometry analysis.[58] The iodinated contrast agents used in CT are filtered at the glomerulus and not re-absorbed by the tubules and have pharmacokinetics comparable to inulin. Physiological indices such as contrast clearance per unit volume, which is closely related to glomerular filtration rate per unit renal volume of kidney, can be measured.[59] Ultrasonography (US) can identify hydronephrosis, provide an accurate measurement of overall kidney size, evaluate parenchyma thickness, and differentiate cystic masses.[60] Nuclear scintigraphy can quantify renal function.[61] MRI can be used to characterize kidney structural changes in renal conditions such as polycystic kidney disease.[62]

GFR changes that develop before the onset of renal injury indicate the probability of prerenal (hemodynamic) factors as the source of the renal injury. If the onset of GFR change occurs after an overt renal injury, it is an indication that the GFR change is the result of the primary renal injury. Xenobiotic effects on renal arteriolar vascular resistance are indicated by changes in the GFR, RPF and filtration fraction (FF = GFR/RPF). For example, vasoconstrictive effects of compounds on the afferent arteriole will be reflected as decreased GFR and RPF without any change in FF, and on the efferent arteriole as decreased RPF and increased GFR and FF.

### 20.2.3 Biomarkers to Predict Kidney Injury

In the context of drug development, a safety biomarker has been defined as any analyte that can be quantified to indicate an adverse response to a test agent.[63] Drug-induced nephrotoxicity is a potential concern because many pharmacological compounds are filtered through the kidney for excretion, and biomarker development is essential to the field of predictive renal toxicology. In preclinical toxicology studies, microscopic evaluation of kidney remains the gold standard, but its limitation is that it represents one static observation in time. Sensitive and specific biomarkers of renal injury are needed, not only because they can permit repetitious monitoring, but to account for the fact that the practical matrices for monitoring renal injury in humans are restricted to blood and urine. The need for monitoring adverse effects in clinical trials and thereafter is emphasized by a recent study from China in which renal biopsies were taken from 104 patients suffering from acute renal failure in various types of chronic kidney disease. More than one third of those cases appeared to be drug-related.[64]

Among the basic requirements for a renal biomarker are: non-invasiveness, specificity for kidney, reliability, easy and inexpensive measurement, and low inter-animal or inter-individual variability. An ideal marker would also: reveal the location of tubule segment or compartment where the injury occurred (*e.g.* cortical renal tubules, *pars recta*, renal pelvis, or interstitium); provide a quantitative reflection discriminating different pathophysiologic processes (*e.g.* sepsis, ischemia, tubule necrosis, inflammation, chronic kidney disease); predict injury progression; and monitor response to therapeutic intervention with prognostic significance.[72,85,86] The utility of reliable biomarkers extends beyond the context of toxicity testing of chemicals in general, for it has important applications in a cross-sectional sense regarding human kidney disease. Thus, it is equally important to develop biomarkers to diagnose and predict clinical outcomes in diverse clinical settings, for example, patients with acute kidney injury due to ischemia from sepsis or hypoperfusion, contrast medium-induced nephropathy, stabilizer-induced osmotic nephrosis, post-operative renal complication of cardiac surgery, and such specific diseases as diabetic nephropathy, IgA nephropathy, lupus nephritis, and several types of renal cancer. Table 20.7 summarizes application of different renal biomarkers to predict location of renal injury. Development and utilization of traditional and novel biomarkers of renal injury prediction are discussed below.

#### *20.2.3.1 Traditional Biomarkers*

Traditional biomarkers of renal injury used for many years in laboratory animals and humans have included total urinary protein and albumin, BUN, sCr, glucose, and certain enzymes including NAG and glutathione-*S*-transferases (GST) or low-molecular-weight proteins such as β2-microglobulin. These analytes can be evaluated in routinely collected serum and urine samples.

**Table 20.7** Predictive relevance of renal biomarker to the site of injury.

| *Biomarker* | *Sample type* | *Injury related to* | *Status* |
|---|---|---|---|
| Albumin | U | Glomerulus and tubule | Pre-clinical & clinical |
| Microalbumin | U | Proximal tubule | Pre-clinical & clinical |
| Blood urea nitrogen (BUN) | S | General kidney injury and disease | Pre-clinical & clinical |
| Creatinine | S | General kidney injury and disease | Pre-clinical & clinical |
| Urinary *N*-acetyl-β-(D)-glucosaminidase (NAG) | U | Proximal tubule | Pre-clinical & clinical |
| Total protein | U | Glomerulus and tubule | Pre-clinical & clinical |
| Kidney injury molecule 1 (KIM-1) | U, K | General kidney injury and disease | Pre-clinical & Clinical |
| β2-microglobulin | U | Proximal tubule | Pre-clinical & clinical |
| Lipocalin 2 (NGAL) | U, K | Proximal tubule | Pre-clinical & clinical |
| Trefoil factor-3 (TFF3) | U, K | Tubule dedifferentiation in response to injury | Pre-clinical/clinical |
| Cystatin C | U | Tubule dysfunction | Pre-clinical/clinical |
| Clusterin | U, K | Tubule epithelial regenerative response | Pre-clinical/clinical |
| Renal papillary antigen 1 (RPA) | U, K | Renal papilla & collecting duct injury | Pre-clinical |
| GSH-π | U, K | Distal tubule injury | Pre-clinical |
| GSH-α | U, K | Proximal tubule injury | Pre-clinical |
| Podocin | U, K | Glomerulus injury | Validation needed |
| Interleukin-18 | U | Inflammatory marker | Validation needed |

U = urine; S = serum; K = Kidney tissue fixed in formalin.

**Proteinuria and Albuminuria.** The classical paradigm of glomerular capillary leakage as the primary cause of proteinuria/albuminuria is currently being challenged by increasing recognition that the glomerulus exerts mainly size selectivity in the process of protein filtration, implying that physiological levels of filtered protein such as albumin have been significantly underestimated in the past.[65–69] Beyond the glomerulus, albumin is retrieved through megalin/cubulin binding into proximal tubule cells where the protein is fragmented to small peptides, some of which are then secreted back into the urine. Thus, increase in albumin in the urine can signal impairment of the degradation pathway when there is proximal tubule injury. Consequently, proteinuria is now regarded as a reflection of two separate mechanisms 1) abnormal transglomerular passage of large proteins due to increased permeability of the glomerular capillary wall, and 2) the subsequent impaired resorption of proteins by epithelial cells of the proximal tubules.[70]

**BUN and Serum Creatinine.** The traditional biomarkers, sCr and BUN are late indicators of renal injury, and do not become significantly elevated until at least one half of the kidney has been compromised.[71] Furthermore, they do not provide any indication concerning the region of kidney affected.

This late flagging of renal involvement is generally regarded as being due to the functional reserve of the kidney. In addition, normal sCr levels are affected by multiple non-renal factors, including age, gender, muscle mass, hydration status, nutritional status, and in humans, medications.[72] Despite this, measurement of sCr remains the universal parameter for monitoring and assessing kidney health in clinical practice.

**β2-Microglobulin (β2-M):** β2-M is a single polypeptide chain of 12 kDa that represents the light chain of the major histocompatibility class (MHC) molecule. It is expressed on the surface of all nucleated cells and is freely filtered through the glomerulus, and almost entirely re-absorbed and catabolized in the PCTs.[73,74] An increase in its urinary excretion has been considered to reflect impairment of the PCTs resorption process, and thus tubule injury. The usefulness of this polypeptide as a biomarker is limited by its instability in pathological urine due to pH-dependent enzymic degradation.[75] Therefore, great care must be taken to collect urine in an ice-cold, adequately buffered environment with the addition of stabilizers to preserve β2-M levels during the period of collection and in storage. β2-Microglobulin is highly species-specific and its assays may not be readily available for all laboratory animal species.

***N*-acetyl-β-(D)-glucosaminidase (NAG).** NAG is a lysosomal brush-border enzyme of 140 kDa present mainly in the proximal tubule cells.[74] It is the most active glycosidase in proximal tubule cell lysosomes, which tend to be concentrated in the S2 segment of PCTs.[76] As NAG is too large to be filtered through glomeruli, its urinary excretion reflects increased lysosomal activity and tubule cell injury. NAG has proved to be a sensitive biomarker of proximal tubule cell injury associated with a wide variety of drugs and environmental toxins in animals, as well as in a cross-section of human renal conditions.[77–81] In contemporary studies on renal biomarkers, this parameter holds its place for judging the comparative performance of newly developed candidate biomarkers. The advantages of NAG pertain to its sensitivity and to its ease of measurement. Firstly, subtle alterations in proximal tubule cells such as brush-border damage lead to shedding of NAG into the urine as a reflection of the amount of tubule damage. Secondly, the analyte is easily and reproducibly measured and quantified colorimetrically by spectrophotometry. However, NAG may lack the specificity required for a reliable marker of tubule necrosis.

**Glutathione-*S*-Transferases (GSTs):** GSTs are cytosolic dimeric enzymes involved in detoxification of xenobiotic compounds through addition of glutathione. Several isoforms exist but in the kidney there are two main classes, GSTα and GSTπ.[82] GSTα is highly expressed in proximal tubule cells, whereas GSTπ is localized to the distal convoluted tubule, thin limbs of Henle, and the collecting ducts.[83] Therefore, application of these parameters raises the possibility of discriminating between damage to the proximal tubules and damage to the distal nephron and collecting system. In a cross-sectional study of human patients with proteinuria, the highest levels of urinary GSTα were in patients still in an early phase of their proteinuric renal disease, while the highest levels of GSTπ were in patients with more compromised kidneys in renal failure.[84]

### 20.2.3.2 Novel Biomarkers

As noted above, it has become increasingly acknowledged that traditional markers of renal toxicity, which may indicate impaired kidney function rather than tissue injury, do not fulfil the requirements for an efficient biomarker that will predict renal injury in an accurate and timely fashion. First and foremost, a biomarker of renal injury should be predictive in both laboratory animals and in humans, because the intention of safety evaluation studies is to prevent adverse effects occurring during and after the clinical trial phases.

Consequently over the past decade, there has been a concerted effort to identify and develop new biomarkers of kidney injury in both humans and laboratory animal species used in safety evaluation studies. Large-scale collaborative efforts between academic and industrial institutions, and regulatory bodies, have stimulated a search for more predictive methods. As one example, a consortium of industry parties interested in exchanging data and samples regarding a safety biomarker qualification process for drug-induced injury in a variety of target organs formed the *Predictive Safety Testing Consortium* (PSTC) in 2006. Following their submission of a suggested panel of seven assayable biomarkers for drug-induced kidney injury, which included several novel biomarkers identified by ILSI-HESI based on microarray data,[63] the Food and Drug Administration (FDA) and European Medicines Agency (EMEA) published a document on qualification of urinary nephrotoxicity biomarkers in 2008.[87,88] The new urinary biomarkers were kidney injury molecule 1 (KIM-1), clusterin, cystatin C, and trefoil factor 3 (TFF3); the list also included albumin, total protein, and β2-microglobulin. Since those initial surveys, additional markers of interest have received investigative attention, particularly neutrophil gelatinase-associated lipocalin (NGAL), and most recently urinary liver-type fatty acid-binding protein (L-FABP).

**Kidney Injury Molecule 1 (KIM-1):** KIM-1 is a type-1 transmembrane glycoprotein with an immunoglobulin ectodomain containing six cysteine residues, *O*- and *N*-glycosylated mucin sites, and a domain rich in threonine/serine and proline.[89] In toxicity or kidney disease states KIM-1 can be measured in urine with a microsphere-based Luminex xMAP technology using monoclonal or polyclonal antibodies raised against rat or human KIM-1 ectodomain.[90] Dipsticks for assaying KIM-1 in urine have also been developed for rapid diagnosis and monitoring at the bedside or in the clinic.[91]

The substantial amount of work on developing KIM-1 as a potential renal biomarker has been summarized by a pioneer in this area of research activity, Dr J. V. Bonventrie.[85] KIM-1 is not detectable in normal kidney tissue, but increases substantially in kidney following injury. Upon injury to proximal tubule cells, the ectodomain of KIM-1 is proteolytically cleaved by metalloproteinases from damaged cells and released into urine. It is expressed at very high levels in de-differentiated proximal tubule cells in animal and human kidneys after toxic or ischemic renal injury.[89,92,93] It has been suggested that KIM-1 has a central role in the renal tubule repair process by removing dying cells and cell debris from the injured tubule.[94] In one rat study, KIM-1 was tested under conditions of nephrotoxicity induced either by gentamycin, inorganic mercury, or chromium. KIM-1 proved to be more sensitive in detecting proximal tubule damage regardless of whether it affected cortical or outer medullary proximal tubules, and was more rapidly elevated than NAG.[95] In the clinical setting, studies have indicated that KIM-1 is most efficient at distinguishing acute tubular necrosis from other types of renal injury, such as chronic kidney disease.[96] KIM-1 has become the most validated of the potential safety biomarkers to date. It seems to have many of the characteristics preferred for a genuinely useful biomarker, including the fact that it is stable in urine. Further work is required to determine if KIM-1 is a useful marker for long-term renal injury and whether it can be used in combination with other markers to determine site-specific kidney injury.

**Neutrophil Gelatinase-Associated Lipocalin (NGAL).** NGAL, also known as lipocalin-2, is an iron-carrying protein of the lipocalin family. The members of this family consist of eight β-strands forming a β-barrel enclosing a hydrophobic calyx, which binds and transports low-molecular-weight lipophilic molecules.[97] NGAL is a 25 kDa polypeptide chain that is secreted in a bound state with gelatinases from neutrophils, macrophages, and other cells involved in inflammation. Due to its iron-carrying function it is believed to have both antimicrobial activity as well as a role in epithelial growth, differentiation, cell survival and proliferation.[98] Because NGAL was rapidly induced in mouse kidney urine after acute cisplatin tubule necrosis, it was proposed as a sensitive marker of acute kidney injury.[99] Subsequently it has been investigated in a series of studies covering a wide spectrum of human renal disease with promising results,[72,100] but with better predictive ability in pediatric cases than in adults.[72] NGAL, however, is not specific for kidney as serum levels are also raised in the presence of liver injury, acute bacterial infections, and chronic obstructive pulmonary disease.[101] In the recent preclinical study by Hoffmann *et al.*[102] using several nephrotoxicants, the performance of NGAL did not match that of KIM-1 or NAG. Nevertheless, NGAL is considered to have successfully passed through the pre-clinical, assay improvement, and initial clinical testing stages of the biomarker-development process, and has now entered the prospective screening stage.[72]

**Interleukin-18 (IL-18).** IL-18 is a 24 kDa cytokine, the precursor form of which is cleaved by IL-1β converting enzyme to produce the mature form of protein, 18 kDa IL-18.[103] Increased IL-18 activity has been reported in a broad range of tissues in a wide variety of inflammatory diseases.[104] IL-18 has also been shown to be an early indicator of acute tubular necrosis and predictive of human mortality in certain renal disease states.[105] In a cross-sectional comparison of 204 patients with or without acute kidney injury, urinary IL-18 had a sensitivity of 68% and specificity of 95%. Although investigated for its immunological role, this potential biomarker appears to have received little attention at the pre-clinical safety evaluation level.

**Cystatin C.** Cystatin C is produced by all nucleated cells in the body, and is considered to have a housekeeping function.[106] It is a non-glycosylated low-molecular-weight protein freely filtered from the blood through the glomerulus. Unlike serum creatinine, it is not influenced by factors unrelated to kidney function, and has proven to be a genuine candidate for estimating GFR, and thus, a marker for impairment of glomerular function.[107,108] After glomerular filtration, 99.5% of cystatin C is re-absorbed and catabolized by the proximal tubules in rats.[109] Therefore, increased urinary cystatin C has been proposed also as a marker of renal tubule impairment.[110] More importantly, there has been a suggestion to complement the widely used estimate of GFR based on creatinine clearance with serum assay of cystatin C, which, in contrast to creatinine, has no dependence on muscle mass.[111]

**Clusterin.** Clusterin is a 75–80 kDa disulfide-linked heterodimeric glycoprotein consisting of $\alpha$ and $\beta$ units. It is an aggregating factor involved in the clearance of cellular debris and apoptosis.[112] Clusterin is expressed in most mammalian tissues and appears to be associated with a range of conditions in humans. It is elevated in the kidney and urine of rats, dogs, and primates in association with the acute injury induced by ischemia/reperfusion, nephrotoxicants and other causes of renal damage.[113,114] In investigating its potential as a biomarker of nephrotoxicity, Ishii *et al.*[115] demonstrated clusterin $\alpha$ in urine and strong positivity for clusterin $\beta$ in tubule epithelium as early changes in a rat model of unilateral urethral obstruction. Like KIM-1, it is expressed on de-differentiated cells after injury. However, as yet there appears to be no trial demonstrating the use of clusterin as a marker of drug-related renal injury in the clinical setting.

**Liver-type fatty acid binding protein (L-FABP).** L-FABP is a member of a superfamily of lipid-binding proteins that occur intra-cellularly in tissues with active fatty acid metabolism. In the kidney, L-FABP is localized in the cytoplasm of proximal tubule cells. The primary function appears to be facilitation of long-chain fatty acid transport from the plasma membrane to intracellular sites for $\beta$-oxidation. Accordingly, expression of L-FABP has been found in human proximal tubule epithelium where there is dependence on energy derived from fatty acid metabolism for normal cellular transport processes. Based on early animal and clinical studies, the diagnostic performance of urinary L-FBAP is shown to be 0.93 when assessed as area under the receiver operating characteristic (ROC) curve (the curve plotting true-positive against false-positive rates). This measure of performance matches that of other novel biomarkers, including KIM-1, NGAL, IL-18, and NAG.

**Trefoil Factor 3 (TFF3).** TFF3 is a member of a family of small secretory proteins characterized by three intra-chain disulfide bonds constituting the trefoil motif, formerly referred to as the P-domain peptides.[116,117] Synthesis of these proteins has been reported particularly in mucin-producing cells of gastrointestinal tract and respiratory epithelia.[117] Despite inclusion of this protein in the list of potential renal injury biomarkers submitted by EMEA[87] to FDA, there is very little published evidence supporting a renal biomarker role to date. Recently, Yu *et al.*[118] recorded marked reduction of TFF3 protein levels following treatment with several renal toxicants, including cisplatin, gentamycin, and carbapenem (a β-lactam antibiotic). In addition, by utilizing *in situ* hybridization they localized TFF3 expression to tubules of the outer stripe of outer medulla and medullary rays,[118] suggesting that it is localized to S3 segments (*pars recta*) of proximal tubules. Clearly, this protein requires more investigative work-up to justify its inclusion in a list of candidate biomarkers.

**Renal Papillary Antigens (RPAs).** Few biomarkers have been discovered capable of detecting damage to the distal collecting system of the kidney. In particular, it is critical to detect any potential of a newly developed drug for causing renal papillary necrosis, a specific type of kidney injury that has been well documented in humans as a drug-induced entity. It is some years since a first attempt was made to develop monoclonal antibodies to rat renal papillary tissue that could be used as a diagnostic tool for identifying toxic damage to the rat papilla.[119] Two of these antibodies, subsequently termed RPA-1 and RPA-2, exhibited relatively intense localization to the renal papilla. Further work from the same group showed that the amount of RPA-1 increased in rat urine following exposure to classical papillotoxins, including single doses of 2-bromoethanamine, propyleneimine, and single or repeated doses of indomethacin.[120] Recently, RPA-1 was confirmed as a very promising, early biomarker of renal papillary necrosis.[121] The exact molecular identity of RPA-1 has not yet been determined, but it is known to be predominantly a high-molecular-weight (in the MDa range) membrane-bound glycoprotein.[121] RPA-1 is normally present in rat urine, presumably through physiological membrane shedding from collecting ducts, but increases can be measured using a commercially available ELISA kit (Biotrin International, Dublin, Ireland). Renal papillary necrosis is a relatively common form of toxicity encountered in pre-clinical safety testing, and, encompassed under the term analgesic nephropathy, has been a problem in humans habitually consuming NSAIDs, particularly those containing phenacetin.[122] It is therefore most important to continue this line of research in order to develop a biomarker that can be included in the monitoring of drug treatment in humans.

Today, there is an increasing number of studies reporting on the comparative performance of some of the novel kidney biomarkers described above in both the pre-clinical and clinical settings. As an example, one recent study[102] compared the putative kidney markers KIM-1, NGAL, clusterin, tissue inhibitor of metalloproteinases-1 (TIMP-1), osteopontin, and heme oxygenase-1 in both kidney tissue and in urine using quantitative real-time PCR, ELISA, and IHC, following exposure of male Wistar rats to one of several nephrotoxins, including gentamycin. The authors confirmed that KIM-1 and clusterin, in particular, were early and sensitive markers of renal injury, whereas urinary glucose and protein, and a rise in serum creatinine were not. ELISA measurement of the biomarkers appeared to be more sensitive than gene and protein expression, and histopathology.[102] In this study, the performance of NGAL and TIMP-1 as early indicators of proximal tubule damage in rats was inferior to KIM-1 and clusterin. The ROC performances of 12 urinary nephrotoxic biomarkers after exposure to either a tubular injury model (cisplatin) or a glomerular injury model (puromycin aminonucleoside) were also compared by Tonomura *et al.*[123] KIM-1 was the best biomarker for detection of cisplatin-induced tubule injury, while NGAL performed best for detecting puromycin aminonucleoside injury, although the latter may have been related to tubular rather than glomerular injury. These authors further noted that lactate dehydrogenase might prove useful for broad-range screening along the whole nephron.[123]

In summing up the position of this field of intense research activity over the past decade, the most practical outcome will not be reliance on a single utilitarian biomarker of renal tubule damage, but assembly of a battery of reliably predictive markers.[124] At least for detection of post-operative kidney injury in human patients, KIM-1, NGAL, and NAG appear to be among the candidates for this combination approach.[125,126] In order to cover the possibility of papillary necrosis, inclusion of RPA-1 might be considered in this context. Just as in the case of individual biomarkers, the efficacy of combining multiple biomarkers will necessitate rigorous validation. In addition, there is a need to augment the limited data currently available regarding temporal expression patterns of the various biomarkers from the time of onset of renal injury. This is an exciting period in the history of kidney research. As aptly stated by Vaidya *et al.*,[91] improved and accurate biomarkers will help the pharmaceutical industry to make more informed decisions concerning drug development, and guide the design of clinical trials to provide clear information about product benefit and safety.

### 20.2.4 Utility of Sophisticated Technologies to Assess Renal Toxicity

The past 10 years have seen remarkable advances in refinement of *in vitro* and *ex vivo* models of cell/organ cultures and utilization of microarrays and gene expressions in furthering the knowledge of renal cell response to toxic insults. The development of sophisticated technologies has already played an important role in the discovery of novel biomarkers of renal injury. This technology and perhaps antibody-based proteomics in particular will continue to be an essential contribution to unravelling the complexity of the kidney's response to chemically induced toxicity. Furthermore, these high-throughput screening methods of genetic profiling introduce the prospect of developing personalized medical treatment in the future.

### *20.2.4.1 Use of "-omics" in Predicting Renal Toxicity*

Since the advent of some new and sophisticated technologies, the literature on the use of the "-omics" in exploration of the kidney response to chemically induced toxic injury has rapidly expanded. Accordingly only a selection of recent publications will be acknowledged here.[74,127] Examples of sophisticated technologies are summarized in Table 20.5; in particular, microarray technology has promoted the field of toxicogenomics.

Toxicogenomic analysis employing DNA microarray technology for identifying gene expression profiles associated with the effects of pharmaceuticals and other chemicals in tissue and body fluids is generating significant information on potential mechanisms of toxicity, as well as leading to the discovery of new biomarkers of renal injury. Although gene-expression profiling has high-throughput capabilities and generates large amounts of data, it is also a high-cost undertaking. Nevertheless, a retrospective evaluation of routine transcriptional profiling in pre-clinical studies suggested that there was significant value for including toxicogenomics in exploratory studies of drug safety.[128]

The leading biomarker candidate, KIM-1, is one example of productive application of gene expression methodology in kidney. KIM-1 was discovered when screening for genes with increased expression in post-ischemic rat kidney.[89] Indeed, KIM-1 mRNA levels increase more than any other known gene after kidney injury.[91] Subsequently, cDNA arrays have been used to determine the specific localization of up-regulated KIM-1 expression to nephron segment in rats using the renal toxicants potassium chromate (with a specificity for $S_1$ and $S_2$ segments of proximal tubule), cephaloridine ($S_2$ specific), and hexachlorobutadiene ($S_3$ specific). This study confirmed that KIM-1 expression was related to proximal tubule cell injury but did not distinguish between specific segments.[129] Also, the very sensitive capability of clusterin for signaling injury after unilateral urethral obstruction was demonstrated using ISH, RT-PCR, and Western blotting.[115]

Thukral *et al.*[130] applied a toxicogenomics approach, using cDNA microarray technology to investigate gene-expression profiles underlying molecular pathways in chemically induced nephrotoxicity in rats. Because the proximal tubule is well endowed with transporters and transport mechanisms, it was not surprising that Thukral *et al.*[130] observed pronounced down-regulation of gene expression of organic anion and cationic transporters during necrosis. Among the many genes up-regulated were the sodium phosphate co-transporter and certain tissue remodeling genes, including heat-shock genes, osteopontin, and KIM-1.

Proteomics focuses on the products of genes; thus, the proteome of a cell is the set of proteins expressed by a genome under certain conditions of time, space, pathological conditions and external stimuli.[131] The sophisticated techniques mentioned above have also been used to identify protein changes in various regions of the kidney associated with toxicity. High-resolution two-dimensional gel electrophoresis of the human urinary proteome has yielded nearly 1400 distinct protein spots.[132] Other analytical techniques such as SELDI-TOF-MS hold promise for further biomarker discovery in body fluids such as urine.[133] Tissue microarray with its high-throughput capability is a promising tool for investigating protein expression profiles in multiple kidney tissue samples from both normal and pathophysiological conditions in rodents.[134] Furthermore, in humans, new assay development through antibody-based proteomics offers the prospect of introducing an approach to realizing personalized medicine.[160]

Exosomes are small vesicles that are expelled from cell surfaces, usually after fusion of an endocytic vesicle with the cell membrane. Exosomes secreted into the tubule lumen by renal tubule cells under both normal and pathological conditions can contain proteins and functional RNA molecules such as mRNA and MicroRNAs (miRNAs).[135] The miRNAs are short single-stranded RNAs which function to regulate endogenous gene expression by interfering with mRNA expression *via* imprecise base-pairing and inhibition of protein translation.[136] Improvements in MS-based tools and exosome purification have facilitated proteomic analysis of exosomes in urine, and gene-expression profiling has indicated some individual and specific miRNAs that may be implicated in cystic kidney disease and diabetic nephropathy.[90,137] Therefore, attention has been drawn to the future prospect of miRNAs found in urinary exosomes for serving as human renal disease biomarkers and biomarkers of renal injury in laboratory animals.[90,135]

Metobolomics is the determination of alterations in levels of endogenous or exogenous metabolites due to physiological stimuli or other biological modifications.[138] Using a combination of GC-MS and LC-MS, Boudonck *et al.*[139] investigated metabolomic markers of nephrotoxicity in rat urine after exposure to either gentamycin, *cis*-platin or tobramycin and a vehicle control at three successive time points (one, five, and 28 days). By selecting metabolites that showed uni-directional fold-changes common to all three nephrotoxins, the authors identified 39 putative biomarkers of tubule toxicity in urine. Among these were marked increases in branched-chain amino acids, and several polyamines (cadaverine, putrescine, agmatine, and spermidine). The amino acid increase is particularly significant because under normal conditions amino acids are almost completely re-absorbed by the renal tubules.[140] The top five classifiers at day 28 were leucine, hippurate, isoleucine, glucose, and valine, while the trio of amino acids, leucine, isoleucine and valine, also had high predictive performance for distinguishing the drug-treated from the control group.[139]

#### *20.2.4.2* In Vitro *Techniques in Screening and Mechanistic Studies*

*In vitro* models of nephrotoxicity can be used to further understand cellular and molecular mechanisms of renal cell injury and kidney dysfunction. Advantages of using *in vitro* models include, the ability to examine direct effects of chemicals at the cellular level, low cost, short turn-around time, and capabilities for automation. However, *in vitro* to *in vivo* correlation is a major limitation of such models. Key questions to consider before selecting an *in vitro* model include: i) Are the cell types being tested *in vitro* (the segment of nephron, the interstitium, or the collecting duct system) typically exposed *in vivo*? ii) Do these cells behave similarly in culture as they do *in vivo*? iii) Are the endpoints (*e.g.*, enzyme leakage) being tested relevant for what one might expect in the *in vivo* situation? iv) Are there known interspecies differences in the utility of cell types of kidney origin (*e.g.*, transporters)? v) What are the limits of translating *in vitro* data to *in situ* whole-nephron/kidney physiology? and vi) is there need for a high-throughput assay system? The *in vitro* models of nephrotoxicity, potential study endpoints, and xenobiotics examples where these systems have been used are summarized in Table 20.8 and the relevant renal cell lines are summarized in Table 20.9. Kidney cells can further be genetically modified to study specific

**Table 20.8** *In vitro* models of nephrotoxicity.

| *Model* | *Potential applications* | *Potential endpoints* | *Examples of toxicants studied* | *References* |
|---|---|---|---|---|
| Isolated perfused kidney | Renal physiology, xenobiotics disposition and accumulation, organic anion transport studies, renal metabolism | Histology, immunohistochemistry (IHC), gene expression, urine output, GFR (inulin clearance) urinary handling of electrolytes, urinary enzyme leakage, metabolism studies | Aminoglycosides | 147–149 |
| Kidney slices | General toxicity, xenobiotic accumulation, renal metabolism, covalent binding, lipid peroxidation, organic cation and anion uptake, and total glutathione concentrations | Histology, IHC, gene expression, urinary enzyme leakage, metabolism studies | Aminoglycosides, cisplatin, radiocontrast agents, and cephalosporins | 150–153 |
| Isolated nephrons | Toxicity to a specific nephron segment, organic anion transport studies, and renal metabolism | Histology, IHC, gene expression, urinary enzyme leakage, metabolism studies, albumin permeability | Antibiotics, glycosides, radiocontrast dyes | 154–156 |
| Renal cell lines | Cytotoxicity, renal transport mechanisms | Necrosis, apoptosis, enzyme leakage, gene expression | Radiocontrast agents; aminoglycoside antibiotics | 157–159 |

**Table 20.9** Common renal cell lines used in investigative toxicology studies.

| *Cell line used* | *Cell line origin* |
|---|---|
| LLC-$RK_1$ | Rabbit kidney |
| LLC-$PK_1$ | Porcine kidney |
| MDCK | Madin–Darby canine kidney |
| MDBK | Madin–Darby bovine kidney |
| RK-13 | Rabbit kidney |
| LLC-MK-2 | Rhesus monkey kidney |
| Vero | African green monkey kidney |
| RCC | Human renal cell carcinoma |
| TRKE-1 | Rat kidney transformed cell line |

targets of interest. Several laboratories have successfully utilized precision-cut renal slices in toxicity and metabolism studies. Some of the examples where *in vitro* systems have provided useful information include: isolated perfused kidney for protein catabolism studies, isolated perfused nephrons for phosphate transport and oxidative metabolism perturbations, primary cell cultures for assessing phospholipidotic potential of aminoglycoside antibiotics, and tissue slices for establishing local metabolism and for demonstrating transport *via* organic anion transporter or peroxidative injury.

## 20.3 Conclusions

The gold standard method for identification of renal damage with chemicals and drugs remains light microscopic examination of the kidney, supplemented with selected serum and urine analyses in light of species, gender, and age-related differences in response to renal insult. The past 10 years have seen remarkable advances in identification of potential new biomarkers for detecting chemically-induced renal injury in safety evaluation studies, as well as for renal disease states in humans. This effort should eventually culminate in a much safer level of pharmaceutical drug use. The development of sophisticated technology has already played an important role in the discovery of novel biomarkers of renal injury. This technology and perhaps antibody-based proteomics in particular will continue to be an essential contribution to unravelling the complexity of the kidney's response to chemically-induced toxicity. Furthermore, these high-throughput screening methods of "-omics" profiling introduce the prospect of developing personalized medical treatment in the future. There has been little effort invested in seeking a genetically modified mouse model that would be suitable for testing the efficacy of newly developed chemotherapeutic agents or biological modifiers for the treatment of renal cell cancer in humans. This tumor type remains an important medical concern as it appears to be increasing in incidence and represents a significant socioeconomic burden worldwide.

## References


1. A. J. Szabo, V. Muller, G. F. Chen, L. J. Samsell, A. Erdely and C. Baylis, *Nephrol., Dial., Transplant.*, 2008, **23**, 2492–2495.
2. K. N. M. Khan and C. L. Alden, in *Handbook of Toxicologic Pathology*, ed. W. M. Haschek, C. G. Rousseaux and M. A. Wallig, Academic Press, San Diego, CA, 2nd edn, 2002, pp. 255–336.
3. G. C. Hard, I. S. Rodgers, K. P. Baetcke, W. L. Richards, R. E. McGaughy and L. R. Valcovic, *Environ. Health Perspect.*, 1993, **99**, 313–349.
4. M. Zhang, Y. Wang, Q. Wang, J. Yang, D. Yang, J. Liu and J. Li, *Toxicol. Sci.*, 2010, **115**, 295–303.
5. R. Sellers and K. N. M. Khan, in *Toxicology of the Kidney*, ed. J. B. Tarloff and L. H. Lash, CRC Press, Washington DC, 3rd edn, 2004, pp. 1059–1098.
6. R. Sellers and K. N. M. Khan, in *Toxicology of the Kidney*, ed. J. B. Tarloff and L. H. Lash, CRC Press, Washington DC, 3rd edn, 2004, pp. 1099–1132.
7. K. N. M. Khan, S. K. Paulson, K. Verburg, J. Lefkowith and T. J. Maziasz, *Kidney Int.*, 2002, **61**, 1210–1219.
8. R. Sellers, Z. Radi and K. N. M. Khan, *Vet. Pathobiol.*, 2010, **47**, 601–613.
9. P. B. Senese, M. R. Gralinski and K. N. M. Khan, *Contemp. Top. Lab. Anim. Sci.*, 1999, **38**, 41–42.
10. D. Choudhury and Z. Ahmed, *Nat. Clin. Pract. Nephrol.*, 2006, **2**, 80–91.
11. R. Guzman, K. Datta and K. N. M. Khan, *Vet. Pathol.*, 2008, **45**, 945–948.
12. K. N. M. Khan, C. L. Alden, S. Geissner, M. K. Gessford and T. J. Maziasz, *Toxicol. Pathol.*, 1998, **26**, 137–142.
13. G. C. Hard and K. N. Khan, *Toxicol. Pathol.*, 2004, **32**, 171–180.
14. D. C. Wolf and P. C. Mann, *Toxicol. Appl. Pharmacol.*, 2005, **202**, 302–308.
15. G. C. Hard, K. J. Johnson and S. M. Cohen, *Crit. Rev. Toxicol.*, 2009, **39**, 332–346.
16. C. Baylis, *J. Clin. Invest.*, 1994, **94**, 1823.
17. G. C. Hard, *Toxicol. Sci.*, 2002, **69**, 30–41.
18. G. C. Hard, J. C. Seely, L. J. Betz and S. M. Hayashi, *Food Chem. Toxicol.*, 2007, **45**, 600–608.
19. G. C. Hard, *Carcinogenesis*, 1985, **6**, 1551–1558.
20. P. Bannasch, U. Schacht and E. Storch, *Z. Krebsforsch. Klin. Onkol.*, 1974, **81**, 311.
21. G. C. Hard and W. H. Butler, *Cancer Res.*, 1971, **31**, 1496–1505.
22. G. C. Hard, *Carcinogenesis*, 1984, **6**, 1047–1050.
23. B. M. Heatfield, M. M. Lipsky and B. F. Trump, *Am. J. Pathol.*, 1980, **100**, 317–320.
24. H. Tsuda, T. Sakata, S. Tamano, M. Okumura and N. Ito, *Carcinogenesis*, 1983, **4**, 523–528.
25. G. C. Hard, in *Nephrotoxicity in the Experimental and Clinical Situation,* ed. P. H. Bach and E. A. Lock, Martinus Nijhoff Publishers, Dordrecht, 1987, pp. 211–250.

26. M. M. Lipsky and B. F. Trump, *Int. Rev. Exp. Pathol.*, 1988, **30**, 357–383.
27. D. R. Dietrich and J. A. Swenberg, *Mutat. Res.*, 1991, **248**, 239–260.
28. E. Nogueira, A. Cardesa and U. Mohr, *J. Cancer Res. Clin. Oncol.*, 1993, **119**, 190–198.
29. G. C. Hard and J. C. Seely, *Toxicol. Pathol.*, 2005, **33**, 641–649.
30. G. C. Hard and J. C. Seely, *Toxicol. Pathol.*, 2006, **34**, 941–948.
31. G. C. Hard, *Toxicol. Pathol.*, 1998, **26**, 104–112.
32. G. C. Hard, in *Carcinogenicity: Testing, Predicting, and Interpreting Chemical Effects,* ed. K.T. Kitchen, Marcel Dekker, New York, 1999, pp. 439–466.
33. E. A. Lock and G. C. Hard, *Crit. Rev. Toxicol.*, 2004, **34**, 211–299.
34. J. I. Everitt, T. L. Goldsworthy, D. C. Wolf and C. L. Walker, *J. Urol.*, 1992, **148**, 1932–1936.
35. R. S. Yeung, G. H. Xiao, F, Jin, W. C. Lee, J. R. Testa and A. G. Knudson, *Proc. Natl. Acad. Sci.*, 1994, **91**, 11413–11416.
36. T. Kobayashi, Y. Hirayama, E. Kobayashi, Y. Kubo and O. Hino, *Nat. Genet.*, 1995, **9**, 70–74.
37. O. Hino, T. Fukuda, N. Satake, T. Kobayashi, S. Honda, K. Orimoto, Y. Yamashita and Y. Kikuchi, *Prog. Exp. Tumor Res.*, 1999, **35**, 95–108.
38. J. M. Hollingsworth, D. C. Miller, S. Daignault and B. K. Hollenbeck, *J. Natl. Cancer Inst.*, 2006, **98**, 1331–1334.
39. S. Weikert and B. Ljundberg, *World J. Urol.*, 2010, **28**, 247–252.
40. K. Gupta, J. D. Miller, J. Z. Li, M. W. Russell and C. Charbonneau, *Cancer Treat. Rev.*, 2008, **34**, 193–205.
41. G. G. Hillman, in *Tumor Models in Cancer Research*, ed. B. A. Teicher, Humana Press, Totowa, New Jersey, 2006, pp. 493–505.
42. W. Y. Kim and W. G. Kaelin, *J. Clin. Oncol.*, 2004, **22**, 4991–5004.
43. E. B. Rankin, J. E. Tomaszewski and V. H. Haase, *Cancer Res.*, 2006, **66**, 2576–2583.
44. M. P. Waalkes, J. Liu, R. A. Goyer and B. A. Diwan, *Cancer Res.*, 2004, **64**, 7766–7772.
45. M. P. Waalkes, J. Liu, K. S. Kasprzak and B. A. Diwan, *Int. J. Toxicol.*, 2005, **24**, 215–220.
46. M. Vasak, *J. Trace Elem. Med. Biol.*, 2005, **19**, 13–17.
47. Inorganic and Organic Lead Compounds, *Monographs on the Evaluation of the Carcinogenic Risks to Humans,* International Agency for Research on Cancer, Lyon, France, 2006, vol. 87.
48. T. D. Anderson, K. N. Khan, M. S. Tassinari and M. E. Hurtt, *J. Tox. Sci.*, 2009, **34**, SP209.
49. *Carcinogenicity Testing: a Report of the Panel on Carcinogenicity of the Cancer Research Commission of UICC*, ed. I. Berenblum, International Union Against Cancer, Geneva, Switzerland, 1969, vol. 2.
50. K. P. Baetcke, G. C. Hard, I. S. Rodgers, R. E. McGaughy and L. M. Tahan, *Alpha$_{2u}$-Globulin: Association with Chemically Induced Renal Toxicity and Neoplasia in the Male Rat,* Risk Assessment Forum, Environmental Protection Agency, Washington, DC, 1991.

51. *Species Differences in Thyroid, Kidney and Urinary Bladder Carcinogenesis*, ed. C. C. Capen, E. Dybing, J. M. Rice and J. D. Wilbourn, International Agency for Research on Cancer, Lyon, France, 1999, pp. 1–14.
52. J. A. Swenberg and L. D. Lehman-McKeeman, in *Species Differences in Thyroid, Kidney and Urinary Bladder Carcinogenesis,* ed. C. C. Capen, E. Dybing, J. M. Rice and J. D. Wilbourn, International Agency for Research on Cancer, Lyon, France, 1999, pp. 95–118.
53. S. M. Cohen, *Exp. Toxicol. Pathol.*, 2010, **62**, 497–502.
54. A. R. Boobis, S. M. Cohen, N. G. Doerrer, S. M. Galloway, P. J. Haley, G. C. Hard, F. G. Hess, J. S. McDonald, S. Thaibukt, D. C. Wolf and J. Wright, *Toxicol. Pathol.*, 2009, **37**, 714–732.
55. G. S. Travlos, G. C. Hard, L. J. Betz and G. E. Kissling, *Toxicol. Pathol.*, 2010, **39**, 381–389.
56. S. Garwood, *Anesth. Analg.*, 2009, **108**, 1371–1376.
57. L. M. Scoutt, K. J. W. Taylor, in *Clinical Applications of Doppler ultrasound,* ed. K. J. W. Taylor, P. N. Burns, P. N. T. Wells, Raven Press, New York, 2nd edn, 1995, pp. 155–178.
58. J. F. Platt, J. H. Ellis and K. A. Reige, *Acad. Radiol.*, 1996, **3**, 718–723.
59. Y. Tsushima, *Eur. J. Radiol.*, 1999, **30**, 191–197.
60. V. E. Noble and D. F. Brown, *Emerg. Med. Clin. North. Am.*, 2004, **22**, 641–659.
61. T. A. el Maghraby, B. L. van Eck-Smit, J. W. de Fijter and E. K. Pauwels, *Eur. J. Radiol.*, 1998, **28**, 256–269.
62. P. Meier, M. T. Farres, B. Mougenot, L. Jacob, F. Le Goas, C. Antignac and P. Ronco, *Am. J. Kidney Dis.*, 2003, **42**, E5–E10.
63. F. D. Sistare, F. Dieterle, S. Troth, D. J. Holder, D. Gerhold, D. Andrews-Cleavenger, W. Baer, G. Betton, D. Bounous, K. Carl, N. Collins, P. Goering, F. Goodsaid, Y. Z. Gu, V. Guilpin, E. Harpur, A. Hassan, D. Jacobson-Kram, P. Kasper, D. Laurie, B. S. Lima, R. Maciulaitis, W. Mattes, G. Maurer, L. A. Obert, J. Ozer, M. Papaluca-Amati, J. A. Phillips, M. Pinches, M. J. Schipper, K. L. Thompson, S. Vamvakas, J. M. Vidal, J. Vonderscher, E. Walker, C. Webb and Y. Yu, *Nat. Biotechnol.*, 2010, **28**, 446–454.
64. L. Zhang, M. Wang and H. Wang, *Clin. Nephrol.*, 2005, **63**, 346–350.
65. W. D. Comper and E. F. Glasgow, *Kidney Intl.,* 1995, **47**, 1242–1251.
66. T. M. Osicka, L. M. Pratt and W. D. Comper, *Nephrology*, 1996, **2**, 199–212.
67. L. M. Russo, G. L. Bakris and W. D. Comper, *Am. J. Kidney Dis.*, 2002, **39**, 899–919.
68. M. Kamimura and S. R. Orth, *J. Hypertens.*, 2003, **21**, 269–271.
69. W. D. Comper and L. M. Russo, *Curr. Opin. Nephrol. Hypertens.*, 2009, **18**, 336–342.
70. G. D'Amico and C. Bazzi, *Kidney Intl.*, 2003, **63**, 809–825.
71. C. G. Duarte and H. B. Preuss, *Clin. Lab. Med.*, 1993, **13**, 33–52.
72. P. Devarajan, *Nephrology*, 2010, **15**, 419–428.

73. T. Miyata, M. Jadoul, K. Kurokawa and C. van Yperserle de Strihou, *J. Am. Soc. Nephrol.*, 1998, **9**, 1723–1735.
74. F. Dieterle, E. Marrer, E. Suzuki, O. Grenet, A. Cordier and J. Vonderscher, *Curr. Opin. Drug Discovery Develop.*, 2008, **11**, 60–71.
75. P. G. Davey and P. Gosling, *Clin. Chem.*, 1982, **28**, 1330–1333.
76. W. Kriz and B. Kaissling, in *The Kidney: Physiology and Pathophysiology,* ed. D.W. Seldin and G. Giebisch, Lippincott Williams and Wilkins, Philadelphia, 3rd edn, 2000, vol. 1, pp. 587–654.
77. R. Gibey, J. L. Dupond, D. Alber, R. Leconte des Floris and J. C. Henry, *Clin. Chim. Acta*, 1981, **116**, 25–34.
78. M. D. Stonard, C. W. Gore, G. J. Oliver and I. K. Smith, *Fundam. Appl. Toxicol.*, 1987, **9**, 339–351.
79. R. G. Price, *Clin. Nephrol.,* 1992, **38**, S14–S19.
80. F. A. S. Clemo, *Toxicol. Pathol.*, 1998, **26**, 29–32.
81. J. Westhuyzen, Z. H. Endre, G. Reece, D. M. Reith, D. Saltissi and T. J. Morgan, *Nephrol. Dial. Transplant*, 2003, **18**, 543–551.
82. D. J. Harrison, R. Kharbanda, D. S. Cunningham, L. I. McLellan and J. D. Hayes, *J. Clin. Pathol.*, 1989, **42**, 624.
83. A. Sundberg, E. L. Appelkvist, G. Dallner and R. Nilsson, *Environ. Health Perspect.*, 1994, **102**, 293–296.
84. A. J. W. Branten, T. P. J. Mulder, W. H. M. Peters, K. J. M. Assman and J. F. M. Wetzels, *Nephron*, 2000, **85**, 120–126.
85. J. V. Bonventre, *Scan. J. Clin. Lab. Investig.*, 2008, **68**, 78.
86. F. Waanders, G. Navis and H. van Goor, *Am. J. Kidney Dis.*, 2010, **55**, 813–816.
87. *Final Report on the pilot joint EMEA/FDA VXDS Experience on Qualification of Nephrotoxicity Biomarkers,* European Medicines Agency, London, 2008.
88. *European Medicines Agency to Consider Additional Test Results When Assessing New Drug Safety,* Food and Drug Administration, Silver Spring, MD, 2008.
89. T. Ichimura, J. V. Bonventre, V. Bailly, H. Wei, C. A. Hession, R. L. Cate and M. Sanicola, *J. Biol. Chem.*, 1998, **273**, 4135–4142.
90. E. A. Lock, *Toxicol. Sci.*, 2010, **116**, 1–4.
91. V. S. Vaidya, M. A. Ferguson and J. V. Bonventre, *Annu. Rev. Pharmacol.*, 2008, **48**, 463–493.
92. W. K. Han, V. Bailly, R. Abichandani, R. Thadhani and J. V. Bonventre, *Kidney Intl.*, 2002, **62**, 237–244.
93. T. Ichimura, C. C. Hung, S. A. Yang, J. L. Stevens and J. V. Bonventre, *Am. J. Physiol. Renal Physiol.*, 2004, **286**, F552–F563.
94. A. J. Rees and R. Kain, *Nephrol. Dial. Transplant*, 2008, **23**, 3394–3396.
95. Y. Zhou, V. S. Vaidya, R. P. Brown, J. Zhang, B. A. Rosenzweig, K. L. Thompson, T. J. Miller, J. V. Bonventre and P. L. Goering, *Toxicol. Sci.*, 2008, **101**, 159–170.
96. W. K. Han, S. S. Waikar, A. M. Johnson, R. A. Betensky, C. L. Dent, P. Devarajan and J. V. Bonventre, *Kidney Intl.*, 2007, **73**, 863–869.

97. D. R. Flower, A. C. North and C. E. Sansom, *Biochim. Biophys. Acta*, 2000, **1482**, 9–24.
98. K. M. Schmidt-Ott, K. Mori, J. Y. Li, A. Kalandadze, D. J. Cohen, P. Devajaran and J. Barasch, *J. Am. Soc. Nephrol.*, 2007, **18**, 407–413.
99. J. Mishra, K. Mori, Q. Ma, C. Kelly, J. Barasch and P. Devarajan, *Am. J. Nephrol.*, 2004, **24**, 307–315.
100. S. S. Soni, D. Cruz, I. Bobek, C. Y. Chionh, F. Nalesso, P. Lentini, M. de Cal, V. Corradi, G. Virzi and C. Ronco, *Int. Urol. Nephrol.*, 2010, **42**, 141–150.
101. S. Xu and P. Venge, *Biochim. Biophys. Acta*, 2000, **1482**, 298–307.
102. D. Hoffmann, M. Adler, V. S. Vaidya, E. Rached, L. Mulrane, W. M. Gallagher, J. J. Callanan, J. C. Gautier, K. Matheis, F. Staedtler, F. Dieterle, A. Brandenburg, A. Sponsy, P. Hewitt, H. Ellinger-Ziegelbauer, J. V. Bonventre, W. Dekant and A. Mally, *Toxicol. Sci.*, 2010, **116**, 8–22.
103. I. Sugawara, *Microbes Infect.*, 2000, **2**, 1257–1263.
104. J. A. Gracie, S. E. Robertson and I. B. McInnes, *J. Leukocyte Biol.*, 2003, **73**, 213–224.
105. C. R. Parikh, A. Jani, V. Y. Melnikov, S. Faubel and C. L. Edelstein, *Am. J. Kidney Dis.*, 2004, **43**, 405–414.
106. M. Mussap and M. Plebani, *Crit. Rev. Clin. Lab. Sci.*, 2004, **41**, 467–550.
107. V. R. Dharnidharka, C. Kwond and G. Stevens, *Am. J. Kidney Dis.*, 2002, **40**, 221–226.
108. M. Madero, M. J. Sarnak and L. A. Stevens, *Curr. Opin. Nephrol. Hypertens.*, 2006, **15**, 610–616.
109. O. Tenstad, A. B. Roald, A. Grubb and K. Aukland, *Scan. J. Clin. Lab. Invest.*, 1996, **56**, 409–414.
110. S. Herget-Rosenthal, J. A. van Wijk, M. Bröcker-Pruess and A. Bökencamp, *Clin. Biochem.*, 2007, **40**, 946–951.
111. L. A. Stevens, J. Coresh, C. H. Schmid, H. I. Feldman, M. Froissart, J. Kusek, J. Rossert, F. Van Lente, R. D. Bruce, Y. Zhang, T. Greene and A. S. Levey, *Am. J. Kidney Dis.*, 2008, **51**, 395–406.
112. S. E. Jones and C. Jomary, *Int. J. Biochem. Cell Biol.*, 2002, **34**, 427–431.
113. M. E. Rosenberg and M. S. Paller, *Kidney Intl.*, 1991, **39**, 1156–1161.
114. J. W. Davis, F. M. Goodsaid, C. M. Bral, L. A. Obert, G. Mandakas, C. E. Garner, N. D. Collins, R. J. Smith and I. Y. Rosenblum, *Toxicol. Appl. Pharmacol.*, 2004, **200**, 16–26.
115. A. Ishii, Y. Sakai and A. Nakamura, *Toxicol. Pathol.*, 2007, **35**, 376–382.
116. P. Gött, S. Beck, J. C. Machado, F. Carneiro, H. Schmitt and N. Blin, *Eur. J. Human Genet.*, 1996, **4**, 3080315.
117. W. Hoffmann, W. Jagla and A. Wiede, *Histol. Histopathol.*, 2001, **16**, 319–334.
118. Y. Yu, H. Jin, D. Holder, J. S. Ozer, S. Villarreal, P. Shughrue, S. Shi, D. J. Figueroa, H. Clouse, M. Su, N. Muniappa, S. P. Troth, W. Bailey, J. Seng, A. G. Aslamkhan, D. Thudium, F. D. Sistare and D. L. Gerhold, *Nat. Biotechnol.*, 2010, **28**, 470–477.

119. F. W. Falkenberg, H. Hildebrand, L. Lutte, S. Schwengberg, B. Henke, D. Greshake, B. Schmidt, A. Friederich, M. Rinke, G. Schlüter and E. Bomhard, *Arch. Toxicol.*, 1996, **71**, 80–92.
120. H. Hildebrand, M. Rinke, G. Schlüter, E. Bomhard and F. W. Falkenberg, *Arch. Toxicol.*, 1999, **73**, 233–245.
121. S. A. Price, D. Davies, R. Rowlinson, C. G. Copley, A. Roche, F. W. Falkenberg, D. Riccardi and G. R. Betton, *Toxicol. Pathol.*, 2010, **38**, 346–358.
122. M. J. Mihatsch, B. Khanlari and F. P. Brunner, *Nephrol. Dial. Transplant*, 2006, **21**, 3139–3145.
123. Y. Tonomura, N. Tsuchiya, M. Torii and T. Uehara, *Toxicology*, 2010, **273**, 53–59.
124. S. G. Coca, R. Yalavarthy, J. Concato and C. R. Parikh, *Kidney Intl.*, 2008, **73**, 1008–1016.
125. W. K. Han, G. Wagener, Y. Zhu, S. Wang and H. T. Lee, *Clin. J. Am. Soc. Nephrol.*, 2009, **4**, 873–882.
126. O. Liangos, M. C. Perianayagam, V. S. Vaidya, W. K. Han, R. Wald, H. Tighiouart, R. W. MacKinnon, L. Li, V. S. Balakrishnan, B. J. Pereira, J. V. Bonventre and B. L. Jaber, *J. Am. Soc. Nephrol.*, 2010, **18**, 904–912.
127. M. G. Janech, J. R. Raymond and J. M. Arthur, *Am. J. Physiol. Renal Physiol.*, 2007, **292**, F501–F512.
128. W. R. Foster, S. J. Chen, A. He, A. Truong, V. Bhaskaran, D. M. Nelson, D. M. Dambach, L. D. Lehmann-McKeeman and B. D. Car, *Toxicol. Pathol.*, 2007, **35**, 621–635.
129. A. Chiusolo, R. Defazio, E. Zanetti, M. Mongillo, N. Mori, P. Cristofori and A. Trevisan, *Toxicol. Pathol.*, 2010, **38**, 338–345.
130. S. K. Thukral, P. J. Nordone, R. Hu, L. Sullivan, E. Galambos, V. D. Fitzpatrick, L. Healy, M. B. Bass, M. E. Cosenza and C. A. Afshari, *Toxicol. Pathol.*, 2005, **33**, 343–355.
131. V. Sandim, D. A. Pereira, A. A. Ornellas and G. Alves, *Urol. Int.*, 2010, **84**, 373–377.
132. R. Pieper, C. L. Gatlin, A. M. McGrath, A. J. Makusky, M. Mondal, M. Seonarain, E. Field, C. R. Schatz, M. A. Estock, N. Ahmed, N. G. Anderson and S. Steiner *Proteomics,* 2004, **4**, 1159–1174.
133. M. De Bock, D. de Seny, L. A. Meuwis, J. P. Chapelle, E. Louis, M. Malaise, M. P. Merville and M. Fillet, *J. Biomed. Biotechnol.*, 2010, 906082.
134. M. Z. Zhang, Y. Su, B. Yao, W. Zheng, M. deCaestecker and R. C. Harris, *J. Histochem. Cytochem.*, 2010, **58**, 413–420.
135. R. J. Simpson, J. W. Lim, R. L. Moritz and S. Mathivana, *Expert Rev. Proteomics*, 2009, **6**, 267–283.
136. J. C. Carrington and V. Ambros, *Science*, 2003, **301**, 336–338.
137. S. Saal and S. J. Harvey, *Curr. Opin. Nephrol. Hypertens.*, 2009, **18**, 317–323.
138. J. K. Nicholson, J. C. Lindon and E. Holmes, *Xenobiotica*, 1999, **29**, 1181–1189.

139. K. J. Boudonck, M. W. Mitchell, L. Nemet, L. Keresztes, A. Nyska, D. Shinar and M. Rosenstock, *Toxicol. Pathol.*, 2009, **37**, 280–292.
140. M. Van de Poll, P. B. Soeters, N. E. P. Deutz, K. C. H. Fearon and Dejong C. H. C, *Am. J. Clin. Nutr.*, 2004, **79**, 185–197.
141. S. K. Patel, N. Ma, T. J. Monks and S. S. Lau, *Mol. Carcinog.*, 2003, **38**, 141–154.
142. C. G. Duarte, J. Zhang and S. Ellis, *Renal Failure,* 1997, **19**, 723–743.
143. B. Ryffel and M. J. Mihatsch, *Toxicol. Pathol.*, 1986, **14**, 73–82.
144. G. Bledsoe, S. Crickman, J. Mao, C. F. Xia, H. Murakami, L. Chao and J. Chao, *Nephrol. Dial. Transplant*, 2006, **21**, 624.
145. J. P. Fillastre and G. Raguenez-Viotte, *Toxicol. Lett.*, 1989, **46**, 163–175.
146. K. C. Linden, C. L. DeHaan, Y. Zhang, S. Glowacka, A. J. Cox, D. J. Kelly and S. Rogers, *Am. J. Physiol. Renal. Physiol.*, 2006, **290**, F205–F213.
147. V. U. Collier, P. S. Lietman and W. E. Mitch, *J. Pharmacol. Exp. Ther.*, 1979, **210**, 247–251.
148. Z. Ma, J. Wang, R. L. Nation, J. Li, J. D. Turnidge, K. Coulthard and R. W. Milne, *Antimicrob. Agents Chemother.*, 2009, **53**, 2857–2864.
149. J. Wang, R. L. Nation, A. M. Evans and S. Cox, *Clin. Exp. Pharmacol. Physiol.*, 2004, **31**, 29–34.
150. A. E. Vickers and R. L. Fisher, *Expert Opin. Drug Metab. Toxicol.*, 2005, **1**, 687–699.
151. J. G. Zhang and W. E. Lindup, *Biochem. Pharmacol.*, 1993, **45**, 2215–2222.
152. C. H. Kuo, K. Maita, S. D. Sleight and J. B. Hook, *Toxicol. Appl. Pharmacol.*, 1983, **67**, 78–88.
153. R. C. Harmon, S. P. Duffy, M. V. Terneus, J. G. Ball and M. A. Valentovic, *Nephrol. Dial. Transplant*, 2009, **24**, 763–768.
154. A. Lungkaphin, B. Lewchalermwongse and V. Chatsudthipong, *Biochim. Biophys. Acta*, 2006, **1758**, 789–795.
155. A. Vandewalle, N. Farman, J. P. Morin, J. P. Fillastre, P. Y. Hatt and J. P. Bonvalet, *Kidney Int.*, 1981, **19**, 529–539.
156. H. Dan, R. X. Peng, Y. Ao and Y. H. Liu, *J. Biochem. Mol. Toxicol.*, 2008, **22**, 422–428.
157. I. Hizoh and C. Haller, *Invest. Radiol.* 2002, **37**, 428–434.
158. J. P. Morin, S. Marouillat, C. Lendormi and C. Monteil, *Cell Biol. Toxicol.*, 1996, **12**, 275–282.
159. D. H. O'Donnell, M. A. Moloney, D. J. Bouchier-Hayes and M. J. Lee, *Am. J. Roentgenol.*, 2010, **195**, W45–W49.
160. D. J. Brennan, D. P. O'Connor, E. Rexhepaj, F. Ponten and W. M. Gallagher, *Nat. Rev. Cancer*, 2010, **10**, 605–615.

CHAPTER 21
# *Metabolism-Based Toxicology Prediction*

F. PETER GUENGERICH

Vanderbilt University School of Medicine, Department of Biochemistry and Center in Molecular Toxicology, 638 Robinson Research Building, 2200 Pierce Avenue, Nashville, Tennessee 37232-0146, USA

## 21.1 Introduction

Toxicology is not a new field, with reports of the dangers of metals (lead) and natural products (*e.g.*, hemlock) going back to the ancient Greeks. Paracelsus, who provided early insight into basic concepts of toxicity and the importance of the dose (which is often forgotten in some circles today), lived 500 years ago.[1] However, metabolism is a much newer discipline. Little knowledge about biological chemicals and metabolism was available until the 19$^{th}$ Century, and the first examples of transformations of xenobiotic chemicals appeared in the latter half of the 19$^{th}$ Century;[2] *e.g.*, hippuric and mercapturic acids. The concept of enzymes did not really develop until the work of Emil Fischer and others at the beginning of the 20$^{th}$ Century.

Links between metabolism and any type of toxicity were not considered until ~ 1940. James and Elizabeth Miller identified covalent binding of known carcinogens to proteins[3] and later DNA[4] and also identified enzymatic processes involved in the metabolism of some of these carcinogens.[5] R. T. Williams characterized several transformations of drugs.[6,7] Brodie and Gillette also reported a number of transformations of drugs by enzymatic systems[8] and in 1973 published a series of seminal articles on the covalent binding of acetaminophen and bromobenzene.[9–12]

RSC Drug Discovery Series No. 12
New Horizons in Predictive Toxicology: Current Status and Application
Edited by Alan G. E. Wilson

Published by the Royal Society of Chemistry, www.rsc.org

Collectively, these studies have established a number of principles and paradigms. While some carcinogens were known to be mutagens, the relationship had not shown good correlation. The work with carcinogen metabolism led to the development of practical bacterial assays for identifying genotoxic carcinogens by Ames.[13] The continuing studies on drug metabolism, particularly with cytochrome P450 (P450) enzymes, have led to understanding drug–drug interactions and genetic differences in drug action.[14] The information about metabolism has been coupled with other biological systems and is being used to better understand and predict the potential toxicity of drugs, as well as the risks, the major subjects of this chapter.

In this brief review of the history of xenobiotic metabolism, it would be amiss not to mention two areas that have enabled modern science in the field. One is analytical chemistry. The advances in sensitivity and speed have made it possible to determine structures of metabolites and detect them at concentration relevant to exposures. The other driver has been recombinant DNA technology, which has facilitated enzymology and also led to important animal models.

## 21.2 Current Working Paradigms

The simplest relationship between drug metabolism and toxicity is that a chemical can exert toxicity due to its pharmacological activity and that metabolism prevents this by converting a drug to an inactive metabolite. Examples would include drug overdoses, *e.g.*, conjugation of bromobenzene,[15] and also genetic deficiencies in which accumulation of a drug occurs in a subset of the population, *e.g.*, perhexiline neuropathy in individuals devoid of P450 2D6.[16]

We can also consider contexts of toxicity (Table 21.1)[17] and the relevance of metabolism.

1) On-target toxicity is a problematic issue in development, in that all changes made in the chemistry to avoid toxicity also decrease efficacy. However, in some cases, safe drugs can be developed because of tissue selectivity due to transporters, *e.g.*, statins.[18] 2) Another context of drug toxicity is hypersensitivity and immunological reactions. This context is not directly linked to metabolism but is considered in conjunction with metabolism in idiosyncratic reactions (*vide supra*). 3) Off-target pharmacology is probably common as a reason for toxicity; with > 20 000 genes and even more gene products in the

**Table 21.1** Contexts of drug toxicity.[17]

| *Context* | *Example* |
|---|---|
| On-target toxicity (mechanism-based) | Statins |
| Hypersensitivity and immune reactions | Penicillins |
| Off-target pharmacology | Terfenadine |
| Bioactivation to reactive intermediates | Acetaminophen |
| Idiosyncratic toxicity | Halothane |

human body, the difficulty of producing small molecules specific to only one is enormous. In one classic case of drug toxicity, terfenadine was shown to be rapidly oxidized by P450 3A4[19] but deficiencies (due to genetics or drug interactions) blocked the process and led to the accumulation of terfenadine, which blocks hERG channels,[20] explaining at least several of the deaths reported with this drug. 4) Bioactivation will be discussed in more detail later, as will 5) idiosyncratic reactions.

The general concept of bioactivation is that relatively inert chemical structures are converted into radicals or, more often, reactive electrophiles. These electrophiles can be inactivated through interception with small nucleophiles, *e.g.*, glutathione (GSH). However, they can also react with the nucleophilic sites of nucleic acids and proteins. There is clear evidence that the modification of DNA can lead to miscoding and mutations. Modification of proteins can cause inactivation or loss of regulatory control (Figure 21.1). Both the reactions of radicals and also reactions of electrophiles with small and large molecules in cells can exacerbate oxidative stress, a process that may be involved in a number of types of toxicity.[22,23]

A diagram of some of the events linking metabolism and toxicity is shown in Figure 21.1. Not all aspects or possibilities have been discussed or even

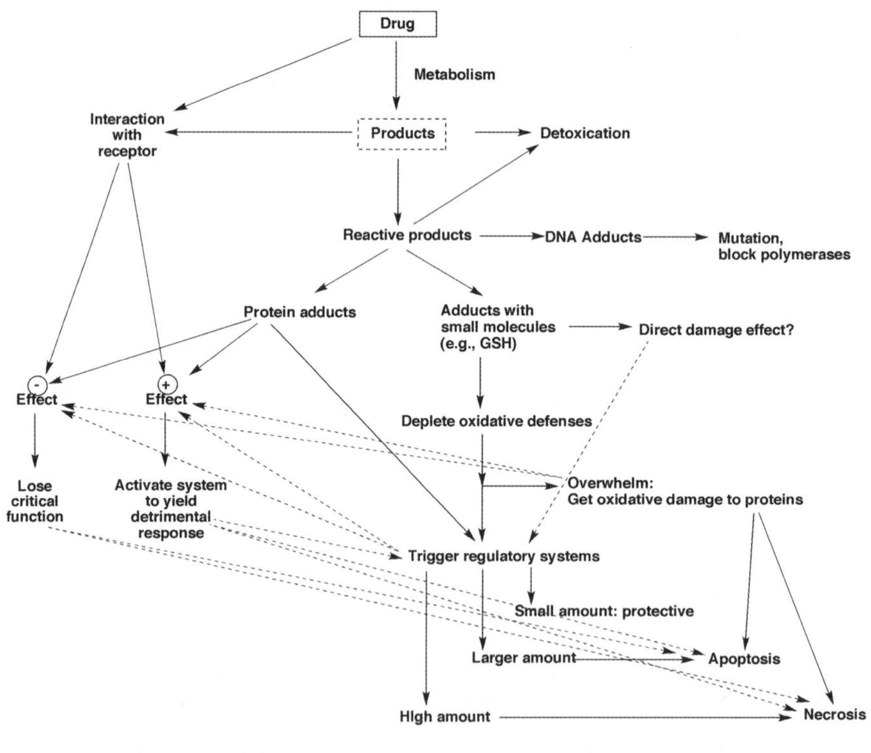


**Figure 21.1** A general scheme of biological events related to the toxicity of drugs and other chemicals.[17,21]

presented. In this working paradigm, covalent binding to macromolecules has a dominant place but not an exclusive one. One complication comes with considerations of dose, which will be discussed later. A small amount of electrophilic damage leads to the induction of protective mechanisms, *e.g.*, Keap1/Nrf2 and GSH transferases. Thus, a small amount of damage can have a protective effect. More extensive damage appears to lead to disruption of important systems and to the process of apoptosis, in which distinct pathways result in cell death in a relatively orderly process. Even more damage leads to cell necrosis, a more disorderly death of cells and tissues. Thus the same chemistry can be involved in all of these processes, and designing simple *in vitro* assays to predict which effects will occur is a challenge, particularly in the face of limited information about what doses and concentrations will be relevant. As can be seen in the diagram (Figure 21.1), there are numerous other ways in which metabolism can yield changes in the concentrations of receptor ligands *etc.* Also, the mitochrondrion has come under increasing interest as a key element of toxicity, particularly hepatotoxicity,[24,25] including oxidative stress.[26,27]

Toxicity is a major reason for failure of new chemical entities to advance in the drug-development process.[28] In one analysis,[28] > 30% of the failures are the result of pre-clinical toxicity and adverse events in clinical trials (also indicative of various toxicities). The question of how often biotransformation has a role in the withdrawal of candidates can be asked. This is not a trivial question, in that most data are proprietary and held within companies, and in many cases the causes are not determined. However, one available estimate from experience at DuPont–Merck and Bristol–Myers Squibb is that 28% of pre-clinical candidate failures are due to metabolism issues (Table 21.2).[21]

Idiosyncratic toxicities are considered individualize responses, classified so because they are too rare to classify well ($1/10^3$–$1/10^4$ frequency). Although they are often considered to be dose-independent, that is probably not the case (Table 21.3), invoking Paracelsus' principles of toxicology.[1] Indeed, Uetrecht has made the point that idiosyncratic liver toxicity is seldom seen with drugs used at $<10$ mg per day.[29,32] A number of hypotheses have been proposed to explain toxicity (Table 21.4).[31,33]

**Table 21.2** Mechanistic causes of toxicology attrition based on experience from DuPont–Merck and Bristol–Myers Squibb, 1993–2006. Information kindly provided by B. D. Car, Bristol–Myers Squibb.

| *Mechanistic cause* | *% Of all advanced molecules*[a] |
|---|---|
| Biotransformation-related | 27 |
| Target-based | 28 |
| Single or multiple ion channel inhibition | 18 |
| Immune-mediated | 7 |
| All other mechanisms | 36 |

[a] $n=88$. Because categories are partially overlapping, the total is > 100%.

**Table 21.3** Intrinsic *vs.* idiosyncratic hepatotoxicity.[17,29–31]

| *Intrinsic* | *Idiosyncratic* |
|---|---|
| Predictable (?) | Unpredictable |
| Relatively common occurrence | Rare occurrence ($<1/10^4$) |
| Detected pre-clinically | Not detected until post-launch |
| Dose-dependent | Occurs at any dose (?) |
| Acute or sub-acute onset | Delayed onset |
| No immune component | Immune/metabolic component (usually see fever, rash, eosinophilia) |
| Animal models useful | Few (any?) animal models available |
| Example: acetaminophen | Examples: isoniazid, halothane |

**Table 21.4** Proposed mechanisms for idiosyncratic toxicity.[31,34]

| *Model* | *Mechanism* |
|---|---|
| Metabolic | Unusual metabolism due to multiple rare alleles |
| Hapten hypothesis | Reactive metabolites act as haptens, probably variations in response genes |
| Inflammagen model | Inflammation or other predisposing episodes render some individuals more sensitive |
| Danger hypothesis | Injured tissue → danger signals → immunological response |
| Pharmacological Intervention hypothesis | Drugs → immunological response as a result of reversible binding |

The issue of bioactivation and reactive metabolites deserves further consideration, if for no other reason than much of the prediction of toxicity is currently based upon this as a principle. Clearly there are correlations of covalent binding and toxicity in pre-clinical studies.[12,35] How much evidence do we really have that this is a major issue in pre-clinical or clinical toxicity, though? As pointed out in Table 21.2, one estimate is that biotransformation was an issue in ~ 28% of the preclinical attrition cases. An extensive analysis was reported by Walgren *et al.* in 2005 (Tables 21.5–21.7).[36]

Two points are striking in considering the data: idiosyncratic toxicity is seen only at higher doses, and a large fraction of the drugs showing toxicity also show covalent binding in either *in vitro* or *in vivo* studies. The use of covalent binding data was advanced as a useful strategy in drug development.[58] In considering these systems, one can ask how well binding would predict clinical issues.

Several efforts have been reported, all with relatively expensive radiolabeled compounds, *i.e.*, drugs with well-documented clinical experience. Masubuchi *et al.*[59] demonstrated good correlation between *in vitro* and *in vivo* covalent binding, although some correction factors were necessary (Figure 21.2).

**Table 21.5** Drugs withdrawn for hepatotoxicity (US).[36]

| *Drug* | *Year* | *Dose (mg per day)* | *Reactive products*[a] | *Reference* |
|---|---|---|---|---|
| Cincophen | 1930 | 300 | No | — |
| Iproniazid | 1959 | 25–150 | Yes | 37 |
| Pipamazine | 1969 | 15 | No | — |
| Fenclozic acid | 1970 | 300 | Yes | 38 |
| Oxyphenisatin | 1973 | 50 | No | — |
| Nialamide | 1974 | 200 | Yes | 39 |
| Tienilic acid | 1980 | 250–500 | Yes | 40 |
| Benoxaprofen | 1982 | 300–600 | Yes | 41 |
| Nomifensine | 1986 | 125 | Yes | 42 |
| Chlormezanone | 1996 | 600 | No | — |
| Bromfenac | 1998 | 25–50 | Yes | — |
| Troglitazone | 2000 | 400 | Yes | 43 |
| Nefazodone | 2004 | 200 | Yes | 44 |
| Pemoline | 2005 | 38–110 | No | — |

[a]9/14 = 64%.

**Table 21.6** Drugs withdrawn for hepatotoxicity (non-US).[36]

| *Drug* | *Year (Country)* | *Dose (mg per day)* | *Reactive products*[a] | *Reference* |
|---|---|---|---|---|
| Alpidem | 1993 (France) | 25–150 | Yes | 45 |
| Amineptine | 1999 (France, Thailand) | 200 | Yes | 46 |
| Bendazac | 1993 (Spain) | 500 | — | — |
| Benzarone | 1992 (Greece) | 300 | Yes | — |
| Benziodarone | 1964 (UK) | 300 | — | — |
| Clomacron | 1982 (UK) | — | — | — |
| Clometacin | 1987 (France) | 450 | — | — |
| Cyclofenil | 1987 (France | 200 | — | — |
| Dilevalol | 1990 (UK) | 200–400 | — | — |
| Ebrotidine | 1998 (Spain) | 400–800 | — | — |
| Exifone | 1989 (France) | 1200 | Yes | — |
| Fipexide | 1991 (France, Greece) | 600 | Yes | — |
| Glafenine | 1984 (France, Greece) | 400 | Yes | — |
| Ibufenac | 1968 (UK) | 2400 | Yes | 47 |
| Isaxonine | 1984 (France) | 1500 | Yes | 48 |
| Mebanazine | 1975 (UK) | 30 | Yes | — |
| Moxisylyte | 1993 (France) | 480 | — | — |
| Niperotidine | 1995 (Italy) | 230–460 | — | — |
| Nitrefazole | 1984 (Greece) | 1200 | — | — |
| Perhexiline | 1985 (UK) | 300 | — | — |
| Phenoxypropazine | 1966 (UK) | 10–20 | Yes | — |
| Pirprofen | 1990 (EU) | 800 | Yes | — |
| Suloctidyl | 1985 (Spain) | 600 | — | — |
| Tolrestat | 1996 (EU) | 400 | — | — |
| Xenazoic acid | 1965 (France) | Unknown | — | — |
| Ximelagatran | 2006 (EU) | 48 | — | — |
| Zimelidine | 1985 (UK) | 100–300 | — | — |

[a]11/11 = 100%.

**Table 21.7** Drugs with Black Box warnings for hepatotoxicity.[36] A "Black Box" warning is the strongest type of warning that the FDA can require for a drug and is generally reserved for warning prescribers about adverse drug reactions that can cause serious injury or death. At issue here is the benefit–risk ratio.

| *Drug* | *Dose (mg per day)* | *Reactive products*[a] | *Reference* |
|---|---|---|---|
| Acitretin | 25–50 | No | — |
| Bosentau | 125–250 | No | — |
| Dacarbazine | 140–315 | Yes | 49 |
| Dantrolene | 300–400 | Yes | 50 |
| Felbamate | 1200 | Yes | 51 |
| Flutamide | 750 | Yes | 52 |
| Gemtuzumab | (9 mg $m^{-3}$) | Yes (?) | 53 |
| Isoniazid | 300 | Yes | 54 |
| Ketoconazole | 200 | Yes | 55 |
| Naltrexone | 50 | No | — |
| Nevirapine | 200 | Yes | — |
| Tolcapone | 300 | Yes | 56 |
| Trovafloxacin | 100–500 | No | — |
| Valporic acid | 1000–2400 | Yes | 57 |

[a]10/14 = 71%

Other studies showed that the level of covalent binding of hepatotoxic drugs was higher than non-hepatotoxic drugs, as a mean, but that there is a wide variation in both classes (Figures 21.3–21.5).[60–62]

Thus one can conclude that the extent of covalent binding of a compound is a factor in (hepato)toxicity, but certainly not the only one. Unfortunately it is still not possible to use a certain level of covalent binding to make a definitive prediction about whether a drug candidate will show toxicity or not (Figures 21.3–21.5).

## 21.3 Predicting Metabolism and Toxicity *In Silico*: State-of-the-Art and Challenges

The large numbers of chemical entities encountered in drug-discovery and drug-development programs and the costs of doing screening, even in high-throughput modes, have made virtual screens attractive in the realms of both metabolism and toxicity.[63–69] Other chapters in this book deal with both of these topics, but some general comments are in order here.

### 21.3.1 Predicting Genotoxicity

Most work with *in silico* prediction of genotoxicity has been done on the basis of the extensive literature available, primarily from Ames tests. Structure–activity relationships (SARs) indicate that certain structures are prone to

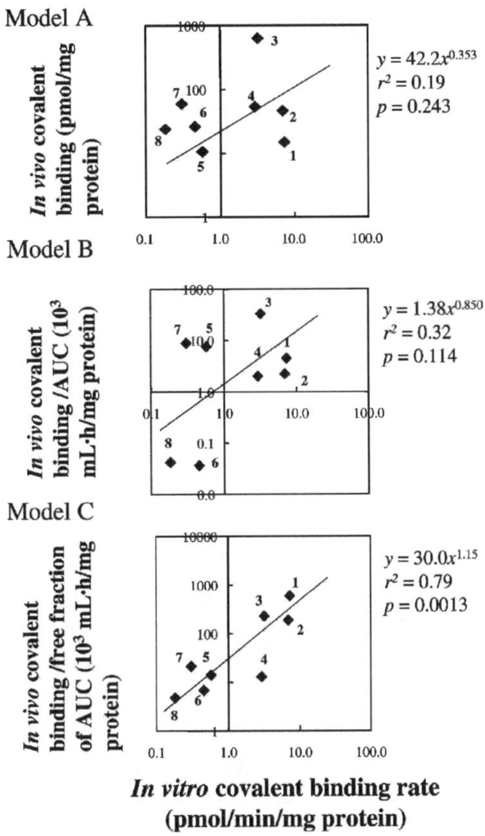


**Figure 21.2** Relationship between *in vitro* covalent binding rate of reactive metabolites to microsomal proteins (10 μM substrate) and *in vivo* covalent binding rate in rat liver tissue after administration of labeled compounds (at 20 mg $kg^{-1}$). Three different models were used.[59] **1**, Furosemide; **2**, tienilic acid; **3**, clozapine, **4**, imipramine; **5**, acetaminophen; **6**, indomethacin; **7**, carbamazepine; **8**, diclofenac.

activation and/or direct reaction with DNA, *e.g.*, aniline-based structures and polycyclic hydrocarbons with 4–5 rings. However, even in good SAR systems there are many exceptions. For instance, the mutagenicity of 2-amino-3,8-dimethylimidazo[4,5-*f*]quinoxaline (MeIQx) and 2-amino-1-methyl-6-phenylimidazo[4,5-*b*]pyridine (PhIP) are *ca.* 10-fold higher in systems with human P450 1A2 than rat P450 1A2, although these two P450 1A2 enzymes have equivalent activity with some model substrates.[70] Even more dramatic are the differences in genotoxicity among a series of heterocyclic amines (Figure 21.6),[71] *e.g.*, deleting an *N*-methyl group lowered the mutagenicity by six orders of magnitude. Replacement of a pyridine-ring nitrogen with a carbon lowered the mutagenicity 50 000-fold, and our own laboratory recently determined that

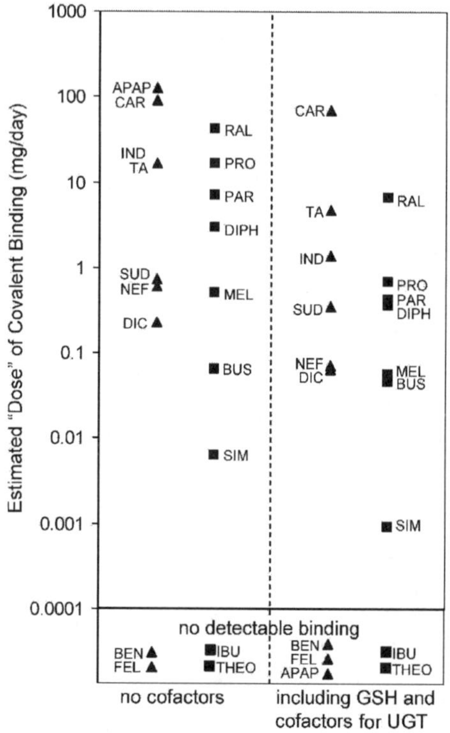


**Figure 21.3** Comparisons of hepatoxins (▲) and non-hepatoxins (■) for estimates of total daily dose of covalently bound material extrapolated from *in vitro* liver microsomal covalent binding and doses.[60] APAP = acetaminiophen; BEN = benoxaprofen; BUS = buspirone; CAR = carbamazepine; DIC = diclofenac; DIPH = diphenhydramine; FEC = felbamate; IBU = ibuprofen; IND = indomethacin; MEL = meloxicam; NEF = nefazodone; PAR = paroxetine; PRO = propranolol; RAL = raloxifene; SIM = simvastatin; SUD = sudoxicam; TA = tienilic acid; THEO = theophylline.

the difference cannot be attributed to rates of oxidation or acetylation or levels of DNA adduct formation but apparently reflects the inherent mutagenicity of the individual DNA adducts.[72]

### 21.3.2 Predicting Metabolism

Some progress has been made in the prediction of sites of metabolism of drugs, at least in the case of P450 oxidations. At least three approaches have been used. One is based on the thermodynamic ease of oxidation at a particular site, *i.e.*, as if the substrate were unrestricted in an enzyme (*e.g.*, MetaSite). Another approach is based upon docking of a molecule within the active site of a crystal structure of a P450 or a homology model, *e.g.*, GLIDE. A third approach ignores the chemistry and structure and approaches the SAR problem on the

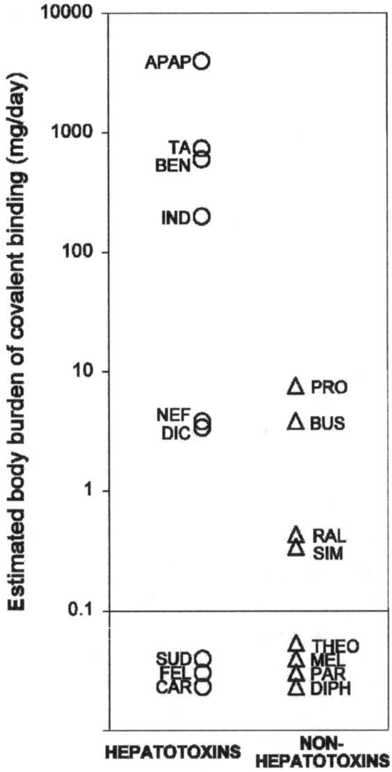


**Figure 21.4** Categorization of hepatoxins (○) and non-hepatotoxins (Δ) based on estimated total daily body burden covalent binding from human hepatocyte data.[61] Drug abbreviations as Figure 21.3.

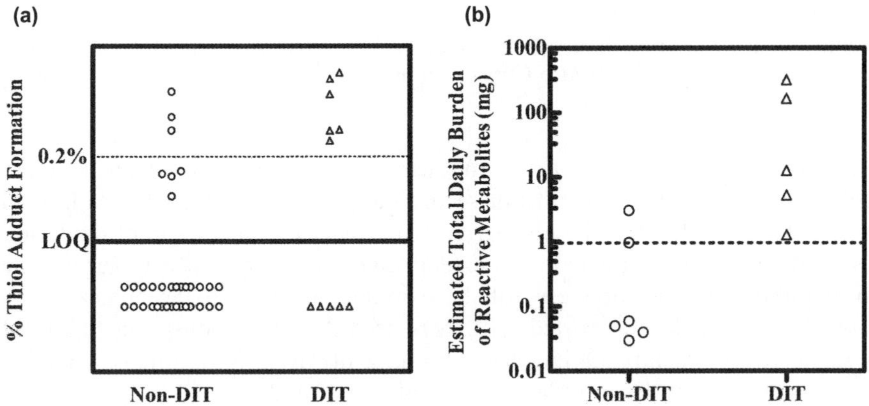


**Figure 21.5** Scatter plots of (a) percentage GSH adduct formation and (b) estimated total daily covalent adduct burden in "drug-induced toxicity" (DIT, Δ) and non-drug-induced toxicity (non-DIT, ○) groups of chemicals.[62] Horizontal lines are drawn at (a) the 0.2% adduct level and (b) the 1 mg body level.

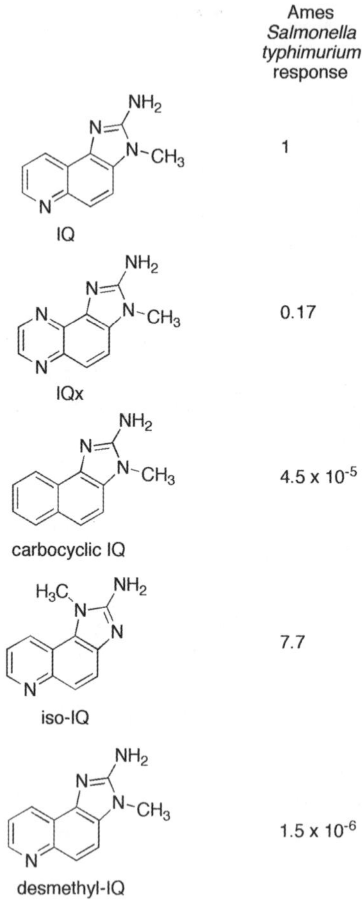


**Figure 21.6** Variation in frameshift mutagenicity among a series of heterocyclic amines.[71] See also Christov *et al.*[72]

basis of previous findings, *i.e.*, a mathematical approach to chemistry (*e.g.*, SPORCALC). Combinations of these approaches are also utilized.[73] At least in some sets of molecules, these programs can select the major site of oxidation $\sim \frac{1}{2}$ of the time. If prediction is extended to three sites on a molecule, the probability that one of these will be a major site rises to as high as 87% approaching the level reported for experienced drug metabolism scientists. Of course, the predictability increases dramatically if information is available about other molecules in the same class of compounds.

With the crystallization of human P450 enzymes and the production of structures, hope developed for routine prediction of P450-dependent metabolism. Indeed, today structures of all the major "drug-metabolizing" P450s are available (*i.e.*, 1A2, 2C9, 2C19, 2D6, 3A4, as well as 1B1, 2A6, 2B6, 2C8, and several involved in steroid oxidations). There are three major reasons why

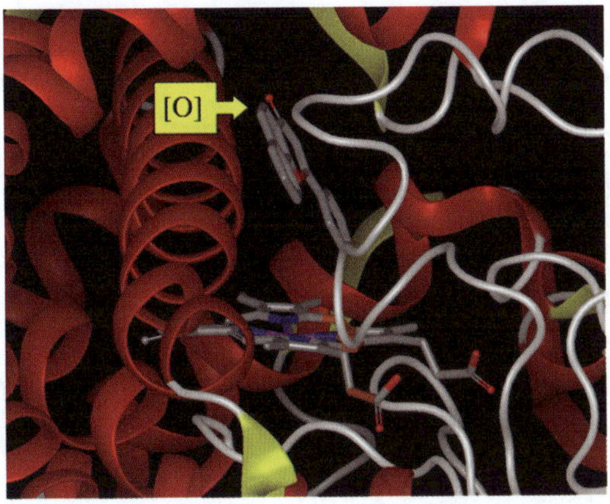


**Figure 21.7** Crystal structure of human P450 1A2 with β-naphthoflavone (β-NF) bound.[76] The arrow shows the only site of oxidation of β-NF by the enzyme,[77,78] which is the furthest from the iron atom.

predicting docking of unknown substrates is still difficult: i) the larger P450s have a considerable amount of space in what is considered the active site. For instance, the estimated size (1385 $\mathring{A}^3$) in P450 3A4 is *ca.* seven times larger than that in P450 2E1.[74,75] Accurately fitting ligands in that much space is problematic, and P450 3A4 is a major player in drug metabolism, in terms of the number of drugs it can be involved with. ii) even when crystal structures of P450–substrate complexes are available, they may not be instructive regarding sites of oxidation. For instance, in the P450 1A2β-naphthoflavone structure[76] (Figure 21.7) the only known site of oxidation of β-naphthoflavone[77,78] is the one most distant from the heme iron atom, indicating that this is not a productive conformation. iii) Another issue is the induced-fit nature of P450s. That is, some P450s adopt different shapes depending on which substrate is bound. This behavior is demonstrated in the P450 3A4 structures of Ekroos and Sjogren.[79] One conformation was determined in the presence of the substrate erythromycin; another structure was solved with two molecules of ketoconazole in the active site and significant changes in the protein structure (Figure 21.8).

Thus, some P450s are capable of undergoing some adjustments in their structures to accommodate a variety of substrates. Johnson[76] has noted that in the more rigid P450s the active site lies along the I-helix but that this is not the case in the more flexible P450s. This flexibility introduces a problem in docking and modeling new (potential) substrates. The question is which structures should be used to begin the modeling. In the author's opinion, ultimately there will be a finite number of major structural motifs of ligand binding to these flexible P450s, and molecular dynamics simulations may be helpful in driving predictions (among these) for future candidates.

Another challenge is prediction of rates of metabolism, specifically with P450s, even if sites of attack can be identified. Such prediction may be possible

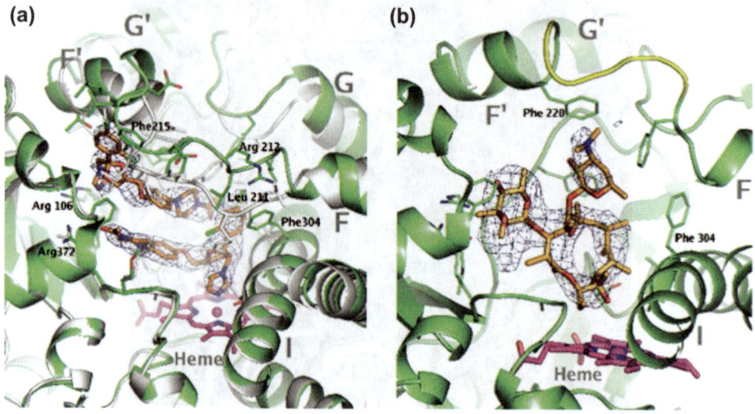


Ketoconazole Erythromycin

**Figure 21.8** Multiple modes of interaction of P450 3A4 with ligands.

with some substrates, *e.g.*, in electrophilic substitution reactions using Hammett plots,[80] if steric constriction is not an issue. The problem is one related to which steps in the enzyme catalytic cycle are rate-limiting. For instance, if steps involved in the activation of oxygen are rate-limiting, then rates of oxygenation of a series of substrates may be invariant.

The characterization of metabolites has become more facile with time but is still not a high- (or even medium-) throughput operation. Virtual suggestions about products will never really replace this process, and the experimental work will be required, even if predictions help restrict the choices. However, experimental screening of rates of disappearance of a drug (in liver microsomes) is routinely used as an experimental method of predicting the half-life and clearance of drugs *in vivo*.

## 21.4 Problems in Extrapolation From *In Vitro* to *In Vivo* Settings in Metabolism and Toxicity

A major goal of *in vitro* work is to predict what could and also what will happen *in vivo*. *In vitro* experiments have two major advantages: i) the cost and time involved are considerably less and ii) mechanistic information results.

The field of drug metabolism has benefited enormously from *in vitro* investigations over the past 30 years. Today we understand the roles that enzymes (including many transporters) play in drug disposition and can explain many *in vivo* clinical phenomena, *e.g.*, grapefruit effects on P450 3A4 and possibly transporters.[81] *In vitro* predictions, however, often fall short in that they predict what can happen but may be quantitatively flawed. For instance, a P450 reaction may be demonstrated *in vitro* but is irrelevant *in vivo* because the substrate is processed by another pathway not represented in the *in vitro* setting. Many efforts have been made to improve the quantitative *in vivo* prediction of drug metabolism, including physiologically based pharmacokinetic modeling. Commercial software systems are available (*e.g.*, SimCyp®) (http://www.simcyp.com/).[82] For instance, if blood flow is not rate-limiting in the clearance of a drug, then intrinsic hepatic clearance ($Cl_H$) can be predicted from *in vitro* $V_{max}/K_m$ ratios, at least to a first approximation.

In general, toxicity is much more difficult to extrapolate than metabolism from *in vitro* settings to *in vivo*. All pharmaceutical industry scientists would favor more *in vitro* work, if possible, in that the differential in resources (cost, time) between *in vitro* and *in vivo* is even greater for drug toxicology than metabolism (Figure 21.9).[21]

Thus, many toxicology studies are done in cell-culture systems. One successful approach is the bacterial "Ames test" for genotoxicity. Even though there are false negatives and positives, the system eliminates most genotoxic chemicals. However, there are also many limitations of *in vitro* mammalian cellular systems, and one can question the general dependence of the scientific community on results obtained in cell culture. In some cases the most relevant cells in a tissue may not be represented in the *in vitro* system, or the *in vivo* phenomena may require the interaction of multiple cell types (*e.g.*, kuppffer cells, neutrophils, monocytes, and lymphocytes interacting with hepatocytes in

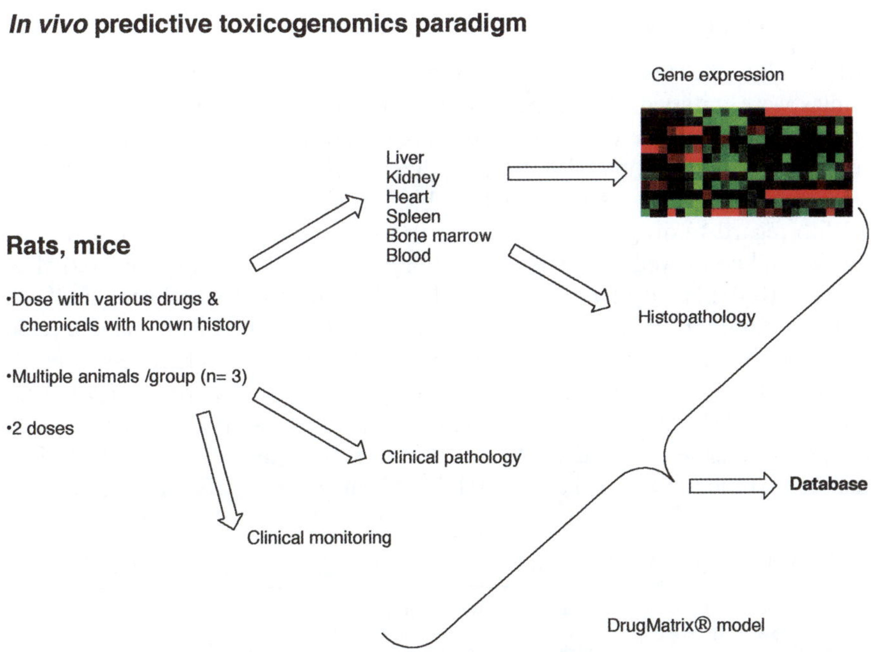


**Figure 21.9** An *in vivo* predictive toxicogenomics paradigm for database development. The model shown here is the DrugMatrix® system developed by Iconix (now part of Entelos).[21]

the liver).[83] In some more complex situations, it is sobering to realize that the toxicity of 2,3,7,8-tetrachloro-*p*-dibenzodioxin (TCDD) has still not been reproduced *in vitro*. Another issue is that cells are prone to de-differentiate in culture and may not reflect their *in vivo* character, *e.g.*, hepatocytes, with regard to some activities. The situation is worse when considering long-term cell culture lines, especially those derived from tumors, *e.g.*, HeLa cells, which have multiple characteristics in different laboratories now. The concern is that some pathways may be altered, simply because the "normal" cells are not adapted to life in culture, and a fine analysis of transcriptomnomics or proteomics may indicate pathway differences irrelevant to *in vivo* situations.

A related example of the disocrdance that can occur between *in vitro* and *in vivo* transcriptomnomics involves a report of Hu *et al.*,[84] in which 59% of the 139 compounds examined induced (rat) P450 1A1 *in vivo* but not *in vitro*.

Nevertheless, there is political pressure in the EU and US to do more *in vitro* testing of chemicals (*e.g.*, REACH, National Toxicology Program), although not necessarily drug candidates, and there is hope that improvements in the methods will develop.[85] Perhaps the biggest challenge is using *in vitro* methods to select against drugs that will show idiosyncratic toxicities (Tables 21.3 and 21.4).

## 21.5 Problems with Extrapolations from Animals to Humans

Historically extensive work was done with animals *in vivo* and then clinical studies were initiated. These studies are still important in predicting toxicity prior to first-in-man research and will probably always continue to be needed to predict clinical problems. However, neither metabolism nor toxicology results can always be directly extrapolated (Table 21.8).

With regard to drug metabolism, the P450s in animals and humans are not always well conserved, and some of the differences have been considered elsewhere.[86] Rodents are particularly notorious for showing unusual gender effects that are minimal in humans. For instance, rat P450 2C11 is a male-specific enzyme only seen during and after puberty and P450 2C12 is female-specific.[87] These and other P450s can provide unusual problems in pre-clinical drug development. Further, even when P450s are relatively well-conserved between species, a considerable difference may exist in structure and properties. For instance, as mentioned earlier, the P450 1A2 enzymes in rats and humans are

**Table 21.8** Applying mechanisms of toxicity to human safety.[21]

| |
|---|
| What is toxic? [parent drug or metabolite(s)] |
| How is it toxic? |
| What is the dose-response relationship? |
| Does toxicity occur in humans? |
| Can a screen be developed to assess the liability? |
| Can the liability be eliminated? |

**Table 21.9** Rodent carcinogenic responses not likely to apply to humans.

| *Tumor site* | *Illustrative chemical agents* |
|---|---|
| Male rat kidney | *d*-Limonene, unleaded gasoline |
| Male bladder | Saccharin, nitrilotriacetic acid |
| Rat thyroid | Goitrogens, some alkylcarbamates, fungicides |
| Forestomach | Butylated hydroxyanisole, propionic acid, ethyl acrylate |
| Mouse liver | Barbiturates, peroxisome proliferators |

$\sim$ 70% identical (primary sequence) and have nearly identical catalytic activity towards the model substrate 7-ethoxyresorufin. However, human P450 1A2 has *ca.* 10-fold more activity than rat P450 1A2 in the *N*-hydroxylation (activation) of the heterocyclic amines MeIQx and PhIP.[70] These differences can have serious implications in considering the interpretation of rat cancer bioassays and their relevance to humans.

Toxicity is even more complicated regarding extrapolation from animal models to humans. A list of animal toxicities now generally regarded to be rather irrelevant to humans is presented in Table 21.9.

Knowledge of the metabolic differences between animal models and humans is useful in understanding differential toxicity. For instance, a gender-specific P450 may produce a metabolite that will only yield a response in one gender of rats.

A further complication is the variation among humans, and there have been efforts to consider the variability in making predictions.[88–90] Thus, it is not enough to only consider extrapolation (*e.g.*, with physiologically-based pharmacokinetic models) of animal data to humans but there is a need to consider the range of the relevant human population.

Another issue is human toxicity problems where animal models are not known. Some classic examples are arsenic- and benzene-related cancers. Thalidomide is often considered in this group, although the teratogenicity is seen in rabbits (but not rats, the original test species). In practice, some would expect to see human problems during clinical trials and then re-evaluate the spectrum of test species used, with the goal of being able to understand the problem and improve the selection in screening for new candidates. One issue here is so-called "human-specific" metabolites (the "MIST" issue).[91] When a certain metabolite is observed at a level of >10% (of all metabolites) only in humans then the guidance (FDA and International Conference on Harmonisation) is to synthesize the metabolites and utilize them in separate animal tests.

## 21.6 The Issue of Dose in Experimental Studies and Applications

One of the complexities in predictions is the dose. An axiom of toxicology is that "the dose makes the poison," going back to Paracelsus.[1] An inherent problem in making predictions is extrapolating to the situation where a certain dose is used in humans, whether *in silico*, *in vitro*, or animal models. One issue is that the projected human dose may not even be estimated early in discover/development. *In vitro* results can be used to make quantitative predictions about *in vivo* human metabolism. Toxicity is more problematic but can be done qualitatively.

## 21.7 Conclusions

Predicting the toxicity of new drug candidates is still very difficult, but is a worthy goal in that even some progress can result in major savings and in improvements in the compounds that reach the market. Predictions are fraught with problems due to the nature of the system. Metabolism is responsible for at least a sizeable fraction of toxicity problems (Table 21.2) and some predictions can be made, with rapid *in vitro* screening being the most widely applied approach. Predicting toxicity is more difficult, and SAR approaches are still limited by our limited understanding of the complex systems involved (Figure 21.1). Earlier (25 years ago) there was a general view in the field that a single "master switch" for toxicity might be identified, but today most scientists in the field would probably agree that there are multiple routes to apoptosis and necrosis (Figure 21.1). Covalent binding data can be of some utility (Figures 21.2–21.5). Some successes in early prediction of potential toxicity have been realized with several approaches, including genomics,[92] transcription profiling,[93–96] and proteomics.[97–101] The next several years should be revealing in terms of how rapid further progress in the area will be, particularly in the context of clinical validation.

## Acknowledgements

Relevant research in the author's laboratory is supported by United States Public Health Service grants R37 CA090426, R01 ES010546, and P30 ES000267. Thanks are extended to K. Trisler for assistance in preparation of the chapter.

## References

1. J. F. Borzelleca, *Toxicol. Sci.*, 2000, **53**, 2.
2. F. P. Guengerich in Biotransformation, *Comprehensive Toxicology*, ed. C. A. McQueen, Elsevier, Oxford, 2nd edn, 2010, vol. 4, p. 1.
3. E. C. Miller and J. A. Miller, *Cancer Res.*, 1947, **7**, 468.
4. J. A. Miller, *Cancer Res.*, 1970, **30**, 559.
5. G. C. Mueller and J. A. Miller, *J. Biol. Chem.*, 1948, **176**, 535.
6. R. T. Williams, *Detoxication Mechanisms*, Wiley, New York, 1947.
7. R. T. Williams, *Detoxication Mechanisms*, Wiley, New York, 2nd edn, 1959.
8. B. B. Brodie, J. R. Gillette and B. N. LaDu, *Annu. Rev. Biochem.*, 1958, **27**, 427.

9. D. J. Jollow, J. R. Mitchell, W. Z. Potter, D. C. Davis, J. R. Gillette and B. B. Brodie, *J. Pharmacol. Exp. Ther.*, 1973, **187**, 195.
10. J. R. Mitchell, D. J. Jollow, W. Z. Potter, D. C. Davis, J. R. Gillette and B. B. Brodie, *J. Pharmacol. Exp. Ther.*, 1973, **187**, 185.
11. W. Z. Potter, D. C. Davis, J. R. Mitchell, D. J. Jollow, J. R. Gillette and B. B. Brodie, *J. Pharmacol. Exp. Ther.*, 1973, **187**, 203.
12. J. R. Mitchell, D. J. Jollow, W. Z. Potter, J. R. Gillette and B. B. Brodie, *J. Pharmacol. Exp. Ther.*, 1973, **187**, 211.
13. B. N. Ames, W. E. Durston, E. Yamasaki and F. D. Lee, *Proc. Natl. Acad. Sci. U. S. A.*, 1973, **70**, 2281.
14. F. P. Guengerich, *in Cytochrome P450: Structure, Mechanism, and Biochemistry*, ed. P. R. Ortiz de Montellano, Plenum Press, New York, 3rd edn, 2005, p. 377.
15. N. Zampaglione, D. J. Jollow, J. R. Mitchell, B. Stripp, M. Hamrick and J. R. Gillette, *J. Pharmacol. Exp. Ther.*, 1973, **187**, 218.
16. R. R. Shah, N. S. Oates, J. R. Idle, R. L. Smith and J. D. F. Lockhart, *Brit. Med. J.*, 1982, **284**, 295.
17. D. C. Liebler and F. P. Guengerich, *Nat. Rev. Drug Discovery*, 2005, **4**, 410.
18. D. P. Zipes, N. J. Zvaifler, R. J. Glassock, S. Gilman, A. Munoz, V. Gogolak, L. Gordis, P. C. Dedon, F. P. Guengerich, S. I. Wasserman, J. L. Witztum and G. N. Wogan, *MedGenMed*, 2006, **8**, 73.
19. C.-H. Yun, R. A. Okerholm and F. P. Guengerich, *Drug Metab. Dispos.*, 1993, **21**, 403.
20. P. K. Honig, D. C. Wortham, K. Zamani, D. P. Conner, J. C. Mullin and L. R. Cantilena, *JAMA, J. Am. Med. Assoc.*, 1993, **269**, 1513.
21. F. P. Guengerich and J. S. MacDonald, *Chem. Res. Toxicol.*, 2007, **20**, 344.
22. M. Valko, C. J. Rhodes, J. Moncol, M. Izakovic and M. Mazur, *Chem.–Biol. Interact.*, 2006, **160**, 1.
23. B. Halliwell, *Biochem. Soc. Trans.*, 2007, **35**, 1147.
24. U. A. Boelsterli and P. L. Lim, *Toxicol. Appl. Pharmacol.*, 2007, **220**, 92.
25. D. P. Jones, J. J. Lemasters, D. Han, U. A. Boelsterli and N. Kaplowitz, *Mol. Interv.*, 2010, **10**, 98.
26. Y. H. Lee, M. C. Chung, Q. Lin and U. A. Boelsterli, *Toxicol. Appl. Pharmacol.*, 2008, **231**, 43.
27. S. Bansal, C.-P. Liu, N. B. V. Sepuri, H. K. Anandatheerthavarada, F. P. Guengerich and N. G. Avadhani, *J. Biol. Chem.*, 2010, **285**, 24609.
28. I. Kola and J. Landis, *Nat. Rev. Drug Discovery*, 2004, **3**, 711.
29. J. P. Uetrecht, *Chem. Res. Toxicol.*, 1999, **12**, 387.
30. J. M. Shenton, J. Chen and J. P. Uetrecht, *Chem.–Biol. Interact.*, 2004, **150**, 53.
31. J. Uetrecht, *Chem. Res. Toxicol.*, 2008, **21**, 84.
32. J. P. Uetrecht, *Curr. Drug Metab.*, 2000, **2**, 133.
33. J. Uetrecht, *Chem. Res. Toxicol.*, 2009, **22**, 24.
34. F. P. Guengerich, *Drug Metab. Pharmacokin.*, 2011, **26**, 3.

35. J. R. Gillette, *Bichem. Pharmacol.*, 1974, **23**, 2785.
36. J. L. Walgren, M. D. Mitchell and D. C. Thompson, *Crit. Rev. Toxicol.*, 2005, **35**, 325.
37. S. D. Nelson, J. R. Mitchell, J. A. Timbrell, W. R. Snodgrass and G. B. Corcoran III, *Science*, 1976, **193**, 901.
38. A. Bradbury, G. M. Powell, C. G. Curtis and C. Rhodes, *Xenobiotica*, 1981, **11**, 665.
39. B. H. Mathison, S. E. Murphy and R. C. Shank, *Toxicol. Appl. Pharmacol.*, 1994, **127**, 91.
40. P. M. Dansette, E. Bonierbale, C. Minoletti, P. H. Beaune, D. Pessayre and D. Mansuy, *Eur. J. Drug Metab. Pharmacokinet.*, 1998, **23**, 443.
41. Y. Qiu, A. L. Burlingame and L. Z. Benet, *Drug Metab. Dispos.*, 1998, **26**, 246.
42. R. S. Obach and D. K. Dalvie, *Drug Metab. Dispos.*, 2006, **34**, 1310.
43. K. Kassahun, P. G. Pearson, W. Tang, I. McIntosh, K. Leung, C. Elmore, D. Dean, R. Wang, G. Doss and T. A. Baillie, *Chem. Res. Toxicol.*, 2001, **14**, 62.
44. A. S. Kalgutkar, I. Gardner, R. S. Obach, C. L. Shaffer, E. Callegari, K. R. Henne, A. E. Mutlib, D. K. Dalvie, J. S. Lee, Y. Nakai, J. P. O'Donnell, J. Boer and S. P. Harriman, *Curr. Drug Metab.*, 2005, **6**, 161.
45. A. Durand, J. P. Thenot, G. Bianchetti and P. L. Morselli, *Drug Metab. Rev.*, 1992, **24**, 239.
46. J. Geneve, D. Larrey, P. Letteron, V. Descatoire, M. Tinel, G. Amouyal and D. Pessayre, *Biochem. Pharmacol.*, 1987, **36**, 323.
47. M. Castillo and P. C. Smith, *Drug Metab. Dispos.*, 1995, **23**, 566.
48. C. Martinat, C. Amar, P. M. Dansette, J. Leclaire, P. Lopez-Garcia, T. D. Cao, H. N. N'Guyen and D. Mansuy, *Eur. J. Pharmacol.*, 1992, **228**, 63.
49. J. M. Reid, M. J. Kuffel, J. K. Miller, R. Rios and M. M. Ames, *Clin. Cancer Res.*, 1999, **5**, 2192.
50. T. H. Arnold Jr., J. M. Epps, III, H. R. Cook and M. E. Hamrick, *Res. Commun. Chem. Pathol. Pharmacol.*, 1983, **39**, 381.
51. C. M. Dieckhaus, W. L. Santos, R. D. Sofia and T. L. Macdonald, *Chem. Res. Toxicol.*, 2001, **14**, 958.
52. A. Berson, C. Wolf, C. Chachaty, C. Fisch, D. Fau, D. Eugene, J. Loeper, J. C. Gauthier, P. Beaune, D. Pompon, P. Maurel and D. Pessayre, *J. Pharmacol. Exp. Ther.*, 1993, **265**, 366.
53. A. D. Cohen, S. M. Luger, C. Sickles, P. A. Mangan, D. L. Porter, S. J. Schuster, D. E. Tsai, S. Nasta, A. M. Gewirtz and E. A. Stadtmauer, *Bone Marrow Transplant.*, 2002, **30**, 23.
54. J. A. Timbrell, J. R. Mitchell, W. R. Snodgrass and S. D. Nelson, *J. Pharmacol. Exp. Ther.*, 1980, **213**, 364.
55. R. J. Rodriguez and D. Acosta Jr, *Toxicology*, 1997, **117**, 123.
56. K. S. Smith, P. L. Smith, T. N. Heady, J. M. Trugman, W. D. Harman and T. L. Macdonald, *Chem. Res. Toxicol.*, 2003, **16**, 123.
57. T. A. Baillie, *Chem. Res. Toxicol.*, 1988, **1**, 195.
58. D. C. Evans, A. P. Watt, D. A. Nicoll-Griffith and T. A. Baillie, *Chem. Res. Toxicol.*, 2004, **17**, 3.

59. N. Masubuchi, C. Makino and N. Murayama, *Chem. Res. Toxicol.*, 2007, **20**, 455.
60. R. S. Obach, A. S. Kalgutkar, J. R. Soglia and S. X. Zhao, *Chem. Res. Toxicol.*, 2008, **21**, 1814.
61. J. N. Bauman, J. M. Kelly, S. Tripathy, S. X. Zhao, W. W. Lam, A. S. Kalgutkar and R. S. Obach, *Chem. Res. Toxicol.*, 2009, **22**, 332.
62. J. Gan, Q. Ruan, B. He, M. Zhu, W. C. Shyu and W. G. Humphreys, *Chem. Res. Toxicol.*, 2009, **22**, 690.
63. D. M. Sanderson and C. G. Earnshaw, *Hum. Exp. Toxicol.*, 1991, **10**, 261.
64. N. Greene, P. N. Judson, J. J. Langowski and C. A. Marchant, *SAR QSAR Environ. Res.*, 1999, **10**, 299.
65. J. C. Dearden, *J. Comput. Aided Mol. Design*, 2003, **17**, 119.
66. L. G. Valerio Jr, *Toxicol. Appl. Pharmacol.*, 2009, **241**, 356.
67. N. Greene, L. Fisk, R. T. Naven, R. R. Note, M. L. Patel and D. J. Pelletier, *Chem. Res. Toxicol.*, 2010, **23**, 1215.
68. R. D. Combes, *Arch. Toxicol.*, 2010, **84**, 333.
69. Anonymous, *Drug Discovery Develop.*, 2010, 29.
70. R. J. Turesky, A. Constable, J. Richoz, N. Vargu, J. Markovic, M. V. Martin and F. P. Guengerich, *Chem. Res. Toxicol.*, 1998, **11**, 925.
71. G. Kaiser, D. Harnasch, M. T. King and D. Wild, *Chem.–Biol. Interact.*, 1986, **57**, 97.
72. P. P. Christov, G. Chowdhury, C. A. Garmendia, F. Wang, J. S. Stover, C. E. Elmquist, P. Christov, A. Kozekova, K. C. Angel, R. J. Turesky, F. P. Guengerich, M. P. Stone and C. J. Rizzo, *Chem. Res. Toxicol.*, 2010, **23**, 1076.
73. L. Afzelius, C. H. Arnby, A. Broo, L. Carlsson, C. Isaksson, U. Jurva, B. Kjellander, K. Kolmodin, K. Nilsson, F. Raubacher and L. Weidolf, *Drug Metab. Rev.*, 2007, **39**, 61.
74. J. K. Yano, M. R. Wester, G. A. Schoch, K. J. Griffin, C. D. Stout and E. F. Johnson, *J. Biol. Chem.*, 2004, **279**, 38091.
75. P. R. Porubsky, K. M. Meneely and E. E. Scott, *J. Biol. Chem.* 2008, **283**, 33698.
76. S. Sansen, J. K. Yano, R. L. Reynald, G. A. Schoch, K. J. Griffin, C. D. Stout and E. F. Johnson, *J. Biol. Chem.*, 2007, **282**, 14348.
77. E. Bauer, Z. Guo, Y.-F. Ueng, L. C. Bell and F. P. Guengerich, *Chem. Res. Toxicol.*, 1995, **8**, 136.
78. C. D. Sohl, E. M. Isin, R. L. Eoff, G. A. Marsch, D. F. Stec and F. P. Guengerich, *J. Biol. Chem.*, 2008, **283**, 7293.
79. M. Ekroos and T. Sjogren, *Proc. Natl. Acad. Sci. U. S. A.*, 2006, **103**, 13682.
80. L. T. Burka, F. P. Guengerich, R. J. Willard and T. L. Macdonald, *J. Am. Chem. Soc.*, 1985, **107**, 2549.
81. D. G. Bailey, G. K. Dresser and J. R. Bend, *Clin. Pharmacol. Ther.*, 2003, **73**, 529.
82. N. J. Proctor, G. T. Tucker and A. Rostami-Hodjegan, *Xenobiotica*, 2004, **34**, 151.

83. D. H. Adams, C. Ju, S. K. Ramaiah, J. Uetrecht and H. Jaeschke, *Toxicol. Sci.*, 2010, **115**, 307.
84. W. Hu, C. Sorrentino, M. S. Denison, K. Kolaja and M. R. Fielden, *Mol. Pharmacol.,* 2007, **71**, 1475.
85. T. A. Moeller, *Drug Discovery Develop.*, 2010, **13**, 10.
86. F. P. Guengerich, *Chem.–Biol. Interact.*, 1997, **106**, 161.
87. D. J. Waxman, G. A. Dannan and F. P. Guengerich, *Biochemistry*, 1985, **24**, 4409.
88. J. L. Dorne, K. Walton, W. Slob and A. G. Renwick, *Food Chem. Toxicol.*, 2002, **40**, 1633.
89. J. L. Dorne, K. Walton and A. G. Renwick, *Food Chem. Toxicol.*, 2003, **41**, 201.
90. J. L. Dorne, *Toxicology*, 2010, **268**, 156.
91. F. P. Guengerich, *Chem. Res. Toxicol.*, 2009, **22**, 237.
92. A. Kindmark, A. Jawaid, C. G. Harbron, B. J. Barratt, O. F. Bengtsson, T. B. Andersson, S. Carlsson, K. E. Cederbrant, N. J. Gibson, M. Armstrong, M. E. Lagerstrom-Fermer, A. Dellsen, E. M. Brown, M. Thornton, C. Dukes, S. C. Jenkins, M. A. Firth, G. O. Harrod, T. H. Pinel, S. M. Billing-Clason, L. R. Cardon and R. E. March, *Pharmacogenom. J.*, 2008, **8**, 186.
93. J. W. Davis and J. A. Kramer, *Expert Opin. Drug Metab. Toxicol.*, 2006, **2**, 95.
94. B. Ganter, R. D. Snyder, D. N. Halbert and M. D. Lee, *Pharmacogenomics*, 2006, **7**, 1025.
95. T. P. Ryan, J. L. Stevens and C. E. Thomas, *Curr. Opin. Pharmacol.*, 2008, **8**, 654.
96. J. L. Smalley, T. W. Gant and S. D. Zhang, *Toxicology*, 2010, **268**, 143.
97. D. E. Amacher, *Toxicol. Appl. Pharmacol.*, 2010, **245**, 134.
98. F. Dieterle, E. Perentes, A. Cordier, D. R. Roth, P. Verdes, O. Grenet, S. Pantano, P. Moulin, D. Wahl, A. Mahl, P. End, F. Staedtler, F. Legay, K. Carl, D. Laurie, S. D. Chibout, J. Vonderscher and G. Maurer, *Nat. Biotechnol.*, 2010, **28**, 463.
99. Y. Yu, H. Jin, D. Holder, J. S. Ozer, S. Villarreal, P. Shughrue, S. Shi, D. J. Figueroa, H. Clouse, M. Su, N. Muniappa, S. P. Troth, W. Bailey, J. Seng, A. G. Aslamkhan, D. Thudium, F. D. Sistare and D. L. Gerhold, *Nat. Biotechnol.*, 2010, **28**, 470.
100. V. S. Vaidya, J. S. Ozer, F. Dieterle, F. B. Collings, V. Ramirez, S. Troth, N. Muniappa, D. Thudium, D. Gerhold, D. J. Holder, N. A. Bobadilla, E. Marrer, E. Perentes, A. Cordier, J. Vonderscher, G. Maurer, P. L. Goering, F. D. Sistare and J. V. Bonventre, *Nat. Biotechnol.*, 2010, **28**, 478.
101. J. S. Ozer, F. Dieterle, S. Troth, E. Perentes, A. Cordier, P. Verdes, F. Staedtler, A. Mahl, O. Grenet, D. R. Roth, D. Wahl, F. Legay, D. Holder, Z. Erdos, K. Vlasakova, H. Jin, Y. Yu, N. Muniappa, T. Forest, H. K. Clouse, S. Reynolds, W. J. Bailey, D. T. Thudium, M. J. Topper, T. R. Skopek, J. F. Sina, W. E. Glaab, J. Vonderscher, G. Maurer, S. D. Chibout, F. D. Sistare and D. L. Gerhold, *Nat. Biotechnol.*, 2010, **28**, 486.

CHAPTER 22

# Impact of Drug Transporters in the Pharmacological and Adverse Reactions of Drugs

HIROYUKI KUSUHARA, KAZUYA MAEDA AND YUICHI SUGIYAMA*

The University of Tokyo, Laboratory of Molecular Pharmacokinetics, Graduate School of Pharmaceutical Sciences, 7-3-1 Hongo, Bunkyo-ku, Tokyo 113-0033, Japan

## 22.1 Introduction

Transporters are membrane proteins mediating influx or efflux of compounds and ions across the lipid membranes. Transporter-mediated membrane transport is characterized by its saturation; whereby its velocity increases along with the substrate concentration at low concentration, but finally reaches a constant value (maximum transport velocity, $V_{max}$). The velocity ($v$) and concentration ($C$) curve follows the Michaelis–Menten equation [eqn (22.1)].

$$v_0 = \frac{V_{max}(C)}{K_m + (C)} \tag{22.1}$$

where $K_m$ represents the Michaelis constant. This assumes the presence of domain-accepting compounds and ions as substrates in the transporter molecule.

Transporters are now classified into two large groups; the solute-carrier (SLC) family and the ATP-binding cassette (ABC) proteins. SLC-type

RSC Drug Discovery Series No. 12
New Horizons in Predictive Toxicology: Current Status and Application
Edited by Alan G. E. Wilson

Published by the Royal Society of Chemistry, www.rsc.org

transporters mediate facilitated diffusion and active transport. Facilitated diffusion is the type of membrane transport which occurs down the electrochemical potential of the substrate drugs, whereas active transport couples with the synport or antiport of ions or other compounds, to drive the transport against the gradient of the electrochemical potential of the substrate drugs. Members of the SLC transporter family are characterized by their bidirectional transport which depends on the gradient of the substrate and the driving force. It is now comprised of 51 sub-families into which 378 genes are classified based on their sequence similarities (http://www.bioparadigms.org/, SLC tables). ABC transporters are characterized by their cytosolic domain which catalyses ATP hydrolysis since the domain is highly conserved across the species. ABC transporters mediate the unidirectional efflux coupled to ATP hydrolysis. They are now classified into seven sub-families (ABCA–ABCG) (special issue (5), 2007 is available in Pflugers Arch).

Some transporters show broad substrate specificity, accepting structurally unrelated compounds as their substrates. Such transporters play key roles in determining the exposure of substrate drugs and toxins to the target molecules, and thereby, modifying their effects. It is well known that the over-expression of ABC transporters, such as P-glycoprotein, MRPs and BCRP confer resistance to anticancer drugs,[1–5] and that the overexpression of MRP4 confers resistance to antivirus drugs[6] by actively extruding the drugs outside the cells. In contrast over-expression of the uptake transporters enhances the accumulation of compounds inside the cells, and consequently sensitizes the cells to the drugs; *e.g.*, OAT1-adefovir,[7] OCT1-metformin,[8] OCT2-platinum agents,[9,10] OCTN1-mitoxantrone and doxorubicin,[11] and OATP1B3-methotrexate.[12] These transporters play pivotal roles as detoxification systems in the body; elimination from the systemic circulation in the liver and kidney, the distribution of drugs to their target organs (*e.g.*, the brain), and oral absorption in the small intestine.[13,14] These transporters include OATPs/*SLCO*, OATs/*SLC22* and OCTs/*SLC22* in the influx process, and P-glycoprotein (P-gp) MDR1/*ABCB1*, BCRP/*ABCG2*, MRPs/ABCC and MATEs/*SLC47* in the efflux process (Table 22.1). Variations in the activities of these transporters, caused by genetic polymorphisms and concomitant drugs, affect the drug exposure, and consequently the pharmacological effects and adverse reactions. Drug transporter-related adverse reactions are classified into three cases based on the mechanism; 1) transporters function in the clearance organs, and intestine so that variation in the transporter activities alter the systemic exposure and thereby, pharmacological action in the target organs, 2) transporters are the determinant of local drug concentrations in non-clearance organs, 3) substrates of the drug transporters include the endogenous one, and disturbance of the drug transporters causes accumulation of such endogenous substrates (Figure 22.1).[14] This chapter describes the drug transporters playing important roles in the systemic elimination, and active barrier at the blood–brain barrier (BBB).

**Table 22.1** Transporters responsible for drug disposition.

| Transporter | Gene name | Alias | OMIM | Tissue distribution | Localization | Substrates | Driving force |
|---|---|---|---|---|---|---|---|
| *Solute-carrier (SLC) family (facilitated transport or secondary active transporters)* | | | | | | | |
| NPT1 | *SLC17A1* | *NaPi-1* | 182308 | Kidney, | ND | *p*-Aminohippurate, benzylpenicillin | Facilitated diffusion |
| NPT4 | *SLC17A3* | — | 611034 | Kidney, | Kidney: BBM | Bumetanide, estrone-sulfate, uric acid | Facilitated diffusion |
| OATP1B1 | *SLCO1B2* | *LST-1 OATP-C OATP2* | 604843 | Liver, | Liver: SM | HMG-CoA Reductase inhibitors (atorvastatin, pravastatin, pitavastatin, rosuvastatain, cerivastatin), angiotensin II receptor antagonist (olmesartan, valsartan), antidiabetic (repaglinidine, nateglinide), bosentan | Active transporter |
| OATP1B3 | *SLCO1B3* | *LST-2 OATP8* | 605495 | Liver, | Liver: SM | CCK-8, angiotensin II receptor antagonist (olmesartan, valsartan, telmisartan), fexofenadine, bosentan | |
| OATP4C1 | *SLCO4C1* | — | 609013 | Kidney, | Kidney: BLM | Digoxin | ND |
| OCT1 | *SLC22A1* | — | 602607 | Liver, | Liver: SM | Tetraethylammonium, metformin, H2 receptor antagonists (cimetidine, ranitidine, famotidine) | Facilitated diffusion |
| OCT2 | *SLC22A2* | — | 602608 | Kidney, | Kidney: BLM | | |
| OCTN1 | *SLC22A4* | — | 604190 | Ubiquitous | ND | Quinidine, verapamil, ergothioneine | $H^+$ antiport (OC) |
| OCTN2 | *SLC22A5* | — | 603377 | Kidney, skeletal muscle | Kidney: BBM(?) | Carnitine | $H^+$ antiport (OC) $Na^+$ symport (carnitine) |
| OAT1 | *SLC22A6* | — | 607582 | Kidney, | Kidney: BLM | *p*-Aminohippurate, 2,4-dichlorophenoxyacetate, diuretics (furosemide, bendroflumethiazide), antiviral drugs (adefovir, tenofovir) | Dicarboxylate antiport |
| OAT2 | *SLC22A7* | — | 604995 | Liver, kidney | Kidney: BLM | cGMP, cAMP, methotrexate, azidothymidine, α-ketoglutarate | ND |
| OAT3 | *SLC22A8* | — | 607581 | Kidney | Kidney: BLM BBB: ALM | *p*-Aminohippurate, 2,4-dichlorophenoxyacetate, diuretics (furosemide, bendroflumethiazide), HMG-CoA reductase inhibitor (pravastatin), angiotensin II receptor antagonist (olmesartan), H2 receptor antagonists (cimetidine, ranitidine, famotidine) | Dicarboxylate antiport |

**Table 22.1** *(Continued)*

| *Transporter* | *Gene name* | *Alias* | *OMIM* | *Tissue distribution* | *Localization* | *Substrates* | *Driving force* |
|---|---|---|---|---|---|---|---|
| *Solute-carrier (SLC) family (facilitated transport or secondary active transporters)* | | | | | | | |
| OAT4 | *SLC22A11* | — | 607097 | Placenta, kidney | Kidney: BBM | DHEAS, estrone-3-sulfate, uric acid | ND |
| URAT1 | *SLC22A12* | *RST* | 607096 | Kidney | Kidney: BBM | Uric acid | Facilitated diffusion |
| MATE1 | *SLC47A1* | — | 609832 | Liver, kidney, skeletal muscle | Liver: CM kidney: BBM | Tetraethylammonium, metformin, cimetidine, creatinine, procainamide, fluoroquinolones | $H^+$ antiport (OC) |
| MATE2-K | *SLC47A2* | — | 609833 | Kidney, | Kidney: LM | | |
| *ABC transporters (primary active transport)* | | | | | | | |
| P-gp | *ABCB1* | *MDR1* | 171050 | Brain, liver, kidney, intestine | Liver: CM kidney: BBM BBB: LM | Anti-cancer drugs (irinotecan, doxorubicin, vinblastine), H1 receptor antagonists (fexofenadine, desloratadine, ebastine), opioid (loperamide), anti-parasitic(ivermectin), asimadoline, $Ca^{2+}$ channel blocker (verapamil), cardiac glycoside (digoxin) | |
| MRP2 | *ABCC2* | *cMOAT cMrp* | 601107 | Liver, kidney, duodenum | Liver: CM kidney: BBM | Glutathione conjugate, glucuronide conjugates, HMG-CoA reductase inhibitors, angiotensin receptor antagonists (valsartan, olmesartan) | |
| MRP3 | *ABCC3* | — | 604323 | Liver, intestine | Liver: SM intestine | Glucuronide conjugates, methotrexate, folic acid | $Mg^{2+}$, ATP |
| MRP4 | *ABCC4* | — | 605250 | Kidney, liver | Kidney: BBM liver, CPx: basal | Dehydroepiandrosterone sulfate, cAMP, cGMP, 6-mercaptopurine, methotrexate, furosemide, trichlorothiazide, adefovir, tenofovir, ceftizoxime, cefazolin, Ro64-0802 | |
| BCRP | *ABCG2* | *MXR* *ABCP* | 603756 | Ubiquitous | Liver: CM, small intestine: BBM BBB: LM | Anti-cancer drugs (mitoxantrone, irinotecan, topotecan, imatinib), phytoestrogenes, fluoroquinolones, HMG-CoA reductase inhibitors, sulfate conjugates of steroid, uric acid | |

ALM, abluminal membrane; BLM, basolateral membrane; BBB, blood–brain barrier; BBM, brush border membrane; CM, canalicular membrane; CPx, choroid plexus; LM, luminal membrane; OC, organic cation; SM, sinusoidal membrane

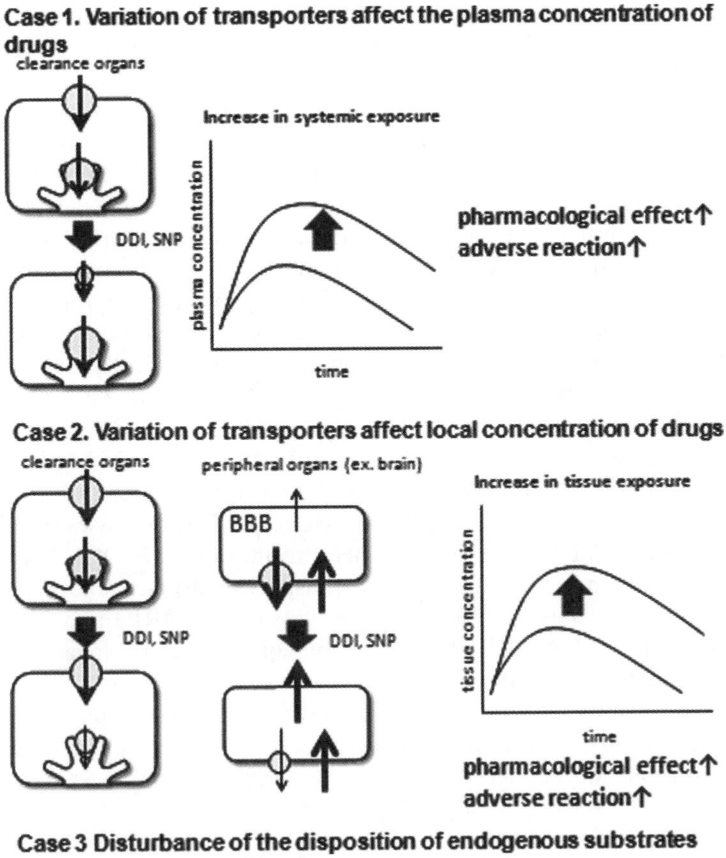


**Figure 22.1** Classification of the effects of a functional change in the transporter activity on the pharmacological effect or adverse reaction of drugs.

## 22.2 Directional Transport across the Monolayers of Epi- and Endothelial Cells

The epithelial cells in the liver, kidney and intestine, and the brain capillary endothelial cells are polarized cells, which are characterized by the directional transport of drugs across the cell monolayers. For lipophilic drugs, the expression of ABC transporters, such as P-gp and BCRP, on the apical membrane, forms directional transport across the cell monolayer. Mizuno *et al.* classified the effect of P-gp on the transcellular transport into three cases: 1) no change in the basal-to-apical transport, marked reduction in the apical-to-basal transport (*e.g.*, grepafloxacin); 2) moderate increase in the basal-to-apical transport, marked reduction in the apical-to-basal transport (*e.g.*, saquinavir and indinavir); 3) marked increase in the basal-to-apical transport, moderate reduction in the apical-to-basal transport (*e.g.*, rhodamine-123, cyclosporin, vinblastine and digoxin).[15] The difference in the impact of P-gp on the transcellular transport is attributable to the magnitude of the efflux activities to the basal and apical sides; case 1 basolateral efflux $>>$ apical efflux, case 2 basolateral efflux $\approx$ apical efflux and case 3 basolateral efflux $<<$ apical efflux.[15] In most cases, the impact of BCRP is classified as case 3.[16,17] Unlike lipophilic drugs, hydrophilic organic cations, and anionic drugs require transporters in their influx process to form efficient directional transport because of their poor membrane permeation (Figure 22.2). This concept has been confirmed by the construction of double transfectants which express both uptake and efflux transporters on the basolateral and apical membranes, respectively. Only cells expressing both uptake and efflux transporters are able to transfer their common substrates to the opposite side of a cell monolayer efficiently. Such double transfectants have been construction in the following combinations; OATP1B1/MRP2,[18] OATP1B1/P-gp,[19] OATP1B1/BCRP,[19] OATP1B3/MRP2,[20,21] OATP1B3/P-gp,[21] OATP1B3/BCRP,[21] OCT1/P-gp,[22] and OATB1B2/MRP2[23] for hepatobiliary transport, and OCT2/MATE1 and OCT2/MATE2-K,[24,25] and OAT3/URAT1[26] for tubular secretion in the kidney. In addition, a quadruple-transfectants, which expresses OATP1B1, OATP1B3 and OATP2B1 in the basolateral membrane of MDCK II cells, was constructed to mimic the hepatobiliary transport of drugs,[27] and triple transfectant, where basolateral ABC transporters, such as MRP3 and MRP4, are over-expressed in OATP1B1/MRP2, were constructed to investigate their impact on the transcellular transport.[28]

The kinetics of the directional transport involving a transporter in the uptake process are complex. The overall flux across a cell monolayer and the intracellular concentration under steady-state conditions are expressed in eqn (22.2)

$$\text{Flux} = CL_{\text{int,seq}} C_{\text{cell}} \qquad (22.2)$$

$$PS_1 C_{\text{basal}} = (PS_2 + PS_3)\ C_{\text{cell}}$$

Therefore, eqn (22.2) can be expressed as follows under steady-state conditions:

$$\text{Flux} = PS_1\ CL_{\text{int,seq}}/(PS_2 + CL_{\text{int,seq}})\ C_{\text{basal}}$$

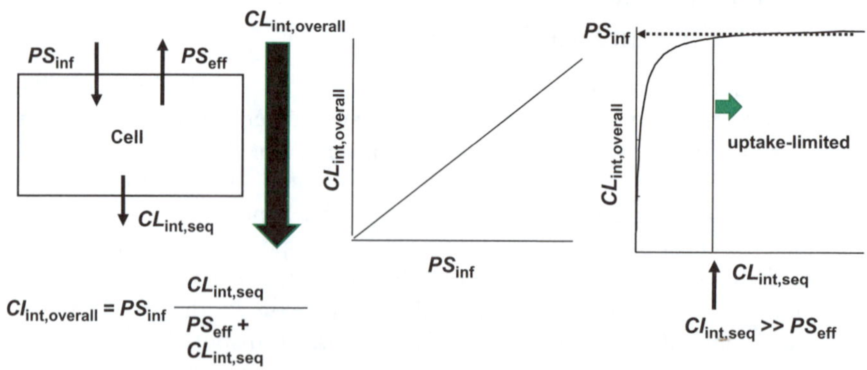


**Figure 22.2** Impact of uptake and sequestration on the overall directional transport of drugs across the monolayers of epi- and endothelial cells.

where $PS_1$, $PS_2$ and $CL_{int,seq}$ represent the uptake on the basolateral side, and the efflux activities on the basolateral and apical sides, respectively (Figure 22.2), and $C_{basal}$ and $C_{cell}$ represent the concentrations in the basal and intracellular compartments, respectively. Eqn (22.2) shows that variations in the uptake transporters affect the overall flux, whereas the impact of subsequent efflux or metabolism depends on the rate-determining process (Figure 22.2). Assuming that $CL_{int,seq}$ is significantly greater than $PS_2$, the overall flux approximates to $PS_1C_{basal}$, and therefore, $CL_{int,seq}$ no longer has any impact on the overall flux. Comparison of overall flux and uptake suggests a rate-determining process. The hepatic elimination of statins and other anionic drugs is similar to the hepatic uptake ability in rats, indicating their elimination is uptake-limited in rats.[29,30] This also holds true for the tubular secretion of anionic drugs, except olmesartan and valsartan, in rats.[31] It has also been suggested that the hepatic elimination of anionic statins is uptake-limited in humans.[29] Under these conditions, $CL_{int,seq}$ affects the intracellular concentration, and thus, variations in $CL_{int,seq}$ modulate the drug response if an intracellular protein is the pharmacological/toxicological target without affecting the overall flux as long as the assumption that $PS_2 << CL_{int,seq}$ is satisfied.

## 22.3 Drug Transporters Playing Key Roles in the Systemic Elimination of Drugs

The liver and kidney are major clearance organs in the liver. Hepatocytes, parenchymal cells in the liver, have an ability to remove drugs from the circulating blood by metabolism and biliary excretion. In the kidney, glomerular filtration, tubular secretion and re-absorption from the lumen determine the renal elimination of drugs. Hepatocytes and the epithelial cells forming the renal proximal tubules are polarized cells and express transporters with different driving forces in the blood-facing sinusoidal and canalicular membranes to form directional transport from the blood into the bile or urine (Figure 22.3). In the proximal tubules, transporters are also involved in the re-absorption of nutrients and some drugs. This section introduces the transporters playing important roles in the hepatic and renal drug transport, and their involvement in the pharmacological effects and adverse reactions.

### 22.3.1 Transporters in the Hepatic Elimination of Anionic Drugs

#### *22.3.1.1 Uptake Transporters in the Sinusoidal Membrane*

Several organic anion transporters have been identified in the sinusoidal membrane. Of these transporters, OATP1B1/*SLCO1B1* and OATP1B3/*SLCO1B3* play important roles in the hepatic uptake of a variety of drugs: their substrates overlap, and include clinically important drugs, such as HMG-CoA reductase inhibitors (statins), angiotensin II receptor antagonists, and angiotensin-converting enzyme inhibitors.[32–36] The importance of the hepatic uptake of a drug has been investigated *in vitro* using cryopreserved human

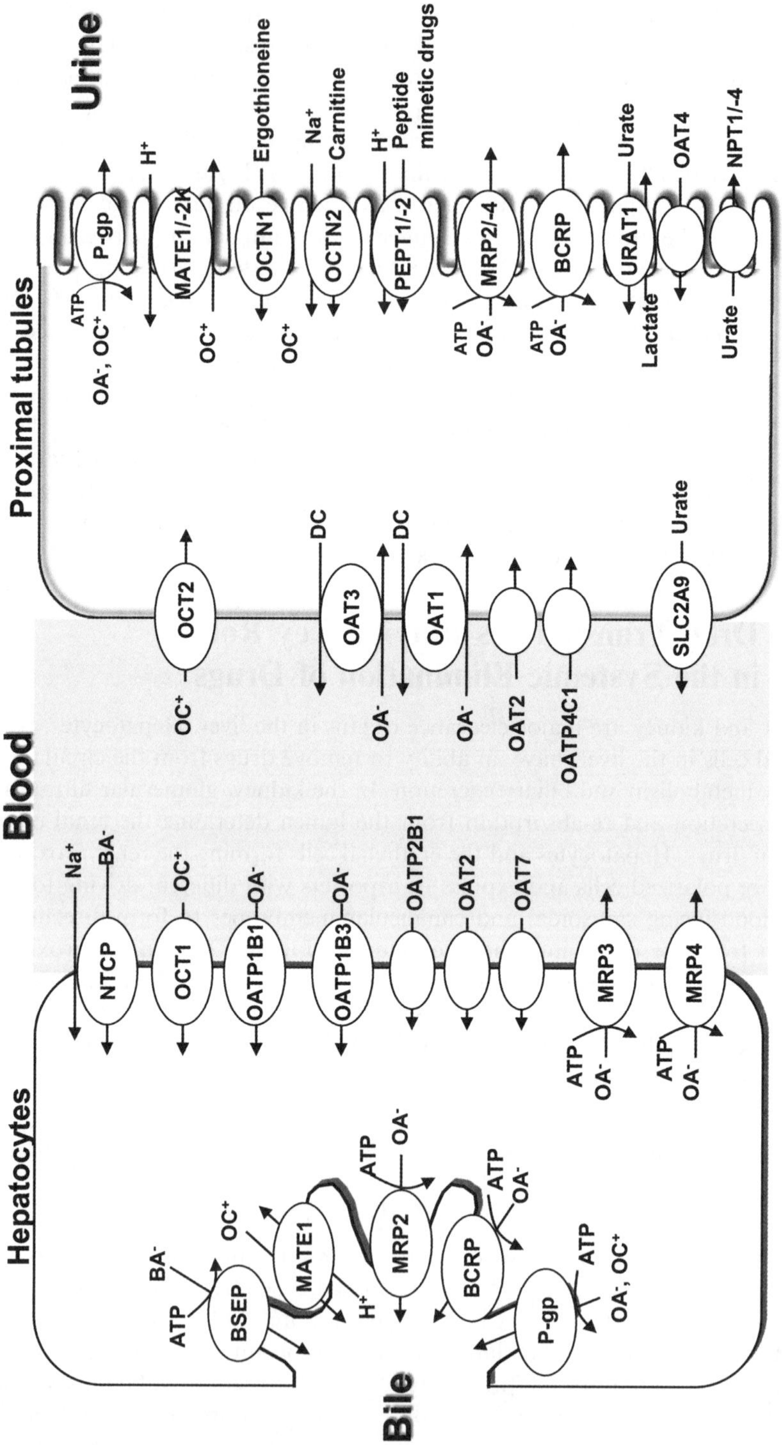


**Figure 22.3** Schematic diagram of the hepatic and renal transport systems.

hepatocytes. Estrone sulfate is an OATP1B1 inhibitor, but does not interact with OATP1B3. The magnitude of inhibition by estrone sulfate suggests the contribution from OATP1B1 to hepatic uptake.[37] Hirano *et al.*[37] proposed two other methods based on the relative activity factor which is defined as the ratio of the uptake of the reference compounds (estrone-3-sulfate for OATP1B1 and cholecystokinin octapeptide for OATP1B3) or the protein expression of the transporters determined in cryopreserved human hepatocytes to that in OATP1B1-HEK and OATP1B3-HEK cells.[37] It was suggested that OATP1B1 plays a major role in the uptake of HMG-CoA reductase inhibitors (pravastatin, pitavastatin, rosuvastatin), and estradiol-17β-glucuronide, whereas the hepatic uptake of fexofenadine, valsartan, olmesartan, and bosentan is mediated by OATP1B1 and OATP1B3, with similar contributions.[36] The hepatic uptake of telmisartan and its glucuronide is mediated predominantly by OATP1B3.[38] It is noteworthy that OATP1B1 makes a significant contribution to the hepatic uptake of drugs the main sequestration pathway of which is metabolism, such as simvastatin and atorvastatin (CYP3A4 substrate), repaglinide and cerivastatin (CYP2C8 substrate), and nateglinide (CYP3A4 and CYP2C9).[29,39–43] OATP1B1 enhances the hepatic elimination of these drugs from the blood circulation by concentrating them inside the hepatocytes.[29,30] The substrate of OATP1B1 and OATP1B3 also includes rifampicin, an agonist of the pregnane-X receptor, a nuclear receptor responsible for the induction of CYP3A4 and P-gp, and thus, OATP1B1 and OATP1B3 expression of which potentiated the PXR reporter gene activity *in vitro*.[44]

Animal studies, using genetically modified mice, have supported the importance of OATP in the hepatic uptake of drugs (Table 22.2). In addition to Oatp1b2, the mouse counterpart of human OATP1B1 and OATP1B3, members of OATP1A family, Oatp1a1 and Oatp1a4 are expressed in the sinusoidal membrane. Defects in Oatp1b2 increase systemic exposure of dibromosulfophthalen, rifampicin and pravastatin,[45,46] and decrease the liver-to-plasma ratio of phalloidin and microcystin-LR,[45] pravastatin and rifampin[46] although the result of pravastatin in Oatp1b2(–/–) mice is controversial.[47] The effect of estradiol-17β-D-glucuronide on the bile flow was partially attenuated in Oatp1b2(–/–) mice, and the hepatotoxicity induced by phalloidin and microcystin-LR was diminished in Oatp1b2(–/–) mice.[45] van de Steeg *et al.*[48,49] produced knockout mice lacking multiple Oatp1a isoforms and Oatp1b2, which exhibited a greater systemic exposure of methotrexate and paclitaxel compared with wild-type mice.[48,49]

Clinical reports of the drug–drug interactions and genetic polymorphisms/mutations of OATP1B1 suggest the importance of OATP1B1 and OATP1B3 in humans. As noted previously (section 22.2), variation in these transporters greatly affects the systemic exposure of their substrate drugs. The systemic exposure of cerivastatin was higher in patients receiving kidney transplantation and cyclosporin A.[50] Shitara *et al.*[43] found that the concentration of cyclosporin A in the portal vein at clinical doses is high enough to inhibit OATP1B1 *in vitro*,[43] but the inhibition mechanism appears to be complex since the inhibition persisted even after cyclosporin A was removed from the buffer.[51]

**Table 22.2** Summary of impact of drug transporters on *in vivo* drug disposition and their effects.

| | *KO mouse* | | |
|---|---|---|---|
| *Transporter* | *Pharmacokinetics* | *Drug/toxin effect* | *Phenotype/disease* |
| *SLC family* | | | |
| Oatp1b2 | Dibromosulfophthalen, rifampicin, pravastatin, phalloidin and microcystin-LR | Lower susceptibility to cholestatic effect of estradiol glucuronide, and hepatotoxic effect of phalloidin and microcystin-LR | Slight accumulation of bilirubin glucuronide |
| Oatp1a/1b2 | Methotrexate, paclitaxel | — | Accumulation of bilirubin glucuronide, and conjugated bile acids |
| Oct1 | TEA, MPP$^+$, metformin, MIBG | Attenuation in metformin effect (lactic acidosis, glucose-lowering effect) | — |
| Oct2 | TEA | — | — |
| Oct1/Oct2 | TEA | Greater susceptibility to nephrotoxic effect of *cis*-platin | — |
| Octn1 | Ergothioneine | — | Greater susceptability to intestinal inflammation under ischemia and reperfusion model |
| Octn2 | Carnitine, acethylcarnitine, TEA, cephaloridine | — | Primary sytemic carnitine deficiency |
| Oat1 | Furosemide, PAH | Attenuation in diuretic effect of frosemide and bendroflumethiazide | Accumulation of endogenous organic anions |
| Oat3 | Benzylpenicillin, methotrexate, ciprofloxacin | Attenuation in diuretic effect of frosemide and bendroflumethiazide | Lower systolic blood pressure |
| Mate1 | Metformin, cephalexin | Potentiate metformin effect in lactic acidosis (by pyrimethamine) senstive to nephrotoxic effect of *cis*-platin | — |
| *ABC transporter* | | | |
| Msr1a/ Mdr1a/1b | Asimadline, loperamide, ivermectin, donperidone, vinblastine, digoxin, dexamethasone, cyclosproin A, verapamil, quinidine | Greater susceptibility to neurotoxic effect of ivermectin potentiate sedative effect of asimadline | — |

**Table 22.2** (*Continued*)

| | *KO mouse* | | |
|---|---|---|---|
| *Transporter* | *Pharmacokinetics* | *Drug/toxin effect* | *Phenotype/disease* |
| *SLC family* | | | |
| Mrp1 | Cobalamin | Greater susceptibility to gastrointestinal toxicity of methotrexate | Reduced DC mobilization |
| Mrp2 | Methotrexate, DBSP, glucuronide conjugates (morphine, acetaminophen and diclofenac) | — | Dubin–Johnson syndrome |
| Mrp3 | Glucuronide conjugates (morphine, acetaminophen, dietary flavonoids), methotrexate | Attenuation in antinociceptive effect of morphine-6-glucuronide | — |
| Mrp4 | Frosemide, hydroclorthiazide, ceftizoxime, cefazolin, adefovir, tenofovir, topotecan, Ro64-0802 | Greater susceptibility to toxic effect by adefovir and 6-mercaptopurine | — |
| Bcrp | PhIP, topotecan, pheophorbide A, sulfasalazine, aflatoxin B1, IQ, Trp-P-1, nitrofurantoin, phytoestrogens, pitavastatin, diclofenac glucuronide | — | Greater susceptability to phototoxicity (pheophorbide A) Protoporphyria |
| Mrp2/ Mrp3/ Bcrp | — | Sensitive to hepatotoxicity of diclofenac glucuronide (mild heptotoxicity) | — |

In addition to cerivastatin, pharmacokinetic interaction with cyclosporin A has been reported for other OATP1B1 substrates, such as atorvastatin, pravastatin,[52] rosuvastatin[53] and repaglinide.[54] Rifampicin is also found to be a clinically relevant inhibitor of OATP1B1, and it greatly increased the systemic exposure of atorvastatin in healthy volunteers.[55]

Pharmacogenomic studies support the importance of OATP1B1 in the hepatic uptake of anionic drugs. To date, 20 single-nucleotide polymorphisms (SNPs) of OATP1B1 have been reported, which form 15 haplotypes.[36,56] In particularly, subjects with OATP1B1*5 (V174A) in the Caucasian population and OATP1B1*15 (N130D, V174A) in the Asian population exhibit the elevated systemic exposure of anionic drugs, such as repaglinide, simvastatin, and atorvastatin, as well as valsartan, temocapril, pravastatin, and pitavastatin,[39–42,57–59] suggesting that these mutations are associated with reduced transport activities compared with the reference haplotype OATP1B1

(OATP1B1*1a). This is in good agreement with *in vitro* data.[56,60] In contrast, homozygoutes of OATP1B1*1b showed smaller systemic exposure of OATP1B1 substrates,[36] it is considered that this SNP is associated with elevated expression and/or transport activity of OATP1B1 in the liver. Pharmacogenomic studies have also demonstrated that the variations in OATP1B1 activity are associated with adverse reactions of drugs. N130D and V174A are associated with the incidence of adverse reaction of irinotecan, grade three diarrhea (18 *versus* 46%) and grade four neutropenia (0 *versus* 15%), respectively.[61] Since patients with the OATP1B1*15 allele showed higher systemic exposure of irinotecan and SN-38 than those with the reference OATP1B1 allele (*1a/*1b or *1b/*1b), but lower exposure of SN-38G,[62] high incidence of grade four neutropenia is attributable to accumulation of SN-38. The higher incidence of grade three diarrhea may be accounted for by elevated secretion of SN-38 into the bile. The glucose-lowering effect of repaglinide is more potent in subjects with V174A through the elevation of systemic exposure to repaglinide.[40] A genome-wide association study (GWAS) using approximately 300 000 markers showed that an intronic SNP of OATP1B1 (rs4363657), which is in nearly complete linkage dis-equilibrium with a non-synonymous SNP (V174A), is associated with the higher risk of the myopathy caused by simavastatin medication (odds ratio of 17 in CC homozygotes compared with TT homozygotes), possibly because of the greater systemic exposure to simvastatin acid of the muscle (Link *et al.*[63]). This is also true for cerivastatin for which the odds ratio was 1.5 in subjects with a non-synonymous SNP (V174A).[64] A GWAS using approximately 500 000 markers also showed that the SNPs located in the SLCO1B1 genes (rs11045879 and rs4149081), which are in linkage dis-equilibrium with a non-synonymous SNP (V174A), are associated with the oral clearance of methotrexate, and the incidence of gastrointestinal (GI) toxicity. The GI toxicity was only observed in the homozygoutes of the TT allele, which showed higher oral clearance of MTX.[65] A SNP (rs11045585) in OATP1B3 is associated with incidence of neutropenia, caused by docetaxel with the odds ratio of 5.4 in heterozygotes for this SNP [66] although the effects of the SNP on the systemic exposure of docetaxel and OATP1B3 expression or transport activity remains to be examined.

### *22.3.1.2 Efflux Transporters in the Canalicular Membrane*

ABC transporters, such as P-gp/*MDR1*, MRP2/*ABCC2*, and BCRP/*ABCG2*, mediate canalicular efflux of drugs into the bile. In particular, the importance of MRP2 has been suggested based on animal studies. Lack of MRP2 impairs the biliary excretion of a variety of anionic drugs, and conjugated metabolites, particularly glutathione- and glucuronide conjugates in rats and mice,[5,67,68] accompanied by prolonged systemic exposure. Those include pravstatin, methotrexate, temocaprilat, and varsartan and olmesartan.[36,67,69,70] The canalicular efflux of some drugs is not influenced by MRP2 deficiency, which is partly explained by BCRP. Lack of BCRP reduces the biliary excretion of pitavastatin and some fluoroquinolones in mice.[71,72] Pharmacogenomic studies have elucidated that a SNP of MRP2 is associated with adverse reactions of drugs. SNPs in the 5′ un-translational region ( − 24 T > C), and coding region (1058 G > A) are associated with greater susceptibility to the hepatotoxic effect of diclofenac (odds ratio of 5 compared with the hospital control), and methotrexate, presumably resulting from the reduced canalicular efflux of diclofenac glucuronide and methotrexate, leading to prolongation of the exposure in the liver.[73,74] Another SNP in the 5′ un-translational region ( − 1019 A > G, ABCC2*2) was associated with lower incidence of the adverse reaction of irinotecan, severe diarrhea (odds ratio of 0.15) only in patients who did not carry UGT1A1*28.[75] Because MRP2 is responsible for the canalicular efflux of SN-38 and its glucuronide conjugate,[76] reduction in the canalicular efflux of these compounds reduces their exposure to the intestine, attenuating the adverse reaction of irinotecan. In a rat study, the inhibition of Mrp2 by probenecid attenuated this adverse reaction.[77]

A non-synonymous SNP of BCRP (Q141K) is associated with lower protein expression in the plasma membrane *in vitro*.[78] Pharmacongenomic studies have demonstrated that this SNP is associated with variations in the pharmacokinetics of BCRP substrate drugs. Systemic exposure of rosuvastatin, atorvastatin and sulfasalazine given orally is higher in healthy subjects with this SNP,[79–81] whereas this effect is not observed for pitavastatin and pravastatin.[57,82] The effect of the BCRP SNP is attributable to the variations in the intestinal absorption and hepatobiliary transport of its substrates. However, the impact of each process on the pharmacokinetic variation remains to be evaluated.

### *22.3.1.3 Efflux Transporters in the Sinusoidal Membrane*

In addition to the canalicular efflux, ABC transporters, such as MRP3 and MRP4, mediate efflux into the sinusoidal space in mice (Table 22.2). Mrp3 (–/–) mice were first characterized by the lower plasma concentrations of glucuronide conjugates of morphine following the administration of morphine.[83] Later studies confirmed that the secretion of the glucuronide conjugates of drugs into the blood circulation is markedly decreased in the liver of Mrp3(–/–) mice compared with that in wild-type mice.[84] Sinusoidal efflux competes with sequestration in the liver, and the magnitude of the sequestration clearance relative to sinusoidal efflux clearance determines the rate-determining process in the overall hepatobiliary transport (see section 22.2). Unless uptake is the rate-determining process, reduced sinusoidal efflux clearance is accompanied by an increase in the overall hepatic elimination. Actually, the systemic elimination of morphine-6-glucuronide and methotrexate is greater in Mrp3(–/–) mice than in wild-type mice,[83,85] and consequently attenuated the antinociceptive effect of morphine-6-glucuronide (10 mg $kg^{-1}$, intraperitoneal) when evaluated by both the hot-plate and the tail-immersion tests.[83] The biliary clearance of methotrexate was 1.6-fold greater in Mrp3(–/–) mice than in wild-type mice although their hepatic uptake and canalicular efflux were unchanged compared with those in wild-type mice.[85] There is only limited information available for Mrp4. It mediates the sinusoidal efflux of sulfate conjugates in the liver, but makes a limited contribution to that of glucuronide conjugates or fexofenadine.[84,86]

### 22.3.2 Transporters in the Hepatic Elimination of Hydrophilic Cationic Drugs

Hepatocytes express the organic cation transporters, OCT1/SLC22A1 and MATE1/SLC47A1 on the sinusoidal and canalicular membranes, respectively. Since the major elimination of their common substrates is generally by renal elimination, the impact of these hepatic transporters on the systemic elimination is limited. However, these transporters are essential for the pharmacological effect/adverse reaction of metformin, a biguanide used for the treatment of hyperglycemia in patients suffering type 2 diabetes. The action of metaformin involves the inhibition of mitochondria respiratory complex I, leading to inhibition of gluconeogenesis from the lactate in the liver,[87,88] and the activation of kinases, such as AMP-activated protein kinase (AMPK) and serine-threonine kinase 11 (STK11/LKB1).[89,90] Therefore, the liver concentration of metformin is the critical factor in its pharmacological action/adverse reaction (lactic acidosis). In Oct1(–/–) mice, which show a marked reduction in the hepatic concentration of metformin compared with that in wild-type mice,[91] the effects of metformin on plasma lactate and the phosphorylation (activation) of AMPK following treatment are attenuated compared with those in wild-type mice.[8,92] MATE1, a proton/organic cation exchanger, mediates the canalicular efflux of metformin in mouse and human liver, but not in rat liver.[93,94] Canalicular membrane vesicles from mouse and human livers show the saturable transport of metformin in the presence of an outward $H^+$ gradient, which is inhibited by pyrimethamine, a potent and competitive inhibitor of MATEs.[95,96] Pyrimethamin (2 μg $kg^{-1}$, intravenous) also inhibits the canalicular efflux of metformin in mice *in vivo*, resulting in a significant increase in the liver concentration of metformin, thereby enhancing its effect on the plasma lactate.[95] Mate1(–/–) mice also show a significant accumulation of metformin in the liver following its intravenous administration compared with the wild-type mice.[97]

The effects of OCT1 and MATE1 on the pharmacological action of metformin are supported by pharmacogenomic studies. In subjects with mutant OCT1 (R61C, G401S, 420del, or G465R), which show lower uptake ability in oocytes,[98] the glucose-lowering effect of metfomin was attenuated compared with those with a reference allele of OCT1.[99] A SNP in the intron (rs2289669) of hMATE1 is associated with a reduction in the pharmacological effect of metformin (hemoglobin A1c reduction) in diabetic patients,[100] whereas it does not alter the systemic exposure of metformin.[101] Because a MATE inhibitor, pyrimethamine did not affect a transient rise in plasma lactate caused by metformin,[96] the effect of the SNP on the pharmacological action of metformin may not be attributable to MATE1 in the liver

### 22.3.3 Transporters in the Tubular Secretion of Anionic Drugs in the Kidney

The organic anion transport system in the kidney consists of two multispecific organic anion transporters, OAT1/*SLC22A6* and OAT3/*SLC22A8* (Figure 22.3).[35,102–104] OAT2/*SLC22A7* and OATP4C1/*SLCO4C1* are also expressed in the basolateral membrane of the proximal tubules, however their functional significance in drug transport remains unknown.[105,106] OAT1 and OAT3 mediate the active transport driven by an outward gradient of dicarboxylate, and thus, they are able to concentrate anionic drugs into the epithelial cells.[35,102–104] The substrate specificities of both OAT1 and OAT3 are broad with a slight overlap. The substrates of OAT1 include *p*-aminohippurate (PAH), antiviral drugs (adefovir, cidofovir and tenofovir) and diuretics (furosemide), whereas those of OAT3 include bulky anionic compounds, which are transported by OATPs, such as estrone-3-sulfate, benzylpenicillin, statins, sartans, zwitterion (fexofenadine) and some cationic drugs (cimetidine, ranitidine and famotidine).[35,102–104] The functional importance of OAT1 and OAT3 has been investigated *in vitro* using rat kidney slices where saturable uptake of PAH, and pravastatin, specific substrates of OAT1 and OAT3, was observed.[107] Based on their contributions evaluated in rat kidney slices, OAT1 and OAT3 are considered to play significant roles in the renal uptake of water-soluble organic anions with low-molecular-weight and bulky ones, respectively.[108] Furthermore, animal studies using knockout mice of OAT1 or OAT3 elucidate their importance in the renal elimination *in vivo*, and effect of diuretics (Table 22.2). Oat1(–/–) mice exhibited delayed elimination of PAH and diuretics (furosemide and bendroflumethiazide),[109,110] and the Oat3(–/–) mice exhibited delayed elimination of benzylpenicillin, methotrexate, diuretics (furosemide and bendroflumethiazide), and ciprofloxacin (only in female mice).[110–113] The lack of OAT1 and OAT3 attenuates the diuretic effects of furosemide and bendroflumethiazide in mice,[110–113] presumably by reducing the effective concentrations in the lumen.

The importance of OAT1 and OAT3 has been supported both clinically and in studies based on human kidney slices. Freshly prepared human kidney slices show a relatively large inter-batch difference. However, since the uptake of typical OAT1 and OAT3 substrate, PAH and benzylpenicillin, respectively, correlated with the mRNA expression of OAT1 and OAT3, respectively, it is considered that the contribution of OAT1 and OAT3 is maintained.[114] The slices showed saturable uptake of typical OAT1 and OAT3 substrates; PAH, benzylpencillin, estrone sulfate, dehydroepiandrosterone sulfate, methotrexate, statins and sartans.[69,114–116] Consistent with the rat kidney slice studies, the effect of PAH on the uptake of OAT3 substrates, such as benzylpenicillin was weaker than expected from its $K_m$ value, whereas the effect of benzylpenicillin for the uptake of OAT1 substrates, such as PAH and 2,4-dichlrophenoxyaceate was weaker than expected from its $K_m$ value.[114] A pharmacokinetic interaction study using probenecid as the inhibitor supports the importance of OAT1 and OAT3 *in vivo*.[13] Probenecid has been used as an *in vivo* inhibitor of renal organic anion transporters, and inhibits tubular secretion of a variety of anionic drugs, and zwitterions such as fexofenadine and Ro64-0802.[103,117,118] Among the H2 receptor antagonists, only the tubular secretion of famotidine is susceptible to probenecid.[119,120] Probenecid is a potent OAT1 and OAT3 inhibitor, but it is a weak inhibitor of OCT2.[121] The clinically relevant concentration of probenecid is high enough to inhibit OAT1 and OAT3, completely,[121] and the magnitude of inhibition by probenecid reflects the contribution of OAT1 and OAT3.

The transporters mediating the luminal efflux have not been fully identified. Classically, transport studies using brush border membrane vesicles (BBMV) have suggested that the luminal transport of organic anions consists of two distinct systems: i) the electroneutral exchange of organic anions and ii) voltage-driven facilitated transport. There are several candidate transporters, including NPT1, NPT4 and mUrat1, which mediate membrane-voltage dependent transport of organic anions[26,122,123] although their significance remains to be investigated. In addition to these transport systems, ABC transporters which mediate primary active transport, such as breast cancer resistance protein (BCRP/*ABCG2*) and multi-drug resistance associated proteins 2 (MRP2/*ABCC2*) and 4 (MRP4/*ABCC4*), have been shown to constitute a third efflux mechanism in the kidney (Figure 22.1). Defect of MRP4 caused a significant increase in the kidney concentrations of trichlorothiazide, cephalosporins (ceftizoxime and cefazolin), and antiviral drugs (adefovir and tenofovir) in mice when they were given intravenously by constant infusion, indicating that MRP4 makes a significant contribution to the luminal efflux of these drugs in the kidney.[125–127] Because the net tubular secretion of these drugs remains intact even in Mrp4(–/–) mice, other transporters are also involved in luminal efflux. A patient who exhibited delayed systemic elimination of methotrexate was heterozygous for the mutation found in Dubin–Johnson syndrome, suggesting that MRP2 also mediates the luminal efflux of methotrexate.[128]

The dose-limiting adverse reaction of adefovir and cidofovir is nephrotoxicity. Renal elimination is the major elimination pathway of adefovir and cidofovir in their unchanged form. The over-expression of OAT1 results in the higher accumulation of these drugs compared with the mock cells, and consequently sensitizes the cells to the cytotoxic effect of adefovir and cidofovir.[7] Therefore, the inhibition of OAT1-mediated uptake protects the kidney from the cytotoxic effects of adefovir and cidofovir. Actually, probenecid attenuates the nephrotoxic effect of cidofovir.[129] MRP4 has been characterized as the efflux transporter of adefovir, and the over-expression of MRP4 confers resistance to adefovir.[6] As described above, MRP4 is suggested to mediate the luminal efflux of adefovir at least in mouse kidney since the kidney concentration was higher in Mrp4(–/–) mice despite its similar plasma concentrations in wild-type and Mrp4(–/–) mice.[127] Unlike adefovir and tenofovir, impaired MRP4 has a negligible effect on the kidney concentration of cidofovir, and the ATP-dependent uptake of cidofovir by MRP4 was not detected in MRP4-expressing vesicles. Since cidofovir undergoes tubular secretion and substrate of OAT1, another transporter is responsible for the luminal efflux of cidofovir. Mrp4(–/–) mice are more sensitive to adefovir than wild-type mice.[130] The toxicity of adefovir was observed in Mrp4(–/–) mice, particularly, in the bone marrow, thymus, spleen and intestine in Mrp4(–/–) mice 72 h after the intraperitoneal injection of adefovir (2 g $kg^{-1}$) with intense aplasia in the bone marrow, diminished lymphoid follicles, lymophcyte depopulation in the cortical region of the thymus, acute mucositis.[130] Since MRP4 is expressed in a variety of organs in the body, MRP4 is a likely determinant of the local concentrations of adefovir since the systemic exposure was unaltered by MRP4 impairment. However, in contrast with clinical observations, the toxicity was not observed in the kidney by histologic analysis in mice given adefovir although the reason for this is unclear.[130]

## 22.3.4 Transporters in the Tubular Secretion of Cationic Drugs in the Kidney

OCT2/*SLC22A1* is the predominant organic cation transporter in the basolateral membrane of the proximal tubules.[131] OCT2 mediates the facilitated diffusion of various cationic drugs, including metformin and cimetidine.[131] The luminal efflux mechanism for hydrophilic organic cations is suggested to be active and driven by an outward concentration gradient of $H^+$.[132] Initially, OCTN1 and OCTN2 were considered candidates because in an expression system, they mediated the antiport of tetraethylammonium (TEA), a typical substrate of renal organic cation transporters with $H^+$.[133,134] Actually, the tubular secretion of gabapentin is decreased in healthy subjects homozygous for L503F from 141 to 110 mL $min^{-1}$,[135] and an OCTN2-deficient mutant mouse showed reduced luminal efflux of cephaloridine.[136] However, except in these cases, the primary role of OCTN1/2 has been considered to be in the reabsorption of ergothioneine and carnitine from the urine.[137–140] MATEs (comprising MATE1 in the rodent kidney and MATE1 and MATE2-K in the human kidney) are now considered to mediate the tubular secretion of cationic drugs in concert with OCT2.[92,141] MATEs mediate the transport of a variety of organic cations with an exchange of $H^+$.[92,141,142] Mate1(–/–) mice and a potent MATE inhibitor pyrimethamine have uncovered the importance of Mate1 as a luminal efflux transporter of organic cations in the kidney. Mate1(–/–) mice show a significant delay in the systemic elimination of metformin and cefalexin, accompanied by their accumulation in the kidney.[96,143] The uptake of metformin by BBMV from the kidney in the presence of an outward $H^+$ gradient was completely inhibited by pyrimethamine with a $K_i$ value similar to that observed in a mMATE1 cDNA transfectant.[95] Furthermore, the kidney concentrations of TEA and metfomin were significantly increased by pyrimethamine (2 μmol $kg^{-1}$, intravenous), but it did not affect the plasma concentration and urinary excretion rate. The increase in their kidney-to-plasma ratio indicates that pyrimethamine inhibited the luminal efflux of these organic cations.[95] Unlike Mate1(–/–) mice, the lack of any effect on the plasma concentration and urinary excretion rate is attributable to its blood-flow limited clearance, and uptake-limited clearance. The inhibition was insufficient to alter the rate-determining process. Pyrimethamine also completely inhibited the metformin uptake in human kidney BBMV with $K_i$ value similar to that observed in hMATE1 and hMATE2-K cDNA transfectants.[95] Notably, the unbound concentration of pyrimethamine at the clinical dose is high enough to inhibit MATE proteins. A pharmacokinetic interaction study between metformin and pyrimethamine in healthy subjects showed that pyrimethamine (50 mg, oral) inhibited renal clearance of metformin by 20–30%, suggesting that hMATE1 and hMATE2-K are involved in metformin transport.[95] Cimetidine has been used as an *in vivo* inhibitor of renal organic cation transporters.[13]

Cimetidine is believed to be an *in vivo* inhibitior of OCT2. However, the clinically relevant concentration is insufficient to inhibit OCT2, and the inhibition of MATE1 is now proposed as the mechanism underlying the drug–drug interactions with cimetidine.[97,144]

Renal organic cation transporters play important roles in the nephrotoxic effect of *cis*-platin. The involvement of transporters in the basolateral uptake of *cis*-platin was suggested in rat kidney slices. The uptake was inhibited by organic cations, but not by PAH.[145] The exogenous expression of OCT2 potentiated the cytotoxic effect of *cis*-platin, which was reversed by an OCT2 substrate/inhibitor.[9,10] *cis*-Platin shows the highest accumulation in the kidney among the platinum anticancer agents (*cis*-platin, carboplatin, oxaliplatin, and nedaplatin). *cis*-Platin is only transported by Oct2, whereas oxaliplatin is transported by Oct2 and Oct3 and Mate1, carboplatin, and nedaplatin are transported by any of the OCT isoforms.[146] The highest accumulation of *cis*-platin is explained by its uptake mediated by Oct2. Although oxaliplatin is also taken up by OCT2, but Mate1 secretes it into the lumen, limiting its accumulation in the kidney.[146] Furthermore, Oct1/2(–/–) mice are resistant to the nephrotoxic effect of *cis*-platin.[147] A non-synonymous SNP in the OCT2 gene (rs316019, A270S) is associated with reduced *cis*-platin-induced nephrotoxicity in patients.[148] Although no functional change was observed *in vitro* when 1-methyl-4-phenylpyridinium ($MPP^+$) was used as the probe,[149] this SNP may affect the transport activities of *cis*-platin. This suggests that inhibition of the OCT2-mediated uptake of *cis*-platin protects the kidney from its nephrotoxic effect. Cimetidine and imatinib attenuate the nephrotoxic effect of *cis*-platin in mice,[147] and rats.[150] The recognition of *cis*-platin by MATE shows a great species difference even in rodents; Mouse Mate1 accepts it as a substrate, but not in rats. Consistent with its substrate specificity, defect of Mate1 sensitizes mice to the nephrotoxic effect of *cis*-platin, attributable to a prolonged systemic exposure and higher accumulation of *cis*-platin in the kidney compared with those in wild-type mice.[151] Pyrimethamine also sensitizes mice to the nephrotoxic effect of *cis*-platin.[151] Whether *cis*-platin is a substrate of MATE1 or MATE2-K is controversial. Yokoo *et al.* reported that neither MATE1 nor MATE2-K accepts *cis*-platin carboplatin, and nedaplatin as a substrate, and MATE2-K accepts oxaliplatin.[146] However, Yonezawa *et al.* reported that *cis*-platin is a substrate of both transporters.[152]

## 22.4 Transporters Limiting the Penetration of Drugs into the Central Nervous System at the Blood–Brain Barrier

ABC transporters act as active barriers that limit the penetration of drugs into the central nervous system (CNS) (Figure 22.4), and thereby, attenuating the effects of drugs in the tissue compartment. ABC transporters, such as P-gp, Bcrp and Mrp4, are expressed on the luminal membranes of the brain capillaries. Their importance has been investigated using knockout mice. Mice lacking Mdr1a, a

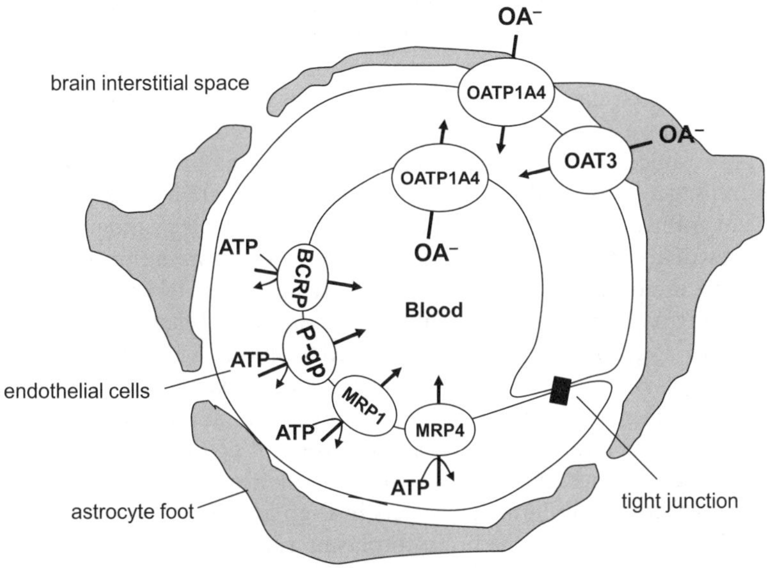


**Figure 22.4** Schematic diagram of the transporters for drugs in the blood–brain barrier.

major mouse P-gp isoform at the blood–brain barrier (BBB), show higher accumulation of a number of drugs compared with wild-type mice.[15,153] A potent P-gp inhibitor GF120918 enhances the antinociceptive effect of morphine in rats, by inhibiting P-gp at the BBB, resulting in a significant increase in its brain concentrations.[154] A defect of Mdr1a sensitizes mice to the neurotoxic effects of ivermectin, and the sedative effect of asimadoline.[155,156] The impact of P-gp on the penetration of P-gp substrates in humans has been investigated with positron emission tomography (PET), a non-invasive high-resolution imaging system using isotopes with short half-lives, such as $^{11}$C, $^{13}$N $^{15}$O and $^{18}$F.[157] In rhesus monkeys, pretreatment with PSC833, a potent P-gp inhibitor, caused a significant increase in the permeation of $^{11}$C-verapamil, determined with an integration plot analysis.[158] The ratio of the area under the curve (AUC) for $^{11}$C-verapamil in the brain and plasma, representing the brain-to-plasma concentration ratio, was 1.9-fold greater in subjects treated with cyclosporin A than that in control subjects.[159] It is worth noting that the inhibition of P-gp by cyclosporin A was not clinically relevant, because an extraordinarily high dose of cyclosporin A was given in that study. Tariquidar increased the K1 of $^{11}$C-*N*-desmethyllopramide dose dependently in healthy subjects. K1, a rate constant for the penetration into the CNS from the blodd, was increased 2- and 4-fold when tariquidar was given at 4 or 6 mg kg$^{-1}$, whereas 2 mg kg$^{-1}$ tariquidar was insufficient to inhibit P-gp at the BBB.[160] Impact of P-gp on the CNS effect of drugs has also been reported in healthy subjects. The CNS effect of a peripheral opioid, loperamide, was observed in subjects treated with quinidine before loperamide administration. Since the systemic exposure of loperamide, when the

CNS effects of loperamide were observed, was similar between subjects with or without quinidine treatment, inhibition of P-gp by quinidine was considered to be the underlying mechanism.[161] A number of studies have examined the effect of SNPs on the pharmacokinetics or drug response.[36] The BBB permeability of $^{11}$C-verapamil was similar in healthy subjects irrespective of their genotypes.[162]

Bcrp(–/–) mice exhibit greater brain concentrations of phytoestrogens such as daidzein, genistein, and coumestrol, food-derived carcinogens such as PhIP, *N*-hydroxyl PhIP, and MeIQx, and drugs such as dantrolene and prazosin.[16,163] It is noteworthy that the impact of BCRP varies depending on the test compound, in spite of their similar transport activities by BCRP, when determined *in vitro* using MDCK cells expressing mouse BCRP.[16] Mice lacking both P-gp and BCRP (P-gp/Bcrp(–/–) mice) exhibited a marked increase in the brain concentrations of their common substrates even compared with knockout mice lacking either P-gp or BCRP.[164–166] When both P-gp- and Bcrp-mediated efflux are significantly greater than the passive diffusion, P-gp or BCRP that remained intact in Bcrp(–/–) or P-gp(–/–) mice still limits the penetration of drugs into the brain.[35] Therefore, simultaneous defects in P-gp and BCRP (P-gp/Bcrp(−/−)) cause a further increase in the brain-to-plasma ratio of the common substrates compared with Bcrp(–/–) and P-gp(–/–) mice, respectively. The contribution of P-gp and BCRP to the net efflux could reasonably explain the increase in the brain-to-plasma ratio of erlotinib, flavopiridol, and mitoxantrone in P-gp/Bcrp(–/–) as well as P-gp(–/–) and Bcrp(–/–) mice.[167] The importance of MRP4 in the efflux transport across the BBB has been suggested for topotecan, adefovir and carboxylate form of oseltamivir (Ro64-0802). Mrp4(–/–) mice exhibit a significant prolongation of the CNS exposure of topteocan and adefovir given by bolus intravenous injection.[130,168] Mrp4(–/–) mice show a significant increase in the brain concentration of Ro64-0802 after a 24 h constant exposure using an osmotic pump embedded beneath the skin, whereas the distribution volume of Ro64-0802 in wild-type mice was limited to the capillary space, and the knockout mice show a delayed elimination of Ro64-0802 from the brain after its microinjection into the cerebral cortex.[169]

## 22.5 Drug Transporters Involved in the Disposition of Endogenous and Food-Derived Compounds

Some drug transporters are involved in the disposition of endogenous compounds, and therefore, any defects cause their accumulation or loss, and some are associated with diseases (Table 22.2). MRP2 is the responsible gene of Dubin–Johnson syndrome, and the symptoms of which arise from the impaired canalicular efflux of bilirubin glucuronide,[170] and OCTN2 is responsible for carnitine deficiency, caused by perturbation of oral and urinary absorption, and tissue distribution of carnitine.[139] Animal studies using knockout mice have identified endogenous substrates of drugs transporters. Bcrp(–/–) mice accumulate pheophorbide A, a metabolite of dietary chlorophyll A, leading to phototoxicity in mice.[171] Furthermore, Bcrp(–/–) mice also show protoporphyria, and erythrocytes transplanted from Bcrp(–/–) mice to wild-type mice accumulate protoprphyrin IX. MRP2-deficient mutant rats and Mrp2(–/–) mice accumulate bilirubin glucuronide because of an impaired canalicular efflux.[68,172,173] Accumulation of bilirubin glucuronide in the plasma is also caused by impaired hepatic uptake. Plasma bilirubin glucuronide is higher in Oatp1b2(–/–) mice than in control mice (0.020 *versus* 0 mg $dL^{-1}$),[45] and the accumulation of plasma bilirubin mono- and diglucuronide was more clearly observed in Oatp1a/1b2(–/–) mice (*ca.* 3 and 0.5 mg $dL^{-1}$) which lack the sinusoidal OATPS.[49] Oatp1a/1b2(–/–) mice also accumulate unconjugated bile acids in the plasma. Association of OATP activity with serum bilirubin and bilirubin glucuronide has also been reported in humans. OATP1B1 accepts both bilirubin and bilirubin glucuronide as substrate[174] although contradictory data is also reported.[175] An SNP of OATP1B1 is associated with serum bilirubin and bilirubin glucuronide.[176] Subjects with a *15 allele show significantly higher serum concentrations of bilirubin and bilirubin glucuronide compared with those with reference alleles (*1a and *1b) (13 *versus* 8.2, and 7.7 *versus* 4.9 μM, respectively). It is worth noting that this effect shows a great ethnic difference; there was no association in the Caucasian population, whereas SNPs of OATP1B3 (rs17680137 and rs2117032) are found to be associated with plasma bilirubin concentration.[177]

MRP2 is responsible for the canalicular efflux of folate and its derivatives,[178] and MRP2- deficient mutant rats show a reduced canalicular efflux of folate and its derivatives, accompanied with higher plasma concentration of 5-methytetrahydrofolate and reduced folate compared with normal rats. MRP3 mediates the intestinal absorption of folic acid and leucovorin in concert with the uptake transporter in the duodenum, but its impact is less pronounced on the absorption of 5-methyltetrahydrofolate.[179] Plasma concentration of folic acid and leucovorin was significantly lower in Mrp3(–/–) mice compared with wild-type mice when they were given orally. However, endogenous 5-methytetrahydrofolic acid did not differ between wild-type and Mrp3(–/–) mice and Mrp3(–/–) mice did not manifest folate deficiency as long as they were maintained under normal conditions.

### 22.5.1 Drug–Creatinine Interactions

Creatinine is a metabolite of creatine phosphate, and is used as an index of kidney function. It is generally believed that the major elimination mechanism of creatinine in the kidney is glomerular filtration since the renal clearance of creatinine is apparently similar to or somewhat greater than the glomerular filtration rate (GFR). It is also suggested that creatinine undergoes tubular secretion. Kabat-Koperska *et al.* showed that cimetidine administration reduced the renal clearance of creatinine to the GFR determined by inulin clearance.[180] Creatinine was found to be an endogenous substrate of renal organic cation transporters, hOCT2 and MATE1.[142,181] In addition to cimetidine, another MATE inhibitor, pyrimethamine also inhibits the renal elimination of creatinine, accompanied by the elevation of serum creatinine in healthy subjects, without affecting the GFR.[96,182] Mate1(–/–) mice also show higher serum creatinine;[97] these transporters are potential sites of drug–creatinine interactions. Namely, creatinine can be used to suggest the drug–drug interaction involving renal organic cation transporters in a retrospective way. DX-619, a novel des-fluoro(6)-quinolone antibacterial agent, was found to be a potent inhibitor of OCT2,[183] and MATEs,[184] and the maximum unbound concentration of DX-619 in plasma at the clinical dose is high enough to inhibit transporters.[184] Actually, DX-619 was reported to elevate the serum creatinine in healthy subjects, but not the GFR determined by iohexol clearance,[185] and pharmacokinetic modeling which assumes its competitive inhibition of OCT2 (Model 1) or OCT2 and MATEs (Model 2) (Figure 22.5) could reasonably explain the elevation of serum creatinine during DX-619 administration, and suggested that the tubular secretion makes a 30–60% contribution to the renal elimination.[184]

## 22.5.2 Drug–Uric Acid Interactions

Uric acid is the end product of purine metabolism in humans. It has anti-oxidant activity, whereas its higher serum level is a risk factor of gout. Uric acid undergoes extensive reabsorption from the urine in the kidney mediated by URAT1/*SLC22A12*, and defect of URAT1 causes hypouricaemia.[186] In addition to uricosuric drugs, such as probenecid and benzbromarone, some drugs are known to influence serum uric acid. Rasburicase,[187] losartan,[188]

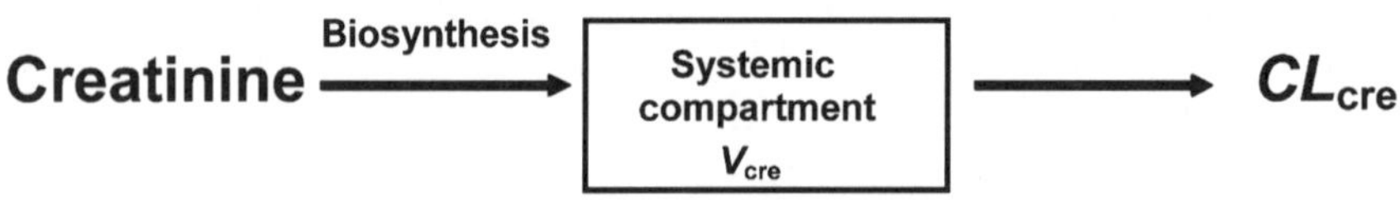


Model 1

$$CL_{cre} = (1-FR)\left( GFR + \frac{\dfrac{RPF\ CL_{rs,intall}}{1+\dfrac{C_{DX\text{-}619}(t)\, f_{p,DX\text{-}619}}{K_{i,hOCT2}}}}{RPF + \dfrac{CL_{rs,intall}}{1+\dfrac{C_{DX\text{-}619}(t)\, f_{p,DX\text{-}619}}{K_{i,hOCT2}}}} \right)$$

Model 2

$$CL_{cre} = (1-FR)\left( GFR + \frac{\dfrac{RPF\ CL_{rs,intall}}{\left(1+\dfrac{C_{DX\text{-}619}(t)\, f_{p,DX\text{-}619}}{K_{i,hOCT2}}\right)\left(1+\dfrac{C_{DX\text{-}619}(t)\, f_{p,DX\text{-}619}}{K_{i,hMATE1\ or\ hMATE2\text{-}K}}\right)}}{RPF + \dfrac{CL_{rs,intall}}{\left(1+\dfrac{C_{DX\text{-}619}(t)\, f_{p,DX\text{-}619}}{K_{i,hOCT2}}\right)\left(1+\dfrac{C_{DX\text{-}619}(t)\, f_{p,DX\text{-}619}}{K_{i,hMATE1\ or\ hMATE2\text{-}K}}\right)}} \right)$$

**Figure 22.5** Kinetic models for drug–creatinine interactions in the tubular secretion involving OCT2 and MATEs.

atorvastatin,[189] fenofibrate[190] and irtemazole[191] increases the urinary excretion of uric acid, whereas torasemide[192] and thiazide[193] decreases it. Of these drugs, losartan and fenofibric acid (metabolite of fenofibrate) have been shown to inhibit URAT1 *in vitro*.[194] Furthermore, the effect of losartan on serum uric acid was diminished in patients whose URAT1 was deficient,[188] supporting that uricosuric effect of losartan is explained by an inhibition of URAT1. It is also known that the renal elimination of losartan involves tubular secretion mediated by organic anion transporters,[195] which may potentiate the inhibitory effect of losartan on URAT1 *in vivo*. The mechanism underlying the hyperuricaemia caused by torasemide and thiazide remains unclear. Hagos *et al.* speculated *trans*-stimulation of OAT4-mediated uptake of uric acid by torasemide or its metabolites as the underlying mechanism.[192]

In addition to URAT1, a GWAS has identified SNPs in some transporters which are associated with serum uric acid.[196–198] Those include OAT4/*SLC22A11*, BCRP, GLUT9/*SLC2A9*, NPT1/*SLC17A1*, NPT4/*SLC17A3* and SLC16A9 although depending on the report, the transporters, SNPs of which produce statistically significant effects, differ somewhat. OAT4, BCRP, GLUT9 and NPT1 are found in all the papers. Among these transporters, SNPs of BCRP and GLUT9 are significantly associated with gout.[198–200] A later study elucidated that GLUT9 is a primary candidate transporter mediating the basolateral efflux of uric acid into the blood.[201,202] NPT1 is known as a facilitated transporter for organic anions.[122] *In vitro* transport studies demonstrated that NPT4 is also a facilitated transporter for organic anions such as PAH, E1S and bumetanide.[123] These transporters may mediate the efflux of their substrate drugs as well as uric acid into the urine.

### 22.5.3 Metabonomic Analysis to Identify the Endogenous Substrates of Drug Transporters

Metabonomics deals with the comprehensive analysis of low-molecular-weight components in biological samples. Targeted and un-targeted metabonomic analysis helps to identify the endogenous substrates of drug transporters. Eraly *et al.* applied this technique to the phenotyping of plasma and urine samples from Oat1(–/–) mouse to measure sixty organic anions, and demonstrated that eighteen organic anions, such as 3-hydroxyisobutylate, are accumulated in the plasma because of reduction of their urinary excretion.[109] A global metabonomic analysis elucidated that defect of OAT3 also causes the accumulation of unknown compounds in the plasma which are different from those accumulated in Oat1(–/–) mice.[110] Those include thymidine and flavin mononucleotide. They also reported that Oat3(–/–) mice show lower blood pressure compared with wild-type mice, which is attributable to the accumulation of thymidine, an endogenous substrate of OAT3.[110] Administration of thymidine or OAT3 inhibitors, such as esosin Y and probenecid, lowered the systolic blood pressure of mice. Kato *et al.* performed comprehensive comparison of endogenous nucleotides, and anionic and cationic metabolites between wild-type mice and

Ocnt1(–/–) mice, and elucidated that the concentration of ergothioneine, an antioxidant absorbed from the diet in the heart, intestine, kidney and red blood cells was markedly fell in Ocnt1(–/–) mice compared with wild-type mice.[138] Pharmacokinetic analysis uncovered the impact of OCNT1 in the intestinal absorption, and the uptake by non-parenchymal liver cells.[203] van de Wetering *et al.*[204] performed a comprehensive investigation of the impact of MRP3 on the disposition of glucuronide conjugates by targeted metabonomics, surveying compounds which lose 176 Da in mass, the molecular weight of a glucuronic acid moiety with a collision-induced dissociation (CID) technique. They identified some dietary flavonoids the glucuronide conjugates of which show lower plasma concentrations in Mrp3(–/–) mice compared with wild-type mice, indicating the importance of MRP3 in the disposition of glucuronide conjugates of a variety of compounds.

## 22.6 Conclusions

In this chapter we described the impact of drug transporters on the pharmacokinetics of drugs, and their effects. Clinical data support the significance of uptake transporters in the pharmacokinetics of drugs in humans. When the target molecule of a drug is inside the cell, the efflux transporter determines their pharmacological effect or adverse reactions even though it has a negligible impact on the plasma concentration. Because of difficulty in quantitative evaluation of the efflux process, the transporters playing key roles in the efflux process remains unclear in humans. Development of probe substrates applicable to the PET/SPECT imaging will clarify the quantitative relationship between the transport activities and drug response. It is now clear that drug transporters are also important in the disposition of endogenous and food-derived compounds. Metabonomic analysis have successfully identified such compounds in animals, and will also shed a light on any additional roles of drug transporters in humans.

## References


1. P. Borst, R. Evers, M. Kool and J. Wijnholds, *J. Natl. Cancer Inst.*, 2000, **92**, 1295–1302.
2. L. A. Doyle and D. D. Ross, *Oncogene,* 2003, **22**, 7340–7358.
3. M. M. Gottesman, T. Fojo and S. E. Bates, *Nat. Rev. Cancer*, 2002, **2**, 48–58.
4. T. Ishikawa and H. Nakagawa, *J. Exp. Ther. Oncol.*, 2009, **8**, 5–24.
5. D. Keppler, in *Drug Transporters*, ed. M. F. Fromm and R. B. Kim, *Handbook of Experimental Pharmacology,* Springer, New York, 2011, vol. 201, pp. 299–323.
6. J. D. Schuetz, M. C. Connelly, D. Sun, S. G. Paibir, P. M. Flynn, R. V. Srinivas, A. Kumar and A. Fridland, *Nat. Med.*, 1999, **5**, 1048–1051.

7. E. S. Ho, D. C. Lin, D. B. Mendel and T. Cihlar, *J. Am. Soc. Nephrol.*, 2000, **11**, 383–393.
8. Y. Shu, S. A. Sheardown, C. Brown, R. P. Owen, S. Zhang, R. A. Castro, A. G. Ianculescu, L. Yue, J. C. Lo, E. G. Burchard, C. M. Brett and K. M. Giacomini, *J. Clin. Invest.*, 2007, **117**, 1422–1431.
9. G. Ciarimboli, T. Ludwig, D. Lang, H. Pavenstadt, H. Koepsell, H. J. Piechota, J. Haier, U. Jaehde, J. Zisowsky and E. Schlatter, *Am. J. Pathol.*, 2005, **167**, 1477–1484.
10. A. Yonezawa, S. Masuda, K. Nishihara, I. Yano, T. Katsura and K. Inui, *Biochem. Pharmacol.*, 2005, **70**, 1823–1831.
11. M. Okabe, G. Szakacs, M. A. Reimers, T. Suzuki, M. D. Hall, T. Abe, J. Weinstein and M. M. Gottesman, *Mol. Cancer Ther.*, 2008, **7**, 3081–3091.
12. T. Abe, M. Unno, T. Onogawa, T. Tokui, T. N. Kondo, R. Nakagomi, H. Adachi, K. Fujiwara, M. Okabe, T. Suzuki, K. Nunoki, E. Sato, M. Kakyo, T. Nishio, J. Sugita, N. Asano, M. Tanemoto, M. Seki, F. Date, K. Ono, Y. Kondo, K. Shiiba, M. Suzuki, H. Ohtani, T. Shimosegawa, K. Iinuma, H. Nagura, S. Ito and S. Matsuno, *Gastroenterology*, 2001, **120**, 1689–1699.
13. K. M. Giacomini, S. M. Huang, D. J. Tweedie, L. Z. Benet, K. L. Brouwer, X. Chu, A. Dahlin, R. Evers, V. Fischer, K. M. Hillgren, K. A. Hoffmaster, T. Ishikawa, D. Keppler, R. B. Kim, C. A. Lee, M. Niemi, J. W. Polli, Y. Sugiyama, P. W. Swaan, J. A. Ware, S. H. Wright, S. W. Yee, M. J. Zamek-Gliszczynski and L. Zhang, *Nat. Rev. Drug Discovery*, 2010, **9**, 215–236.
14. K. M. Giacomini and Y. Sugiyama, in *Goodman & Gilman's The Pharmacological Basis of Therapeutics*, ed. L. L. Brunton, J. S. Lazo and K. L. Parker, McGraw-Hill Professional Publishing, New York, 11th edn, 2005, pp. 41–70.
15. N. Mizuno, T. Niwa, Y. Yotsumoto and Y. Sugiyama, *Pharmacol. Rev.*, 2003, **55**, 425–461.
16. J. Enokizono, H. Kusuhara, A. Ose, A. H. Schinkel and Y. Sugiyama, *Drug Metab. Dispos.*, 2008, **36**, 995–1002.
17. J. W. Jonker, J. W. Smit, R. F. Brinkhuis, M. Maliepaard, J. H. Beijnen, J. H. Schellens and A. H. Schinkel, *J. Natl. Cancer Inst.*, 2000, **92**, 1651–1656.
18. M. Sasaki, H. Suzuki, K. Ito, T. Abe and Y. Sugiyama, *J. Biol. Chem.*, 2002, **277**, 6497–6503.
19. S. Matsushima, K. Maeda, C. Kondo, M. Hirano, M. Sasaki, H. Suzuki and Y. Sugiyama, *J. Pharmacol. Exp. Ther.*, 2005, **314**, 1059–1067.
20. Y. Cui, J. Konig and D. Keppler, *Mol. Pharmacol.*, 2001, **60**, 934–943.
21. N. Ishiguro, K. Maeda, A. Saito, W. Kishimoto, S. Matsushima, T. Ebner, W. Roth, T. Igarashi and Y. Sugiyama, *Drug Metab. Dispos.*, 2008, **36**, 796–805.
22. A. T. Nies, E. Herrmann, M. Brom and D. Keppler, *Naunyn-Schmiedebergs Arch. Pharmakol.*, 2008, **376**, 449–461.

23. M. Sasaki, H. Suzuki, J. Aoki, K. Ito, P. J. Meier and Y. Sugiyama, *Mol. Pharmacol.*, 2004, **66**, 450–459.
24. J. Konig, O. Zolk, K. Singer, C. Hoffmann and M. Fromm, *Br. J. Pharmacol.*, 2011, **163**, 546–555.
25. T. Sato, S. Masuda, A. Yonezawa, Y. Tanihara, T. Katsura and K. Inui, *Biochem. Pharmacol.*, 2008, **76**, 894–903.
26. T. Imaoka, H. Kusuhara, S. Adachi-Akahane, M. Hasegawa, N. Morita, H. Endou and Y. Sugiyama, *J. Am. Soc. Nephrol.*, 2004, **15**, 2012–2022.
27. K. Kopplow, K. Letschert, J. Konig, B. Walter and D. Keppler, *Mol. Pharmacol.*, 2005, **68**, 1031–1038.
28. M. Hirouchi, H. Kusuhara, R. Onuki, B. W. Ogilvie, A. Parkinson and Y. Sugiyama, *Drug Metab. Dispos.*, 2009, **37**, 2103–2111.
29. T. Watanabe, H. Kusuhara, K. Maeda, H. Kanamaru, Y. Saito, Z. Hu and Y. Sugiyama, *Drug Metab. Dispos.*, 2010, **38**, 215–222.
30. T. Watanabe, H. Kusuhara, K. Maeda, Y. Shitara and Y. Sugiyama, *J. Pharmacol. Exp. Ther.*, 2009, **328**, 652–662.
31. T. Watanabe, K. Maeda, T. Kondo, H. Nakayama, S. Horita, H. Kusuhara and Y. Sugiyama, *Drug Metab. Dispos.*, 2009, **37**, 1471–1479.
32. I. Ieiri, S. Higuchi and Y. Sugiyama, *Expert Opin. Drug Metab. Toxicol.*, 2009, **5**, 703–729.
33. A. Kalliokoski and M. Niemi, *Br. J. Pharmacol.*, 2009, **158**, 693–705.
34. J. Kindla, M. F. Fromm and J. Konig, *Expert Opin. Drug Metab. Toxicol.*, 2009, **5**, 489–500.
35. H. Kusuhara and Y. Sugiyama, *Drug Metab. Pharmacokinet.*, 2009, **24**, 37–52.
36. K. Maeda and Y. Sugiyama, *Drug Metab. Pharmacokinet.*, 2008, **23**, 223–235.
37. M. Hirano, K. Maeda, Y. Shitara and Y. Sugiyama, *J. Pharmacol. Exp. Ther.*, 2004, **311**, 139–146.
38. N. Ishiguro, K. Maeda, W. Kishimoto, A. Saito, A. Harada, T. Ebner, W. Roth, T. Igarashi and Y. Sugiyama, *Drug Metab. Dispos.*, 2006, **34**, 1109–1115.
39. A. Kalliokoski, M. Neuvonen, P. J. Neuvonen and M. Niemi, *J. Clin. Pharmacol.*, 2008, **48**, 311–321.
40. M. Niemi, J. T. Backman, L. I. Kajosaari, J. B. Leathart, M. Neuvonen, A. K. Daly, M. Eichelbaum, K. T. Kivisto and P. J. Neuvonen, *Clin. Pharmacol. Ther.*, 2005, **77**, 468–478.
41. M. K. Pasanen, H. Fredrikson, P. J. Neuvonen and M. Niemi, *Clin. Pharmacol. Ther.*, 2007, **82**, 726–733.
42. M. K. Pasanen, M. Neuvonen, P. J. Neuvonen and M. Niemi, *Pharmacogenet. Genomics*, 2006, **16**, 873–879.
43. Y. Shitara, T. Itoh, H. Sato, A. P. Li and Y. Sugiyama, *J. Pharmacol. Exp. Ther.*, 2003, **304**, 610–616.
44. R. Tirona, B. F. Leake, A. W. Wolkoff and R. B. Kim, *J. Pharmacol. Exp. Ther.*, 2003, **304**, 223–228.

45. H. Lu, S. Choudhuri, K. Ogura, I. L. Csanaky, X. Lei, X. Cheng, P. Z. Song and C. D. Klaassen, *Toxicol. Sci.*, 2008, **103**, 35–45.
46. H. Zaher, H. E. zu Schwabedissen, R. G. Tirona, M. L. Cox, L. A. Obert, N. Agrawal, J. Palandra, J. L. Stock, R. B. Kim and J. A. Ware, *Mol. Pharmacol.*, 2008, **74**, 320–329.
47. C. Chen, J. L. Stock, X. Liu, J. Shi, J. W. Van Deusen, D. A. DiMattia, R. G. Dullea and S. M. de Morais, *Drug Metab. Dispos.*, 2008, **36**, 1840–1845.
48. E. van de Steeg, A. van Esch, E. Wagenaar, C. M. van der Kruijssen, O. van Tellingen, K. E. Kenworthy and A. H. Schinkel, *Clin. Cancer Res.*, 2010, **17**, 294–301.
49. E. van de Steeg, E. Wagenaar, C. M. van der Kruijssen, J. E. Burggraaff, D. R. de Waart, R. P. Elferink, K. E. Kenworthy and A. H. Schinkel, *J. Clin. Invest.*, 2010, **120**, 2942–2952.
50. W. Muck, I. Mai, L. Fritsche, K. Ochmann, G. Rohde, S. Unger, A. Johne, S. Bauer, K. Budde, I. Roots, H. H. Neumayer and J. Kuhlmann, *Clin. Pharmacol. Ther.*, 1999, **65**, 251–261.
51. Y. Shitara, Y. Nagamatsu, S. Wada, Y. Sugiyama and T. Horie, *Drug Metab. Dispos.*, 2009, **37**, 1172–1178.
52. Y. Shitara, T. Horie and Y. Sugiyama, *Eur. J. Pharm. Sci.*, 2006, **27**, 425–446.
53. S. G. Simonson, A. Raza, P. D. Martin, P. D. Mitchell, J. A. Jarcho, C. D. Brown, A. S. Windass and D. W. Schneck, *Clin. Pharmacol. Ther.*, 2004, **76**, 167–177.
54. L. I. Kajosaari, M. Niemi, M. Neuvonen, J. Laitila, P. J. Neuvonen and J. T. Backman, *Clin. Pharmacol. Ther.*, 2005, **78**, 388–399.
55. Y. Y. Lau, Y. Huang, L. Frassetto and L. Z. Benet, *Clin. Pharmacol. Ther.*, 2007, **81**, 194–204.
56. R. G. Tirona, B. F. Leake, G. Merino and R. B. Kim, *J. Biol. Chem.*, 2001, **276**, 35669–35675.
57. I. Ieiri, S. Suwannakul, K. Maeda, H. Uchimaru, K. Hashimoto, M. Kimura, H. Fujino, M. Hirano, H. Kusuhara, S. Irie, S. Higuchi and Y. Sugiyama, *Clin. Pharmacol. Ther.*, 2007, **82**, 541–547.
58. K. Maeda, I. Ieiri, K. Yasuda, A. Fujino, H. Fujiwara, K. Otsubo, M. Hirano, T. Watanabe, Y. Kitamura, H. Kusuhara and Y. Sugiyama, *Clin. Pharmacol. Ther.*, 2006, **79**, 427–439.
59. Y. Nishizato, I. Ieiri, H. Suzuki, M. Kimura, K. Kawabata, T. Hirota, H. Takane, S. Irie, H. Kusuhara, Y. Urasaki, A. Urae, S. Higuchi, K. Otsubo and Y. Sugiyama, *Clin. Pharmacol. Ther.*, 2003, **73**, 554–565.
60. M. Iwai, H. Suzuki, I. Ieiri, K. Otsubo and Y. Sugiyama, *Pharmacogenetics*, 2004, **14**, 749–757.
61. J. Y. Han, H. S. Lim, Y. H. Park, S. Y. Lee and J. S. Lee, *Lung Cancer*, 2009, **63**, 115–120.
62. X. Xiang, S. R. Jada, H. H. Li, L. Fan, L. S. Tham, C. I. Wong, S. C. Lee, R. Lim, Q. Y. Zhou, B. C. Goh, E. H. Tan and B. Chowbay, *Pharmacogenet. Genomics*, 2006, **16**, 683–691.

63. E. Link, S. Parish, J. Armitage, L. Bowman, S. Heath, F. Matsuda, I. Gut, M. Lathrop and R. Collins, *N. Engl. J. Med.*, 2008, **359**, 789–799.
64. K. D. Marciante, J. P. Durda, S. R. Heckbert, T. Lumley, K. Rice, B. McKnight, R. A. Totah, B. Tamraz, D. L. Kroetz, H. Fukushima, R. Kaspera, J. C. Bis, N. L. Glazer, G. Li, T. R. Austin, K. D. Taylor, J. I. Rotter, C. E. Jaquish, P. Y. Kwok, R. P. Tracy and B. M. Psaty, *Pharmacogenet. Genomics*, 2011, **21**(5), 280–288.
65. L. R. Trevino, N. Shimasaki, W. Yang, J. C. Panetta, C. Cheng, D. Pei, D. Chan, A. Sparreboom, K. M. Giacomini, C. H. Pui, W. E. Evans and M. V. Relling, *J. Clin. Oncol.*, 2009, **27**, 5972–5978.
66. K. Kiyotani, T. Mushiroda, M. Kubo, H. Zembutsu, Y. Sugiyama and Y. Nakamura, *Cancer Sci.*, 2008, **99**, 967–972.
67. H. Suzuki and Y. Sugiyama, *Semin. Liver Dis.*, 1998, **18**, 359–376.
68. M. L. Vlaming, K. Mohrmann, E. Wagenaar, D. R. de Waart, R. P. Elferink, J. S. Lagas, O. van Tellingen, L. D. Vainchtein, H. Rosing, J. H. Beijnen, J. H. Schellens and A. H. Schinkel, *J. Pharmacol. Exp. Ther.*, 2006, **318**, 319–327.
69. A. Yamada, K. Maeda, E. Kamiyama, D. Sugiyama, T. Kondo, Y. Shiroyanagi, H. Nakazawa, T. Okano, M. Adachi, J. D. Schuetz, Y. Adachi, Z. Hu, H. Kusuhara and Y. Sugiyama, *Drug Metab. Dispos.*, 2007, **35**, 2166–2176.
70. W. Yamashiro, K. Maeda, M. Hirouchi, Y. Adachi, Z. Hu and Y. Sugiyama, *Drug Metab. Dispos.*, 2006, **34**, 1247–1254.
71. T. Ando, H. Kusuhara, G. Merino, A. I. Alvarez, A. H. Schinkel and Y. Sugiyama, *Drug Metab. Dispos.*, 2007, **35**, 1873–1379.
72. M. Hirano, K. Maeda, S. Matsushima, Y. Nozaki, H. Kusuhara and Y. Sugiyama, *Mol. Pharmacol.*, 2005, **68**, 800–807.
73. A. K. Daly, G. P. Aithal, J. B. Leathart, R. A. Swainsbury, T. A. Dang and C. P. Day, *Gastroenterology*, 2007, **132**, 272–281.
74. P. Ranganathan, R. Culverhouse, S. Marsh, A. Mody, T. J. Scott–Horton, R. Brasington, A. Joseph, V. Reddy, S. Eisen and H. L. McLeod, *J. Rheumatol.*, 2008, **35**, 572–579.
75. F. A. de Jong, T. J. Scott-Horton, D. L. Kroetz, H. L. McLeod, L. E. Friberg, R. H. Mathijssen, J. Verweij, S. Marsh and A. Sparreboom, *Clin. Pharmacol. Ther.*, 2007, **81**, 42–49.
76. X. Y. Chu, Y. Kato and Y. Sugiyama, *Cancer Res.*, 1997, **57**, 1934–1938.
77. M. Horikawa, Y. Kato and Y. Sugiyama, *Pharm. Res.*, 2002, **19**, 1345–1353.
78. C. Kondo, H. Suzuki, M. Itoda, S. Ozawa, J. Sawada, D. Kobayashi, I. Ieiri, K. Mine, K. Ohtsubo and Y. Sugiyama, *Pharm. Res.*, 2004, **21**, 1895–1903.
79. J. E. Keskitalo, O. Zolk, M. F. Fromm, K. J. Kurkinen, P. J. Neuvonen and M. Niemi, *Clin. Pharmacol. Ther.*, 2009, **86**, 197–203.
80. Y. Yamasaki, I. Ieiri, H. Kusuhara, T. Sasaki, M. Kimura, H. Tabuchi, Y. Ando, S. Irie, J. Ware, Y. Nakai, S. Higuchi and Y. Sugiyama, *Clin. Pharmacol. Ther.*, 2008, **84**, 95–103.

81. W. Zhang, B. N. Yu, Y. J. He, L. Fan, Q. Li, Z. Q. Liu, A. Wang, Y. L. Liu, Z. R. Tan, J. Fen, Y. F. Huang and H. H. Zhou, *Clin. Chim. Acta*, 2006, **373**, 99–103.
82. R. H. Ho, L. Choi, W. Lee, G. Mayo, U. I. Schwarz, R. G. Tirona, D. G. Bailey, C. M. Stein and R. B. Kim, *Pharmacogenet. Genomics*, 2007, **17**, 647–656.
83. N. Zelcer, K. van de Wetering, M. Hillebrand, E. Sarton, A. Kuil, P. R. Wielinga, T. Tephly, A. Dahan, J. H. Beijnen and P. Borst, *Proc. Natl. Acad. Sci. U. S. A.*, 2005, **102**, 7274–7279.
84. M. J. Zamek-Gliszczynski, K. Nezasa, X. Tian, A. S. Bridges, K. Lee, M. G. Belinsky, G. D. Kruh and K. L. Brouwer, *J. Pharmacol. Exp. Ther.*, 2006, **319**, 1485–1491.
85. Y. Kitamura, M. Hirouchi, H. Kusuhara, J. D. Schuetz and Y. Sugiyama, *J. Pharmacol. Exp. Ther.*, 2008, **327**, 465–473.
86. X. Tian, B. Swift, M. J. Zamek-Gliszczynski, M. G. Belinsky, G. D. Kruh and K. L. Brouwer, *Drug Metab. Dispos.*, 2008, **36**, 911–915.
87. M. Y. El-Mir, V. Nogueira, E. Fontaine, N. Averet, M. Rigoulet and X. Leverve, *J. Biol. Chem.*, 2000, **275**, 223–228.
88. M. R. Owen, E. Doran and A. P. Halestrap, *Biochem. J.*, 2000, **348**, 607–614.
89. R. J. Shaw, K. A. Lamia, D. Vasquez, S. H. Koo, N. Bardeesy, R. A. Depinho, M. Montminy and L. C. Cantley, *Science*, 2005, **310**, 1642–1646.
90. G. Zhou, R. Myers, Y. Li, Y. Chen, X. Shen, J. Fenyk-Melody, M. Wu, J. Ventre, T. Doebber, N. Fujii, N. Musi, M. F. Hirshman, L. J. Goodyear and D. E. Moller, *J. Clin. Invest.*, 2001, **108**, 1167–1674.
91. D. S. Wang, J. W. Jonker, Y. Kato, H. Kusuhara, A. H. Schinkel and Y. Sugiyama, *J. Pharmacol. Exp. Ther.*, 2002, **302**, 510–515.
92. D. S. Wang, H. Kusuhara, Y. Kato, J. W. Jonker, A. H. Schinkel and Y. Sugiyama, *Mol. Pharmacol.*, 2003, **63**, 844–848.
93. M. Otsuka, T. Matsumoto, R. Morimoto, S. Arioka, H. Omote and Y. Moriyama, *Proc. Natl. Acad. Sci. U. S. A.*, 2005, **102**, 17923–17928.
94. T. Terada, S. Masuda, J. Asaka, M. Tsuda, T. Katsura and K. Inui, *Pharm. Res.*, 2006, **23**, 1696–1701.
95. S. Ito, H. Kusuhara, Y. Kuroiwa, C. Wu, Y. Moriyama, K. Inoue, T. Kondo, H. Yuasa, H. Nakayama, S. Horita and Y. Sugiyama, *J. Pharmacol. Exp. Ther.*, 2010, **333**, 341–350.
96. H. Kusuhara, S. Ito, Y. Kumagai, M. Jiang, T. Shiroshita, Y. Moriyama and Y. Sugiyama, *Clin. Pharmacol. Ther.*, 2011, **89**, 837–844.
97. M. Tsuda, T. Terada, T. Mizuno, T. Katsura, J. Shimakura and K. Inui, *Mol. Pharmacol.*, 2009, **75**, 1280–1286.
98. Y. Shu, M. K. Leabman, F. Feng, L. M. Mangravite, C. C. Huang, D. Stryke, M. Kawamoto, S. J. Johns, J. DeYoung, E. Carlson, T. E. Ferrin, I. Herskowitz and K. M. Giacomini, *Proc. Natl. Acad. Sci. U. S. A.*, 2003, **100**, 5902–5907.

99. Y. Shu, C. Brown, R. A. Castro, R. J. Shi, E. T. Lin, R. P. Owen, S. A. Sheardown, L. Yue, E. G. Burchard, C. M. Brett and K. M. Giacomini, *Clin. Pharmacol. Ther.*, 2008, **83**, 273–280.
100. M. L. Becker, L. E. Visser, R. H. van Schaik, A. Hofman, A. G. Uitterlinden and B. H. Stricker, *Diabetes*, 2009, **58**, 745–749.
101. M. V. Tzvetkov, S. V. Vormfelde, D. Balen, I. Meineke, T. Schmidt, D. Sehrt, I. Sabolić, H. Koepsell and J. Brockmöller, *Clin. Pharmacol. Ther.*, 2009, **86**, 299–306.
102. A. A. El-Sheikh, R. Masereeuw and F. G. Russel, *Eur. J. Pharmacol.*, 2008, **585**, 245–255.
103. R. Masereeuw and F. G. Russel, *Pharmacol. Ther.*, 2010, **126**, 200–216.
104. T. Sekine, H. Miyazaki and H. Endou, *Am. J. Physiol. Renal Physiol.*, 2006, **290**, F251–F261.
105. T. Mikkaichi, T. Suzuki, T. Onogawa, M. Tanemoto, H. Mizutamari, M. Okada, T. Chaki, S. Masuda, T. Tokui, N. Eto, M. Abe, F. Satoh, M. Unno, T. Hishinuma, K. Inui, S. Ito, J. Goto and T. Abe, *Proc. Natl. Acad. Sci. U. S. A.*, 2004, **101**, 3569–3574.
106. H. Motohashi, Y. Sakurai, H. Saito, S. Masuda, Y. Urakami, M. Goto, A. Fukatsu, O. Ogawa and K. Inui, *J. Am. Soc. Nephrol.*, 2002, **13**, 866–874.
107. M. Hasegawa, H. Kusuhara, D. Sugiyama, K. Ito, S. Ueda, H. Endou and Y. Sugiyama, *J. Pharmacol. Exp. Ther.*, 2002, **300**, 746–753.
108. M. Hasegawa, H. Kusuhara, H. Endou and Y. Sugiyama, *J. Pharmacol. Exp. Ther.*, 2003, **305**, 1087–1097.
109. S. A. Eraly, V. Vallon, D. A. Vaughn, J. A. Gangoiti, K. Richter, M. Nagle, J. C. Monte, T. Rieg, D. M. Truong, J. M. Long, B. A. Barshop, G. Kaler and S. K. Nigam, *J. Biol. Chem.*, 2006, **281**, 5072–5083.
110. V. Vallon, T. Rieg, S. Y. Ahn,W. Wu, S. A. Eraly and S. K. Nigam, *Am. J. Physiol. Renal. Physiol.*, 2008, **294**, F867–F873.
111. A. L. Vanwert, R. M. Bailey and D. H. Sweet, *Am. J. Physiol. Renal Physiol.*, 2007, **293**, F1332–F1341.
112. A. L. Vanwert, C. Srimaroeng and D. H. Sweet, *Mol. Pharmacol.*, 2008, **74**, 122–131.
113. A. L. Vanwert and D. H. Sweet, *Pharm. Res.*, 2008, **25**, 453–462.
114. Y. Nozaki, H. Kusuhara, T. Kondo, M. Hasegawa, Y. Shiroyanagi, H. Nakazawa, T. Okano and Y. Sugiyama, *J. Pharmacol. Exp. Ther.*, 2007, **321**, 362–369.
115. Y. Nozaki, H. Kusuhara, T. Kondo, M. Iwaki, Y. Shiroyanagi, H. Nakayama, S. Horita, H. Nakazawa, T. Okano and Y. Sugiyama, *J. Pharmacol. Exp. Ther.*, 2007, **322**, 1162–1170.
116. T. Watanabe, H. Kusuhara, T. Watanabe, Y. Debori, K. Maeda, T. Kondo, H. Nakayama, S. Horita, B. W. Ogilvie, A. Parkinson, Z. Hu and Y. Sugiyama, *Drug Metab. Dispos.*, 2011, **39**, 1031–1038.
117. G. Hill, T. Cihlar, C. Oo, E. S. Ho, K. Prior, H. Wiltshire, J. Barrett, B. Liu and P. Ward, *Drug Metab. Dispos.*, 2002, **30**, 13–19.

118. N. Yasui-Furukori, T. Uno, K. Sugawara and T. Tateishi, *Clin. Pharmacol. Ther.*, 2005, **77**, 17–23.
119. N. Inotsume, M. Nishimura, M. Nakano, S. Fujiyama and T. Sato, *J. Clin. Pharmacol.*, 1990, **30**, 50–56.
120. H. Tahara, H. Kusuhara, M. Chida, E. Fuse and Y. Sugiyama, *J. Pharmacol. Exp. Ther.*, 2006, **316**, 1187–1194.
121. H. Tahara, H. Kusuhara, H. Endou, H. Koepsell, T. Imaoka, E. Fuse and Y. Sugiyama, *J. Pharmacol. Exp. Ther.*, 2005, **315**, 337–345.
122. P. Jutabha, N. Anzai, K. Kitamura, A. Taniguchi, S. Kaneko, K. Yan, H. Yamada, H. Shimada, T. Kimura, T. Katada, T. Fukutomi, K. Tomita, W. Urano, H. Yamanaka, G. Seki, T. Fujita, Y. Moriyama, A. Yamada, S. Uchida, M. F. Wempe, H. Endou and H. Sakurai, *J. Biol. Chem.*, 2005, **285**, 35123–35132.
123. H. Uchino, I. Tamai, K. Yamashita, Y. Minemoto, Y. Sai, H. Yabuuchi, H. Miyamoto, E. Takeda and A. Tsuji, *Biochem. Biophys. Res. Commun.*, 2000, **270**, 254–259.
124. A. E. Busch, A. Schuster, S. Waldegger, C. A. Wagner, G. Zempel, S. Broer, J. Biber, H. Murer and F. Lang, *Proc. Natl. Acad. Sci. U.S.A.*, 1996, **93**, 5347–5351.
125. L. Ci, H. Kusuhara, M. Adachi, J. D. Schuetz, K. Takeuchi and Y. Sugiyama, *Mol. Pharmacol.*, 2007, **71**, 1591–1597.
126. M. Hasegawa, H. Kusuhara, M. Adachi, J. D. Schuetz, K. Takeuchi and Y. Sugiyama, *J. Am. Soc. Nephrol.*, 2007, **18**, 37–45.
127. T. Imaoka, H. Kusuhara, M. Adachi, J. D. Schuetz, K. Takeuchi and Y. Sugiyama, *Mol. Pharmacol.*, 2007, **71**, 619–627.
128. J. S. Hulot, E. Villard, A. Maguy, V. Morel, L. Mir, I. Tostivint, D. William-Faltaos, C. Fernandez, S. Hatem, G. Deray, M. Komajda, V. Leblond and P. Lechat, *Pharmacogenet. Genomics*, 2005, **15**, 277–285.
129. K. C. Cundy, *Clin. Pharmacokinet.*, 1999, **36**, 127–143.
130. M. G. Belinsky, P. Guo, K. Lee, F. Zhou, E. Kotova, A. Grinberg, H. Westphal, I. Shchaveleva, A. Klein-Szanto, J. M. Gallo and G. D. Kruh, *Cancer Res.*, 2007, **67**, 262–268.
131. H. Koepsell, K. Lips and C. Volk, *Pharm. Res.*, 2007, **24**, 1227–1251.
132. K. Inui, H. Saito and R. Hori, *Biochem. J.*, 1985, **227**, 199–203.
133. I. Tamai, H. Yabuuchi, J. Nezu, Y. Sai, A. Oku, M. Shimane and A. Tsuji, *FEBS Lett.*, 1997, **419**, 107–111.
134. X. Wu, P. D. Prasad, F. H. Leibach and V. Ganapathy, *Biochem. Biophys. Res. Commun.*, 1998, **246**, 589–595.
135. T. J. Urban, C. Brown, R. A. Castro, N. Shah, R. Mercer, Y. Huang, C. M. Brett, E. G. Burchard and K. M. Giacomini, *Clin. Pharmacol. Ther.*, 2008, **83**, 416–421.
136. T. Kano, Y. Kato, K. Ito, T. Ogihara, Y. Kubo and A. Tsuji, *Drug Metab. Dispos.*, 2009, **37**, 1009–1016.
137. D. Grundemann, S. Harlfinger, S. Golz, A. Geerts, A. Lazar, R. Berkels, N. Jung, A. Rubbert and E. Schomig, *Proc. Natl. Acad. Sci. U. S. A.*, 2005, **102**, 5256–5261.

138. Y. Kato, Y. Kubo, D. Iwata, S. Kato, T. Sudo, T. Sugiura, T. Kagaya, T. Wakayama, A. Hirayama, M. Sugimoto, K. Sugihara, S. Kaneko, T. Soga, M. Asano, M. Tomita, T. Matsui, M. Wada and A. Tsuji, *Pharm. Res.*, 2010, **27**, 832–840.
139. J. Nezu, I. Tamai, A. Oku, R. Ohashi, H. Yabuuchi, N. Hashimoto, H. Nikaido, Y. Sai, A. Koizumi, Y. Shoji, G. Takada, T. Matsuishi, M. Yoshino, H. Kato, T. Ohura, G. Tsujimoto, J. Hayakawa, M. Shimane and A. Tsuji, *Nat. Genet.*, 1999, **21**, 91–94.
140. I. Tamai, R. Ohashi, J. Nezu, H. Yabuuchi, A. Oku, M. Shimane, Y. Sai and A. Tsuji, *J. Biol. Chem.*, 1998, **273**, 20378–20382.
141. S. Masuda, T. Terada, A. Yonezawa, Y. Tanihara, K. Kishimoto, T. Katsura, O. Ogawa and K. Inui, *J. Am. Soc. Nephrol.*, 2006, **17**, 2127–2135.
142. Y. Tanihara, S. Masuda, T. Sato, T. Katsura, O. Ogawa and K. Inui, *Biochem. Pharmacol.*, 2007, **74**, 359–371.
143. S. Watanabe, M. Tsuda, T. Terada, T. Katsura and K. Inui, *J. Pharmacol. Exp. Ther.*, 2010, **334**, 651–656.
144. S. Matsushima, K. Maeda, K. Inoue, K. Y. Ohta, H. Yuasa, T. Kondo, H. Nakayama, S. Horita, H. Kusuhara and Y. Sugiyama, *Drug Metab. Dispos.*, 2009, **37**, 555–559.
145. R. Safirstein, P. Miller and J. B. Guttenplan, *Kidney Int.*, 1984, **25**, 753–758.
146. S. Yokoo, A. Yonezawa, S. Masuda, A. Fukatsu, T. Katsura and K. Inui, *Biochem. Pharmacol.*, 2007, **74**, 477–487.
147. R. M. Franke, A. M. Kosloske, C. S. Lancaster, K. K. Filipski, C. Hu, O. Zolk, R. H. Mathijssen and A. Sparreboom, *Clin. Cancer Res.*, 2010, **16**, 4198–4206.
148. K. K. Filipski, R. H. Mathijssen, T. S. Mikkelsen, A. H. Schinkel and A. Sparreboom, *Clin. Pharmacol. Ther.*, 2009, **86**, 396–402.
149. M. K. Leabman, C. C. Huang, M. Kawamoto, S. J. Johns, D. Stryke, T. E. Ferrin, J. DeYoung, T. Taylor, A. G. Clark, I. Herskowitz and K. M. Giacomini, *Pharmacogenetics*, 2002, **12**, 395–405.
150. Y. Tanihara, S. Masuda, T. Katsura and K. Inui, *Biochem. Pharmacol.*, 2009, **78**, 1263–1271.
151. T. Nakamura, A. Yonezawa, S. Hashimoto, T. Katsura and K. Inui, *Biochem. Pharmacol.*, 2010, **80**, 1762–1767.
152. A. Yonezawa and K. Inui, *Biochem. Pharmacol.*, 2010, **81**, 563–568.
153. J. M. Scherrmann, *Expert Opin. Drug Metab. Toxicol.*, 2005, **1**, 233–246.
154. S. P. Letrent, G. M. Pollack, K. R. Brouwer and K. L. Brouwer, *Drug Metab. Dispos.*, 1999, **27**, 827–834.
155. J. W. Jonker, E. Wagenaar, L. van Deemter, R. Gottschlich, H. M. Bender, J. Dasenbrock and A. H. Schinkel, *Br. J. Pharmacol.*, 1999, **127**, 43–50.
156. A. H. Schinkel, J. J. Smit, O. van Tellingen, J. H. Beijnen, E. Wagenaar, L. van Deemter, C. A. Mol, M. A. van der Valk, E. C. Robanus-Maandag, H. P. te Riele, A. J. M. Berns and P. Bors, *Cell*, 1994, **77**, 491–502.

157. P. H. Elsinga, N. H. Hendrikse, J. Bart, W. Vaalburg and A. van Waarde, *Curr. Pharm. Des.*, 2004, **10**, 1493–1503.
158. Y. J. Lee, J. Maeda, H. Kusuhara, T. Okauchi, M. Inaji, Y. Nagai, S. Obayashi, R. Nakao, K. Suzuki, Y. Sugiyama and T. Suhara, *J. Pharmacol. Exp. Ther.*, 2006, **316**, 647–653.
159. L. Sasongko, J. M. Link, M. Muzi, D. A. Mankoff, X. Yang, A. C. Collier, S. Shoner and J. D. Unadkat, *Clin. Pharmacol. Ther.*, 2005, **77**, 503–514.
160. W. C. Kreisl, J. S. Liow, N. Kimura, N. Seneca, S. S. Zoghbi, C. L. Morse, P. Herscovitch, V. W. Pike and R. B. Innis, *J. Nucl. Med.*, **51**, 2010, 559–566.
161. A. J. Sadeque, C. Wandel, H. He, S. Shah and A. J. Wood, *Clin. Pharmacol. Ther.*, 2000, **68**, 231–237.
162. A. Takano, H. Kusuhara, T. Suhara, I. Ieiri, T. Morimoto, Y. J. Lee, J. Maeda, Y. Ikoma, H. Ito, K. Suzuki and Y. Sugiyama, *J. Nucl. Med.*, 2006, **47**, 1427–1433.
163. J. Enokizono, H. Kusuhara and Y. Sugiyama, *Mol. Pharmacol.*, 2007, **72**, 967–975.
164. R. L. Oostendorp, T. Buckle, J. H. Beijnen, O. van Tellingen, J. H. Schellens, *Invest. New Drugs*, 2009, **27**, 31–40.
165. J. W. Polli, K. L. Olson, J. P. Chism, L. S. John-Williams, R. L. Yeager, S. M. Woodard, V. Otto, S. Castellino and V. E. Demby, *Drug Metab. Dispos.*, 2009, **37**, 439–442.
166. L. Zhou, K. Schmidt, F. R. Nelson, V. Zelesky, M. D. Troutman and B. Feng, *Drug Metab. Dispos.*, 2009, **37**, 946–955.
167. H. Kodaira, J. Kusuhara, J. Ushiki, E. Fuse and Y. Sugiyama, *J. Pharmacol. Exp. Ther.*, 2010, **333**, 788–796.
168. M. Leggas, M. Adachi, G. L. Scheffer, D. Sun, P. Wielinga, G. Du, K. E. Mercer, Y. Zhuang, J. C. Panetta, B. Johnston, R. J. Scheper, C. F. Stewart and J. D. Schuetz, *Mol. Cell Biol.*, 2004, **24**, 7612–7621.
169. A. Ose, M. Ito, H. Kusuhara, K. Yamatsugu, M. Kanai, M. Shibasaki, M. Hosokawa, J. D. Schuetz and Y. Sugiyama, *Drug Metab. Dispos.*, 2009, **37**, 315–321.
170. S. Toh, M. Wada, T. Uchiumi, A. Inokuchi, Y. Makino, Y. Horie, Y. Adachi, S. Sakisaka and M. Kuwano, *Am. J. Hum. Genet.*, 1999, **64**, 739–746.
171. J. W. Jonker, M. Buitelaar, E. Wagenaar, M. A. Van der Valk, G. L. Scheffer, R. J. Scheper, T. Plosch, F. Kuipers, R. P. Elferink, H. Rosing, J. H. Beijnen and A. H. Schinkel, *Proc. Natl. Acad. Sci. U. S. A.*, 2002, **99**, 15649–15654.
172. R. P. Elferink, R. Ottenhoff, W. Liefting, J. de Haan and P. L. Jansen, *J. Clin. Invest.*, 1989, **84**, 476–483.
173. H. Kurisu, K. Kamisaka, T. Koyo, S. Yamasuge, H. Igarashi, H. Maezawa, T. Uesugi and O. Tagaya, *Life Sci.*, 1991, **49**, 1003–1011.
174. Y. Cui, J. Konig, I. Leier, U. Buchholz and D. Keppler, *J. Biol. Chem.*, 2001, **276**, 9626–9630.

175. P. Wang, R. B. Kim, J. R. Chowdhury and A. W. Wolkoff, *J. Biol. Chem.*, 2003, **278**, 20695–20699.
176. W. Zhang, Y. J. He, Z. Gan, L. Fan, Q. Li, A. Wang, Z. Q. Liu, S. Deng, Y. F. Huang, L. Y. Xu and H. H. Zhou, *Clin. Exp. Pharmacol. Physiol.*, 2007, **34**, 1240–1244.
177. S. Sanna, F. Busonero, A. Maschio, P. F. McArdle, G. Usala, M. Dei, S. Lai, A. Mulas, M. G. Piras, L. Perseu, M. Masala, M. Marongiu, L. Crisponi, S. Naitza, R. Galanello, G. R. Abecasis, A. R. Shuldiner, D. Schlessinger, A. Cao and M. Uda, *Hum. Mol. Genet.*, 2009, **18**, 2711–2718.
178. H. Kusuhara, Y. H. Han, M. Shimoda, E. Kokue, H. Suzuki and Y. Sugiyama, *Am. J. Physiol.*, 1998, **275**, G789–G796.
179. Y. Kitamura, H. Kusuhara and Y. Sugiyama, *Pharm. Res.*, 2010, **27**, 665–672.
180. J. Kabat–Koperska, W. Motyl, L. Domanski, K. Safranow, E. Golembiewska, K. Kedzierska and K. Ciechanowski, *Acta Med. Austriaca*, 2004, **31**, 51–55.
181. Y. Urakami, N. Kimura, M. Okuda and K. Inui, *Pharm. Res.*, 2004, **21**, 976–981.
182. M. Opravil, G. Keusch and R. Luthy, *Antimicrob. Agents Chemother.*, 1993, **37**, 1056–1060.
183. M. Okuda, N. Kimura and K. Inui, *Drug Metab. Pharmacokinet.*, 2006, **21**, 432–436.
184. Y. Imamura, N. Murayama, N. Okudaira, A. Kurihara, O. Okazaki, T. Izumi, K. Inoue, H. Yuasa, H. Kusuhara and Y. Sugiyama, *Clin. Pharmacol. Ther.*, 2011, **89**, 81–88.
185. N. Sarapa, P. Wickremasingha, N. Ge, R. Weitzman, M. Fuellhart, C. Yen and J. Lloyd-Parks, *Antimicrob. Agents Chemother.*, 2007, **51**, 1912–1917.
186. A. Enomoto, H. Kimura, A. Chairoungdua, Y. Shigeta, P. Jutabha, S. H. Cha, M. Hosoyamada, M. Takeda, T. Sekine, T. Igarashi, H. Matsuo, Y. Kikuchi, T. Oda, K. Ichida, T. Hosoya, K. Shimokata, T. Niwa, Y. Kanai and H. Endou, *Nature*, 2002, **417**, 447–452.
187. M. Malaguarnera, M. Vacante, C. Russo, G. Dipasquale, M. P. Gargante and M. Motta, *Expert Opin. Pharmacother.*, 2009, **10**, 737–742.
188. T. Hamada, K. Ichida, M. Hosoyamada, E. Mizuta, K. Yanagihara, K. Sonoyama, S. Sugihara, O. Igawa, T. Hosoya, A. Ohtahara, C. Shigamasa, Y. Yamamoto, H. Ninomiya and I. Hisatome, *Am. J. Hypertens.*, 2008, **21**, 1157–1162.
189. H. J. Milionis, A. I. Kakafika, S. G. Tsouli, V. G. Athyros, E. T. Bairaktari, K. I. Seferiadis and M. S. Elisaf, *Am. Heart J.*, 2004, **148**, 635–640.
190. M. D. Feher, A. L. Hepburn, M. B. Hogarth, S. G. Ball and S. A. Kaye, *Rheumatology*, 2003, **42**, 321–325.
191. U. Gresser, I. Kamilli, U. Kronawitter and N. Zollner, *Eur. J. Clin. Pharmacol.*, 1990, **38**, 489–491.

192. Y. Hagos, A. Bahn, S. V. Vormfelde, J. Brockmoller and G. Burckhardt, *J. Am. Soc. Nephrol.*, 2007, **18**, 3101–3109.
193. S. Shahinfar, R. L. Simpson, A. D. Carides, B. Thiyagarajan, Y. Nakagawa, J. G. Umans, J. H. Parks and F. L. Coe, *Kidney Int.*, 1999, **56**, 1879–1885.
194. D. Uetake, I. Ohno, K. Ichida, Y. Yamaguchi, H. Saikawa, H. Endou and T. Hosoya, *Intern. Med.*, 2010, **49**, 89–94.
195. R. M. Edwards, E. J. Stack and W. Trizna, *J. Pharmacol. Exp. Ther.*, 1999, **290**, 38–42.
196. A. Dehghan, A. Kottgen, Q. Yang, S. J. Hwang, W. L. Kao, F. Rivadeneira, E. Boerwinkle, D. Levy, A. Hofman, B. C. Astor, E. J. Benjamin, C. M. van Duijn, J. C. Witteman, J. Coresh and C. S. Fox, *Lancet*, 2008, **372**, 1953–1961.
197. M. Kolz, T. Johnson, S. Sanna, A. Teumer, V. Vitart, M. Perola, M. Mangino, E. Albrecht, C. Wallace, M. Farrall, A. Johansson, D. R. Nyholt, Y. Aulchenko, J. S. Beckmann, S. Bergmann, M. Bochud, M. Brown, H. Campbell, J. Connell, A. Dominiczak, G. Homuth, C. Lamina, M. I. McCarthy, T. Meitinger, V. Mooser, P. Munroe, M. Nauck, J. Peden, H. Prokisch, P. Salo, V. Salomaa, N. J. Samani, D. Schlessinger, M. Uda, U. Volker, G. Waeber, D. Waterworth, R. Wang-Sattler, A. F. Wright, J. Adamski, J. B. Whitfield, U. Gyllensten, J. F. Wilson, I. Rudan, P. Pramstaller, H. Watkins, A. Doering, H. E. Wichmann, T. D. Spector, L. Peltonen, H. Volzke, R. Nagaraja, P. Vollenweider, M. Caulfield, T. Illig and C. Gieger, *PLoS Genet.*, 2009, **5**, e1000504.
198. Q. Yang, A. Kottgen, A. Dehghan, A. V. Smith, N. L. Glazer, M. H. Chen, D. I. Chasman, T. Aspelund, G. Eiriksdottir, T. B. Harris, L. Launer, M. Nalls, D. Hernandez, D. E. Arking, E. Boerwinkle, M. L. Grove, M. Li, W. H. Linda Kao, M. Chonchol, T. Haritunians, G. Li, T. Lumley, B. M. Psaty, M. Shlipak, S. J. Hwang, M. G. Larson, C. J. O'Donnell, A. Upadhyay, C. M. van Duijn, A. Hofman, F. Rivadeneira, B. Stricker, A. G. Uitterlinden, G. Pare, A. N. Parker, P. M. Ridker, D. S. Siscovick, V. Gudnason, J. C. Witteman, C. S. Fox and J. Coresh, *Circ. Cardiovasc. Genet.*, 2010, **3**, 523–530.
199. H. Matsuo, T. Takada, K. Ichida, T. Nakamura, A. Nakayama, Y. Ikebuchi, K. Ito, Y. Kusanagi, T. Chiba, S. Tadokoro, Y. Takada, Y. Oikawa, H. Inoue, K. Suzuki, R. Okada, J. Nishiyama, H. Domoto, S. Watanabe, M. Fujita, Y. Morimoto, M. Naito, K. Nishio, A. Hishida, K. Wakai, Y. Asai, K. Niwa, K. Kamakura, S. Nonoyama, Y. Sakurai, T. Hosoya, Y. Kanai, H. Suzuki, N. Hamajima and N. Shinomiya, *Sci. Transl. Med.*, 2009, **1**, 5ra11.
200. O. M. Woodward, A. Kottgen, J. Coresh, E. Boerwinkle, W. B. Guggino and M. Kottgen, *Proc. Natl. Acad. Sci. U. S. A.*, 2009, **106**, 10338–10342.
201. N. Anzai, K. Ichida, P. Jutabha, T. Kimura, E. Babu, C. J. Jin, S. Srivastava, K. Kitamura, I. Hisatome, H. Endou and H. Sakurai, *J. Biol. Chem.*, 2008, **283**, 26834–26838.

202. V. Vitart, I. Rudan, C. Hayward, N. K. Gray, J. Floyd, C. N. Palmer, S. A. Knott, I. Kolcic, O. Polasek, J. Graessler, J. F. Wilson, A. Marinaki, P. L. Riches, X. Shu, B. Janicijevic, N. Smolej-Narancic, B. Gorgoni, J. Morgan, S. Campbell, Z. Biloglav, L. Barac-Lauc, M. Pericic, I. M. Klaric, L. Zgaga, T. Skaric-Juric, S. H. Wild, W. A. Richardson, P. Hohenstein, C. H. Kimber, A. Tenesa, L. A. Donnelly, L. D. Fairbanks, M. Aringer, P. M. McKeigue, S. H. Ralston, A. D. Morris, P. Rudan, N. D. Hastie, H. Campbell and A. F. Wright, *Nat. Genet.*, 2008, **40**, 437–442.
203. T. Sugiura, S. Kato, T. Shimizu, T. Wakayama, N. Nakamichi, Y. Kubo, D. Iwata, K. Suzuki, T. Soga, M. Asano, S. Iseki, I. Tamai, A. Tsuji and Y. Kato, *Drug Metab. Dispos.*, 2010, **38**, 1665–1672.
204. K. van de Wetering, W. Feddema, J. B. Helms, J. F. Brouwers and P. Borst, *Gastroenterology*, 2009, **137**, 1725–1735.

CHAPTER 23
# Toxicokinetics

DENNIS A. SMITH

Pfizer Global Research and Development, Ramsgate Road, Sandwich, Kent, CT13 9NJ, UK

## 23.1 Introduction

Toxicokinetics has been defined as pharmacokinetic studies performed at the doses used in toxicity studies. Although now an essential component of most multiple-dose toxicity studies, its common adoption only occurred about two decades ago. Initially the need for some form of pharmacokinetic analysis was to answer the simple but vital question: does absence of a response in the test mean the substance is "safe" or does it mean simply the absence of the test article from the circulation. Plasma concentration analysis is now routinely part of safety assessment. The original premise has expanded into two prime reasons for determining the plasma concentrations in toxicology studies:

1) To allow interpretation of dose response within a study. Due to the processes of dissolution, absorption and metabolism plasma concentrations may not be linear with dose resulting in exaggerated dose–response curves.
2) To allow comparison across species by correcting for pharmacokinetic differences and thereby allow some prediction of the possible therapeutic window in humans.

Sampling of pre-clinical studies is usually sparse and not easily amenable to true pharmacokinetics/pharmacodynamics (PK/PD) exploration. Moreover the dynamic measurements show considerable variation in effects between

RSC Drug Discovery Series No. 12
New Horizons in Predictive Toxicology: Current Status and Application
Edited by Alan G. E. Wilson

Published by the Royal Society of Chemistry, www.rsc.org

individuals. These factors should not discourage maximum use of toxicokinetic information in safety assessment.

## 23.2 Sparse Sampling and Quality Data

In these studies the actual animals on test are sampled or the study employs small groups of satellite animals.[1] Toxicokinetic data therefore is generated with certain limitations: number of samples, size of sample, *etc.* Although sparse sampling has limitations, it is possible to generate plasma concentration profiles fairly representative of a 24 h dosing period with a relatively small number of samples. This is illustrated in Figure 23.1. Sampling schedules such as 1, 2, 4, 6 or 8 and 24 h will in most cases be effective. At steady state during multiple dosing a 24 h sample is also effectively a time 0 sample in describing the curve.[1]

The need for small sample volumes with rodents, or if the larger species used are actually the subject of the test, means that assay sensitivity is important. Modern technology has answered this problem with mass spectrometric methods providing almost a universal answer. In fact the sensitivity of these methods has allowed the use of technologies borrowed from other disciplines to allow a reproducible ultra-low-volume methodology to be applied. One technique is the collection of whole blood samples on paper, known as dried blood spot. This dates back to the early 1960s in newborn screening for inherited metabolic disorders, but has been advanced by new absorbents developed for DNA analysis. Dried blood spots offer a less invasive sampling method, simpler sample collection and storage and easier transfer, combined with a smaller blood volumes. The technique is readily compatible with LC-MS/MS methods.[2]

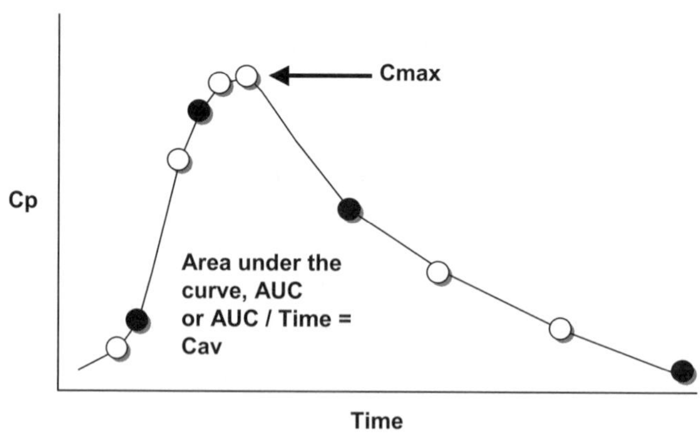


**Figure 23.1** Typical plasma concentration profile with multiple sampling and sparse sampling. For the purposes of a toxicokinetic study the effects on key parameters are usually insignificant.

## 23.3 Plasma Concentration–Dose Relationships in a Single Species

Once the first principle of presence or absence of the test article is met, a natural follow-on is the question 'what is happening at each dose level used in the study to the concentrations of the test article?' To achieve systemic concentrations of a drug in animals and man *via* the oral route requires that the drug dissolves in the contents of the gastro-intestinal tract (GIT). Absorption occurs mainly in the upper gastrointestinal tract, following emptying from the stomach, thus aqueous drug concentrations need to be maintained sufficiently highly to facilitate absorption in this environment (near-neutral pH, *etc.*). Drug absorption can continue in the large intestine but this process is not so efficient due to decreasing surface area, smaller aqueous pore area and a lowering of aqueous content. The drug can cross the GIT by aqueous pore (paracellular) or cell membrane (transcellular routes). The former route applies to small hydrophilic drug molecules such as atenolol, the latter route is the major route for most (lipophilic) drugs. As the drugs pass through the GIT membrane they can be subject to metabolism by both oxidative and conjugative enzyme systems. Also providing a barrier, which may be complimentary, are efflux transporters such as Pg-p. Once in the portal circulation the drug moves through the liver (major site of enzymatic and transporter processes) before entering the systemic circulation. Once in the systemic circulation the drug can distribute and is now cleared by the kidney (if hydrophilic) or the liver.

This route to the systemic circulation means an oral drug can exert effects on the GIT, blood and liver without appearing in the systemic circulation. More realistically, effects on these organs may be disproportionate or unrelated to systemic plasma concentrations.

Moreover, systemic plasma concentrations are separated from administered dose by a variety of processes that can attenuate the appearance of drug in the systemic circulation. Dissolution is dependent on the form of the drug (crystal structure, wettable area) and its intrinsic solubility. Many drugs have comparatively low solubilities and increasing dose levels may not undergo complete dissolution. This effect means that the relationship between dose and plasma concentrations is not linear and is in fact sub-proportional. This type of behaviour can lead to shallow dose–response curves, even when large dose ranges are used.

An example of this is provided by sulfasalazine[3] a poorly soluble drug. The drug was dosed orally by gavage to male and female B6C3F mice at dose levels ranging from 67.5 to 2700 mg $kg^{-1}$. Plasma concentrations of the parent drug and its metabolites sulfapyridine and acetylated sulfapyridine did not increase at dose levels above 675 mg $kg^{-1}$ regardless of dose size (Figure 23.2). This example uses total drug concentrations, another cause of sub-proportional total concentration–dose relationships will be discussed in the section on plasma protein binding.

Once dissolution has been achieved, actual transfer across the membrane is a linear process. The other processes described are enzymatic or transporter-assisted and they are subject to Michaelis–Menten or pseudo Michaelis–Menten kinetics

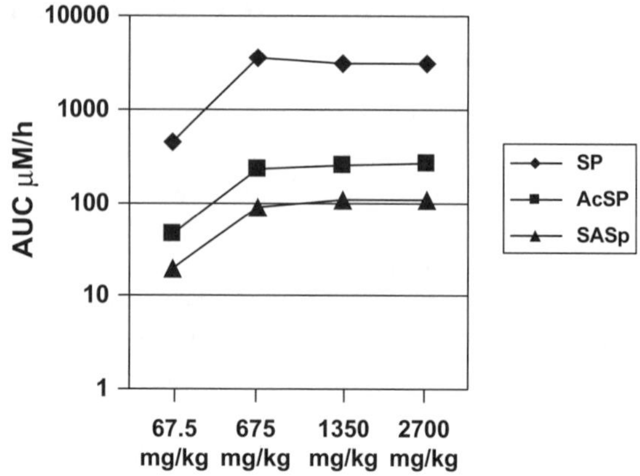


**Figure 23.2** Plasma concentrations of sulfasalazine (SP) and its metabolites, sulfapyridine (SASP) and acetylated sulfapyridine (AcSP) after oral dosage to male mice.

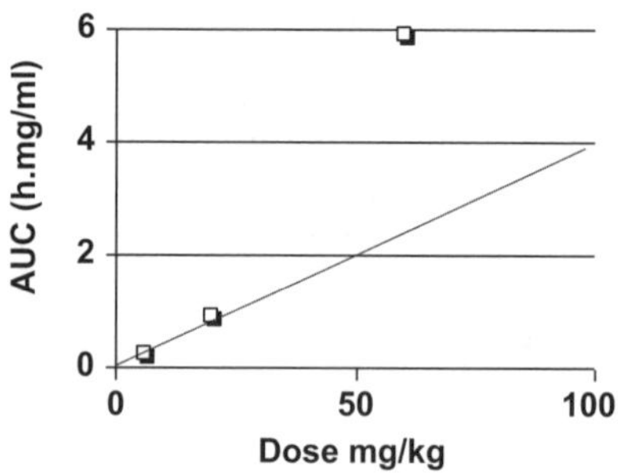


**Figure 23.3** Total plasma concentrations (shown as AUC) of proxicromil after oral administrations in dogs.

and are saturable. Thus the attenuating effects may be witnessed at low doses but not seen at higher doses. This behavior leads again to a non-linear relationship between dose and plasma concentration: in this case the relationship is super-proportional. This behaviour can lead to steep dose–response curves where sharply escalating effects are seen over a comparatively narrow dose range. Super-proportional increases in plasma concentration with dose were observed for proxicromil, a drug demonstrating capacity-limited elimination with increasing dose in dog.[4] This super-proportional increase related to a steep dose–response curve in which no effects were observed at 20 mg kg$^{-1}$ but marked hepatotoxicity was observed in all dogs at 60 mg kg$^{-1}$ (Figure 23.3).

### 23.3.1 Variation in the Pharmacodynamic Phase in a Single Species

Plasma concentration data across a series of different tests is a valuable tool in understanding toxicity dose–response particularly when the measured outcome is different between tests. The use of outbred rather than inbred strains of rodents and dogs, however, means that there is a constant drift in the genetic pool of animals used for pre-clinical testing. Thus it cannot be assumed that identical plasma concentrations guarantees identical dose response in a single species from animal to animal or toxicity test to toxicity test, particularly if there is a time gap between the various tests. Often toxicity studies show similar concentrations between animals in a particular dose group, but varying response in terms of severity and numbers of animals affected. An example of this is an anti-cholinergic compound which underwent toxicology testing in Pfizer laboratories. One-month studies showed the compound generally well tolerated by the Beagle dog at 10 mg $kg^{-1}$. Six-month toxicology studies were commenced at 4 mg $kg^{-1}$, the lower dose to compensate for increased duration of dosing. The animals rapidly demonstrated anti-cholinergic effects sufficient to warrant a further decrease in dose. Normalisation of plasma concentration (including protein-binding) data for dose showed bioavailability of drug to be identical with the plasma concentrations linearly related to administered dose. Thus the dogs used in the later six-month study were considerably more sensitive to the anti-cholinergic effects than the dogs used in the earlier one-month study.

### 23.3.2 Variation in the Plasma Concentration against Time Curve—Influence of Formulation

During a full safety evaluation programme various formulations of the drug will be used to evaluate the efficacy and safety. Early safety studies may be conducted with a different cryatalline form than that used later with possible pharmacokinetic implications. It is common practice to perform short-term rodent studies by gavage and then change to dietary administration for longer term studies. For soluble, permeable compounds the plasma concentration curve will show a rapid rise to a peak and then a subsequent decline. Such curves are common and show high variation between $C_{max}$ and $C_{min}$ over the (daily) dosage interval. Rodents eat throughout the day and night (some diurnal rhythm is apparent in some cases) and the daily dietary dose is ingested throughout the 24 h resulting in a near constant plasma concentration throughout the 24 h with minimal variation between $C_{max}$ and $C_{min}$. Thus dietary administration results usually in lower, more sustained plasma concentrations of drug than gavage. Dietary administration can decrease the bioavailability of drugs subjected to first-pass metabolism due to this slower rate of presentation resulting in concentrations below the $K_m$ of the various clearance processes. The combination of the solid drug and diet may not be as favourable as suspension dosing to dissolution also resulting in lower plasma concentrations.

The effects of a change in the mode of administration are variable. The HMG-CoA reductase inhibitor CI-981, showed reduced bioavailability after dietary administration compared to gavage.[5] Dietary plasma concentrations (AUC) were between two- and eight-fold lower over the dose range (20 to 250 mg $kg^{-1}$) than in gavage toxicology studies. These lowered plasma concentrations resulted in a lowered incidence and severity of adverse effects in the dietary group compared to gavage. Large increases in alanine aminotransferase (AST) levels were observed at 70 and 250 mg $kg^{-1}$ in gavage-treated animals, but only moderate changes were seen at 250 mg in animals receiving the drug in diet. Similarly aspartate aminotransferase (ALT) was only elevated in gavage-treated animals (70 and 250 mg $kg^{-1}$). These changes in transaminases paralleled histopathological findings in the liver. Likewise fluperlapine,[6] an anti-psychotic compound, shows lower plasma concentrations of the parent drug after dietary administration compared to gavage, but with a different toxicity outcome. The drug showed liver toxicity (hyperlipidosis) when administered to rats in the diet at 40 mg $kg^{-1}$ and 80 mg $kg^{-1}$ but not by gavage at 80 mg $kg^{-1}$. The increased sensitivity of the animals to the compound in the diet was postulated to reflect a higher proportional formation of various hydroxylated metabolites when administered in the diet.

## 23.4 Species Differences in the Pharmacokinetic Phase and Drug Effect

Considerable effort has focused on detecting and rationalising species differences in the pharmacokinetic phase. Although differences are seen in the extent of absorption: water-soluble compounds are more extensively absorbed by the dog than other species; it is the clearance processes which have received the most attention. Species differences can give rise to differences in clearance of the parent molecule and also differences in the metabolites formed. Greater enzyme activity and blood flows result in a general observation for weight-normalized clearance (mL $min^{-1}$ $kg^{-1}$) to be of the order of mouse $\geq$ rat $>$ dog $>$ human.

Under closer examination these general observations show many exceptions and these relate to the expression in the various species of the actual enzymes and transporters involved in drug clearance. For instance cytochrome P450 enzymes show differences across the species. These enzymes catalyse the primary clearance of the majority of compounds. Moreover a number of these first-generation metabolites are pharmacologically active. Among the P450 enzymes,[7] the CYP2 family (especially 2C) shows a great deal of divergence across species. Humans express CYP2C8, 2C9, and 2C19, dogs CYP2C21 and 2C41, and rats CYP2C6, 2C11, 2C12, and 2C13 (with the latter three being gender-specific). Human CYP2C9 substrates such as diclofenac and tolbutamide are handled differently in dogs. The major metabolite of tolbutamide in dogs is the cleaved product *p*-tolylsulfonylurea rather than the 4-hydroxy and 4-carboxytolbutamide metabolites observed in humans and rats. For diclofenac, dogs primarily generate the taurine conjugate and very little of the 4′-hydroxydiclofenac metabolite that is major in humans.[7] The consequences of such differences can be sometimes relatively easy to interpret. For instance centrilobular necrosis was seen in dogs after repeated dosing of proxicromil at 60 mg $kg^{-1}$, whilst other species such as baboon, cynomolgus monkey and rat showed no evidence of hepatotoxicity at comparable or greater dose levels. The toxicity was ascribed to the inability of the dog to metabolise proxicromil and the resultant high concentrations of the detergent-like parent molecule in the biliary canaliculus. The hydroxylated metabolites formed in other species including man were water-soluble and non-detergent.[4]

Paracetamol is a hepatotoxic drug and there is evidence that the different species-specificity may relate to formation and clearance of the metabolite implicated in the drugs toxicity. The toxicity of paracetamol and its putative toxic metabolite, *N*-acetyl-*p*-benzoquinoneimine (NAPQI) have been investigated in hepatocytes.[8] Clear conclusions were drawn from some earlier studies in that paracetamol triggered cell blebbing and a loss of viability in hepatocytes from mouse and hamster in contrast to human and rat hepatocytes, which were much more resistant to these effects. When NAPQUI itself was studied, there were no significant differences in the sensitivity of the cells from any species to the toxic effects. This suggested that species differences in sensitivity to the hepatotoxicity of paracetamol were due almost entirely to differences in the rate of formation of NAPQI, and not to any intrinsic differences in sensitivity or in any difference in the fate of NAPQI once formed. Later studies[9] have seen some correlations but without such clear-cut conclusions. Measuring all the metabolites and separating those into those downstream of NAPQUI (glutathione, cysteinylglycine, cysteine, and mercapturate) and detoxication/clearance pathway metabolites, such as the glucuronide and sulphate may help explain species sensitivities. The ratio of toxication/detoxication pathway metabolites excreted was (2.2, 1.0, 0.25, 0.1 and 0.08 for hamsters, mice, rabbits, rats and guinea pigs respectively) and inversely related to the hepatotoxic dose reported for these species. This is supportive of species sensitivity being partly determined by the balance between toxification and detoxication metabolic pathways.[10]

It is likely that species differences in paracetamol toxicity are due to a combination of pharmacokinetic (metabolism) differences and other biological variations. There is a natural inclination to believe that metabolism differences explain different responses, but the evidence in many cases is lacking. This is particularly true where the products of metabolism differ along with species responses.

Rosiglitazone is metabolized primarily by *N*-demethylation and *p*-hydroxylation by CYP2C8 and 2C9.[7] All metabolic products are similar between species but a minor route of metabolism is deamination of the 2-aminomethylpyridine moiety to a carboxylic acid metabolite (SB-271258). This is present as only 3.7% of the dose in urine and was not observable in plasma. However, in dogs, SB-271258 represents 24% of the dose *in excreta* and 9% of circulating drug-related material.[5] Rosiglitazone causes cardiac hypertrophy in dogs at high doses. SB-271258 shows a small to moderate trophic effect on cardiac myocytes possibly suggesting some involvement in the toxicity.[7] However, studies of insulin receptors in cardiomyocyte-restricted knockout mice demonstrate that the effects are general for other peroxisome proliferator-activated receptor (PPAR-$\gamma$) agonists and are likely due to the consequences of the plasma volume expansion witnessed in response to this class of compounds.

In addition to differences in CYP2C family enzymes, other notable species differences that could generate different metabolite profiles between humans and animals include greater activity of CYP2D orthologues in rats. The substrate selectivity and level of expression of CYP2D1 in rats explains some of the classic early species differences cited 30 years ago including the abundant aromatic hydroxylations of amphetamine, lidocaine and diazepam[7] in rats and consequent higher clearance of the parent molecule in this species compared to humans.

## 23.5 Species Differences in Plasma Protein Binding: the Need to Correct for Free Fraction

Species differences are observed in plasma protein binding leading to the need to correct total drug for free fraction in each species. It is the unbound drug that interacts with proteins in the body, changing their conformation and leading to pharmacodynamic (including toxicity) effects. Zamifenacin, a selective M3 anti-muscarinic agent[11] illustrates this need. The compound produced no histopathological evidence of toxicology. Reduction in body weight was the general adverse effect in rats and dogs, often associated with reduced food intake. Various graded pharmacological effects were observed across the animal species all relating to anti-muscarinic effects. Consistently (in animals and humans) one of the first side-effects noted as doses or concentrations increased was a decrease in salivary flow and a loss of adaption of the eye to light (mydriasis) and ability to focus. The concentration response based on total drug suggested that rats were much more sensitive to these effects than humans. Figure 23.4 shows the relationship between dose, total drug concentration and anti-muscarinic side-effect. The rodent and human data reveal large differences in the total drug $C_{max}$ at which the onset of these anti-muscarinic side-effects occurs. Plasma protein binding was shown to be 99.80%

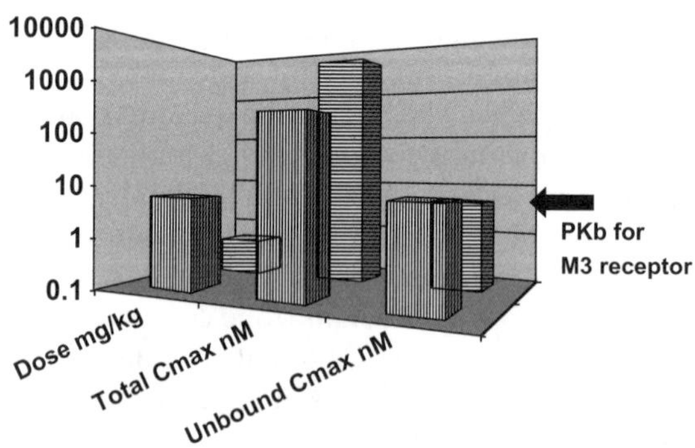


**Figure 23.4** Relationship between administered dose, total plasma concentration and the free drug concentration of zamifenacin producing threshold side-effects in humans and animals. Horizontal bars refer to humans and vertical bars rats. The affinity of zamifencin for the M3 receptor is illustrated relative to the unbound drug concentrations.

in rats compared to 99.98% in humans, a difference in free fraction of 20 fold. Correction of $C_{max}$ for free drug, as depicted in the figure, showed a high consistency in the relationship between free concentration and dynamic response across the species.

It is difficult to make any firm predictions on species differences in protein binding in terms of linking particular structures to expected protein binding differences. Zanifenacin is a basic compound. Likewise, tolteridine is a basic compound which shows broadly similar differences between humans and rodents.[12] Tolteridine exhibited high protein binding in human plasma with an unbound fraction of 3.7%. The unbound fraction was slightly lower in dog plasma (2.1%,) but much higher in rodent and lagomorph (rat, 22%; mouse, 16–17%; rabbit, 39%). Similar findings were made for another basic compound remoxipride[13] (with an overall lower binding than tolteridine) showing a free fraction lowest in dog and humans (20%) and greatest in rodent plasma 70–80%. In contrast for another basic compound, sildenafil[14] the unbound fraction was 4–6% in mouse, rat, rabbit and human, but 16% in dog. It is possible these differences reflect variations in binding to α-1-acid glycoprotein in addition to albumin. However this reinforces the need to study protein binding in each species over the concentration range seen in all the studies. This data can then allow the extrapolation of total drug concentrations to unbound drug concentrations.

### 23.5.1 Linear and Non-Linear Plasma Protein Binding

For many drugs plasma protein binding is essentially linear. The major protein binding drugs in the plasma is albumin. This is present in plasma at about 550 μM. The other major binding protein is α-1-acid glycoprotein (AAG) present in plasma at around 12 μM. Albumin binds acidic, neutral and basic drugs with the highest affinity for acidic compounds. AAG binds mainly basic drugs. Assuming a single binding site, total drug concentrations need to be in excess of these values to show non-linear binding. This generalisation is largely true but endogenous ligand such as fatty acids may lower these numbers somewhat. Clinically therefore only a few drugs show this phenomena, but it is obviously more likely to occur in toxicity studies with exaggerated doses and concentrations. The phenomena may represent itself as a sub-proportional relationship between dose and total concentration. In the simplest setting if free drug concentration is calculated, the relationship between dose and free drug concentration will be linear since unbound drug concentrations depend on intrinsic clearance.[15] The saturation may be made more complex by saturation of clearance pathways, leading to a linear total, but super-proportional relationship. This complexity is illustrated by a study on the effects of age and dose on the pharmacokinetics of naproxen in young and senescent male Fischer-344 rats.[16] When pharmacokinetic parameters, after 2.5 and 25 mg $kg^{-1}$ doses, were based on total drug concentration, clearance and steady-state volume of distribution were indistinguishable between young and old rats. However, when based on free naproxen concentrations there was a significant decrease in free clearance (related to intrinsic clearance by metabolising enzymes) and free steady-state volume of distribution in the aged rats (related to albumin binding). *In vitro* enzyme kinetic studies confirmed the decline in the metabolism rate (intrinsic clearance) for naproxen in the aged rats. Plasma protein binding studies revealed a larger free fraction of drug in the plasma of senescent rats. The binding of naproxen to plasma proteins was also dependent on drug concentration. Total plasma clearance and volume of distribution increased with increasing dose, due to this non-linear protein binding whereas free clearance and free volume of distribution decreased as dose increased. By concentrating on the important unbound pharmacokinetic parameters rather than the total, the complexities are simplified and allow the dose response to any effect to be properly evaluated.

## 23.6 Metabolites and Toxicokinetics

Circulating metabolites and whether they should be routinely incorporated into toxicokinetic studies is an area of debate. Three clear situations can be described when there is a need to provide concentration data on a metabolite:

1) When the drug is a pro-drug and the active principle is a metabolite: best practice is to determine the concentrations of both.
2) When metabolites are contributing to the primary pharmacology of the drug. This may be an iterative procedure. In general *in vitro* studies are predictive of primary metabolites and these are the ones most likely to be active.[17] The vast majority of active metabolites are of similar structure to the parent and arise from metabolic steps such as hydroxylation, reduction and *N*-demethylation.[7,18,19] Moreover, these metabolites display similar selectivity to the parent molecule in terms of off-target pharmacology. Primary metabolites identified in *in vitro* screens should therefore be tested for pharmacological activity. Preliminary *in vivo* studies can identify those that circulate at concentrations which when combined with potency and free-fraction data will contribute to the pharmacological activity. The measurement of these allows dose–response curves to be assessed in terms of receptor occupancy. Metabolites which do not change the ionised properties of the molecule will generally show similar or higher free fraction to the parent due to the change in lipophilicity. For example tolteridine described in the section on protein binding has an active metabolite (5-hydroxymethyltolteridine) of similar receptor potency to the parent. The unbound fraction of 5-hydroxymethyltolteridine[12] was much higher than the parent in plasma from humans (36%) and all animal species investigated (mouse, 72%; rabbit, 68%; cat, 32%; dog, 45%). These differences would need to be incorporated to understand fully the dose response in the species tested.

3) Recent guidelines around metabolism such as the ICHM3(R2) guidance stress the need to qualify metabolites formed in humans in disproportionate amounts relative to animals. These are identified usually from single-dose $^{14}C$-radiolabelled studies. Such studies are often conducted at doses which may not reflect the highest no-effect dose level in safety assessment. Similarly the human component of the studies may be conducted before the range of human clinical doses is firmly established. The consequence of this is it is prudent to investigate the animal species used in safety evaluation at the correct doses at steady state after multiple dosing to determine if sufficient safety qualification has been provided.[7] Although empirical and based on pragmatism, similar concentrations of the metabolite in one of the species used in a comprehensive toxicity study (one month or greater) will generally be accepted as qualifying the metabolite.
4) One problem in interpreting the need to monitor metabolites and which ones should be monitored is a lack of published examples of known stable toxic metabolites. Some guidelines refer anecdotally to examples without providing further details. For further progression of the science in this area the need to publish information on this topic is paramount.

## 23.7 Differences in the Dynamic Response across Species

The process of evolution ensures that just as the enzymes of drug metabolism will differ across species, as to their selectivities and affinities for different substrates or ligands so will the "receptors" that govern the dynamic response of drugs. It is illuminating to look at a modern example of evolution: the appearance of warfarin-resistant strains of rat. A number of different strains have developed and each demonstrates differences in the way they have responded to the environment. The Welsh resistant strain, compared to normal strain, has vitamin K epoxide reductase and vitamin K quinone reductase enzymes with greatly reduced sensitivity to inhibition by warfarin. The Scottish resistant strain has epoxide and quinone reductases with similar sensitivities compared to normal strain. However, in contrast to normal strain, the inhibition of both reductases by warfarin is readily reversible. The Chicago resistant strain shows similarities to the Scottish strain in this pharmacodynamic adaptation.[20] What is striking is that pharmacokinetic or other drug metabolism adaptions are not found to be significant.[21] Similar observations can be made for a variety of toxicity outcomes and strain differences. Complex interrelationships are similarly involved. Taking the example of nephrotoxicity, sensitivity can vary widely. Daunomycin nephrotoxicity, as judged by urinary albumin excretion, was found to be strain specific in eight inbred murine strains, after intravenous injection.[22] This specificity did not relate to the plasma clearance of the drug. The sensitivity ranged from two strains A/J and BALB/c which were highly susceptible to the drug in contrast to three strains

C57BL/6J, DBA-2 and B10D2/o which were completely resistant to it. Acetaminophen shows similar pharmacokinetics in male Fischer-344 (F-344) and Sprague–Dawley (SD) rats, moreover urinary metabolites are also similar.[23] In contrast to these similarities in disposition parameters male F-344 rats are susceptible to acetaminophen nephrotoxicity whereas SD rats are resistant to the toxicity.

These strain differences are not unsurprisingly mirrored by species difference. For instance, daunomycin (referred to above) is more renally toxic to rats compared to rabbits at comparative doses.[24] Many receptors, ion channels and enzymes which are potential or actual targets for therapeutic agents have been reported to show marked species differences in affinity or response, to agonists or antagonists, due to the structure of the protein or the level of its expression.[25] It is important to note that the differences in affinity and actual dynamic response can be of the order of 3–4 orders of magnitude between the species, and such differences may dwarf pharmacokinetic differences. An example of such differences is the $Na^+/K^+$ ATPase enzymes and their sensitivity to cardiac glycosides.[26] The human, dog and sheep cardiac enzymes are a thousand times more sensitive than the corresponding major ones from adult rat and mouse. This difference in sensitivity is due to an increase in the dissociation rate of drug from the binding site on the enzyme. Site-directed mutagenesis has shown that only two amino acid substitutions convert the sensitive form to the resistant form. Thus, the rat enzymes lack of affinity is bestowed by the presence of the charged amino acids arginine and aspartic acid, instead of glutamine and asparagine, on the amino and carboxyl end of the H1–H2 extracellular domain of the $Na^+/K^+$ ATPase.[26] These changes have been modelled and demonstrated that each amino acid change is additive in changing the consensus orientation binding mode of human and sheep $Na^+/K^+$ ATPase to one in which the cardiac glycoside is completely dislodged from the consensus orientation.[27] Such relatively small changes (mutations) in a drug target (receptor) should be contrasted with what would be required to alter drug clearance to a similar extent, bearing in mind the plethora of clearance systems available to any compound.

Large differences are also seen in affinity between species for anti-platelet agents[28] targeting glycoprotein $\alpha$IIb$\beta$3 integrin (GPII/IIIa). For instance DMP 802 binds with high affinity to both inactivated and activated human platelets ($K_d = 0.61$ and 0.57 nM, respectively). When this is investigated functionally DMP 802 demonstrates species specificity in potently inhibiting platelet aggregation in human, guinea pig, dog, swine and hamster with $IC_{50}$ values ranging from 0.025 to 0.092 μM in contrast to the weak effect in rabbit and rat where $IC_{50}$ values were up to 40-fold higher (0.88–1.0 μM). Other antagonists show different species specificity but still exhibit a broad range of potencies across the species.[29] For instance the non-peptide anti-parasite agent pentamidine is a broad spectrum anti-platelet agent with an $IC_{50}$ of 1.1 μM in ADP-induced platelet aggregation in human platelet rich plasma. It has been shown to be an inhibitor of fibrinogen binding to GPIIb/IIIa. Pentamidine, compared with human, has similar anti-platelet activity in monkey and dog platelet-rich plasma but very low activity in guinea pig, rabbit, rat and mouse platelet rich plasma. These differences were shown to be dependent on the species of platelets and independent of the species of fibrinogen.

Species specificity may not only be dependent on actual structural differences between the targets across the species but may reflect the actual amount. Thus the specific activity of HMG-CoA reductase in hamster and rabbit liver is some 10–200 times lower than that in rat, mouse, monkey or dog. These differences probably play a role in rendering these species more susceptible to the hepatotoxic effect of HMG-CoA reductase inhibitors. Oral doses of lovastatin, a specific inhibitor of the rate-limiting enzyme in cholesterol biosynthesis, HMG-CoA (3-hydroxy-3-methylglutaryl CoA) reductase, that were tolerated by dogs, rats and mice were found to be lethal to rabbits in sub-acute studies.[30] Post-mortem findings in rabbits consisted of centrilobular hepatic necrosis, frequently accompanied by renal tubular necrosis and occasionally gallbladder necrosis. The liver lesions were associated with up to 300-fold elevations in serum aspartate and alanine aminotransferase activities. The histopathogical and serum biochemistry changes were prevented by co-administration of mevalonate, the product of the inhibited HMG-CoA reductase enzyme. Simvastatin, another HMG-CoA reductase inhibitor was hepatotoxic in male Syrian hamsters[31] and likewise the elevated biochemical changes and morphological alterations were prevented by co-administration of mevalonate.

The toxicity of these drugs could indeed result from the low basal activity of HMG-CoA reductase in these species coupled with a prolonged inhibition of mevalonate synthesis. However, supplementation of the animal diets or with oral doses of cholesterol (the major product of mevalonate metabolism) enhanced the liver damage, indicating that depletion of a non-sterol metabolite(s) of mevalonate may be important in the toxicity findings. It is not too surprising, therefore, that PK/PD responses across strains or species may vary widely.

More profound changes to biochemical pathways are behind the marked species-specific responses to agonists of the PPAR (PPARα) have been observed in rats and dogs.[32] The dog shows evidence of single-cell necrosis in the liver but not the rat. Dog hepatocytes, but not rat hepatocytes, treated with LY465608, a PPARα agonist demonstrate abnormalities in the regulation of cell renewal and death, oxidative stress, and mitochondrial bioenergetics. At a biochemical level these differences can be understood. Rat hepatocytes respond to PPAR agonists with an induction of both peroxisomal and mitochondrial β-oxidation (PBox and MBox) activities. Dog hepatocytes treated with both PPAR agonists, however, do not show increased PBox activity but demonstrate increased MBox activity. PPAR agonists induce the peroxisomal enzymes, acyl-CoA oxidase, enoyl-CoA hydratase/L-3-hydroxyacyl-CoA dehydrogenase, and 3-ketoacyl-CoA thiolase at the transcriptional level in rat hepatocytes, but not dog hepatocytes. Expression of mRNA for the mitochondrial β-oxidation, gene hydroxyacyl-CoA dehydrogenase/3-ketoacyl-CoA thiolase, however, increases in both rat and dog hepatocytes.

Plasma concentration comparisons across species, whether corrected for free fraction not, cannot be viewed therefore as a general reliable method for determining safety margin unless considerable understanding of the biological variation of the actual toxicity is available across the species tested.

## 23.8 Future Refinements: the use of $C_{av}$

It has become standard practice to summarise the plasma concentration data from toxicity studies by calculating $C_{max}$ and AUC, usually as stated above in terms of unbound concentration. Because of the limited sampling these terms may be expressed as $C_t$ (which refers to the highest concentration measured and the time it occurs, rather than a true $C_{max}$) and $AUC_t$ (which calculates AUC out to the last time point at which drug is detectable). These summary calculations are the reference terms cited in guidelines such as the ICH *S3A: Note for guidance on toxicokinetics: the assessment of systemic exposure in toxicity studies*. $C_{max}$ is a pharmacokinetic measure of the acute stress on the system a drug may impose. It can obviously be related to rapid onset and reversible effects, perhaps cardioavascular (*e.g.*, rhythm disturbances) and CNS (*e.g.*, drowsiness). AUC is viewed as a measure of the chronic stress imposed. $C_{max}$ will have units, often of ng $ml^{-1}$ or µg $ml^{-1}$. Much more direct information is provided if molar units are used, particularly when unbound drug data is presented because this can be directly related to the units normally used to describe the potency and selectivity of the drug obtained during *in vitro* testing. AUC has complex units such as ng $mL^{-1}$ min or µg $mL^{-1}$ min. The units do not allow easy visualisation and reduce AUC values to numbers that can be compared between doses to look at linearity or between species to understand relative "systemic exposure" but do not impart any extra information. $C_{av}$[33] is the average concentration across time and can be calculated by dividing AUC by time. The value therefore gives identical information to AUC, but now the units are the same as $C_{max}$. $C_{av}$ gives therefore a way of rapidly understanding the behaviour of a drug against the potency and selectivity of the drug obtained during *in vitro* testing. This is useful in guiding the researcher to understand if the toxicology observed relates to the target or off-target receptors. For a permeable compound or one acting on cell-surface receptors once concentrations exceed 10 times the $K_i$, $K_b$ or even $EC_{50}$ the target receptor is likely to be fully occupied. When toxic effects are not seen at this concentration but observed at higher concentrations the effects are unlikely to be associated with the known pharmacology. This can help the researcher determine if "class effects" are a problem of a particular target. $C_{av}$ can be subdivided readily into periods such as 0–6 h and 6–24 h to give a numerical description of the plasma concentration–time curve. Dose elevation in toxicity studies often results in different shapes to the plasma concentration curves. A drug can be rapidly dissolved in the GIT at the low doses of a toxicology study, but at the highest have solubility-limited dissolution. Under these conditions the drug may still show linear AUC values. Under these conditions as doses increase so a broader flatter concentration curve is observed. This will be reflected in decreasing $C_{max}$ : dose ratios but will not be reflected in AUC. When the data is presented as $C_{av}$ such trends as a flatter curve will be apparent and reflected in a decreased $C_{av}$ 0–6 h per dose and an increased $C_{av}$ 6–24 h per dose. These types of effects explain some dose–response curves where the effects seen at the higher doses correlate to high occupancy of the target receptor for the complete dosing period. This is illustrated with zatosetron a 5HT3 receptor with a high affinity ($K_b$ = 1.5 nM) against the human receptor. The metabolites are not thought to contribute to the pharmacology of the drug.[34] Studies in man[35] showed that the drug at steady state gave rise to unbound concentrations of 3.5, 12 and 20 nM at 5, 10 and 20 mg day. Doses up to 5 mg were well tolerated although some minor side-effects such as constipation have been noted. Chronic toxicity of the drug was studied in Rhesus monkeys at dose levels of 3, 10 and 25 mg $kg^{-1}$. Depressed appetite[36] was seen in all treatment groups accompanied by salivation, diarrhea, soft stools and emesis at 10 and 25 mg $kg^{-1}$. 5HT3 antagonists have effects on gastric motility. Alostron, dolasetron, ondasetron and palostron all cause some or all of the effects: salivation, vomiting and a mixture of diarrhoea and constipation. Figure 23.5 shows the toxicokinetic data expressed as $C_{max}$ and $C_{av}$ values and illustrates how the progression from lowered appetite to actual visible clinical signs with dose probably reflects increased duration of high-receptor occupancy of the 5HT3 receptor throughout the dosing period. There is little occupancy at 3 mg $kg^{-1}$ during the 6–24 h period in contrast to the high

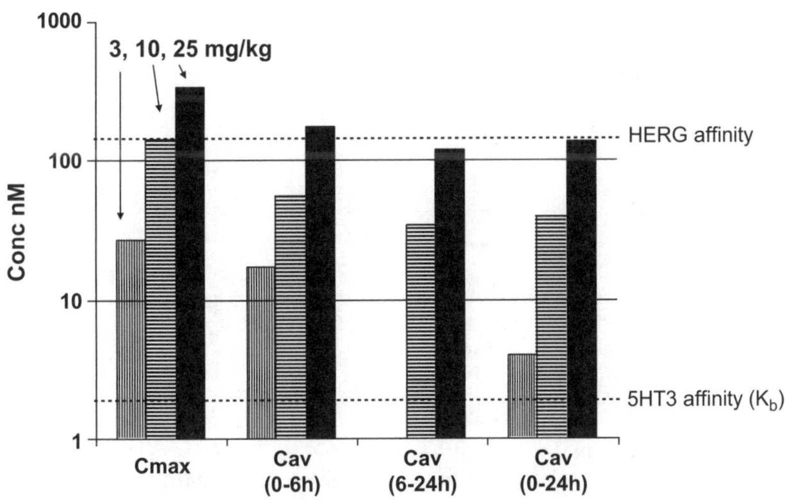


**Figure 23.5** Toxicokinetic data for zatosetron presented as unbound concentrations compared to the affinity of zatostraon for its target receptor 5HT3 and off-target affinity for the HEG channel. The data assumes a plasma protein binding of 75% (the same as in humans). The portrayal of all the data as simple concentrations allows immediately the receptor occupancy of 5HT3 and other ion channels (see text) to be understood in a dynamic fashion.

occupancy in the two higher dose groups. Q-Tc interval was increased at 4 h post treatment at 10 and 25 mg kg$^{-1}$ an effect that persisted throughout the 24 h at the top-dose level. Figure 23.3 illustrates how these effects cannot be correlated with 5HT3 receptor antagonism. The threshold effect at the end of the 24 h period at 25 mg kg$^{-1}$ and the absence of effect at 3 g kg$^{-1}$ suggests the compound has affinity for another receptor. Data from other antagonists both *in vitro* and *in vivo* suggest 5HT3 antagonists block sodium channels (hH1) and potassium channels (HERG). Comparative studies with ondasetron and zatosetron indicate that the affinity of zatosetron for the HERG potassium channel is around 200 nM. Figure 23.3 illustrates how $C_{av}$ values allow this order of potency and the plasma concentration data to allow a correlation with effect.

Sildenalfil is a PDE5 inhibitor used for the treatment of erectile dysfunction and pulmonary hypertension. This compound also has some activity against PDE6 which is present in the retina and plays a role in vision. Therefore there is a need to demonstrate that any slight inhibition of PDE6 was without pathological implications.[37] Figure 23.6 presents the data as $C_{max}$ and $C_{av}$ values with concentrations in molar units of unbound drug, at the dose levels which produced no significant toxicological effects and the clinical dose in man. This is compared with the primary *in vitro* pharmacological potencies against PDE5 (4 nM), PDE6 (40 nM). Inhibition of the rapidly activating delayed rectifier potassium current (IKr) activity is too weak to portray (100 000 nM) on the plot correlating with the complete lack of effect in any *in vivo* experiment or situation. The data clearly show the multiples between man and animals in terms of systemic exposure. Importantly the concentration data exactly matches the transient inhibition of PDE6 in man (around the time of $C_{max}$),

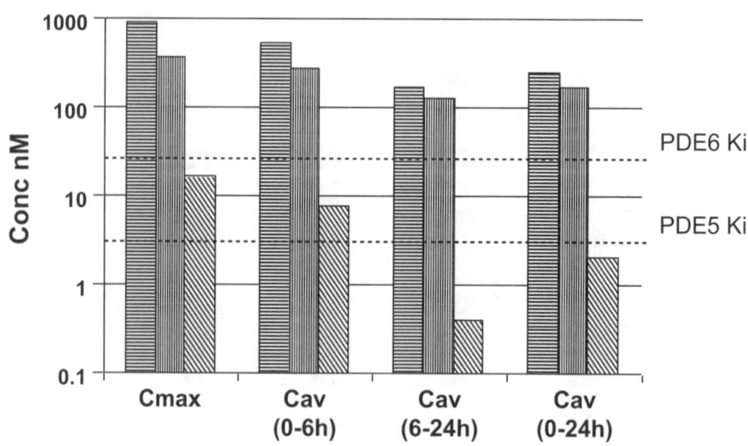


**Figure 23.6** Toxicokinetic data for sildenafil presented as unbound concentrations compared to the potency against the target PDE5 and off-target potency for PDE6. The portrayal as simple concentrations allows immediately the understanding of safety data concerning PDE6 to be understood in a dynamic fashion. The horizontal bars represent rat, the vertical bars, dog and the diagonal, man.

particularly at the highest clinical dose of 100 mg (or 1.4 mg $kg^{-1}$) which accounts for the blue tinge to vision experienced by some patients. This is most marked at the highest clinical dose of 100 mg (or 1.4 mg $kg^{-1}$). The graphical or tabular use of $C_{max}$ and $C_{av}$ demonstrates that PDE6 inhibition was robustly tested in animals (experiments included extensive retinal examination) both in terms of maximal degree of inhibition and the chronicity of the inhibition. Importantly the potency of sildenafil against PDE5 and PDE6 in human and dog is known to be similar.

### 23.8.1 Induction and Toxicokinetics—the Liver as a Target Organ

In many cases mild induction is seen for many compounds at the elevated dose levels used in toxicity tests. The relevance for man is small due to differences in the various receptors associated with induction and the fact that induction follows a classical dose and concentration response relationship.[38] Most clinical inducers are high-dose drugs, either due to weak interactions with the primary target ($Na^+$ blockers such as phenytoin and carbamezepine) or the need to dose to achieve an $IC_{90}$ as for an anti-infective (*e.g.*, rifampicin).[39] When auto-induction occurs this is often without undue consequence, with the dose levels used still providing (unbound) plasma concentrations which are relevant (greater than) to the (unbound) plasma concentrations achieved in the clinic. In certa*in situ*ations the clearance route of a compound or series in the rodent (rat and mouse) combined with a marked sensitivity to induction to the compound or series makes standard toxicokinetic measures and interpretations misleading. UK-453,061 is a non-nucleoside reverse transcriptase inhibitor.[40] High clearance in rodents, made even more marked by autoinduction, limits systemic exposure to very low concentrations when compared to other species like dog and man receiving comparable doses. When comparing dose response between species, some account of the dose the liver is receiving needs to be incorporated, rather than relying on systemic concentrations alone. For instance although systemic plasma concentrations (both total and unbound) may be below those seen clinically, a dose of 300 mg $kg^{-1}$ to a rodent represents a dose of 7.7 mg $g^{-1}$ to the liver which can be compared to a liver dose of 0.67 mg $kg^{-1}$ for a 100 mg clinical dose. Such factors need to be incorporated if say the liver is a target organ in carcinogenicity testing.[38] That the liver becomes a target organ, of course, is accentuated by the induction effects.

## 23.9 Conclusions

This chapter has explored the prime reasons for toxicokinetic analysis:

1) To allow interpretation of dose response within a study. Due to the processes of dissolution, absorption and metabolism plasma concentrations may not be linear with doses resulting in exaggerated dose–response curves.

2) To allow comparison across species and to correct for pharmacokinetic differences and thus to understand dose–response relationships sufficiently to allow some prediction of possible therapeutic windows in humans.

A key to utilising toxicokinetic data is to correct for unbound concentrations. The use of total concentration can distort understanding due to species differences in free fraction and the possibility of saturable non-linear protein binding.

Sampling of pre-clinical studies is usually sparse and not easily amenable to true PK/PD exploration. Moreover the dynamic measurements show considerable variation in effects between individuals. Improvements in toxicokinetic/toxicodynamic (TK/TD) analysis are provided by converting AUC into $C_{av}$ (average concentration over specified time) values. $C_{av}$ units are identical to $C_{max}$ and allow immediate comparison with this value and thus the ability to numerically describe a plasma concentration curve. Moreover these values allow easy direct comparison with the potency and selectivity of the drug obtained during *in vitro* testing. Candidate drugs are now screened against a large panel of proteins (receptors, ion channels, enzymes *etc.*) alongside their intended target. This data can be exploited to its full by the use of $C_{max}$ and $C_{av}$ comparisons in TK/TD analysis. The use of this type of analysis will become more valuable as screening panels are expanded, possibly involving more proteins implicated in toxic events.

Circulating metabolites may contribute to TK/TD relationships and a much clearer picture is now available of the form of metabolites likely to contribute to TK/TD outcomes in terms of physicochemistry, structure and concentration. Information about metabolites is again best conveyed by the use of $C_{max}$ and $C_{av}$ values.

## References

1. D. A. Smith, M. J. Humphrey and C. Charuel, *Xenobiotica*, 1990, **20**, 1187.
2. W. Li and F. L. S. Tse, *Biomed. Chromatogr.*, 2010, **24**, 49.
3. W. Zheng, S. M. Winter, M. Mayersohn, J. B. Bishop and I. G. Sipes, *Drug Metab. Dispos.*, 1993, **21**, 1091.
4. B. Clark and D. A. Smith, *Crit. Rev. Toxicol.*, 1984, **12**, 343.
5. J. H. Lin, I. W. Chen and J. King, *J. Pharmacol. Exp. Ther.*, 1992, **263**, 105.
6. R. L. Susick and T. Woolf, in *Drug Toxicokinetics*, ed. P. G. Welling and F. A. de la Iglesia, Marcel Dekker, New York, 1992, p. 305.
7. D. A. Smith and R. S. Obach, *Chem. Res. Toxicol.*, 2009, **22**, 267.
8. L. B. Tee, D. S. Davies, C. E. Seddon and A. R. Boobis, *Biochem. Pharmacol.*, 1987, **36**, 1041.
9. K. Jemnitz, Z. Veres, K. Monostory, L. Kobori and L. Vereczkey, *Toxicol. in vitro*, 2008, **22**, 961.
10. Z. Gregus, C. Madhu and C. D. Klaassen, *J. Pharmacol. Exp. Ther.*, 1988, **244**, 91.

11. K. C. Beaumont, A. G. Causey, P. E. Coates and D. A. Smith, *Xenobiotica*, 1996, **26**, 459.
12. I. Pahlman and P. Gozzi, *Biopharm. Drug Dispos.*, 1999, **20**, 91.
13. M. Widman, L. B. Nilsson, B. Bryske and J. Lundstrom, *Arzneim. Forsch.*, 1993, **43**, 287.
14. D. K. Walker, M. J. Ackland, G. C. James, G. J. Muirhead, D. J. Rance, P. Wastall and P. A. Wright, *Xenobiotica*, 1999, **29**, 297.
15. L. Z. Benet and B.-A. Hoener, *Clin. Pharmacol. Ther.,* 2002, **71**, 115.
16. J. H. Satterwhite and F. D. Boudinot, *J. Gerontol., Ser. B*, 1991, **46**, 222.
17. D. Dalvie, R. S. Obach, P. Kang, C. Prakash, C. M. Loi, S. Hurst, A. Nedderman, L. Goulet, E. Smith, H. Z. Buz and D. A. Smith, *Chem. Res. Toxicol.*, 2009, **22**, 357.
18. D. A. Smith and R. S. Obach, *Drug. Metab. Dispos.*, 2005, **33**, 1409.
19. D. A. Smith and R. S. Obach, *Chem. Res. Toxicol.*, 2006, **19**, 1570.
20. J. H. Fenton and J. R. Fry, *Comp. Biochem. Physiol., Part C: Toxicol. Pharmacol.*, 1993, **104**, 1.
21. M. G. Townsend, E. M. Odam and J. M. J. Page, *Biochem. Pharmacol.*, 1975, **24**, 729.
22. M. Kimura, H. Takahashi, T. Ohtake, T. Sako, A. Hishida, M. Nishimura and N. Honda, *Nephron*, 1993, **63**, 193.
23. J. B. Tarloff, R. S. Goldstein and J. B. Hook, *Toxicology*, 1989, **56**, 167.
24. D. Deprez-DeCampeneere, R. Jaenke and A. Trouet, *Cancer Treat. Rep.*, 1982, **66**, 395.
25. D. A. Smith, *Eur. J. Drug Metab. Pharmacokinet.*, 1993, **18**, 31.
26. E. M. Price and J. B. Lingrel, *Biochemistry*, 1988, **27**, 8400.
27. S. M. Keenan, R. K. DeLisle, W. J. Welsh, S. Paula and W. J. Ball, *J. Mol. Graphics Modell.*, 2005, **23**, 465.
28. S. A. Mousa, R. E. Olson, J. M. Bozarth, W. Lorelli, M. S. Forsythe, A. Racanelli, S. Gibbs, K. Schlingman, T. Bozarth, R. Kapil, J. Wityak, T. M. Sielecki, R. R. Wexler, M. J. Thoolen, A. Slee, T. M. Reilly, P. S. Anderson and P. A. Friedman, *J. Cardiovasc. Pharmacol.*, 1998, **32**, 169.
29. D. Cox, Y. Motoyama, J. Seki, T. Aoki, M. Dohi, K. Yoshida, *Thromb. Haemostasis*, 1992, **68**, 731.
30. D. J. Kornbrust, J. S. MacDonald, C. P. Peter, D. M. Duchai, J. R. Stubbs, J. I. Germershausen and A. W. Alberts, *J. Pharmacol. Exp. Ther.*, 1989, **248**, 498.
31. Y. Horsmans, J. P. Desager, and C. Harvengt, *Pharmacol. Toxicol.*, 1990, **67**, 336.
32. Y. Guo, R. A. Jolly, B. W. Halstead, T. K. Baker, J. P. Stutz, M. Huffman, J. N. Calley, A. West, H. Gao, G. H. Searfoss, S. Li, A. R. Irizarry, H. Qian, J. L. Stevens and T. P. Ryan, *Toxicol. Sci.*, 2007, **96**, 294.
33. D. A. Smith, P. Morgan, W. M. Vogel and D. K. Walker, *Regul. Toxicol. Pharmacol.*, 2010, **57**, 70.
34. M. L. Cohen, W. Bloomquist, C. R. Schmid, D. W. Robertson and D. T. Wong, *Drug Develop. Res.*, 1993, **29**, 209.

35. W. T. Ward, P. D. Londborg, S. L. Blomgren, G. D. Tollefson and M. E. Sayler, *J. Clin. Psychopharmacol.*, 1999, **19**, 125.
36. A. Bendele, J. Means, J. Shoufler, C. Schmalz, G. Hanasono, J. Symanowski and E. Adams, *Drug Chem. Toxicol.*, 1995, **18**, 61.
37. D. Abbott, P. Comby, C. Charuel, P. Graepel, G. Hanton, B. Leblanc, A. Ladola, L. Longeart, G. Paulus, C. Peters and J. Stadler, *Int. J. Impotence Res.*, 2004, **16**, 498.
38. D. A. Smith, M. Dickins, O. A. Fahmi, K. Iwasaki, C. Lee, R. S. Obach, G. Padbury, S. M. De Morais, S. L. Ripp, J. Stevens, R. Voorman and K. Youdim, *Drug Metab. Dispos.*, 2007, **35**, 697.
39. D. A. Smith, *Eur. J. Pharm. Sci.*, 2000, **11**, 185.
40. D. K. Walker, J. Davis, C. Houle, I. B. Gardner and R. Webster, *Xenobiotica*, 2009, **39**, 534.

CHAPTER 24

# *The Role of Computational Systems Biology Models in Toxicity Testing in the 21$^{st}$ Century: an Example with Predictive Multi-Scale Models of the Liver*

SUDIN BHATTACHARYA,[a] QIANG ZHANG,[a] ROBERT A. ROTH[b] AND MELVIN E. ANDERSEN*,[a]

[a] The Hamner Institutes for Health Sciences, Program in Chemical Safety Sciences, Research Triangle Park, NC 27709- 2137, USA;
[b] Michigan State University, Department of Pharmacology and Toxicology, East Lansing, MI 48824, USA

## 24.1 Introduction

In the recent report *Toxicity Testing in the 21st Century: a Vision and a Strategy*,[1] the National Research Council of the US National Academies of Science (NRC) has laid out a vision where in the near future most toxicity testing will be carried out *in vitro*, with a gradual reduction of reliance on high-dose animal studies. This new approach to toxicity testing and risk assessment, abbreviated ***TT21C***, would be based on perturbation of cellular responses using a carefully selected suite of *in vitro* assays. Central to this vision is the idea of

RSC Drug Discovery Series No. 12
New Horizons in Predictive Toxicology: Current Status and Application
Edited by Alan G. E. Wilson

Published by the Royal Society of Chemistry, www.rsc.org

"toxicity pathways"—the innate cellular signaling pathways that are perturbed by chemicals, and the determination of chemical concentration ranges where those perturbations are likely to be excessive, thereby leading to adverse health effects if present for a prolonged duration in an organism. A key element of the proposed approach is the use of computational systems biology models as a tool to generate hypotheses based on existing data sets, and to identify data and knowledge gaps in order to help guide the design of *in vitro* assays and focused animal studies.

A computational or mathematical model is "a formal hypothesis about how the elements of a system are mathematically related, which will typically include multiple sources of data and algorithms".[2] Computational models already play a vital and ever-growing role in risk assessment, providing a quantitative framework to proceed from "uncertain information to a hypothetical view of the physical world to a rational, regulatory decision".[2] Well-designed models can: 1) provide a more rigorous conceptual understanding of a problem than is possible from a reliance on intuition alone; 2) synthesize a broad range of available information into a single analytical tool for shared understanding across disciplines and multiple actors; and 3) help quantify sources of uncertainty in data and hypotheses.[2–4]

The US Environmental Protection Agency's (EPA) Strategic Plan for Evaluating the Toxicity of Chemicals,[5] published in response to the NRC report, also envisions dynamic mathematical modeling as a key component of risk assessment, linking toxicity pathways to dose response (Figure 24.1). This plan calls for computational models that can predict organ injury from chemical exposure through simulation of: 1) the dynamic characteristics of exposure and dose; 2) perturbations to molecular pathways; 3) the link between these perturbations and alterations to cell state; and 4) integration of molecular and cellular responses into a physiological "virtual tissue" model.[5]

Despite their potential as a robust tool in the regulatory decision-making process, computational models are too often used as black-box "answer machines"[6] without proper understanding of the assumptions, data sets and algorithms on which they are based. This discrepancy is in part due to the somewhat different priorities of policy makers and the modelers themselves. In addition, computational modeling is a relatively new field, as yet lacking an established set of best practice principles available to modelers. Consensus has not yet been achieved about appropriate characterization of the various sources of uncertainty in a model, or the general principles for comparing multiple modeling approaches, further impeding successful dialog among modelers and

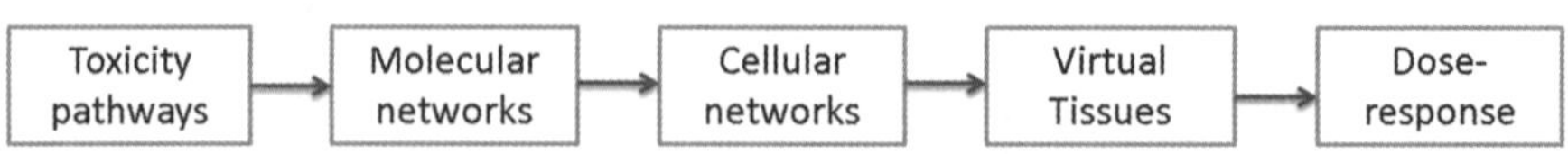


**Figure 24.1** EPA risk-assessment paradigm linking toxicity pathways to dose–response. Adapted from US EPA with permission. (Adapted from ref. 5, copyright EPA, 2009).

regulatory decision makers.[2,7] The modeling approaches implemented in the new toxicity testing paradigm will have to account for these deficiencies.

Here we provide an introduction to some concepts relevant to developing computational systems biology models of intracellular toxicity pathways. We then use the example of toxicant action in the liver to outline the process of developing a multi-scale spatial model of the liver lobule and interactions among multiple hepatic cell types consequent to exposure to toxic agents. These modeling approaches, applied across different pathways and tissues, will be pivotal in creating 21$^{st}$ Century *in vitro* toxicology testing strategies that are capable of determining likely pathway targets (*i.e.*, the hazards associated with the chemicals at high exposures) and the risks associated with specific use conditions.

## 24.2 Toxicity Pathways Underlying Biological Response to Chemicals

The biological effects of a chemical or hazardous substance in individual cells are mediated by cognate "receptor" molecules and downstream signaling and transcriptional networks, which together comprise the intracellular toxicity pathways. The subsequent changes in the state and dynamic behavior of these networks form the basis of the particular shape of the dose–response curve for specific phenotypic end points. A finite, small number of core stress–response pathways mediate the response of cells to various chemical stimuli to maintain homeostasis, or to make specific cell-fate decisions, such as apoptosis.[8] These include the oxidative stress response, heat-shock response, DNA-damage response, hypoxia, and endoplasmic reticulum stress pathways. All of these stress–response pathways feature a common architecture consisting of a transcription factor, a "sensor," and a "transducer", and are present in all cell types of an organism (Figure 24.2).[8] This suite of pathways is typically activated at concentrations of chemicals significantly lower than those that lead to adverse effects at the organism level, and can be assayed as a group to serve as predictors of potential cell damage.[8,9] The signaling networks related to activation of specific endogenous receptor pathways, such as estrogen, androgen, and thyroid hormone signaling form a second group of toxicity pathways.

The canonical stress–response pathways are in turn made up of a core set of functional *regulatory network motifs* that underlie cellular homeostasis, decision making, and phenotypic transitions.[10] Discovered from detailed investigation of transcriptional regulatory networks in the bacterium *Escherichia coli*[11] and the budding yeast *Saccharomyces cerevisiae*,[12] each of these motifs has a characteristic structure and the capacity to perform specific information-processing functions (Figure 24.3).[10,13,14] Some examples of response motifs are: i) *negative feedback*, which enables homeostasis and acceleration of response time in gene circuits;[15,16] ii) *positive feedback*, which generates switching behavior between multiple phenotypic states;[17] iii) the *coherent feed-forward loop*, which can introduce a time delay in activation as well as detect

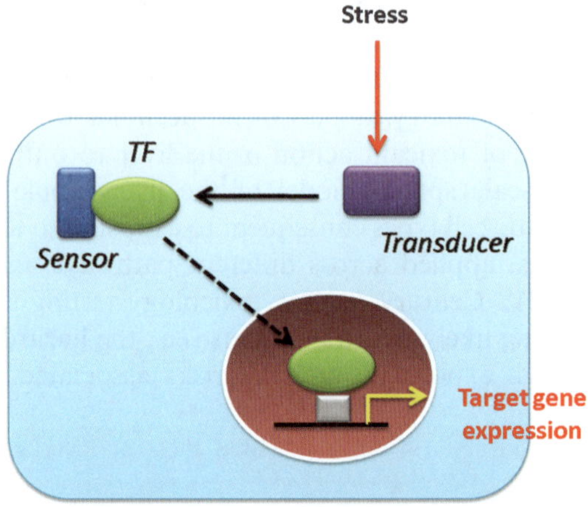


**Figure 24.2** Typical structure of a stress–response pathway. The eight so-called canonical stress–response pathways, conserved broadly across eukaryotes, have a common structure for sensing damage and mounting a transcriptional response to counteract the stress. Adapted from ref. 8 with permission. Copyright Oxford University Press, 2009.

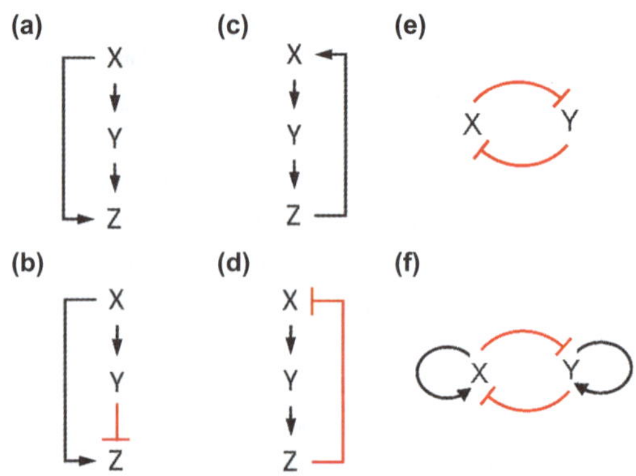


**Figure 24.3** Common network motifs in intracellular response pathways. Three elements (genes/proteins) X, Y, and Z, in a pathway can regulate each other to form: (a) a coherent feed-forward loop where X activates Y, and both X and Y activate Z; (b) an incoherent feed-forward loop where X activates both Y and Z, but Y suppresses Z; (c) a positive feedback loop; and (d) a negative feedback loop. Two transcription factors X and Y can regulate each other through, for instance: (e) a double-negative feedback loop; or (f) a double-negative feedback loop with positive autoregulation. Black sharp arrows denote activation; red flat arrows denote suppression.

persistence in the activating signal;[18] and iv) the *incoherent feed-forward loop*, which can function as a pulse generator and response accelerator.[18,19] These motifs often act in combination to generate more complex regulatory patterns in transcriptional networks.[10] Similar response motifs have been identified in the cells of higher organisms—for example in the circuits that control gene expression in the pancreas and the liver[20] as well as the regulatory circuits of human embryonic[21] and hematopoietic[22,23] stem cells. Response motifs are likely to be key components underlying toxic response, and a better understanding of their organization and quantitative behavior should lead to improved prediction of the cellular outcome of specific perturbations introduced by various chemicals.

## 24.3 Computational Systems Biology Models to Understand Perturbations in Toxicity Pathways

The advent of the "*-omics*" era has enabled detailed characterization of the molecular signatures associated with perturbations associated with chemical treatments or disease states. However, rigorous quantitative analysis of specific pathways and network motifs derived from these large-scale molecular signatures will be required for a mechanistic understanding of the underlying biological processes.[24] In particular, understanding the dynamic behavior of toxicity pathways will require stimulation of these pathways at a number of time points and at various concentrations of the activating chemical, rather than static snapshots of the molecular state.[25]

Computational systems biology pathway (CSBP) models are expected to play a key role in this process, allowing mechanistic prediction of the dose response based on pathway dynamics. Crucially, these models need to include the molecular circuits responsible for the basal operation of toxicity pathways in the absence of an external chemical stressor. The basal dynamics set up the background state from which additional perturbations will occur as the stress level increases. A properly implemented CSBP model would take such changes into account to predict the range of concentrations of stressors that would not produce appreciable adversity. A key aspect of the applicability of such models is the quantitative characterization of the underlying network circuits from appropriately designed *in vitro* assays. CSBP models can also allow the assessment of pathway components that display polymorphisms in the human population to help identify sensitive sub-populations.

The most common approach to modeling dynamical systems like intracellular signaling circuits involves deterministic simulations using ordinary differential equations (ODEs). This approach assumes that the molecular components of the network of interest exist in a well-mixed volume such as the cytosol or nucleus and that the amounts or concentrations of all molecular species in the network can be approximated by continuous variables. A typical deterministic model consists of a set of coupled first-order ODEs, each describing the rate of change in the concentration or abundance of a molecular component.[26] The ODEs contain terms that specify the way one molecular species regulates the others based on known biochemical interactions. Once the numerical values of parameters and initial conditions are assigned based on existing literature and *in vitro* data, the time evolution of the system can be followed using a variety of numerical ODE solvers. Although this ODE-based approach does not take into account spatial diffusion or stochastic fluctuation, it is a valuable computational tool that has provided many insights into the intricate design of molecular circuits underlying a variety of biological processes like cell cycle regulation, signal transduction, cell differentiation, stress response, and biological rhythms.[27–31]

The ODE-based modeling approach does not take into account stochastic fluctuation in gene expression and intracellular components, which may play an important role in cellular response by generating non-genetic phenotypic variability among an isogenic cell population.[32] The random fluctuations in mRNA and protein concentrations can be modeled by stochastic simulation algorithms like Gillespie's direct method and first-reaction method.[33,34] Gillespie's algorithm is essentially a Monte Carlo simulation technique where the number of reacting molecules in the model system and the reaction rate constants are used to generate two probability density functions, one of which predicts the time interval between successive reaction events, while the other function identifies which one among all possible reactions is likely to occur next. The time variable in the simulation is then updated by the calculated time interval, and the copy numbers of the reactants and products of the predicted reaction are updated according to the reaction stoichiometry. Several modified versions of the original Gillespie algorithm have been developed to improve its computational efficiency, including the next-reaction method, tau-leaping, and hybrid models.[35–38] Most of these are approximate methods, but greatly reduce the simulation time. In some cases, stochastic simulations are performed simply by adding "white noise" terms to the most variable species in ODE equations.

Developmental processes are usually characterized by discrete, all-or-none changes in the expression of lineage-specific genes belonging to a large gene regulatory network. The Boolean network modeling paradigm is often a good approximation of the gene expression patterns in these processes. In this approach, each gene in the model system is assumed to take one of only two values, 0 (off) and 1 (on). The state of each gene is updated according to its current state and that of other regulatory genes it is connected to in the network, as governed by a pre-set Boolean logical rule table. This binary-state assumption reduces the dependence on various kinetic parameters in a model, instead making full use of the large available database of qualitative protein–protein and protein–gene interactions. As with deterministic and stochastic models, a simulation of a Boolean network model is expected to converge to an attractor state representing the binary gene expression pattern of a particular phenotypic state.[39] For chemicals that exhibit developmental toxicity, a Boolean network model can be used to predict low-dose effects based on high-throughput screening, which would allow comparison of gene expression profiles between the undisturbed and disrupted states of the transcriptional regulatory network.

In evaluating *in vitro* results for safety assessment pathway modeling in individual cells, especially primary cells or in organotypic cell cultures, should suffice to provide results for establishing acceptable exposure standards for low-dose environmental exposures.[40] However, pathway analysis in single cells is unlikely to be adequate for assessing risks at higher exposures, such as those expected with pharmaceuticals that are used at sufficient doses to cause therapeutic responses. In these cases, network perturbations need to be evaluated in the context of intercellular interactions arising in more complex tissue matrices. The modeling techniques discussed above, based on a topological representation of cellular signaling networks, ignore the spatial relationship among intracellular molecular species as well as the spatial heterogeneity inside a cell. In reality, the cytosol, nucleus and organelles such as mitochondria and endoplasmic reticulum segregate the intracellular space into a number of discrete compartments. To account for the difference in concentrations of molecules between these compartments and inter-compartment molecular traffic, simple compartmental models can be established where each compartment is still assumed to behave as a well-mixed sub-system. However, in cases where the spatial aspect of molecular diffusion within cellular compartments is of biological importance, the diffusion process must be explicitly considered. Examples include pattern formation in the animal body in response to a concentration gradient of morphogens, effects of chemicals on different dermal layers when absorbed by the skin, and propagating waves of signaling molecules in the cytosol. In these circumstances, spatial–temporal models based on partial differential equations may be employed.[41,42] Another way to incorporate space in a model is by modeling the motion and interaction of distinct molecular species as discrete particles, for example with agent-based spatial modeling. Agent-based models can also address another problem arising from the lack of a spatial component in network models: incorporating multicellular or tissue-level interactions.

## 24.4 The Agent-Based Modeling Approach

Agent-based modeling (ABM), also referred to as "individual-based modeling"[43–45] is more intuitive than traditional equation-based modeling formalisms. As such, this approach can be helpful in model development, interpretation and use by a variety of stakeholders. The "agents" in an ABM may be individual molecules, cells or other entities that populate a virtual "world" (a discrete lattice), with each agent represented as a distinct data structure (or "object") in the computational model (see Figure 24.4). Agents can move in the physical space of the world, and interact with neighboring agents according to a pre-defined set of rules. Over a large number of iterations, these local interactions generate macroscopic, sometimes counterintuitive, phenomena of interest'— sometimes referred to as "emergent properties" of the system being modeled.

Agents in an ABM are modeled as discrete entities located in a physical space—therefore the assumption of a well-mixed continuous system, essential in differential-equation-based dynamic modeling approaches, is no longer required. The reliance on averaged aggregate parameters is thus reduced in favor of an emphasis on strict definition of rules governing agent behavior and

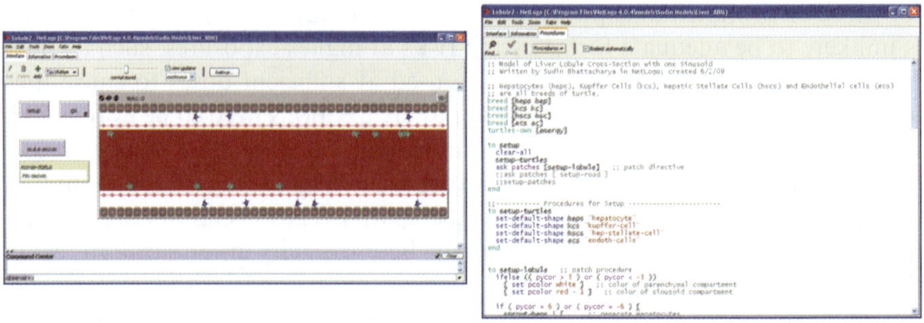

**Figure 24.4** The NetLogo agent-based modeling platform with an integrated visualization/programming interface.

interactions. Decisions regarding such explicit rules for agent behavior are typically more intuitive than the choice and estimation of abstract parameters in equation-based models, making it easier for decision makers to interpret and use the model. ABM platforms like NetLogo[46] use an integrated visualization/programming interface (Figure 24.4), which facilitates evaluation of how modifications to the "engine" of the model may affect model behavior.

First used in models in social science and ecology, ABMs have been applied to a wide range of biological problems in recent years, particularly for modeling pathophysiological processes with a significant spatial component.[43] These include tumor formation,[47–50] inflammation,[51,52] wound healing,[53–55] T-cell activation and proliferation within a lymph node,[56] and stromal cell trafficking during acute skeletal muscle ischemia.[57] In these "virtual tissue" models agents represent the behavior of individual cells—the natural functional unit in tissue-level biological phenomena. In the toxicology context, virtual tissues can be thought of as multicellular models of tissue microenvironment that attempt to reconstruct the *in vivo* milieu of target organs to simulate the physiological consequences of toxicity pathway activation by specific chemicals. As such they represent an extension of traditional compartmental models to the scale of individual cells in a tissue.[58]

## 24.5 Motivation for Multi-Scale Liver Models

### 24.5.1 The Effects of TCDD in the Liver

In the discussion below, we lay out the motivation for, and an approach to, developing a multi-scale agent-based model of the liver lobule, using the persistent environmental contaminant 2,3,7,8-tetrachlorodibenzo-*p*-dioxin (TCDD) as a case study. This modeling framework would also be adaptable to the study of toxic effects of other environmental or pharmaceutical agents. TCDD belongs to a class of toxicants known as halogenated aromatic hydrocarbons (HAHs), which produce toxic effects in mammals through binding to the aryl hydrocarbon receptor (AhR).[59–61] The toxic effects of

TCDD and other AhR agonists, which feature prominently in the list of high-risk substances associated with hazardous sites on the NPL compiled by the US EPA and the Agency for Toxic Substances and Disease Registry (ATSDR), are of interest to the environmental health research community. The liver is one of the most sensitive organs for toxicity induced by TCDD. A spatial agent-based "virtual tissue" model of the liver lobule that incorporates a mechanistic dose–response model of the activation of the AhR toxicity pathway in individual hepatocytes can be used to investigate the sequence of events leading from early activation of the AhR pathway through subsequent cellular effects to cell proliferation, and culminating in liver cancer as an endpoint. The structure of the AhR pathway is well studied (Figure 24.5), and as such could serve as a good case study for multi-scale, quantitative dose–response model development based on information from *in vitro* assays and *in vivo* biomarkers, as envisioned in the 2007 NAS report.[1]

Key steps in the hepatic exposure–dose–response continuum of TCDD culminating in liver cancer can be summarized as follows:[62]

1) Accumulation of TCDD in the target tissue.
2) Formation of a complex with AhR.

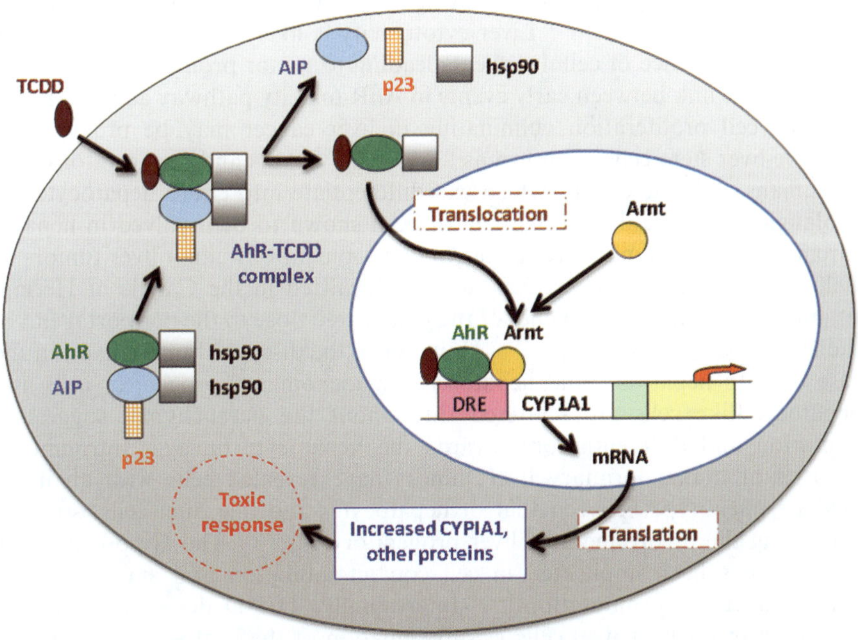


**Figure 24.5** Key components and events in AhR signaling pathway activation. AIP: Aryl hydrocarbon receptor interacting protein; hsp90: heat-shock protein 90; Arnt: aryl hydrocarbon receptor nuclear translocator; DRE: dioxin-responsive element.

3) Activation of growth-regulatory genes by the AhR–TCDD complex.
4) Cellular responses to the altered expression of growth-regulatory gene products.
5) The effect of these cellular events on tumor promotion and progression.

However the mechanistic and causal links connecting steps 3) to 5) are not fully understood.

The carcinogenic effects of TCDD are believed to be mediated by tumor promotion rather than initiation.[63] Based on this assumption, a "negative selection" model of tumor promotion has been proposed where specifically mutated cells acquire a proliferative advantage in the presence of persistent mitosuppression.[64] TCDD suppresses apoptosis induced in rat hepatocytes by DNA-damaging agents, suggesting that it could result in selective expansion of clones evading growth arrest and apoptosis.[65,66] The traditional benchmark-dose calculation for low-dose hepatotoxic effects of TCDD has been based on centrilobular induction of cytochromes P450 1A1 (CYP1A1) and 1A2 (CYP1A2). However the link between these early centrilobular gene expression events, and subsequent cell proliferation events which originate in the periportal region of the liver lobule, is unclear. Specifically, cytochrome P450 activity and cell proliferation follow different dose–response patterns, with CYP1A1 activity appearing to be reversible following prolonged TCDD exposure, whereas the selective growth of altered hepatic foci and cell proliferation are persistent.[67–71] Liver cytotoxicity is likely to be an intermediate step in the sequence of cellular events leading to tumor promotion.[67,70–72]

A possible link between early events in AhR toxicity pathway activation and eventual cell proliferation culminating in liver cancer may be provided by putative liver stem cells— known as "oval cells" in rats and "progenitor cells" in humans.[73,74] These cells, which can differentiate into either hepatocytes or cholangiocytes (bile duct cells),[75] have been shown to be involved in hepatocarcinogenesis, and may have a role in development of human liver tumors as well.[74] In a quiescent liver, oval cells are localized in the Canals of Hering, situated in the smallest branches of the biliary tree close to the periportal end of the liver lobule (Figure 24.6).[76–78] However in the diseased human liver, in the case of both hepatitis[79] and hepatocellular adenomas,[74] progenitor cells and hepatocyte-like cells are scattered throughout the parenchyma, suggesting migration and differentiation towards the hepatocyte lineage. Intriguingly, biopsies of human primary liver tumors have revealed cells with an intermediate phenotype between that of hepatocytes and bile duct cells, strongly suggesting the involvement of liver progenitor cells.[80,81] The Hippo signaling pathway has been implicated in cell contact inhibition and suppression of hepatic oval cell proliferation.[82,83] Interestingly, TCDD deregulates contact inhibition in rat liver oval cells *via* upregulation of the proto-oncogene cyclin A,[84] suggesting a possible role for this pathway in TCDD-induced tumor promotion. Several other non-parenchymal cells (*e.g.*, hepatic stellate cells and Kupffer cells) are also involved in regulation of oval cell activity.[85] Loss of cell–cell contact and enhanced cell proliferation including oval cell

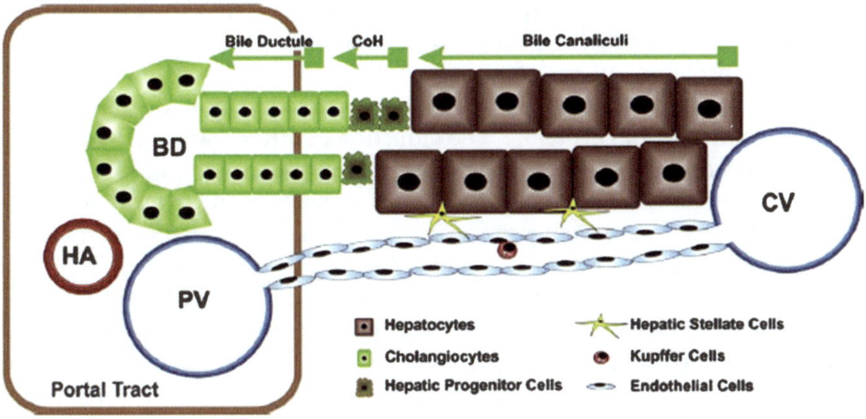


**Figure 24.6** Location of hepatic progenitor cells in the liver. Progenitor cells are located in the Canals of Herring (CoH), the connection between bile canaliculi and bile ducts. Reproduced from ref. 77 with permission. Copyright Elsevier, 2009.

hyperplasia has been noted in livers of rats treated with TCDD and other AhR agonists.[86–90]

In spite of the large number of empirical studies with TCDD, there is no agreement on a unifying hypothesis to connect these observations into a mechanistic description linking AhR toxicity pathway activation to liver cancer. Spatial multicellular agent-based modeling of the liver lobule incorporating parenchymal (hepatocytes) and non-parenchymal cells (hepatic stellate cells and Kupffer cells), along with oval cell proliferation, appear necessary to serve as an ontological tool to assemble diverse *in vitro* and *in vivo* observations and compare alternative hypotheses for TCDD-induced tumor promotion. Research teams at The Hamner are pursuing ABM approaches with TCDD and in examining pathways perturbed by therapeutic molecules that cause drug-induced liver injury (DILI).

## 24.5.2 Pharmacokinetic Models for Dioxin and Regional Hepatic Induction of Cytochromes Require Expanding Liver Compartments

Accumulation of TCDD in the liver causes increased expression of several proteins, including cytochrome P450 (CYP) 1A2 which binds TCDD and leads to its dose-dependent sequestration in the liver. Physiologically based pharmacokinetic (PBPK) and pharmacodynamic (PBPD) models of TCDD and related compounds therefore need to account for induction of the binding protein to describe tissue time courses. The earliest PBPK models for TCDD used fractional occupancy of a transcriptionally active receptor to provide an instantaneous adjustment of the protein levels depending on occupancy of the

DNA-response elements for AhR in the CYP 1A1/2 genes.[91] This approach lumped together complex steps associated with transcription and translation, and ignored protein synthesis and degradation rates. Second-generation PBPK/PBPD models provided explicit rates for production and degradation of CYP1A1/2 mRNA and protein.[92] The induction of mRNA was modeled with a Hill relationship that allowed for co-operative promoter binding. In all these efforts, the liver was modeled as a single homogeneous compartment, and data from whole-liver homogenates were used to compare model simulations to variables such as levels of CYP1A1 and CYP1A2 or sequestration of TCDD in the liver. However, immunohistochemical staining[93] revealed that levels of CYP proteins induced by TCDD in the liver were not uniformly distributed across the liver acinus. At low-inducing doses, induction occurs in the centrilobular region and progresses to the periportal areas as dose increases. Responses of individual cells appear to be dichotomous: cells are either in a basal non-induced phenotype or maximally stained, suggestive of a switch-like transition from a normal to an induced phenotype. Similar behavior, all-or-none induction, had been reported for methylcholanthrene induction of CYP1A1/2 *in vitro*.[94]

Geometric models have been developed to describe and explain this regional induction of CYP1A1/2 in the liver acinus by TCDD.[95,96] In this model structure, it was assumed that differential sensitivity to induction in each zone occurs due to the different affinity of the DNA-binding sites for the Ah-TCDD complex; Hill-coefficients for induction were kept high to insure steepness in the induction in each separate region. Andersen *et al.*[95] implemented this structure with five zones within the liver: a concentric peritportal zone, a fenestrated periportal region that interconnected multiple functional units, and three concentric centrilobular areas [Figure 24.7(a)]. Estimates of regional induction were calculated by a PBPK/PD model and then converted into color intensities to compare model output with immunohistochemical data [Figure 24.7(b)]. The five-subcompartment liver model reproduced sharp boundaries between induced and non-induced regions as seen with the immunochemistry of the liver. However, the model structure used is primitive in describing the molecular interactions controlling induction of batteries of genes, and the biological consequences of altered protein patterns in different regions of the liver and on different cells within these regions.

Development of PBPD models for transcript and protein induction still present many challenges since the cellular processes involved in induction of single genes and battery of genes are under active investigation with the new methods of cellular and molecular biology.[97] An important step in regard to evaluating the adverse responses to chemicals (both toxicants and drugs) is the need to understand and create quantitative PD models of the innate biology. With TCDD, the process of tissue binding and liver sequestration is intimately associated with signaling mediated *via* receptor-activation and transcriptional enhancement. Current findings on involvement of protein kinase cascades and histone modification in transcriptional activation of gene expression may underlie aspects of the transcriptional switch.[17,27] Yet the characterization of

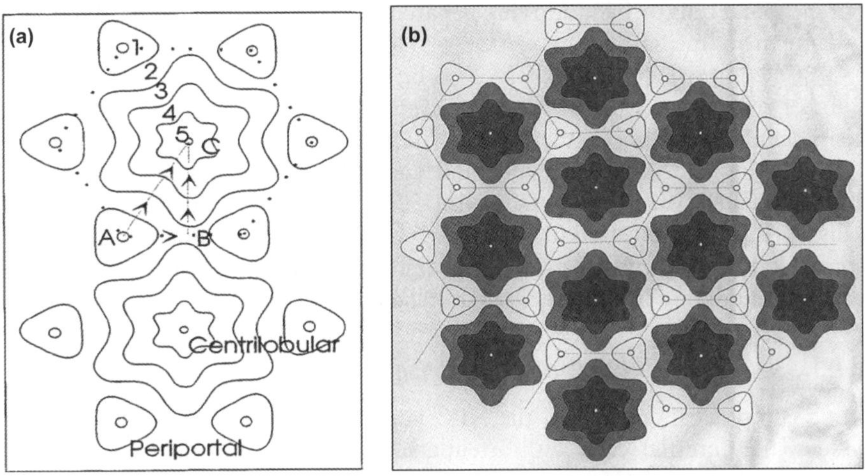


**Figure 24.7** A geometric model for the liver acinus. (a) The liver acinus is depicted as consisting of five regions whose surface areas and volumes were estimated by least distance and greatest distance flow lines from periportal to centrilobular. Polar coordinate descriptions allowed tools to calculate the zonal boundaries and volumes. Reproduced from ref. 96 with permission. (b) Regional induction was estimated colorimetrically by simulating extent of induction in various regions and using the values to specify intensity of staining.

the molecular mechanisms of non-linear induction is only the first step in understanding tissue response. The alterations in cellular phenotype (*i.e.*, the change from a basal to an induced phenotype) and the extent of the change in protein expression in relation to liver dose of TCDD need to be linked to responses of various cells in the different regions of the liver. The liver does not consist of hepatocytes alone and other cell types are located in specific regions of the liver. For instance, oval cells are found in the periportal region and give rise to both hepatocytes and biliary epithelium.[98,99] An agent-based model of liver responses to TCDD needs to account for the consequences of gene battery induction of each cell type in the liver. Before outlining the structure of an agent-based description for the liver, we need a sense of the "cast of characters" to include in a quantitative assessment of toxicity induced by TCDD and other chemicals in this tissue.

### 24.5.3 Involvement of Non-Parenchymal Cells in Liver Toxicity

It has become increasingly clear over the past two decades that the liver is not just a bag of hepatic parenchymal cells ("hepatocytes," HPCs), and that non-parenchymal cells (NPCs) also play important roles in hepatotoxic response. It is now appreciated by most hepatotoxicologists that studies employing only hepatocytes *in vitro* are unlikely to capture the nature and complexity of *in vivo* hepatotoxic responses and may lead to erroneous conclusions about modes and mechanisms of action. NPCs influence responses by directly injuring parenchymal cells or by modifying hepatocellular injury through production of inflammatory mediators.

NPCs comprise approximately 20% of liver volume and about 35% of the number of liver cells. Most reside in liver sinusoids, but the NPC population also includes bile duct epithelial cells (BDECs) and cells of conducting blood vessels (*e.g.*, smooth muscle cells and endothelium). Sinusoidal cells include endothelial cells (SECs), Kupffer cells (KCs), stellate cells (StCs), natural killer cells (NKCs) and natural killer T-cells (NKTCs). Under certain circumstances, some blood-borne cells can be considered liver cells when they arrest in this organ and migrate into the hepatic parenchyma.

### *24.5.3.1 Sinusoidal Endothelial Cells*

SECs comprise about half of the NPC population. Like endothelium in other tissues, they are flat cells with attenuated cytoplasm, and they comprise the sinusoidal lining.[100] However, unlike capillary endothelium of other tissues, liver SECs are fixed to an attenuated basement membrane, with small (100 nm) pores, or fenestrae, traversing these cells, allowing them to function as a biofilter between the Space of Disse (the space between the SECs and HPCs; see Figure 24.8) and the sinusoidal lumen. These fenestrae impart selective barrier properties to SECs. In addition, these cells are involved in scavenging macromolecules such as lipoproteins and glycosaminoglycans, in antigen clearance and presentation, and in tissue regeneration after liver injury.

### *24.5.3.2 Kupffer Cells*

KCs account for about one third of the NPC population. They are the resident macrophages of the liver and reside in sinusoids on the luminal side of the SECs

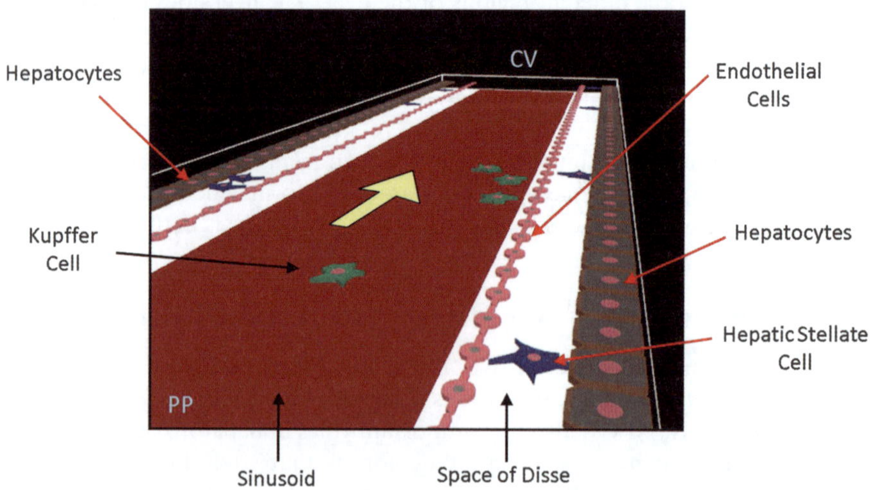


**Figure 24.8** Agent-Based model of liver lobule section (representational unit: one sinusoid).

(Figure 24.8). Cellular projections from KCs through SEC fenestrae put these cells in close physical contact with HPCs. They are anatomically and functionally heterogeneous, and occur in greater numbers in the periportal regions of liver lobules, where they are also more active. KCs phagocytose bacteria and circulating cell debris and have the capacity to kill foreign as well as host cells. They remove and degrade bacterial products *e.g.*, bacterial lipopolysaccharide (LPS) from the circulation and modulate immune responses by clearing and presenting antigen to T-cells. They also regulate fibroblast proliferation and HPC function and, when activated, produce a variety of inflammatory mediators and undergo a respiratory burst that results in the production of potentially damaging reactive oxygen species (ROS). Activators of KCs include various microbes and microbial products (*e.g.*, LPS, zymosan) as well as endogenous agents (*e.g.*, estrogen). Moreover, KCs become activated during hepatotoxic responses caused by agents such as ethanol, acetaminophen and carbon tetrachloride. KCs can participate in hepatotoxic responses either directly through the release of ROS or other cytotoxic factors, or indirectly through the release of mediators that control HPC function or that activate other NPCs to promote HPC killing.

#### *24.5.3.3 Bile Duct Epithelial Cells*

BDECs also called cholangiocytes, form bile ducts within the liver through which bile secreted by HPCs is conducted to the small intestine. Intra-hepatic bile ducts are located in periportal regions of liver lobules and ultimately coalesce into a common bile duct that exits the liver. BDECs that form the ducts are epithelial cells with a microvillar surface and comprise about 2% of liver cells. They modulate bile fluidity and pH by reabsorbing solutes (*e.g.*, amino acids) and secreting water and electrolytes (*e.g.*, chloride and bicarbonate). Under conditions of insult, BDECs can produce chemokines that recruit and activate inflammatory cells. A number of toxicants produce BDEC injury, including aflatoxin B1, 1-nitronaphthylene, methylenedianiline and α-naphthylisothiocyanate (ANIT). ANIT, for example, is concentrated in the bile and causes release of chemotactic factors from BDECs that recruit neutrophils, which become activated and damage these cells. TCDD can induce a combination of hepatocellular carcinoma/adenomas and cholangiocarcinomas.[101]

#### *24.5.3.4 Stellate Cells*

StCs (Figure 24.8) comprise about 20% of the NPC population. As the name suggests, they have a star-like shape and contain cytoplasmic droplets comprising fat-soluble substances like vitamin A. They are found in the Space of Disse, with their stellate processes wrapped around the layer of SECs that forms the sinusoidal lumen. In their usual, contractile phenotype they are ideally positioned to control sinusoidal diameter and thereby regulate local blood flow. Like other NPCs they can become stimulated acutely to release various biologically active meditators, including transforming growth factor-β (TGF-β) and colony stimulating factor-1 (CSF-1).

#### *24.5.3.5 Natural Killer Cells and Natural Killer T-Cells*

NKCs and NKTCs comprise about 15% of circulating blood lymphocytes and about 3% of the sinusoidal NPC population. These are large, granular lymphocytes that are considered innate immune cells capable of lysing virus-infected host cells or tumor cells without prior sensitization. The cell surface of NKCs houses receptors that recognize molecules on neighboring cells that are induced by cell stress and other, inhibitory receptors that recognize class I major histocompatibility complex molecules expressed by healthy cells. When HPCs or are infected or otherwise damaged, the balance of ligands they express for these NKC receptors is altered in a way that activates a killing response. NKCs secrete cytokines (*e.g.*, interferon-γ) that can prompt release of bioactive factors by other cells (*e.g.*, KCs) and proteases that kill target cells. Conversely, NKCs are activated by cytokines (*e.g.*, interleukin 12) released from other NPC types.

#### *24.5.3.6 Neutrophils*

Neutrophils are normally considered to be circulating white blood cells. However, during many forms of liver pathogenesis, these cells become trapped in liver sinusoids and migrate through the SEC barrier into the parenchyma, effectively becoming part of the liver's NPC population. Activated neutrophils release ROS and toxic proteases that can injure other liver cells, and are clearly involved in the pathogenesis of liver injury from microbial products such as LPS.

Overall, NPCs can play a major role in the pathogenesis of liver injury from various xenobiotic agents as both effectors and targets. An agent-based model of liver tissue structure and development of injury would have to explicitly include these various cell types (*i.e.*, various 'agents'). Each of these agents has a complement of networks and pathways that are expected to respond either directly to specific receptor agonists or indirectly through intercellular signaling from other neighboring cells.

## 24.6 Agent-Based Model of the Human Liver

It should be clear from the discussion above that a realistic model of the liver lobule and toxic effects therein should have to account for:

1) cellular heterogeneity across the lobule;
2) multiple cell types in the liver lobule that participate in liver injury.

The virtual tissue formalism can be used to develop a spatial agent-based model of the human liver lobule (the "lobule ABM"), with individual hepatocytes represented by single agents. There have been some initial efforts towards

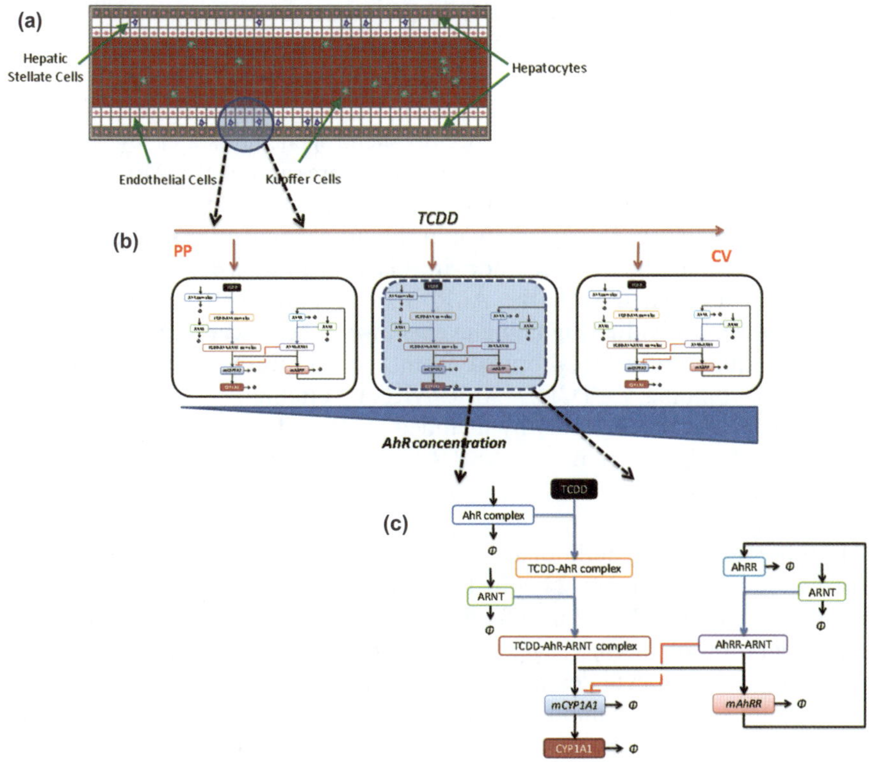


**Figure 24.9** Implementation of multi-scale agent-based model (ABM) of liver lobule. (a) ABM of the lobule showing distinct cell types, with kinetics from PBPK model used as input for TCDD flow rate through the lobule. (b) Individual agents (hepatocytes) along the lobule, with heterogeneous states (*e.g.*, with graded AhR concentration), will be exposed to TCDD molecules flowing through lobule sinusoid, which determines the dose for each agent (PP: periportal end; CV: central-vein end). (c) Each agent (hepatocyte) is implemented as a molecular network: in this case the intra-hepatocyte cascade of events linking ligand (TCDD)—activation of the the Ah receptor to expression of cytochrome (CYP) P450 proteins. Panel (c) was adapted from Ref. 115, 2010 with permission. Copyright Oxford University Press, 2010.

development of agent-based representations of the liver.[102–104] Here we lay out the steps towards developing a multi-scale model, where the lobule ABM is coupled with an intra-hepatocyte ODE-based kinetic model of AhR pathway activation for TCDD dose–response prediction (Figure 24.9). A preliminary version of such a model, incorporating hepatocytes, liver endothelial cells, hepatic stellate cells and Kupffer cells, is shown in Figure 24.8. Other components, including oval cells, can be added in the course of model development.

A multi-scale dose–response model of AhR toxicity pathway activation in the human liver may be implemented in the following manner.

1) Output from a standard TCDD PBPK model (*e.g.*, Leung *et al.*[91,105]) can be used to estimate disposition of TCDD in the liver lobule: the input dose for the lobule agent-based model [Figure 24.9(a)].
2) This TCDD input dose would act upon the individual agents (hepatocytes) in the model, which occupy heterogeneous states by virtue of differential gene exposure: *e.g.*, graded expression of the AhR along the lobule (higher at the centrilobular end)[106] [Figure 24.9(b)].
3) The agents (hepatocytes) would be implemented essentially as an intracellular signaling cascade: in this case all molecular events known to be associated with the AhR toxicity pathway [Figures 24.5 and 24.9(c)]. Individual signaling events along the cascade can be modeled and quantitatively calibrated from the literature, including TCDD–AhR binding,[59] TCDD–AhR–ARNT binding,[60,107] activation of AhRR (AhR repressor) by liganded AhR and reciprocal inhibition of AhR binding activity by AhRR,[108,109] and cytochrome (CYP) P450 protein induction.[110–112]

In subsequent steps, additional events can be incorporated into the signaling cascade shown in Figure 24.9(c), for example crosstalk between the AhR pathway and cell cycle/cell proliferation.[90,113] This would be accompanied by implementation of specific "agent rules", *e.g.*, hepatocyte proliferation (agent addition), or hepatocyte death (agent deletion), at specific doses of TCDD or downstream signaling components/metabolites. The model structure would be extensible to other chemicals besides TCDD: however the implementation of the agent structure (*i.e.*, the signaling cascade shown in Figure 24.9(c) would vary from case to case, depending on the specific toxicity pathways stimulated). In addition, a variety of interactions between diverse cell types/agents would need to be specified to account for pharmacodynamic responses, including necrosis, apoptosis, proliferation and tumor promotion.

## 24.7 Conclusions

Toxicity pathway identification and computational systems biology modeling of these pathways are key components of the ***TT21C***[1] initiative to develop *in vitro*, mode-of-action based assays for toxicity testing and risk assessment for low-level exposure to chemicals in the general environment. Prediction of organism-level responses for drugs requires linking these cell-based pathway models to intercellular interactions expected within target organs. "Virtual liver" projects[58,114] are being designed to implement computational systems approaches for assessing liver toxicity. These projects require a starting point of defining normal function in the tissue as a basis for quantitatively defining deviations in function associated with drug and chemical perturbations. The normal tissue behavior will be common across platforms and across chemical treatments. Chemical-specific information will then inform pharmacokinetics of delivery to the cells within the organ and the pathway targets of the chemical in cells within the tissue. As described here, a combination of modeling tools will be essential in making the ***TT21C*** vision a reality and extending the vision from low-dose risk assessment for environmental chemicals on to pharmaceuticals, foodstuffs, and consumer products.

## References


1. NAS/NRC, *Toxicity Testing in the 21st Century: A Vision and a Strategy*, 2007.
2. W. Wagner, E. Fisher and P. Pascual, *New York University Environmental Law Journal*, 2010, **18**, 293.
3. F. A. G. den Butter and M. S. Morgan, What makes the models-policy interaction successful?, in *Empirical models and policy-making: interaction and institutions. Edited by F. A. G. d. Butter and M. S. Morgan*, Routledge, New York, 2000, 222-224.
4. N. Oreskes, Why believe a computer? Models, measures, and meaning in the natural world, in *The Earth Around Us: Maintaining a Livable Planet.* Edited by J. S. Schneiderman, W.H. Freeman and Co., San Francisco, 2000, 70-82.
5. U.S.EPA., *The U.S. Environmental Protection Agency's Strategic Plan for Evaluating the Toxicity of Chemicals. EPA100/K-09/001,* 2009.
6. J. L. King and K. L. Kraemer, *Models, Facts, and the Policy Process: The Political Ecology of Estimated Truth (Working Paper #URB-006)*, undated.
7. NAS/NRC, *Models in Environmental Regulatory Decision Making*, 2007.
8. S. O. Simmons, C. Y. Fan and R. Ramabhadran, *Toxicol. Sci.*, 2009, **111**, 202–225.
9. D. Kultz, *Annu. Rev. Physiol.*, 2005, **67**, 225–257.
10. U. Alon, *Nat. Rev. Genet.*, 2007, **8**, 450–461.
11. S. S. Shen-Orr, R. Milo, S. Mangan and U. Alon, *Nat. Genet.*, 2002, **31**, 64–68.
12. T. I. Lee, N. J. Rinaldi, F. Robert, D. T. Odom, Z. Bar-Joseph, G. K. Gerber, N. M. Hannett, C. T. Harbison, C. M. Thompson, I. Simon, J. Zeitlinger, E. G. Jennings, H. L. Murray, D. B. Gordon, B. Ren, J. J. Wyrick, J. B. Tagne, T. L. Volkert, E. Fraenkel, D. K. Gifford and R. A. Young, *Science*, 2002, **298**, 799–804.
13. U. S. Bhalla and R. Iyengar, *Science*, 1999, **283**, 381–387.
14. J. J. Tyson, K. C. Chen and B. Novak, *Curr. Opin. Cell Biol.*, 2003, **15**, 221–231.
15. N. Rosenfeld, M. B. Elowitz and U. Alon, *J. Mol. Biol.*, 2002, **323**, 785–793.
16. Q. Zhang and M. E. Andersen, *PLoS Comp. Biol.*, 2007, **3**, 345–363.
17. J. E. Ferrell, Jr., *Curr. Opin. Cell Biol.*, 2002, **14**, 140–8.
18. S. Mangan, A. Zaslaver and U. Alon, *J. Mol. Biol.*, 2003, **334**, 197–204.

19. S. Mangan, S. Itzkovitz, A. Zaslaver and U. Alon, *J. Mol. Biol.*, 2006, **356**, 1073–1081.
20. D. T. Odom, N. Zizlsperger, D. B. Gordon, G. W. Bell, N. J. Rinaldi, H. L. Murray, T. L. Volkert, J. Schreiber, P. A. Rolfe, D. K. Gifford, E. Fraenkel, G. I. Bell and R. A. Young, *Science*, 2004, **303**, 1378–1381.
21. L. A. Boyer, T. I. Lee, M. F. Cole, S. E. Johnstone, S. S. Levine, J. R. Zucker, M. G. Guenther, R. M. Kumar, H. L. Murray, R. G. Jenner, D. K. Gifford, D. A. Melton, R. Jaenisch and R. A. Young, *Cell*, 2005, **122**, 947–956.
22. E. V. Rothenberg, *Nat. Immunol.*, 2007, **8**, 441–444.
23. G. Swiers, R. Patient and M. Loose, *Dev. Biol.*, 2006, **294**, 525–540.
24. R. P. Araujo, L. A. Liotta and E. F. Petricoin, *Nat. Rev. Drug Discov.*, 2007, **6**, 871–880.
25. E. A. Danna and G. P. Nolan, *Curr. Opin. Chem. Biol.*, 2006, **10**, 20–27.
26. B. B. Aldridge, J. M. Burke, D. A. Lauffenburger and P. K. Sorger, *Nat. Cell Biol.*, 2006, **8**, 1195–203.
27. U. S. Bhalla, P. T. Ram and R. Iyengar, *Science*, 2002, **297**, 1018–1023.
28. H. H. Chang, P. Y. Oh, D. E. Ingber and S. Huang, *BMC Cell Biol.*, 2006, **7**, 11.
29. H. El-Samad and M. Khammash, *Biophys. J.*, 2006, **90**, 3749–3761.
30. D. B. Forger and C. S. Peskin, *Proceedings of the National Academy of Sciences of the United States of America*, 2003, **100**, 14806–14811.
31. B. Novak and J. J. Tyson, *Biochem. Soc. Trans.*, 2003, **31**, 1526–1529.
32. M. Kaern, T. C. Elston, W. J. Blake and J. J. Collins, *Nat. Rev. Genet.*, 2005, **6**, 451–464.
33. D. T. Gillespie, *J. Comput. Phys.*, 1976, **22**, 403–434.
34. D. T. Gillespie, *J. Phys. Chem.*, 1977, **81**, 2340–2361.
35. M. A. Gibson and J. Bruck, *J. Phys. Chem. A*, 2000, **104**, 1876–1889.
36. D. T. Gillespie, *J. Chem. Phys.*, 2000, **113**, 297–306.
37. M. Rathinam, L. R. Petzold, Y. Cao and D. T. Gillespie, *J. Chem. Phys.*, 2003, **119**, 12784–12794.
38. H. Salis and Y. Kaznessis, *J. Chem. Phys.*, 2005, **122**, 54103.
39. R. Albert and H. G. Othmer, *J. Theor. Biol.*, 2003, **223**, 1–18.
40. K. Boekelheide and M. E. Andersen, *Altex*, 2010, **27**, 243–252.
41. B. N. Kholodenko, *Nat. Rev. Mol. Cell Biol.*, 2006, **7**, 165–176.
42. B. N. Kholodenko, J. F. Hancock and W. Kolch, *Nat. Rev. Mol. Cell Biol.*, 2010, **11**, 414–426.
43. G. An, Q. Mi, J. Dutta-Moscato and Y. Vodovotz, *Wiley Interdisciplinary Reviews: Systems Biology and Medicine*, 2009, **1**, 159–171.
44. E. Bonabeau, *Proceedings of the National Academy of Sciences of the United States of America*, 2002, **99**, 7280–7287.
45. V. Grimm, E. Revilla, U. Berger, F. Jeltsch, W. M. Mooij, S. F. Railsback, H. H. Thulke, J. Weiner, T. Wiegand and D. L. DeAngelis, *Science*, 2005, **310**, 987–991.
46. U. Wilensky, NetLogo. http://ccl.northwestern.edu/netlogo/. Center for Connected Learning and Computer-Based Modeling, Northwestern University, Evanston, IL, 1999.

47. J. A. Engelberg, G. E. P. Ropella and C. A. Hunt, *BMC Syst. Biol.*, 2008, **2**, 110.
48. P. Gerlee and A. R. A. Anderson, *J. Theor. Biol.*, 2009, **259**, 67–83.
49. L. Zhang, C. G. Strouthos, Z. Wang and T. S. Deisboeck, *Mathematical and Computer Modelling*, 2009, **49**, 307–319.
50. L. Zhang, Z. H. Wang, J. A. Sagotsky and T. S. Deisboeck, *J. Math. Biol.*, 2009, **58**, 545–559.
51. G. An, *Shock*, 2001, **16**, 266–273.
52. G. An, *Theoretical Biology and Medical Modelling*, 2008, **5**, 11.
53. T. Sun, P. McMinn, S. Coakley, M. Holcombe, R. Smallwood and S. MacNeil, *J. Royal Soc. Interface*, 2007, **4**, 1077–1092.
54. Y. Vodovotz, *Immunol. Res.*, 2006, **36**, 237–245.
55. D. C. Walker, G. Hill, S. M. Wood, R. H. Smallwood and J. Southgate, *IEEE Trans. NanoBiosci.*, 2004, **3**, 153–163.
56. G. Bogle and P. R. Dunbar, *Immunol. Cell Biol.*, 2010, **88**, 172–179.
57. A. M. Bailey, M. B. Lawrence, H. Shang, A. J. Katz and S. M. Peirce, *PLoS Comp. Biol.*, 2009, **5**, e1000294.
58. I. Shah and J. Wambaugh, *J. Toxicol. Environ. Health, Pt. B Crit. Rev.*, 2010, **13**, 314–328.
59. A. Poland and J. C. Knutson, *Annu. Rev. Pharmacol. Toxicol.*, 1982, **22**, 517–554.
60. J. C. Rowlands and J. A. Gustafsson, *Crit. Rev. Toxicol.*, 1997, **27**, 109–134.
61. J. V. Schmidt and C. A. Bradfield, *Annu. Rev. Cell. Dev. Biol.*, 1996, **12**, 55–89.
62. J. J. Mills and M. E. Andersen, *Toxicol. Lett.*, 1993, **68**, 177–189.
63. H. C. Pitot, T. Goldsworthy, H. A. Campbell and A. Poland, *Cancer Res.*, 1980, **40**, 3616–3620.
64. M. E. Andersen, J. J. Mills, R. L. Jirtle and W. F. Greenlee, *Toxicology*, 1995, **102**, 223–237.
65. W. Worner and D. Schrenk, *Cancer Res.*, 1996, **56**, 1272–1278.
66. K. W. Bock and C. Kohle, *Biochem. Pharmacol.*, 2005, **69**, 1403–1408.
67. R. R. Maronpot, J. F. Foley, K. Takahashi, T. Goldsworthy, G. Clark, A. Tritscher, C. Portier and G. Lucier, *Environ. Health Perspect.*, 1993, **101**, 634–42.
68. C. H. Sewall, D. A. Bell, G. C. Clark, A. M. Tritscher, D. B. Tully, J. V. Heuvel and G. W. Lucier, *Clin. Chem.*, 1995, **41**, 1829–1834.
69. A. M. Tritscher, G. C. Clark, C. Sewall, R. C. Sills, R. Maronpot and G. W. Lucier, *Carcinogenesis*, 1995, **16**, 2807–2811.
70. J. Whysner and G. M. Williams, *Pharmacol. Ther.*, 1996, **71**, 193–223.
71. M. Viluksela, Y. Bager, J. T. Tuomisto, G. Scheu, M. Unkila, R. Pohjanvirta, S. Flodstrom, V. M. Kosma, J. Maki-Paakkanen, T. Vartiainen, C. Klimm, K. W. Schramm, L. Warngard and J. Tuomisto, *Cancer Res.*, 2000, **60**, 6911–6920.
72. M. T. Busser and W. K. Lutz, *Carcinogenesis*, 1987, **8**, 1433–7.
73. J. M. Lemire, N. Shiojiri and N. Fausto, *Am. J. Pathol.*, 1991, **139**, 535–552.

74. L. Libbrecht, R. De Vos, D. Cassiman, V. Desmet, R. Aerts and T. Roskams, *Am. J. Surgical Pathol.*, 2001, **25**, 1388–1396.
75. T. A. Roskams, L. Libbrecht and V. J. Desmet, *Seminars in Liver Disease*, 2003, **23**, 385–396.
76. N. Fausto and J. S. Campbell, *Mechanisms of Development*, 2003, **120**, 117–130.
77. N. Fausto, J. S. Campbell and K. J. Riehle, *Hepatology*, 2006, **43**, S45–S53.
78. E. Gaudio, G. Carpino, V. Cardinale, A. Franchitto, P. Onori and D. Alvaro, *Digestive and Liver Disease*, 2009, **41**, 455–462.
79. L. Libbrecht, V. Desmet, B. Van Damme and T. Roskams, *J. Pathol.*, 2000, **192**, 373–378.
80. C. Robrechts, R. De Vos, M. Van den Heuvel, E. Van Cutsem, B. Van Damme, V. Desmet and T. Roskams, *Liver*, 1998, **18**, 288–293.
81. H. Kim, C. Park, K. -H. Han, J. Choi, Y. B. Kim, J. K. Kim and Y. N. Park, *J. Hepatology*, 2004, **40**, 298–304.
82. Q. Zeng and W. Hong, *Cancer Cell*, 2008, **13**, 188–192.
83. K.-P. Lee, J.-H. Lee, T.-S. Kim, T.-H. Kim, H.-D. Park, J.-S. Byun, M.-C. Kim, W.-I. Jeong, D. F. Calvisi, J.-M. Kim and D.-S. Lim, *Proceedings of the National Academy of Sciences*, 2010, **107**, 8248–8253.
84. C. Weiss, D. Faust, I. Schreck, A. Ruff, T. Farwerck, A. Melenberg, S. Schneider, B. Oesch-Bartlomowicz, J. Zatloukalova, J. Vondracek, F. Oesch and C. Dietrich, *Oncogene*, 2008, **27**, 2198–2207.
85. W. Zhang, X.-P. Chen, W.-G. Zhang, F. Zhang, S. Xiang, H.-H. Dong and L. Zhang, *World Journal of Gastroenterology*, 2009, **15**, 552–560.
86. K. Chramostová, J. Vondráèek, L. Šindlerová, B. Vojtìšek, A. Kozubík and M. Machala, *Toxicol. Appl. Pharmacol.*, 2004, **196**, 136–148.
87. NTP, *NTP technical report on the toxicology and carcinogenesis studies of 2,2′,4,4′,5,5′-hexachlorobiphenyl (PCB 153) (CAS No. 35065-27-1) in female Harlan Sprague-Dawley rats (Gavage studies)*, 2006.
88. NTP, *NTP Toxicology and Carcinogenesis Studies of a Mixture of 2,3,7,8-Tetrachlorodibenzo-p-Dioxin (TCDD) (CAS No. 1746-01-6), 2,3,4,7,8-Pentachlorodibenzofuran (PeCDF) (CAS No. 57117-31-4), and 3,3′,4,4′, 5-Pentachlorobiphenyl (PCB 126) (CAS No. 57465-28-8) in Female Harlan Sprague-Dawley Rats (Gavage Studies)*, 2006.
89. Z. Andrysík, J. Vondráèek, M. Machala, P. Krèmáø, L. Švihálková-Šindlerová, A. Kranz, C. Weiss, D. Faust, A. Kozubík and C. Dietrich, *Mutat. Res.-Fundamental and Molecular Mechanisms of Mutagenesis*, 2007, **615**, 87–97.
90. C. Dietrich and B. Kaina, *Carcinogenesis*, 2010, **31**, 1319–1328.
91. H. W. Leung, R. H. Ku, D. J. Paustenbach and M. E. Andersen, *Toxicol. Lett.*, 1988, **42**, 15–28.
92. M. C. Kohn, G. W. Lucier, G. C. Clark, C. Sewall, A. M. Tritscher and C. J. Portier, *Toxicol. Appl. Pharmacol.*, 1993, **120**, 138–154.
93. A. M. Tritscher, J. A. Goldstein, C. J. Portier, Z. McCoy, G. C. Clark and G. W. Lucier, *Cancer Res.*, 1992, **52**, 3436–3442.

94. R. G. Bars, A. M. Mitchell, C. R. Wolf and C. R. Elcombe, *Biochem. J.*, 1989, **262**, 151–8.
95. M. E. Andersen, C. R. Eklund, J. J. Mills, H. A. Barton and L. S. Birnbaum, *Toxicol. Appl. Pharmacol.*, 1997, **144**, 135–144.
96. M. E. Andersen, L. S. Birnbaum, H. A. Barton and C. R. Eklund, *Toxicol. Appl. Pharmacol.*, 1997, **144**, 145–155.
97. M. E. Andersen, Q. Zhang and S. Bhattacharya, Modeling Gene and Protein Expression-Nested Motifs in Cellular and Tissue Response Networks, in *Quantitative Modeling in Toxicology*. Edited by K. Krishnan and M. E. Andersen, John Wiley & Sons, Hoboken, NJ, 2010.
98. D. C. Hixson, R. A. Faris and N. L. Thompson, *Pathobiology*, 1990, **58**, 65–77.
99. N. Shiojiri, J. M. Lemire and N. Fausto, *Cancer Res.*, 1991, **51**, 2611–2620.
100. E. Wisse, F. Braet, D. Luo, R. De Zanger, D. Jans, E. Crabbe and A. Vermoesen, *Toxicol. Pathol.*, 1996, **24**, 100–111.
101. NTP, *NTP technical report on the toxicology and carcinogenesis studies of 2,3,7,8-tetrachlorodibenzo-p-dioxin (TCDD) (CAS No. 1746-01-6) in female Harlan Sprague-Dawley rats (Gavage Studies)*, 2006.
102. A. A. Davila and G. An, *J. Surg. Res.*, 2010, **158**, 411.
103. C. A. Hunt, G. E. P. Ropella, L. Yan, D. Y. Hung and M. S. Roberts, *J. Pharmacokinetics and Pharmacodynamics*, 2006, **33**, 737–772.
104. J. Wambaugh and I. Shah, *PLoS Comp. Biol.*, 2010, **6**, e1000756.
105. H. W. Leung, D. J. Paustenbach, F. J. Murray and M. E. Andersen, *Toxicol. Appl. Pharmacol.*, 1990, **103**, 399–410.
106. K. O. Lindros, T. Oinonen, I. Johansson and M. Ingelman-Sundberg, *J. Pharmacol. Exp. Ther.*, 1997, **280**, 506–511.
107. J. C. Rowlands, I. J. McEwan and J. Ã. Gustafsson, *Mol. Pharmacol.*, 1996, **50**, 538–548.
108. J. Mimura, M. Ema, K. Sogawa and Y. Fujii-Kuriyama, *Genes and Development*, 1999, **13**, 20–25.
109. B. R. Evans, S. I. Karchner, L. L. Allan, R. S. Pollenz, R. L. Tanguay, M. J. Jenny, D. H. Sherr and M. E. Hahn, *Mol. Pharmacol.*, 2008, **73**, 387–398.
110. P. B. C. Jones, D. R. Galeazzi, J. M. Fisher and J. P. Whitlock Jr, *Science*, 1985, **227**, 1499–1502.
111. J. M. Fisher, K. W. Jones and J. P. Whitlock Jr, *Mol. Carcinog.*, 1989, **1**, 216–221.
112. D. W. Nebert, T. P. Dalton, A. B. Okey and F. J. Gonzalez, *J. Biol. Chem.*, 2004, **279**, 23847–23850.
113. C. J. Elferink, *Progress in cell cycle research*, 2003, **5**, 261–267.
114. S. Hohme, J. G. Hengstler, M. Brulport, M. Schafer, A. Bauer, R. Gebhardt and D. Drasdo, *Chem.-Biol. Interact.*, 2007, **168**, 74–93.
115. J. Gim, H. S. Kim, J. Kim, M. Choi, J. R. Kim, Y. J. Chung and K. H. Cho, *Bioinformatics*, 2010, **26**, 2169–2175.

CHAPTER 25

# Animal Models of Idiosyncratic, Drug-Induced Liver Injury

CHRISTINE M. DUGAN,[a] PATRICIA E. GANEY[b] AND ROBERT A. ROTH*[b]

[a] Michigan State University, Cell and Molecular Biology Program, East Lansing, MI 48824, USA; [b] Michigan State University, Department of Pharmacology and Toxicology, Center for Integrative Toxicology, East Lansing, MI 48824, USA

## 25.1 Introduction

Idiosyncratic, adverse drug reactions (IADRs) are a significant cause of morbidity and mortality. IADR liability evades detection during preclinical testing for drug safety, and modes of action remain unknown. Using hepatic IADRs as examples, current hypotheses regarding mechanisms of pathogenesis and supporting experimental animal models are discussed, with an emphasis on immune-mediated and risk-based models.

## 25.2 Hepatic Adverse Drug Reactions

Hepatic adverse drug reactions (ADRs) are the leading cause of acute liver failure in the US,[1] and drug-induced hepatotoxicity is the most common cause of withdrawal of FDA-approved drugs from the pharmaceutical market.[2] In 2002, the global incidence of hepatic ADRs was estimated to be $13.9 \pm 2.4$ per 100 000 inhabitants.[3] Results of a prospective study of the French general

RSC Drug Discovery Series No. 12
New Horizons in Predictive Toxicology: Current Status and Application
Edited by Alan G. E. Wilson

Published by the Royal Society of Chemistry, www.rsc.org

population suggested that symptomatic cases of hepatic ADRs were under-reported and that the actual incidence might be 16 times greater than that reported.[3] Furthermore, the detection and identification of hepatic ADRs in clinics is hindered by the reliance on plasma transaminase activity as a biomarker for hepatic injury, which might not detect drugs for which hepatotoxicity progresses slowly. This is the case, for example, for the selective serotonin re-uptake inhibitor, nefazodone, which was removed from the market following reports of hepatotoxicity that developed after several weeks of treatment.[4] Accordingly, it is possible that the incidence and seriousness of hepatic ADRs in the general population is underestimated.

## 25.3 Liver as a Target Organ

The liver is the first organ to be exposed to ingested drugs and other xenobiotic agents. The liver is also a common site for drug-induced toxicity because it is the major organ of xenobiotic metabolism and is also involved with carrier-mediated elimination into the bile. Whereas metabolic transformation and elimination of xenobiotics is a normal function of the liver, the resulting metabolites can be more toxic than the parent compounds, as in the case of acetaminophen. Acetaminophen is metabolically bioactivated by several cytochrome P450 (CYP) isoforms, with the major contribution coming from CYP2E1[5] and minor contributions from CYP1A2, CYP3A4, and CYP2D6 isoforms.[5,6] The product is the reactive metabolite, *N*-acetyl-*p*-benzoquinoneimine (NAPQI). When acetaminophen is given at nontoxic doses, NAPQI is detoxified by reduced glutathione forming an NAPQI–glutathione conjugate.[7] At toxic doses, NAPQI depletes glutathione stores and subsequently binds covalently to proteins.[7] The amount of covalent binding correlates with hepatotoxicity.[8] The centrilobular distribution of CYP enzymes is consistent with the pattern of liver injury seen in patients with acetaminophen-induced hepatotoxicity. The liver is often a target of toxicity because of its greater exposure to ingested drugs and its role in metabolizing them.

In addition to its central role in metabolism and disposition of nutrients, the liver is also involved in systemic and local immune responses. Acute-phase proteins and many circulating cytokines and growth factors are synthesized in the liver.[9] The liver is also enriched in cells capable of mediating immune surveillance and innate defense (*i.e.*, Kupffer cells, natural killer (NK) cells and NKT cells)[9]. These qualities that characterize the liver as an organ of innate immunity likely contribute to the sensitivity of the liver to drug toxicity, as noted below.

## 25.4 Intrinsic *versus* Idiosyncratic ADRs

In 1978, drugs causing adverse reactions were categorized as "intrinsic" or "non-predictable" by Zimmerman,[10] and the reactions caused by these drugs were classified as Type A or Type B, respectively, by Pirmohamed *et al.*[11]

Intrinsic drug reactions are dose-dependent and are generally predictable. Most, if not all, patients exposed to toxic doses of these drugs develop liver damage. In contrast, the dose dependency of "non-predictable", or idiosyncratic reactions is usually not obvious, and these reactions often occur in a small minority of patients. Despite their relatively rare occurrence, IADRs account for up to 20% of cases of severe liver injury requiring hospitalization.[12] Accordingly, these responses represent a significant health concern. A recent report indicated that drugs for which patients consume $\geq$50 mg daily are more likely to be associated with idiosyncratic liver injury than drugs for which the dose is smaller,[13] suggesting that IADRs are not dose-independent. Another characteristic of IADRs is that the temporal relationship between the onset of injury and drug administration is not consistent among drugs and can often vary even among patients exposed to the same drug.

Idiosyncratic liability of a drug is typically not discovered until it has been used in a large number of people. One likely reason for this is that most of these drugs do not cause hepatotoxicity in animals under current preclinical drug testing paradigms. Animal models in which IADRs occur with much greater frequency than in the human patient population would facilitate prediction and allow studies designed to understand underlying mechanisms that produce IADRs. Understanding mechanisms could lead to even better predictive models, including *in vitro* and high-throughput systems. In this chapter we describe the current hypotheses about mechanisms of idiosyncratic, drug-induced liver injury (IDILI) and present in greater depth some of the animal models that address immune-mediated modes of action with a focus on the potential predictive value of these models.

## 25.5 Mechanisms of Idiosyncratic Drug-Induced Liver Injury

Little is known about mechanisms by which drugs cause idiosyncratic drug-induced liver injury (IDILI). Until the last 10 years, these reactions were thought to arise from differences in metabolism or from acquired immune responses. More recently, several other hypotheses have arisen. Each hypothesis has supporting rationale, but for the majority of drugs associated with idiosyncratic reactions, no mechanism of pathogenesis has been proven.

### 25.5.1 Metabolic Idiosyncrasy

One proposed mechanism of hepatic IADR pathogenesis is variation in drug metabolism. For example, a polymorphism in a metabolic enzyme necessary for drug metabolism might lead to the accumulation of harmful reactive metabolites. Such appears to be the case for the anti-tuberculosis drug isoniazid (INH). INH can be acetylated to acetyl-isoniazid or biotransformed by CYP2E1 to hydrazine, the major toxic reactive metabolite.[14] Patients are categorized as rapid or slow acetylators based on the rate at which the INH is acetylated. Slow acetylation leads to greater plasma INH and hydrazine concentrations during chronic administration of the drug, with associated increased risk of toxicity. A meta analysis of clinical studies reported that genetic polymorphisms in the metabolic enzymes *N*-acetyltransferase 2, CYP2E1, and glutathione-*S*-transferase are associated with increased risk for INH-induced hepatotoxicity in human patients afflicted with tuberculosis.[15] These polymorphisms are thought to contribute to the wide intra- and inter-ethnic variability in INH-induced hepatotoxicity. Nonetheless, genetic polymorphisms are not likely the sole explanation for most idiosyncratic reactions. Interestingly, it has recently been suggested that large plasma concentrations of INH inhibit the activity of CYP2E1[16] and the formation of hydrazine. Therefore, several pharmacokinetic and other factors might contribute to the unpredictable nature of INH-induced liver injury. Although metabolism is a common feature considered in models developed to study IDILI, animal models in which liver injury occurs and that address specific metabolic idiosyncracies are lacking.

### 25.5.2 Failure to Adapt

At the start of therapy with some drugs associated with IDILI, mild hepatic injury that resolves without the necessity of drug withdrawal occurs in 5–15% of patients. For example, the proportion of patients treated with INH who develop asymptomatic transaminase elevations is approximately 10–20%,[17] whereas symptomatic hepatotoxicity (fever, jaundice, abdominal pain) and fatal hepatitis occurs in 0.1–1% of patients.[18,19] It has been hypothesized that the IDILI patients experiencing severe hepatotoxicity represent a subset whose livers "fail to adapt" to the minor, initial enzyme elevations and progress to severe injury.[20]

Results consistent with this hypothesis can be seen in clinical trials with troglitazone, an anti-diabetic drug that was removed from use because of hepatic IADRs. In clinical trials, troglitazone caused increases in plasma alanine aminotransferase (ALT) activity that mirrored the timing and pattern of acute liver injury initially but then resolved for most patients.[21,22] Liver injury became more severe in a smaller number of patients. It is not known why some patients developed liver failure whereas the majority did not. It is possible that failure to adapt might result from the inhibition of hepatocellular regenerative processes or an accumulation of intracellular stresses. No animal models using drugs that cause IADRs in humans have appeared based on this hypothesis.

### 25.5.3 Mitochondrial Toxicity

Drug-induced mitochondrial toxicity might underlie some IDILI responses, and variability in the rate at which individuals accumulate dysfunctional mitochondria could explain variations in sensitivity and in times to onset of overt toxicity.[23] Mitochondrial toxicity can manifest as decreased production of adenosine triphosphate, disruption of the mitochondrial membrane potential or production of reactive oxygen species within the mitochondria.

This hypothesis derives support from the observation that a number of drugs that cause IDILI in people also cause mitochondrial dysfunction in hepatocytes *in vitro*. Among these drugs are trovafloxacin, troglitazone, isoniazid, diclofenac, tolcapone, and valproic acid.[23–29] Cell death of human hepatoma cells (HepG2) from either troglitazone or diclofenac is dependent on mitochondria.[30,31] On the other hand, drugs that cause mitochondrial alterations *in vitro* rarely cause hepatic injury in healthy experimental animals.[23] This might be explained by the several-fold greater drug doses used for *in vitro* systems and plasma protein binding to drug *in vivo*.[23]

Support for the hypothesis that mitochondrial toxicity contributes to IDILI for some drugs is garnered from studies using superoxide dismutase 2 heterozygous mice (Sod2$^{+/-}$). These mice represent a model of silent mitochondrial abnormality in which deficiency in Sod2 results in excessive oxidant stress in the mitochondria. Chronic treatment of these mice with troglitazone resulted in mild hepatocellular necrosis, whereas no injury was observed in wild-type mice.[32] Similar results have been observed upon treatment of Sod2$^{+/-}$ mice with flutamide[33] or nimesulide.[34]

#### *25.5.3.1 Predictive Value of Models of IDILI Based on the Mitochondrial Toxicity Hypothesis*

It is likely that mitochondrial toxicity contributes to some instances of IDILI, and drugs for which this is true might be revealed by performing experiments in Sod2$^{+/-}$ or other sensitive mice. It should be noted that in studies using Sod2$^{+/-}$ mice, sometimes liver injury was mild or lacking and/or characterized by apoptotic necrosis. This is not usually true for human cases of IDILI, in which hepatotoxicity can be severe and often characterized by oncotic necrosis. On the other hand, since mitochondrial dysfunction can be caused by a variety of independent factors, such as inflammation, hypoxia or concurrent xenobiotic exposure, it is possible that alterations in mitochondrial function play a role in other hypothesized modes of action of IADRs.

### 25.5.4 Hypotheses Involving the Immune System

#### *25.5.4.1 The Acquired Immune Response in IDILI Reactions*

It has been proposed that an acquired immune response to drug administration is responsible for some IADRs. The antibiotic penicillin elicits anaphylactic shock in those patients who develop an immune response to the parent drug. Classically, for immune-mediated, drug-induced adverse reactions there is a close temporal relationship between the drug exposure and onset of the reaction. Also, the adverse reaction resolves upon removal of the offending drug. In contrast, many presumably immune-mediated IADRs demonstrate a delayed temporal relationship between drug exposure and the adverse reaction, and the reaction does not resolve upon removal of the drug. These characteristics present an obstacle for clinicians attempting to identify the causative agent. Despite this inconsistency with classical allergic reactions, the hypothesis that some cases of IDILI are driven by an acquired immune response has gained favor due to the rarity of these reactions and the finding that multiple exposures can be a risk factor for toxicity.

Most drugs are too small ($<1000$ Da) to be recognized by the immune system; however, drugs or their metabolites can act as haptens and bind covalently to endogenous proteins to form immunogenic conjugates.[35] These neoantigens elicit an acquired immune reaction upon a subsequent (or continued) drug exposure. Often the immune response targets the carrier protein, and this initiates an autoimmune response.

In 2002, Matzinger suggested that the driving force of the immune system is the recognition of danger signals from dying or damaged cells. This represents a shift from the previous paradigm in which recognition of "self or not-self" was the principal driving force.[36] Within this construct, tissue injury as well as foreign material can direct the immune system to mediate deleterious and/or beneficial events leading to progression or resolution of injury, respectively. Several groups have attempted to apply this hypothesis to the pathogenesis of acquired immune-mediated IADRs,[37,38] in which cytokines, such as Kupffer cell-derived tumor necrosis factor-α (TNF-α), exacerbate T- and B-lymphocyte activity to develop a specific adaptive immune response.

**Nevirapine as an example of acquired immune-mediated adverse reactions.** Nevirapine (NVP) is a non-nucleoside reverse transcriptase inhibitor (NNRTI) used to treat patients with human immunodeficiency virus (HIV) infection or acquired immune deficiency syndromes (AIDS). Since virus mutation and resistance occur quickly in monotherapy, NVP is administered as a component of combination anti-retroviral therapy (ART) with nucleoside reverse transcription inhibitors and protease inhibitors. Like other NNRTI drugs, rash is a common adverse reaction to NVP, with 32% to 48% of treated patients developing a rash within the first month of exposure.[39,40] Severe mucocutaneous or cutaneous reactions are more rare, with incidence of 1% and 8% of patients, respectively.[41]

Asymptomatic liver toxicity (liver enzyme elevations without concurrent symptoms of abdominal pain, nausea, vomiting, malaise, rash, or fever) has been noted in 5–10% of HIV-positive patients treated for more than six months with combination ART therapy.[42] Symptomatic clinical hepatic events during ART therapy are associated with NVP use, as well as other factors.[43] NVP in particular has been associated with several cases of liver failure.[44–47] Retrospective studies report symptomatic liver injury in 5% of patients administered NVP;[48] whereas two prospective studies found this incidence to be 6–10% to 17% of patients within the first month of dosing.[49] In 2000, the FDA issued a black box warning for NVP due to reports of acute hepatotoxicity and liver failure associated with NVP therapy.

The adverse reactions to NVP therapy in humans can be either cutaneous, hepatic or both, and usually occur within 14–21 days of treatment.[42,48] These adverse reactions are also reported to be more severe upon NVP re-administration.[50] Delayed onset and increased severity upon rechallenge are common characteristics of acquired immune reactions.[51] Hepatic and cutaneous reactions to NVP share risk factors and the characteristic that the reaction is delayed in onset relative to initial exposure. Furthermore, occasionally a patient presents with both reactions. These observations suggest a common, immune hypersensitivity mechanism for hepatic and cutaneous NVP-induced reactions; however, there is no conclusive evidence to support this.

Since NVP-induced adverse reactions do not occur in some patients at any dose, they are considered idiosyncratic.[50] The human risk factors for NVP-induced hepatotoxicity are female sex,[49] plasma NVP concentration,[52,53] length of time on the drug,[54] concurrent hepatitis C or B infection,[55] and genetics.[56] A higher CD4+ T cell count has been reported to be a risk factor for NVP-induced hepatotoxicity,[56,57] however, other reports refute this claim.[58,59]

One of the first rodent models of an IADR that clearly indicates an adaptive immune mechanism is the NVP-induced rash model in rats. NVP-induced rash was found in 100% of female, Brown–Norway rats and 21% of female, Sprague–Dawley rats, whereas no cutaneous adverse reactions were noted in male, Brown–Norway or Sprague–Dawley rats, or Lewis rats regardless of sex.[60]

The female Brown–Norway rats developed red ears on days 7–10 and skin lesions on days 10–21 after the initiation of the NVP regimen. Upon re-challenge, the rats had a shorter time to onset of rash, increased CD4+ and CD8+ cellular infiltrate in their skin lesions, and appeared generally less well than after the initial exposure.[60] The initial delay in toxicity, the earlier onset of toxicity upon rechallenge, and the increased T-cells in the tissue specimens are suggestive of an acquired immune response.[61] Adoptive transfer of splenocytes from rechallenged rats conferred a shorter time of rash onset, and T-cell depletion decreased the incidence of NVP-induced rash in this rat model.[62]

**Predictive value of models of IDILI based on the acquired immune response hypothesis.** The NVP rat model presented above is the first animal model that accurately depicts the idiosyncratic NVP-induced mild rash seen in some patients by sharing the characteristic delayed time of onset and increased severity on NVP rechallenge, as well as having the histological features seen in patients with NVP-associated adverse reactions. Importantly, liver injury did not occur in the animals under conditions that produced skin rash. This observation raises questions about whether the cutaneous effects of NVP are related mechanistically to the hepatic effects. Similarly, most models that have been developed in an effort to reproduce IDILI from sensitization and challenge have failed to produce liver damage (see below in the discussion of halothane).

### 25.5.4.2 The Innate Immune Response in IDILI Reactions

The innate immune response also has the potential to contribute to the pathogenesis of IADRs.[63] Liver lesions from patients who have experienced IDILI often contain inflammatory infiltrates, including neutrophils[33,64–66] In addition, in laboratory animals, coexposure to inflammatory agents increases sensitivity to the hepatotoxic effects of a number of xenobiotic agents (reviewed in Ganey *et al.*[67]), raising the possibility that this might also be true for drugs.

In people, inflammation can occur due to a variety of chronic, adverse health conditions such as arthritis and atherosclerosis, from infection with bacteria or viruses, or from increased exposure to products of indigenous microorganisms, such as gut-derived endotoxins from gram-negative bacteria. Mild endotoxemia resulting from intestinal translocation is a normal but episodic occurrence in people, and numerous conditions enhance endotoxin concentration in the plasma (reviewed in Ganey *et al.*[67] and Roth *et. al.*[68]). The magnitude of exposure from intestinal translocation of endotoxin is typically too small to cause overt illness but might be sufficient to initiate a modest inflammatory response in tissues.

Lipopolysaccharide (LPS), the principal active component of bacterial endotoxin, binds to Toll-like receptor 4 (TLR4) on mammalian cells, activates signaling mechanisms and results in expression and release of numerous proinflammatory mediators. These mediators include reactive oxygen and nitrogen species, lipid metabolites (*e.g.*, prostaglandins), cytokines, and toxic proteases.[69–71] Although important in defense against pathogens, these mediators can be deleterious by altering homeostasis of host cells and thereby increasing the sensitivity to develop injury to subsequent stressful insults.

The inflammatory stress hypothesis of IDILI reactions proposes that when an inflammatory episode of sufficient magnitude occurs during drug therapy, the threshold for toxicity from drugs decreases.[67] Large doses of LPS alone can damage liver; accordingly, it is also possible that some drugs or their metabolites might increase the responsiveness of the liver to LPS or other inflammatory mediators, thereby rendering an otherwise nontoxic exposure to them hepatotoxic.[72] This hypothesis has been supported by the development of several rodent models in which cotreatment with a modestly inflammatory dose of LPS and one of several drugs with human idiosyncratic liability (*e.g.*, chlorpromazine, sulindac, trovafloxacin, amiodarone, ranitidine, diclofenac, halothane and doxorubicin) results in liver injury, whereas treatment with either the drug alone or LPS alone does not.[73–78] The liver injury in these animal models ranges from moderate to severe necrosis and occurs reproducibly in a large fraction of drug-treated animals. In these models, coupling LPS exposure with drugs from the same class that lack idiosyncratic potential (*e.g.*, famotidine for ranitidine, levofloxacin for trovafloxacin) does not produce injury,[73,74] lending credence to this mechanism for hepatic IADRs (for a review, see Deng *et al.*[79] and Shaw *et al.*[80]). With at least some drugs, inflammagens other than LPS that activate TLRs other than TLR4 also synergize with drug treatment to result in hepatotoxicity. For example, a peptidoglycan/

lipoteichoic acid combination that activates TLR2 caused a hepatotoxic response in trovafloxacin-cotreated mice similar to that caused by LPS.[81] Similarly, halothane synergizes not only with LPS[82] but also with polyinosinic-poly-cytidylic acid [poly(I:C)], which activates TLR9.[83] Since different TLRs activate somewhat different intracellular signaling pathways, exploring several TLR agonists for a particular drug might lead to identification of a common aspect of the signaling pathways at which the drug interacts to produce hepatotoxicity.

A variety of inflammatory mediators contributes to liver injury from LPS/drug exposure. In particular, interference with TNF or depletion of neutrophils reduces liver damage, suggesting a critical role for each of these mediators.[79,80] With some drugs, the coagulation system is activated, the fibrinolytic system is impaired, and fibrin deposits in hepatic sinusoids.[75,84–86] These events are accompanied by hepatic hypoxia. Interestingly, the anticoagulant heparin ameliorates liver injury under these circumstances, indicating that alterations in the hemostatic system are also important to these responses[75,84–86] Other inflammatory mediators shown to be involved in some IDILI-like responses in animal models include IFN-$\gamma$, reactive oxygen species and interleukin-18. [87–89]

Whether inflammatory stress contributes to hepatic IADRs in people is unknown; however the presence of viral hepatitis (*i.e.*, hepatic inflammation) is a risk factor for idiosyncratic hepatotoxicity from anti-retroviral combination therapy,[42] and many patients experience signs consistent with a concurrent inflammatory response.[80] It may also be significant that the drug classes responsible for most IDILI are antibiotics and NSAIDs, *i.e.*, drugs that are used in patients with inflammatory conditions.[79]

The inflammatory stress hypothesis is attractive because it can account for all of the characteristics of idiosyncratic reactions (for a brief review, see Roth and Ganey[72]). Acute inflammatory episodes occur occasionally and erratically in most people, which might explain why IDILI reactions display an inconsistent temporal relationship to drug exposure and why they often affect only a small fraction of people during drug therapy. An additional feature of this hypothesis is the possibility that polymorphisms in human genes that govern the magnitude of an individual's response to inflammagens could contribute a genetic component to susceptibility and could explain why some people respond with hepatotoxicity whereas most do not.[90] The observation that an interaction of several IDILI-causing drugs with inflammatory stress causes liver injury in animals is consistent with the liver being a frequent target of IADRs in human patients.

**Predictive value of models of IDILI based on the innate immune response hypothesis.** The animal models of LPS–drug interaction described above are the first to mimic pronounced liver injury seen in human patients with IDILI, employing drugs from a variety of pharmacologic classes. The liver injury is reproducible and occurs in most animals that are treated, affording a distinct advantage for the exploration of mechanisms, because changes in factors putatively involved in the response can be evaluated in the context of this clinically relevant endpoint. Nonetheless, the models developed so far based on this hypothesis are not ideal for use in pharmaceutical safety evaluation, for which standard dosing regimens are advantageous, if not requisite. The development of liver injury depends not only on doses of LPS and drug but also on the timing of their administrations relative to each other. The optimal regimens seem to be different for different drugs. Furthermore, the biologic activity of LPS differs for different serotypes, and even among lots within a serotype. Accordingly, the current inflammation–drug interaction models would be cumbersome in a preclinical testing situation with liver injury as the endpoint. On the other hand, they could be valuable for discovering mechanisms that could lead to cell-based, *in vitro* assays adaptable to high-throughput screening of drug candidates. Efforts have begun to apply the knowledge gained from these animal models to cell-based systems.[91–94]

## 25.6 A Risk-Based Approach to Development of Animal Models of IDILI using Halothane as an Example

Halothane is an anesthetic that was introduced in the US in 1958. By 1963, the drug manufacturer issued a warning due to clinical reports of fatal hepatic necrosis following halothane administration. In 1966, a large retrospective study was unable to establish or refute a causal relationship between halothane and fulminant liver injury due to an incidence rate that was rarer than 1 in 10 000. The report also indicated that halothane had a good safety record compared to other anesthetic options available at the time (*e.g.*, ether).[95] Although the number of reports of halothane-associated liver failure continued to increase, and ultimately the use of halothane was curtailed in the US, it is still used in other countries and is included on the current "World Health Organization's Model List of Essential Medicine" released in March 2009. Careful assessment of the risk factors for halothane-associated liver failure, such as female sex, genetics, age (the young are resistant), and multiple exposures,[96,97] should provide useful guidelines for physicians trying to avoid halothane-associated injury in patients.

### 25.6.1 Clinical Spectrum of Halothane Hepatotoxicity

Halothane produced a non-icteric, mild liver injury in one in five patients.[98,99] A more severe idiosyncratic liver injury, termed "halothane hepatitis," was observed in 1 in 6000–30 000 adult patients who received the drug.[95,100,101] The clinical signs of halothane hepatitis are fever, jaundice, vomiting, and coma.[102] The laboratory findings are characteristic of hepatocellular injury, with increase in plasma liver enzyme activity, hyperbilirubinemia, and decrease in prothrombin time.[102] Fever is usually the first sign of halothane hepatitis, with onset between 8 and 14 days;[101,103] however, not all patients present with fevers. Retrospective studies indicate a shortened time until onset of fever presentation to four days following non-primary halothane administration.[101] Another prominent clinical sign is the onset of jaundice. Kline and colleagues[103] noted that patients became icteric 10–28 days following the primary exposure of halothane and 3–17 days following a non-primary exposure. The shortened latency of symptoms following a non-primary exposure might indicate that the primary halothane exposure sensitized patients to the subsequent halothane exposures. In contrast, other groups reported that patients developed jaundice eight and seven days following primary and non-primary halothane exposures, respectively.[101]

Transaminase activity and bilirubin concentration are elevated in patients with halothane hepatitis and indicate damage to the liver parenchyma. Bottiger and colleagues[101] found that patients who had serum bilirubin concentrations that were greater than 10 mg $dL^{-1}$ had a 60% mortality rate, whereas there were no deaths in patients who had serum bilirubin concentrations less than 5 mg $dL^{-1}$. The most prominent histological feature seen in liver biopsies from patients who had halothane hepatitis is centrilobular necrosis.[104] Other histopathological findings in postmortem liver specimens include fatty degeneration, vacuolation, and inflammatory infiltrates.[102,105] Eosinophilia was a minor finding and was a feature in only 10% of halothane hepatitis patients.

### 25.6.2 Metabolism of Halothane

Approximately 20% of absorbed halothane is metabolized in humans.[106] In mice given $^{14}$C-halothane intravenously, the liver was the primary site of metabolism and accumulation of halothane metabolites.[107,108] Since halothane is widely dispersed in the body, and the major site of the adverse reaction is the site of metabolism, it is likely that a reactive metabolite of halothane is involved in the initiation of pathogenesis. It was subsequently demonstrated that pretreament of rats with phenobarbital, an inducer of some CYP enzymes, increased the covalent binding of halothane metabolites in the liver.[109] CYP is responsible for both anaerobic and aerobic metabolism of halothane.[110] Under aerobic conditions, the reductive pathway is inhibited, and aerobic metabolism predominates.[110] Under aerobic conditions, halothane is oxidized by CYP, mainly the isoform 2E1,[111] to a halohydrin intermediate which spontaneously loses hydrobromic acid to form trifluoroacetyl (TFA-)chloride.[112] TFA-chloride interacts with nucleophiles to form TFA-adducts.[113]

The sera of some halothane hepatitis patients contains antibodies that react with at least five polypeptides that were chemically altered by TFA-chloride and were approximately 100, 76, 59, 57 and 54 kDa.[114,115] These TFA-adducted proteins were predominately localized to the microsomal subcellular fraction of the livers.[114] TFA-adducts can persist for at least seven days in rat hepatocytes in culture[115] and 21 days in guinea pig livers.[116] Although the contribution of specific TFA-adducted proteins to the pathogenesis of halothane-induced hepatotoxicity is not clear, evidence from animal studies suggests that oxidative metabolism of halothane to TFA and subsequent adduction to proteins are necessary events for toxicity.[117,118]

## 25.6.3 Animal Models of Halothane-Induced Hepatotoxicity

Many attempts have been made to develop animal models of halothane-induced hepatotoxicity. These are summarized in Table 25.1.

Rats, mice and guinea pigs have served as models, the drug has been administered by intraperitoneal injection or by inhalation, and a variety of co-treatments have been employed. For example, rats have been pretreated with phenobarbital, isoniazid, triiodothyronine, or a mixture of polychlorinated biphenyls (Aroclor 1254) to induce drug-metabolizing enzymes.[109,119–125] In some studies, animals were coexposed to hypoxia in an effort to mimic the presumed clinical condition under which exposure occurred. Each of these conditions produced some liver damage, although not usually to the extent seen in clinical cases of halothane hepatitis. Also, the usefulness of this model was called into question upon the discovery that hypoxia itself could produce liver injury in treated rats.[126,127] Pretreament with buthionine sulfoxamine to decrease stores of reduced glutathione resulted in liver damage in all guinea pigs exposed to a subanesthetic dose of halothane and lethality in about half of the animals exposed to a larger dose.[128,129]

The prevailing hypothesis for the mechanism of halothane hepatotoxicity is that halothane induces liver damage through an acquired immune-mediated mechanism,[130] and some animal models have been developed in an attempt to reproduce these events. Accordingly, efforts have involved multiple exposures to halothane.[118,122,131] Hughes *et al.*[132] demonstrated that inhaled halothane administered in 100% oxygen at two-week intervals induced hepatocellular injury in 7 of 50 treated guinea pigs in a dose-dependent fashion. Unfortunately, no relationship with single halothane exposure was tested, so it is unknown whether halothane sensitized mice to subsequent halothane challenge. Another report indicated that guinea pigs exposed to halothane at six-day or five-week intervals responded similarly upon re-exposure regardless of the number of exposures or interval of administration.[133] Other attempts to develop a model involved sensitizing animals to proteins containing a TFA moiety prior to exposure to halothane.[116,132,134] This produced an enhanced humoral immune response to TFA or halothane but lacked an associated increase in liver pathology. Therefore, the dearth of evidence that halothane immunologically sensitizes guinea pigs to halothane-induced liver injury upon subsequent exposure and the lack of any animal model in which liver injury occurs from a sensitization-and-challenge paradigm challenges the role of acquired immunity as the sole mechanism of halothane-mediated IDILI.

More recently, a mouse model has been developed in which halothane administration induced mild hepatotoxicity that was sex- and strain-dependent, with BALB/c being a sensitive strain.[135] Results of this investigation indicated that the mild form of halothane hepatotoxicity was dependent on

**Table 25.1** Animal models of halothane-induced hepatotoxicity.

| *Species/gender* | *Pretreatment* | *Halothane route of exposure* | *Necrosis?* | *Approximate ALT (units/L)* | *Reference* |
|---|---|---|---|---|---|
| Rat/male | Aroclor 1254, fasted | Inhalation | Y | 150 at 1 day | 123 |
| Rat/male | Phenobarb + hypoxia (some fasted) | Inhalation | Y | 100 at 6 h<br>150–800 at 1 day | 109, 119–122 |
| Rat/male | Isoniazid | Inhalation | Y | 800 at 1 day | 124 |
| Rat/male | Triiodothyronine | Inhalation | Y | (NR) | 125 |
| GP/male | +/– TFA-immunization | Inhalation | — | AST <150 | 131 |
| GP/male | — | Inhalation | Y | <100–600 at 2–3 days<br>135–935 at 3 days<br>250 at 2 days<br>200–2000 | 118, 128, 135, 142–146 |
| GP/male | Buthionine sulfoxamine | Inhalation | Y | Up to ICDH 6000 | 128, 129 |
| GP/male | — | Intraperitoneal | — | 50–400 at 2 days | 117, 147 |
| Mouse/male and female | — | Intraperitoneal | Y | 10–1200 at 2 days (strain- and gender-dependent) | 137 |
| | | | | 10 000 at 12 h (strain- and gender-dependent) | 82 |
| Mouse/male | LPS | Intraperitoneal | Y | 3000 at 24 h | 82 |
| Mouse/female | Poly (I:C) | Intraperitoneal | Y | 12 000 at 24 h | 83 |
| Mouse/male | IL-10 knockout | Intraperitoneal | Y | 800 at 1 day | 148 |

ALT = alanine aminotransferase; GP = guinea pig; LPS = lipopolysaccharide
NR = not reported; ICDH = isocitrate dehydrogenase; AST = aspartate aminotransferase; Phenobarb = phenobarbital; TFA = trifluoroacetyl; IL = interleukin; Poly (I:C) - polyinosinic : polycytidylic acid

neutrophil activity. A subsequent study demonstrated that poly(I:C) exacerbated halothane-induced hepatotoxicity,[83] indicating that inflammation can exacerbate halothane-induced hepatotoxicity in BALB/c mice.

In summary, most of the attempts to produce animal models of halothane hepatotoxicity have either not resulted in consistent liver damage or have mimicked the mild injury seen in 20% of patients exposed to halothane,[117,135–137] which is of less clinical concern than the more severe, halothane hepatitis. Low incidence of responders and/or lack of severe hepatotoxicity limit the usefulness of many of these as models for studying the mechanism(s) of pathogenesis.

## 25.6.4 A Risk-based Approach to Animal Model Development

The model of mild liver damage in BALB/c mice served as a platform to develop a model of severe halothane hepatotoxicity[135] in which known and possible human risk factors were imposed simultaneously. Severe halothane-induced hepatotoxicity is more common in women than men[138] and less common in the young.[139,140] Accordingly, mature, female BALB/c mice were used. In addition, since most patients are required to fast prior to surgery (during which halothane would be used as anesthesia), mice were fasted overnight. Using these conditions, mice developed severe and reproducible hepatotoxicity (plasma ALT ~10 000 units/L) that was characterized by centrilobular necrosis, steatosis and hepatic accumulation of neutrophils,[82] *i.e.*, pathology similar to that observed in human cases. As in humans, male, BALB/c mice developed less severe liver damage. Younger, female BALB/c mice were also resistant to halothane-induced liver damage. Moreover, C57BL6 mice were completely resistant to halothane-induced liver injury, indicating a strong genetic predisposition. This is consistent with observations in human patients of heightened sensitivity to halothane hepatitis among closely related family members.[141]

Potential modes of toxicity were investigated using this model of severe halothane-induced liver damage. Liver injury did not develop in ovariectomized, halothane-treated mice, suggesting that ovarian hormones are involved in the sex difference in susceptibility. The inflammatory response also appears to be critical for severe liver injury, since 1) female, halothane-treated mice had a more robust inflammatory response than similarly treated male mice, 2) inhibition of neutrophil function or of natural killer cell function reduced the hepatotoxic response, and 3) mice deficient in interferon-$\gamma$ did not develop liver damage from halothane.[82,89] Accordingly, the innate immune response and ovarian hormones appear to be important determinants of susceptibility to halothane-induced severe hepatotoxicity in mice.

There are several characteristics of this mouse model of halothane hepatitis that closely parallel the idiosyncratic response seen in humans. The histopathologic picture of centrilobular necrosis, steatosis, and cellular infiltrate is similar. The desired effects of anesthesia and sedation, as well as the undesired effects of respiratory depression and liver injury are evident in humans and the BALB/cJ mice. There are also some notable differences. In the mouse model, halothane was administered intraperitoneally, whereas humans inhale volatilized halothane. The intraperitoneal administration of halothane in the animals was chosen to eliminate variation in dose due to differences in rates of respiration among individual mice, as well as the pharmacologically induced variation due to respiratory depression from halothane. Respiratory depression limited the halothane dose that was administered in these studies. Mice exposed to sublethal halothane doses by inhalation did not develop liver injury. It is possible that the high respiratory rate in mice, lower halothane availability in the liver, or lower rate of metabolism underlie the greater halothane sensitivity of mice exposed by intraperitoneal route rather than by inhalation.

### 25.6.5 Predictive Value of This Approach to Model Development

With respect to the particular model of severe, halothane-induced liver damage, this approach provided a model that mimics the spectrum of response seen in humans who suffered from halothane hepatitis. Accordingly, this model may be useful to study mechanisms by which halothane causes severe hepatotoxicity. But does it have broader applicability? This approach requires knowledge of risk factors in humans for specific drugs that cause IDILI responses, and for many IDILI-associated drugs, those are not known. Certainly, they are not known for new drugs for which IDILI liability has not been identified. On the other hand, if this approach is used for those drugs for which risk factors have been identified, results might suggest some susceptibility factors that prevail for a variety of drugs. If this is the case, these factors could then be incorporated into predictive evaluation of new drugs. For example, as is the case for halothane, a number of drugs are more likely to cause IDILI in women than in men. Perhaps the mechanistic information gleaned from studies of sex-specificity of the hepatotoxic response to halothane will provide a path for prediction of these responses.

## 25.7 Conclusions

IADRs are associated with a high human health and economic cost as well as the loss of efficacious drugs for use in combating disease. Although there is no universal agreement as to the cause(s) of these reactions, several tenable hypotheses have emerged. Due to the rarity of the reactions, their unpredictable nature, and their presentation late in the course of injury, studies of hepatic IADRS in human patients are not likely to provide unequivocal proof of underlying mechanisms of pathogenesis. Nonetheless, it is from human data that drugs with IDILI liability are identified and hypotheses about mechanisms

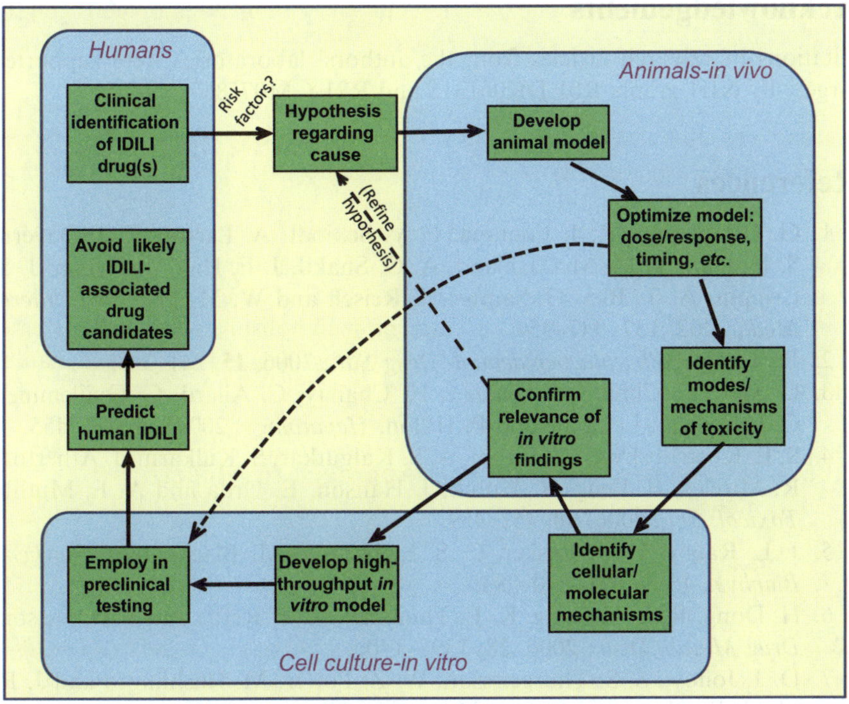


**Figure 25.1** An approach to prediction of drugs with IDILI potential. The approach involves identifying potential risk factors and developing hypotheses based on clinical data. These then drive the development of animal models in which risk factors are considered. Modes of action revealed in animal models can then be used to develop *in vitro* and high-throughput models that can be employed in preclinical testing.

are developed, and these are necessary steps in the approach to prediction of these reactions (Figure 25.1). Animal models in which genetic and/or environmental conditions are adjusted to enable a reproducible hepatotoxic response to an IDILI-associated drug have perhaps the greatest potential to improve understanding of these reactions. A good animal model of IDILI should have reproducible liver injury as an endpoint and be based on a plausible hypothesis for causality in humans. Animal models based on some of these hypotheses are currently being developed. Although at present none of these models is easily adapted to a standardized testing modality needed for routine safety evaluation of drug candidates, they have begun to provide support for some modes of action of idiosyncratic responses (Figure 25.1). Importantly, results from animal models are increasing our understanding of biologic factors and events potentially involved in human IDILI, and this understanding could lead in the not-too-distant future to cell-based and *in silico* systems that could have predictive value as well as value in furthering our understanding of mechanisms of action.

## Acknowledgements

Citations of research articles from the authors' laboratories were supported largely by NIH grants R01 DK061315 and R21 GM075865.

## References

1. G. Ostapowicz, R. J. Fontana, F. V. Schiodt, A. Larson, T. J. Davern, S. H. Han, T. M. McCashland, A. O. Shakil, J. E. Hay, L. Hynan, J. S. Crippin, A. T. Blei, G. Samuel, J. Reisch and W. M. Lee, *Ann. Intern. Med.*, 2002, **137**, 947–954.
2. R. Temple, *Pharmacoepidemiol. Drug Saf.*, 2006, **15**, 241–243.
3. C. Sgro, F. Clinard, K. Ouazir, H. Chanay, C. Allard, C. Guilleminet, C. Lenoir, A. Lemoine and P. Hillon, *Hepatology*, 2002, **36**, 451–455.
4. S. E. Kostrubsky, S. C. Strom, A. S. Kalgutkar, S. Kulkarni, J. Atherton, R. Mireles, B. Feng, R. Kubik, J. Hanson, E. Urda and A. E. Mutlib, *Toxicol. Sci.*, 2006, **90**, 451–459.
5. J. L. Raucy, J. M. Lasker, C. S. Lieber and M. Black, *Arch. Biochem. Biophys.*, 1989, **271**, 270–283.
6. H. Dong, R. L. Haining, K. E. Thummel, A. E. Rettie and S. D. Nelson, *Drug Metab. Disp.*, 2000, **28**, 1397–1400.
7. D. J. Jollow, S. S. Thorgeirsson, W. Z. Potter, M. Hashimoto and J. R. Mitchell, *Pharamacology*, 1974, **12**, 251–271.
8. D. J. Jollow, J. R. Mitchell, W. Z. Potter, D. C. Davis, J. R. Gillette and B. B. Brodie, *J. Pharmacol. Exp. Ther.*, 1973, **187**, 195–202.
9. E. Nemeth, A. W. Baird and C. O'Farrelly, *Semin. Immunopathol.*, 2009, **31**, 333–343.
10. H. J. Zimmerman, *Drugs*, 1978, **16**, 25–45.
11. M. Pirmohamed, A. M. Breckenridge, N. R. Kitteringham and B. K. Park, *BMJ*, 1998, **316**, 1295–1298.
12. W. M. Lee, *Semin. Liver Dis.*, 2008, **28**, 142–152.
13. C. Lammert, S. Einarsson, C. Saha, A. Niklasson, E. Bjornsson and N. Chalasani, *Hepatology*, 2008, **47**, 2003–2009.
14. P. Preziosi, *Curr. Drug Metab.*, 2007, **8**, 839–851.
15. F. Sun, Y. Chen, Y. Xiang and S. Zhan, *Int. J. Tuberc. Lung Dis.*, 2008, **12**, 994–1002.
16. D. O'Shea, R. B. Kim and G. R. Wilkinson, *Br. J. Clin. Pharmacol.*, 1997, **43**, 99–103.
17. E. J. Forget and D. Menzies, *Expert Opin. Drug Saf.*, 2006, **5**, 231–249.
18. C. M. Nolan, S. V. Goldberg and S. E. Buskin, *JAMA, J. Am. Med. Assoc.*, 1999, **281**, 1014–1018.
19. D. E. Kopanoff, D. E. Snider Jr and G. J. Caras, *Am. Rev. Respir. Dis.*, 1978, **117**, 991–1001.
20. P. B. Watkins, *Semin. Liver Dis.*, 2009, **29**, 393–399.
21. P. B. Watkins, *Toxicol. Pathol.*, 2005, **33**, 1–5.
22. P. B. Watkins and R. W. Whitcomb, *N. Engl. J. Med.*, 1998, **338**, 916–917.

23. U. A. Boelsterli and P. L. Lim, *Toxicol. Appl. Pharmacol.*, 2007, **220**, 92–107.
24. K. Haasio, K. Lounatmaa and A. Sukura, *Exp. Toxicol. Pathol.*, 2002, **54**, 9–14.
25. B. J. Keller, H. Yamanaka and R. G. Thurman, *Toxicology*, 1992, **71**, 49–61.
26. I. Petrescu and C. Tarba, *Biochim. Biophys. Acta*, 1997, **1318**, 385–394.
27. C. E. Schwab and H. Tuschl, *Hum. Exp. Toxicol.*, 2003, **22**, 607–615.
28. D. Pessayre, A. Mansouri, A. Berson and B. Fromenty, in Adverse Drug Reactions, ed. J. P. Uetrecht, *Handbook of Experimental Pharmacology,* Springer, New York, 2010, vol. 196, pp. 311–365.
29. S. Shishido, H. Koga, M. Harada, H. Kumemura, S. Hanada, E. Taniguchi, R. Kumashiro, H. Ohira, Y. Sato, M. Namba, T. Ueno and M. Sata, *Hepatology*, 2003, **37**, 136–147.
30. U. A. Boelsterli, *Toxicol. Appl. Pharmacol.*, 2003, **192**, 307–322.
31. M. A. Tirmenstein, C. X. Hu, T. L. Gales, B. E. Maleeff, P. K. Narayanan, E. Kurali, T. K. Hart, H. C. Thomas and L. W. Schwartz, *Toxicol. Sci.*, 2002, **69**, 131–138.
32. M. M. K. Ong, C. Latchoumycandane and U. Boelsterli, *Toxicol. Sci.*, 2007, **97**, 205–213.
33. R. Kashimshetty, V. G. Desai, V. M. Kale, T. Lee, C. L. Moland, W. S. Branham, L. S. New, E. C. Chan, H. Younis and U. A. Boelsterli, *Toxicol. Appl. Pharmacol.*, 2009, **238**, 150–159.
34. M. M. Ong, A. S. Wang, K. Y. Leow, Y. M. Khoo and U. A. Boelsterli, *Free Radic. Biol. Med.*, 2006, **40**, 420–429.
35. P. G. Gell, C. R. Harington and R. P. Rivers, *Br. J. Exp. Pathol.*, 1946, **27**, 267–286.
36. P. Matzinger, *Ann. N. Y. Acad. Sci.*, 2002, **961**, 341–342.
37. B. Seuguin and J. P. Uetrecht, *Curr. Opin. Allergy Clin. Immunol.*, 2003, **3**, 235–242.
38. J. P. Uetrecht, *Chem. Res. Toxicol.*, 1999, **12**, 387–395.
39. A. Carr, S. Vella, M. D. de Jong, F. Sorice, A. Imrie, C. A. Boucher and D. A. Cooper, *AIDS*, 1996, **10**, 635–641.
40. D. Havlir, S. H. Cheeseman, M. McLaughlin, R. Murphy, A. Erice, S. A. Spector, T. C. Greenough, J. L. Sullivan, D. Hall, M. Myers, M. Lamson and D. D. Richman, *J. Infect. Dis.*, 1995, **171**, 537–545.
41. K. J. Warren, D. E. Boxwell, N. Y. Kim and B. A. Drolet, *Lancet*, 1998, **351**, 567.
42. J. O. Stern, P. A. Robinson, J. Love, S. Lanes, M. S. Imperiale and D. L. Mayers, *J. Acquir. Immune Defic. Syndr.*, 2003, **34**, S21–S33.
43. F. W. Wit, G. J. Weverling, J. Weel, S. Jurriaans and J. M. Lange, *J. Infect. Dis.*, 2002, **186**, 23–31.
44. B. E. Sha, L. A. Proia and H. A. Kessler, *JAMA, J. Am. Med. Assoc.*, 2000, **284**, 2722–2723.
45. A. M. Cattelan, E. Erne, A. Salatino, M. Trevenzoli, F. Meneghetti and P. Candrobbi, *Clin. Infect. Dis.*, 1999, **29**, 455–456.

46. J. K. Maniar, S. R. Shah, R. Verma, R. Kamath, P. Gupte and A. Maniar, *J. Assoc. Physicians India*, 2006, **54**, 957–958.
47. P. J. Piliero and B. Purdy, *AIDS Read.*, 2001, **11**, 379–382.
48. D. Dieterich, P. Robinson, J. Love and J. O. Stern, *Clin. Infect. Dis.*, 2004, **38**, S80–S89.
49. I. Sanne, H. Mommeja-Marin, J. Hinkle, J. A. Bartlett, M. M. Lederman, G. Maartens, C. Wakeford, A. Shaw, J. Quinn, R. G. Gish and F. Rousseau, *J. Infect. Dis.*, 2005, **191**, 825–829.
50. J. Uetrecht, *Curr. Drug Metab.*, 2000, **1**, 133–141.
51. M. Popovic, J. M. Shenton, J. Chen, A. Baban, T. Tharmanathan, B. Mannarqudi, D. Abdulla and J. P. Uetrecht, in Adverse Drug Reactions, ed. J. P. Uetrecht, *Handbook of Experimental Pharmacology,* Springer, New York, 2010, vol. 196, pp. 437–451.
52. D. González de Requena, M. Núñez, I. Jiménez-Nácher and V. Sorino, *AIDS*, 2002, **16**, 290–291.
53. L. M. Almond, M. Boffito, P. G. Hoggard, S. Bonora, R. Raiteri, H. E. Reynolds, S. Garazzino, A. Sinicco, S. H. Khoo, D. J. Back and G. DiPerri, *AIDS Res. Hum. Retroviruses*, 2004, **20**, 716–722.
54. J. M. McKoy, C. L. Bennett, M. H. Scheetz, V. Differding, K. L. Chandler, K. K. Scarsi, P. R. Yarnold, S. Sutton, F. Palella, S. Johnson, E. Obadina, D. W. Raisch and J. P. Parada, *Drug Saf.*, 2009, **32**, 147–158.
55. J. B. T. Mbougua, C. Laurent, C. Kouanfack, A. Bourgeois, L. Ciaffi, A. Calmy, H. Gwet, S. Koula-Shiro, J. Ducos and E. Mpoudi-Ngolé, *BMC Public Health*, 2010, **1**, 105.
56. A. M. Martin, D. Nolan, I. James, P. Cameron, J. Keller, C. Moore, E. Phillips, F. T. Christiansen and S. Mallal, *AIDS*, 2005, **19**, 97–99.
57. B. O. Taiwo, *Int. J. STD AIDS*, 2006, **17**, 364–370.
58. A. M. Kesselring, F. W. Wit, C. A. Sabin, J. D. Lundgren, M. J. Gill, J. M. Gatell, A. Rauch, J. S. Montaner, F. de Wolf, P. Reiss and A. Mocroft, *AIDS*, 2009, **23**, 1689–1699.
59. A. Antela, A. Ocampo, R. Gómez, M. J. López, A. Mariño, E. Losada, R. Rodríguez, R. Fernández, J. C. Corredoira, G. Naval, A. Rodríguez, C. Miralles, A. Prieto and the Galician HIV Study Group, *HIV Clin. Trials*, 2010, **11**, 11–17.
60. J. M. Shenton, M. Teranishi, M. S. Abu-Asab, J. A. Yager and J. P. Uetrecht, *Chem. Res. Toxicol.*, 2003, **16**, 1078–1089.
61. J. Chen, B. M. Mannargudi, L. Xu and J. Uetrecht, *Chem. Res. Toxicol.*, 2008, **21**, 1862–1870.
62. J. M. Shenton, M. Popovic, J. Chen, M. J. Masson and J. P. Uetrecht, *Chem. Res. Toxicol.*, 2005, **18**, 1799–1813.
63. R. A. Roth, J. P. Luyendyk, J. F. Maddox and P. E. Ganey, *J. Pharmacol. Exp. Ther.*, 2003, **307**, 1–8.
64. M. Fukano, S. Amano, J. Sato, K. Yamamoto, H. Adachi, H. Okabe, Y. Fujiyama and T. Bamba, *Hum. Pathol.*, 2000, **31**, 250–253.
65. M. R. Khouri, S. H. Saul, A. A. Dlugosz and R. D. Soloway, *Dig. Dis. Sci.*, 1987, **32**, 1207–1211.

66. E. J. Murphy, T. J. Davern, A. O. Shakil, L. Shick, U. Masharani, H. Chow, C. Freise, W. M. Lee and N. M. Bass, *Dig. Dis. Sci.*, 2000, **45**, 549–553.
67. P. E. Ganey, J. P. Luyendyk, J. F. Maddox and R. A. Roth, *Chem.–Bio. Interact.*, 2004, **150**, 35–51.
68. R. A. Roth, J. R. Harkema, J. P. Pestka and P. E. Ganey, *Toxicol. Appl. Pharmacol.*, 1997, **147**, 300–311.
69. A. Banerjee and S. Gerondakis, *Immunol. Cell Biol.*, 2007, **85**, 420–424.
70. C. M. Blatteis, *Pharmacol. Ther.*, 2006, **111**, 194–223.
71. X. Li, S. Jiang and R. I. Tapping, *Cytokine*, 2010, **49**, 1–9.
72. R. A. Roth and P. E. Ganey, *J. Pharmacol. Exp. Ther.*, 2010, **332**, 692–697.
73. P. J. Shaw, M. J. Hopfensperger, P. E. Ganey and R. A. Roth, *Toxicol. Sci.*, 2007, **100**, 259–266.
74. J. Luyendyk, G. Cosma, P. E. Ganey, G. L. Cockerell and R. A. Roth, *J. Pharmacol. Exp. Ther.*, 2003, **307**, 9–16.
75. W. Zou, S. S. Devi, E. Sparkenbaugh, H. S. Younis, R. A. Roth and P. E. Ganey, *Toxicol. Sci.*, 2009, **108**, 184–193.
76. R. C. Lind, A. J. Gandolfi, I. G. Sipes and B. R. Brown Jr, *Anesthesiology* 1984, **61**, 544–550.
77. F. Hassan, A. Morikawa, S. Islam, G. Tumurkhuu, J. Dagvadorj, N. Koide, Y. Naiki, I. Mori, T. Yoshida and T. Yokochi, *Clin. Exp. Immunol.*, 2008, **151**, 334–340.
78. J. P. Buchweitz, P. E. Ganey, S. J. Bursian and R. A. Roth, *J. Pharmacol. Exp. Ther.*, 2002, **300**, 460–467.
79. X. Deng, J. Luyendyk, P. E. Ganey and R. A. Roth, *Pharmacol. Rev.*, 2009, **61**, 262–282.
80. P. J. Shaw, P. E. Ganey and R. A. Roth, *Toxicol. Sci.*, 2010, **118**, 7–18.
81. P. J. Shaw, P. E. Ganey and R. A. Roth, *J. Pharmacol. Exp. Ther.*, 2009, **330**, 72–78.
82. C. M. Dugan, A. E. MacDonald, R. A. Roth and P. E. Ganey, *J. Pharmacol. Exp. Ther.*, 2010, **333**, 364–372.
83. L. Cheng, Q. You, H. Yin, M. Holt, C. Franklin and C. Ju, *Hepatology*, 2009, **49**, 215–226.
84. J. P. Luyendyk, J. F. Maddox, C. D. Green, P. E. Ganey and R. A. Roth, *Hepatology*, 2004, **40**, 1342–1351.
85. J. P. Luyendyk, P. J. Shaw, C. D. Green, J. F. Maddox, P. E. Ganey and R. A. Roth, *J. Pharmacol. Exp. Ther.*, 2005, **314**, 1023–1031.
86. P. J. Shaw, A. M. Fullerton, M. A. Scott, P. E. Ganey and R. A. Roth, *Toxicol. Appl. Pharmacol.*, 2009, **236**, 293–300.
87. P. J. Shaw, A. C. Ditewig, J. F. Waring, M. J. Liguori, E. A. Blomme, P. E. Ganey and R. A. Roth, *Toxicol. Sci.*, 2009, **107**, 270–280.
88. T. K. Chang and F. S. Abbott, *Drug Metab. Rev.*, 2006, **38**, 627–639.
89. C. M. Dugan, A. M. Fullerton, R. A. Roth and P. E. Ganey, *Toxicol. Sci.*, 2011, **120**, 507–518.

90. N. C. Arbour, E. Lorenz, B. C. Schutte, J. Zabner, J. N. Kline, M. Jones, K. Frees, J. L. Watt and D. A. Schwartz, *Nat. Genet.*, 2000, **25**, 187–191.
91. B. D. Cosgrove, B. M. King, M. A. Hasan, L. G. Alexopoulos, P. A. Farazi, B. S. Hendriks, L. G. Griffith, P. K. Sorger, B. Tidor, J. J. Xu and D. A. Lauffenburger, *Toxicol. Appl. Pharmacol.*, 2009, **237**, 317–330.
92. P. J. Shaw, K. M. Beggs, E. M. Sparkenbaugh, C. M. Dugan, P. E. Ganey and R. A. Roth, *Toxicol. Sci.*, 2009, **111**, 288–301.
93. F. F. Tukov, J. F. Maddox, D. E. Amacher, W. F. Bobrowski, R. A. Roth and P. E. Ganey, *Toxicol. in Vitro*, 2006, **20**, 1488–1499.
94. W. Zou, K. M. Beggs, E. M. Sparkenbaugh, A. D. Jones, H. S. Younis, R. A. Roth and P. E. Ganey, *J. Pharmacol. Exp. Ther.*, 2009, **331**, 114–121.
95. Subcommittee on the National Halothane Study of the Committee on Anesthesia, National Academy of Sciences–National Research Council, *JAMA, J. Am. Med. Assoc.*, 1966, **197**, 775–788.
96. W. Inman and W. Mushin, *BMJ*, 1974, **1**, 5; correction, *BMJ*, 1974 **1**, 254.
97. M. Cousins, J. Plummer and P. M. de la Hall, *Can. Anaesth. Soc. J.*, 1985, **32**, S52–S55.
98. J. Trowell, R. Peto and A. C. Smith, *Lancet*, 1975, **305**, 821–824 .
99. R. Wright, M. Chisholm, B. Lloyd, J. C. Edwards, O. E. Eade, M. Hawksley, T. M. Moles and M. J. Gardner, *Lancet*, 1975, **305**, 817–820.
100. W. W. Mushin, M. Rosen and E. V. Jones, *BMJ*, 1971, **3**, 18–22.
101. L. E. Bottiger, E. Dalen, B. Hallen, *Acta Anaesthesiol. Scand.*, 1976, **20**, 40–46.
102. W. R. Blackburn, S. H. Ngai and J. Lindenbaum, *Anesthesiology*, 1964, **25**, 270–283.
103. F. M. Klion F. Schaffner and H. Popper, *Ann. Intern. Med.*, 1969, **71**, 467–477.
104. R. L. Peters, H. A. Edmondson, T. B. Reynolds and J. C. Meister, *Am. J. Med.*, 1969, **47**, 748–764.
105. E. J. Wills and B. A. Walton, *Am. J. Pathol.*, 1978, **91**, 11–32.
106. K. Rehder, *Anesthesiology*, 2003, **99**, 1220–1221.
107. E. N. Cohen, *Anesthesiology*, 1969, **31**, 560–565.
108. E. N. Cohen and N. Hood, *Anesthesiology*, 1969, **31**, 553–559.
109. G. McLain, I. G. Sipes and B. R. Brown Jr, *Anesthesiology*, 1979, **51**, 321–326.
110. K.Fujii, N. Miki, T. Sugiyama, M. Morio, T. Yamano and Y. Miyake, *Biochem. Biophys. Res. Commun.,* 1981, **102**, 507–512.
111. K. D. Gruenke, K. Konopka, D. R. Koop and L. A. Waskell, *J. Pharmacol. Exp. Ther.*, 1988, **246**, 454–459.
112. J. Gut, U. Christen and J. Huwyler, *Pharmacol. Ther.*, 1993, **58**, 133–155.
113. R. A. Van Dyke and A. J. Gandolfi, *Drug Metab. Dispos.*, 1974, **2**, 469–476.
114. J. G. Kenna, J. Neuberger and R. Williams, *J. Pharmacol. Exp. Ther.*, 1987, **242**, 733–740.

115. J. G. Kenna, H. Satoh, D. D. Christ and L. R. Pohl, *J. Pharmacol. Exp. Ther.*, 1988, **245**, 1103–1109.
116. M. Chen and A. J. Gandolfi, *Drug Metab. Rev.*, 1997, **29**, 103–122.
117. M. Bourdi, H. R. Amouzadeh, T. H. Rushmore, J. L. Martin and L. R. Pohl, *Chem. Res. Toxicol.*, 2001, **14**, 362–370.
118. C. A. Lunam, M. J. Cousins and P. M. de la Hall, *J. Pharmacol. Exp. Ther.*, 1985, **232**, 802–809.
119. M. H. Harper, P. Collins, B. Johnson, E. I. Edgard II and C. Biava, *Anesthesiology*, 1982, **56**, 14–17.
120. R. A. Van Dyke, *Anesth. Analg.*, 1982, **61**, 812–819.
121. Y. Odaka, T. Takahashi, A. Yamasaki, T. Suzuki, T. Fujiwara, T. Yamada, M. Hirakawa, H. Fujita, E. Ohmori and R. Akagi, *Biochem. Pharmacol.*, 2000, **59**, 871–880.
122. J. L. Plummer, P. M. de la Hall, M. A. Jenner and M. J. Cousins, *Anesthesiology*, 1987, **67**, 355–360.
123. E. S. Reynolds and M. T. Moslen, *Anesthesiology*, 1977, **47**, 19–27.
124. S. A. Rice, M. Maze, C. M. Smith, J. C. Kosek and R. I. Mazze, *Toxicol. Appl. Pharmacol.*, 1987, **87**, 411–419.
125. M. L. Berman, L. Kuhnert, J. M. Phythyon and D. A. Holaday, *Anesthesiology*, 1983, **58**, 1–5.
126. K. Shingu, E. I. Eger and B. H. Johnson, *Anesth. Analg.*, 1982, **61**, 824–827.
127. K. Shingu, E. I. Eger and B. H. Johnson, *Anesth. Analg.*, 1982, **61**, 820–823.
128. R. C. Lind, A. J. Gandolfi and P. M. de la Hall, *Anesthesiology*, 1992, **77**, 721–727.
129. R. C. Lind, A. J. Gandolfi and P. M. de la Hall, *Anesthesiology*, 1994, **81**, 478–487.
130. L. R. Pohl, H. Satoh, D. D. Christ and J. G. Kenna, *Annu. Rev. Pharmacol. Toxicol.*, 1988, **28**, 367–387.
131. A. Mathieu, D. DiPadua, B. Kahan, J. J. Galdabini and J. Mills, *Anesth. Analg.*, 1975, **54**, 332–339.
132. H. C. Hughes Jr. and C. M. Lang, *Anesthesiology*, 1972, **36**, 466–471.
133. C. A. Lunam, M. J. Cousins and P. M. de la Hall, *Anesth. Analg.*, 1986, **65**, 1143–1148.
134. K. L. Hastings, C. Thomas, A. P. Brown and A. J. Gandolfi, *Immunopharmacol. Immunotoxicol.*, 1995, **17**, 201–213.
135. Q. You, L. Cheng, T. P. Reilly, D. Wegmann and C. Ju, *Hepatology*, 2006, **44**, 1421–1431.
136. S. Furst, D. Luedke, H.-H. Gaw, R. Reich and A. J. Gandolfi, *Toxicol. Appl. Pharmacol.*, 1997, **143**, 245–255.
137. R. Lind, A. J. Gandolf and P. M. de la Hall, *Anesthesiology*, 1990, **73**, 1208–1213.
138. P. Eghtesadi-Araghi, A. Sohrabpour, H. Vahedi and M. Saberi-Firoozi, *World J. Gastroenterol.*, 2008, **14**, 5322–5326.
139. F. M. T Carney and R. A. Van Dyke, *Anesth. Analg.*, 1972, **51**, 135–160.

140. L. O. Warner, T. P. Beach, J. P. Garvin and E. J. Warner, *Anesth. Analg.*, 1984, **63**, 838–840.
141. R. H. Hoft, J. P. Bunker, H. I. Goodman and P. B. Gregory, *N. Eng. J. Med.*, 1981, **304**, 1023–1024.
142. G. C. Farrell, J. Mahoney, M. Bilous and L. Frost, *J. Pharmacol. Exp. Ther.*, 1988, **247**, 751–756.
143. R. C. Lind, A. J. Gandolfi and P. M. de la Hall, *Anesthesiology*, 1989, **70**, 649–653.
144. L. Frost, J. Mahoney, J. Field and C. G. Farrell, *Hepatology*, 1996, **23**, 80–86.
145. G. C. Farrell, L. Frost, M. Tapner, J. Field, M. Weltman and J. Mahoney, *J. Gastroenterol. Hepatol.*, 1996, **11**, 594–601.
146. R. C. Lind and A. J. Gandolfi, *Toxicol. Appl. Pharmacol.*, 1997, **142**, 201–207.
147. M. Bourdi, T. P. Reilly, A. G. Elkahloun, J. W. George and L. R. Pohl, *Biochem. Biophys. Res. Commun.*, 2002, **294**, 225–230.
148. Y. Feng, Q. Yang, J. Xu, G. Qian and Y. Liu, *Exp. Mol. Pathol.*, 2008, **85**, 214–222.

# Subject Index